INFECTIOUS AGENTS AND PATHOGENESIS

Series Editors: Allen L. Honeyman and
                   Herman Friedman, *University of South Florida*
                                    College of Medicine
                   Mauro Bendinelli, *University of Pisa*

W9-DFZ-181

Recent volumes in this series:

DNA TUMOR VIRUSES
Oncogenic Mechanisms
    Edited by Giuseppe Barbanti-Brodano, Mauro Bendinelli,
    and Herman Friedman·

ENTERIC INFECTIONS AND IMMUNITY
    Edited by Lois J. Paradise, Mauro Bendinelli, and Herman Friedman

HERPESVIRUSES AND IMMUNITY
    Edited by Peter G. Medveczky, Herman Friedman,
    and Mauro Bendinelli

HUMAN RETROVIRAL INFECTIONS
Immunological and Therapeutic Control
    Edited by Kenneth E. Ugen, Mauro Bendinelli,
    and Herman Friedman

MICROORGANISMS AND AUTOIMMUNE DISEASES
    Edited by Herman Friedman, Noel R. Rose, and Mauro Bendinelli

OPPORTUNISTIC INTRACELLULAR BACTERIA AND IMMUNITY
    Edited by Lois J. Paradise, Herman Friedman, and Mauro Bendinelli

PSEUDOMONAS AERUGINOSA AS AN OPPORTUNISTIC PATHOGEN
    Edited by Mario Campa, Mauro Bendinelli, and Herman Friedman

PULMONARY INFECTIONS AND IMMUNITY
    Edited by Herman Chmel, Mauro Bendinelli, and Herman Friedman

RAPID DETECTION OF INFECTIOUS AGENTS
    Edited by Steven Specter, Mauro Bendinelli, and Herman Friedman

RICKETTSIAL INFECTION AND IMMUNITY
    Edited by Burt Anderson, Herman Friedman, and Mauro Bendinelli

STAPHYLOCOCCUS AUREUS INFECTION AND DISEASE
    Edited by Allen L. Honeyman, Herman Friedman,
    and Mauro Bendinelli

A Continuation Order Plan is available for this series. A continuation order will bring delivery of each new volume immediately upon publication. Volumes are billed only upon actual shipment. For further information please contact the publisher.

Staphylococcus aureus
Infection and Disease

Staphylococcus aureus
Infection and Disease

Edited by

Allen L. Honeyman and
Herman Friedman
University of South Florida College of Medicine
Tampa, Florida

and

Mauro Bendinelli
University of Pisa
Pisa, Italy

Kluwer Academic / Plenum Publishers
New York, Boston, Dordrecht, London, Moscow

Library of Congress Cataloging-in-Publication Data

Staphylococcus aureus infection and disease/edited by Allen Honeyman, Herman Friedman and Mauro Bendinelli.
    p.   ; cm. — (Infectious agents and pathogenesis)
    Includes bibliographical references and index.
    ISBN 0-306-46591-4
    1. Staphylococcus aureus infections. I. Honeyman, Allen. II. Friedman, Herman, 1931– III. Bendinelli, Mauro. IV. Series.
    [DNLM: 1. Staphylococcus aureus—pathogenicity. 2. Staphylococcal Infections. QW 142.5.C6 S7938 2001]
    QR201.S68 S85 2001
    616′.01453—dc21

            2001025358

ISBN: 0-306-46591-4

©2001 Kluwer Academic / Plenum Publishers
233 Spring Street, New York, New York 10013

http://www.wkap.nl/

10 9 8 7 6 5 4 3 2 1

A C.I.P. record for this book is available from the Library of Congress

Printed in the United States of America

Contributors

KENNETH W. BAYLES • Department of Microbiology, Molecular Biology and Biochemistry, University of Idaho, Moscow, ID 83844-3052

ALISON A. BEHARKA • Division of Biology, Kansas State University, and Department of Veterans Affairs, Division of Infectious Disease, University of Iowa, Iowa City, IA 52246

GREGORY A. BOHACH • Department of Microbiology, Molecular Biology and Biochemistry, University of Idaho, Moscow, ID 83844-3052

STEPHEN K. CHAPES • Division of Biology, Kansas State University, Manhattan, KS 66506

AMBROSE L. CHEUNG • Department of Microbiology, Dartmouth Medical School, Hanover, NH 03755

PAUL M. DUNMAN • Infectious Diseases, Wyeth-Ayerst Research, Pearl River, NY 10965

CHRISTOF von EIFF • Institute for Medical Microbiology, Westphalian Wilhelms University, Münster, Germany

LARRY K. FOX • Department of Veterinary Clinical Medicine and Surgery, Washington State University, Pullman, WA 99164

YOSHIYUKI KAMIO • Department of Molecular and Cell Biology, Graduate School of Agricultural Science, Tohoku University, Sendai 981-8555, Japan

JUN KANEKO • Department of Molecular and Cell Biology, Graduate School of Agricultural Science, Tohoku University, Sendai 981-8555, Japan

CHIA Y. LEE • Department of Microbiology, Molecular Genetics and Immunology, University of Kansas Medical Center, Kansas City, KS 66160

JEAN C. LEE • Department of Medicine, Channing Laboratory, Brigham and Women's Hospital and Harvard Medical School, Boston, MA 02115

GWEN LIU • Department of Microbiology and Immunology, UCLA School of Medicine, University of California, Los Angeles, Los Angeles, CA 90095

SARKIS K. MAZMANIAN • Department of Microbiology and Immunology, UCLA School of Medicine, University of California, Los Angeles, Los Angeles, CA 90095

CARL L. NELSON • Department of Orthopaedic Surgery, University of Arkansas for Medical Sciences, Little Rock, AR 72205

VIJAYKUMAR PANCHOLI • Bacterial Pathogenesis and Immunology, The Rockefeller University, New York, NY 10021

GEORG PETERS • Institute for Medical Microbiology, Westphalian Wilhelms University, Münster, Germany

RICHARD A. PROCTOR • Departments of Medicine and Medical Microbiology/Immunology, University of Wisconsin, Madison, WI 53706

STEVEN J. PROJAN • Antibacterial Research, Wyeth-Ayerst Research, Pearl River, NY 10965

PATRICK M. SCHLIEVERT • Department of Microbiology, University of Minnesota Medical School, Minneapolis, MN 55455

OLAF SCHNEEWIND • Department of Microbiology and Immunology, UCLA School of Medicine, University of California, Los Angeles, Los Angeles, CA 90095

MARK S. SMELTZER • Department of Microbiology and Immunology and Department of Orthopaedic Surgery, University of Arkansas for Medical Sciences, Little Rock, AR 72205

GEORGE C. STEWART • Department of Diagnostic Medicine/Pathobiology, College of Veterinary Medicine, Kansas State University, Manhattan, KS 66506

TOSHIO TOMITA • Department of Molecular and Cell Biology, Graduate School of Agricultural Science, Tohoku University, Sendai 981-8555, Japan

HUNG TON-THAT • Department of Microbiology and Immunology,

UCLA School of Medicine, University of California, Los Angeles, Los Angeles, CA 90095

ALBION D. WRIGHT • Division of Biology, Kansas State University, Manhattan, KS 66506

JEREMY M. YARWOOD • Department of Microbiology, University of Minnesota Medical School, Minneapolis, MN 55455

SHUPING ZHANG • Department of Diagnostic Medicine/Pathobiology, College of Veterinary Medicine, Kansas State University, Manhattan, KS 66506

Preface to the Series

The mechanisms of disease production by infectious agents are presently the focus of an unprecedented flowering of studies. The field has undoubtedly received impetus from the considerable advances recently made in the understanding of the structure, biochemistry, and biology of viruses, bacteria, fungi, and other parasites. Another contributing factor is our improved knowledge of immune responses and other adaptive or constitutive mechanisms by which hosts react to infection. Furthermore, recombinant DNA technology, monoclonal antibodies, and other newer methodologies have provided the technical tools for examining questions previously considered too complex to be successfully tackled. The most important incentive of all is probably the regenerated idea that infection might be the initiating event in many clinical entities presently classified as idiopathic or of uncertain origin.

Infectious pathogenesis research holds great promise. As more information is uncovered, it is becoming increasingly apparent that our present knowledge of the pathogenic potential of infectious agents is often limited to the most noticeable effects, which sometimes represent only the tip of the iceberg. For example, it is now well appreciated that pathologic processes caused by infectious agents may emerge clinically after an incubation of decades and may result from genetic, immunologic, and other indirect routes more than from the infecting agent in itself. Thus, there is a general expectation that continued investigation will lead to the isolation of new agents of infection, the identification of hitherto unsuspected etiologic correlations, and, eventually, more effective approaches to prevention and therapy.

Studies on the mechanisms of disease caused by infectious agents demand a breadth of understanding across many specialized areas, as well as much cooperation between clinicians and experimentalists. The series *Infectious Agents and Pathogenesis* is intended not only to document the state of the art in this fascinating and challenging field but also to help lay bridges among diverse areas and people.

M. Bendinelli
H. Friedman

Preface

Staphylococcus aureus is considered a very interesting microorganism causing multiple diseases in man and animals. These include invasive infections, generalized toxemias, and alterations of the host immune response. However, *S. aureus* is generally considered part of the normal flora of its hosts and is typically found in the nares or on the skin of a host. Only following an insult to the normal skin architecture does an invasive infection occur. During this invasive infection, the host's immune response may be altered by the various antigens produced by the organism. In other instances, growth of the organism in food or in a small invasive lesion can lead to a generalized toxemia of the host. Taken all together, *S. aureus* is a wonderful pathogen that attacks its host in a variety of ways that physicians and microbiologists have yet to completely understand.

While one may wonder at the capabilities of *S. aureus*, one must also recognize the seriousness of *S. aureus* infections. During the pre-antibiotic era, many staphylococcal invasive infections resulted in the death of the patient from the systemic effects of toxin or septicemias. This devastating effect was relieved, to a great extent, by the introduction of penicillin in the 1940s. However, by the end of the 1950s, approximately 50% of hospital isolates of this bacterium were penicillin resistant. Subsequently, semi-synthetic derivatives of penicillin (methicillin and others) were used to treat *S. aureus* infections. Once again, within a few years, methicillin resistant *S. aureus* (MRSA) were found in the clinical setting. Today, approximately 60% of clinical isolates are MRSA. This has left vancomycin as the drug of choice to treat MRSA infections. However, strains of *S. aureus* that display intermediate resistance to vancomycin are increasingly being found. Treatment for patients with these infections has been difficult, though possible. We now realize that we are currently using our last lines of defense against this dangerous pathogen and that additional research on its pathogenic process is required.

As previously stated, *S. aureus* is a common inhabitant of the nasal tract and the skin of humans and animals. Approximately 30% of adults are carriers of this organism. Due to this high rate of carriage, both community and nosocomial transmission of *S. aureus* is quite common and leads to the spread of staphylococcal infections in the hospital setting. Since many strains of *S. aureus* associated with hospitals are MRSA, hospital staffs and administrators are extremely concerned with this transmission and are actively attempting to limit this reservoir. In addition, the incidence of vancomycin intermediate-resistant *S. aureus* (VISA) could easily arise from this reservoir. This is why many groups are attempting to produce a vaccine against *S. aureus.*

The invasive diseases caused by *S. aureus* can range from the infection of small cuts and scrapes, which are easily treated, to the very serious cases of bacteremia, endocarditis, and osteomyelitis, which are much more difficult to treat. Toxemias can occur as scaled skin syndrome or toxic shock syndrome, each from an invasive infection, or staphylococcal food poisoning can occur following ingestion of a preformed enterotoxin. Invasive infections of *S. aureus* can modulate the immune response of the host by the production of superantigens. These molecules cause a simulation of the immune response, which in turn causes a deletion of various types of T cells. This process may enhance the invasive nature of the organism. While much of this current discussion centers on human health and disease, one should not forget that *S. aureus* is an important pathogen of many animals, causing similar invasive diseases. This can be simply illustrated by the estimate that 90% of dairy herds may be carriers of the organism, which may be transmitted to humans in various dairy products. This reservoir can serve to reinfect the human carrier population.

This book covers a large area of research on *S. aureus.* Chapters range from animal infections to the production of vaccines for human use to the regulation of virulence factors involved with staphylococcal pathogenesis. This treatise is by no means a complete coverage of the current knowledge or research on staphylococcal infections but should serve as an introduction to an important pathogen and an interesting microorganism.

The chapters in this volume, written by experts in the field of staphylococcal pathogenesis and disease, summarize the current status of work in this area as well as future directions for research and therapeutic development. The first chapter, by Drs. Dunman and Projan, summarizes our knowledge concerning the regulation of virulence in staphylococci. This is followed by the chapter by Drs. von Eiff, Peters, and Proctor concerning the mechanism for production, biology of infection, and clinical significance of small colony variants of *S. aureus,* considered the pathogenic prototype of staphylococci. The third and fourth chapters, written by Drs. Chia

Y. Lee and Jean C. Lee, discuss capsule production by staphylococci and newer developments concerning possible vaccines against staphylococci. The chapters by Drs. Smeltzer and Nelson and by Drs. Fox, Bayles, and Bohach discuss clinical diseases caused by staphylococci including osteomyelitis, septic arthritis, and mastitis. Other chapters discuss production of toxins, cytolysins, hemolysins, leukocidin, and other extracellular enzymes secreted by staphylococci. Others deal with surface protein anchoring and display in staphylococci and superantigen which activates macrophages. The final chapter, by Dr. Cheung, describes the regulation of virulence determinants by these important disease-causing microbes.

It is anticipated by the editors that this volume will be an extremely valuable contribution to the series "Infectious Agents and Pathogenesis." This volume provides a useful summary of the current status of the pathogenesis as well as the immunologic factors involved in the diseases caused by *Staphylococcus aureus*.

The editors thank Ilona Friedman for excellent editorial assistance in coordinating and assisting in the preparation of the manuscripts for this volume.

Allen L. Honeyman
Herman Friedman
Mauro Bendinelli

Contents

11. Osteomyelitis and Septic Arthritis

MARK S. SMELTZER and CARL L. NELSON

12. Internalization of *Staphylococcus aureus* by Nonprofessional Phagocytes

KENNETH W. BAYLES and GREGORY A. BOHACH

The Regulation of Virulence in the Staphylococci

PAUL M. DUNMAN and STEVEN J. PROJAN

1. INTRODUCTION

Staphylococci produce a large number of substances that are involved in promoting the disease state. These "virulence factors" include both exoproteins, such as secreted toxins, and factors that play diverse roles in pathogenesis but don't directly confer toxicity to host tissues, such as surface proteins. As our ability to perform genetic manipulations with the staphylococci has improved, so has our understanding of the roles attributed to the various virulence factors. Yet, that understanding remains incomplete and the roles proposed for most virulence factors remain speculative.

An important fact to be kept in mind is that the staphylococci that cause disease in humans and animals are not inherently pathogenic organisms (unlike the influenzae virus, for example, which must infect to propagate). Rather, the purpose of a given virulence factor is not to cause disease, but to enhance the survival of the bacterium in adverse environments. In that regard, the infected host should be viewed as the environment to which the bacterium must adapt in order to survive. It is widely accepted that few, if any, virulence factors are required for cellular proliferation in an *in vitro* setting (i.e., the laboratory), as a result they are collectively considered to be "accessory" rather than "essential" substances. However, in the context of an infection, many of these virulence factors are apparently as essential as a shot of rum for an avalanche victim.

It is also important to realize that no single virulence factor produced by a staphylococcus has been shown to be either necessary or sufficient for the establishment of an infection (although the infective or lethal

PAUL M. DUNMAN • Infectious Diseases, Wyeth-Ayerst Research, Pearl River, NY 10965. STEVEN J. PROJAN • Antibacterial Research, Wyeth-Ayerst Research, Pearl River, NY 10965.

Staphylococcus aureus *Infection and Disease,* edited by Allen L. Honeyman *et al.* Kluwer Academic/Plenum Publishers, New York, 2001.

dose does vary). This has been evidenced by a number of allelic replacement experiments in which strains that no longer produce specific toxic proteins are still capable of causing disease, this is even true for strains rendered defective in the production of several virulence factors simultaneously. These findings coupled with a wealth of additional studies, have indicated that the pathology of a staphylococcal infection is due not to a single factor, but the coordinate actions of several independent virulence factors. The regulatory functions responsible for this coordinate action are currently a focus of study and a coherent picture is now beginning to emerge.

In this chapter the emerging picture of the coordinate regulation of the expression of these virulence factors is examined and we will endeavor to describe how our understanding of the regulation of production of these virulence factors in vitro relates to the causation of disease.

2. STAPHYLOCOCCAL VIRULENCE FACTORS

The narrowest definition of a virulence factor would be a substance that, when purified to homogeneity and introduced into a test animal, produces a pathogenic effect. Using that definition, most of the virulence factors identified to date, especially those involved in attachment and probably most of the degratory enzymes (lipases, proteases, hyalouronidase, etc.) would not be considered true virulence factors. In the broadest sense, any factor produced by a bacterium that is not essential (or useful) for growth, but allows survival within or on a host organism in a non-symbiotic manner would be considered a virulence factor. This second definition is probably too broad and in many cases, it is possible that the production of at least some of these factors may actually assist the host in combating an infection. For example, a relatively benign cell surface protein may serve as the recognition site for anti-staphylococcal antibodies thereby assisting the host in clearing an infection.

Allelic Replacement Experiments

A now common molecular genetic approach to test for the impact of a given virulence factor (or genetic locus) is to inactivate the gene responsible for production of a virulence factor in question. Generally, in these studies some portion of the target gene being inactivated is cloned onto a plasmid vector, a selectable genetic marker (usually an antibiotic resistance gene) is then inserted within the coding region of the target gene,

presumably inactivating it. This recombinant plasmid is subsequently introduced into the wild type strain (carrying the active gene of interest) and
the genetic marker is selected for. Colonies arising by homologous recom-
bination between the engineered gene on the recombinant plasmid and
the wild type, chromosomal copy can be selected for stable acquisition of
the selected marker. Southern blotting analysis can then verify that the predicted genetic exchange took place. The end result is an isogenic strain
that is genetically identical to its parent with the exception of a single, now
interrupted gene. Using the parent strain and its isogenic mutant in an
animal model, the relative virulence of the two strains can be determined
and the effect of genetic inactivation of the gene encoding the putative
virulence factor can be assessed. There are several important facts to keep
in mind when examining data from these allelic replacement experiments:
A) What is true for one strain of staphylococcus may or may not hold true
for others; B) The inactivation of a gene may have pleiotrophic effects, i.e.,
does not necessarily mean that all the other virulence factors are produced
in the same manner as in the isogenic parent, as the failure to produce
one substance may well affect cellular regulatory circuitry; C) The assay for
virulence may not be sufficiently sensitive or even appropriate for the
virulence factor being examined; D) Disruption of the target gene may not
fully inactivate or may alter the function(s) of the gene in question; and
E) Essential genes may not be investigated using this approach and may,
in fact, account for the observation that all known virulence factors are
accessory (as described above).

While the role(s) of the multitude of individual virulence factors produced by the staphylococci will not be reviewed here, a few will be discussed
in the context of coordinate regulation. In addition the three general
aspects of an infection, attachment, evasion of host defense and tissue invasion, will also be discussed (as depicted in Figure 1).

A general class of proteins that promote the attachment of bacteria to
all manner of extracellular matrices has been named MSCRAMMS (an
acronym for microbial surface components recognizing adhesive matrix
molecules).[1] In addition to MSCRAMMS, staphylococci have other factors
that have been found to bind other extracellular matrix molecules, but
neither a specific protein nor gene has been identified for them. These
include activities which bind to bone sialoprotein,[2] elastin,[3] laminin,[4]
thrombospondin,[5] and vitronectin.[6]

Evasion of the Host Response

Bacterial survival during an infection is dependent on the ability of
the bacterium to circumvent the host's defenses, principally the immune

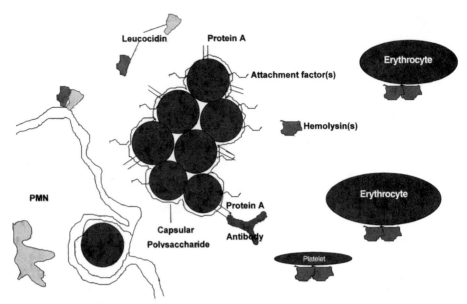

FIGURE 1. Virulence properties of *Staphylococcus aureus.* Filled circles (●) represent individual staphylococci forming an aggregate, which is surrounded by a polysaccharide capsule (composed of hyaluronic acid). Capsid protects the bacterium from complement mediated phagocytic killing and influences attachment to various host tissues.[47] Staphylococci also produce cell surface proteins that are involved in attachment to host cells, including various attachment factors (indicated) and factors that camouflage the bacterium from host defensive mechanisms, such as protein A (∦), as described in text. Following adherence staphylococci are endocytosed into membrane-bound vauoles (shown bottom left), where they may be released into the host cell's matrix, ultimately destroying the cell.[43] At high cell densities exoprotein toxins, such as leukocidin (✸) and hemolysins are produced, which can lyse various host cells (including erythrocytes and platelets).

Attachment: An essential step in the establishment of a staphylococcal infection is attachment of the bacteria to host tissue. It is clear that attachment must play a critical role for either colonization or entrance into the host cell.

system. The critical role the immune system plays in preventing infection is most clearly observed in individuals whose immune systems are compromised; there is no greater risk factor for the development of a bacterial infection than a poorly functioning immune system. Therefore, it should come as little surprise that bacteria in general and staphylococci, in particular, have developed multiple strategies for avoiding host defense systems. Perhaps the most significant immune evasion factor is protein A, which binds to the Fc portion of IgG antibodies, as reviewed by Potter *et al.*[7] It is of note that protein A is produced early in exponential growth in vitro. One can envisage that *S. aureus* cells, present in the bloodstream (at low cell density), are camouflaged with a protective coat of IgG antibodies (which are mis-aligned) and thereby circumventing the action of anti-staphylococcal antibodies. At higher cell densities, the protein A is not expressed *in vitro* and would be superfluous *in vivo* if the bacterium is not part of a biofilm community.

Tissue Invasion

As an infection matures, surrounding tissues may be either a source of nutrients or a physical barrier to the spread of the bacteria; as a result, Staphylococci have developed a number of elaborate mechanisms to degrade host tissues. In the case of *S. aureus*, the predominant extracellular virulence factor is the pore-forming, cytolytic alpha toxin. Like most extracellular virulence factors of the staphylococci, alpha toxin, is produced late during growth in vitro and mutants, generated by allelic replacement, are significantly less virulent in models of invasive staphylococcal disease [e.g., infectious endocarditis[8]].

3. COORDINATE REGULATION OF VIRULENCE

It is fair to assume, a priori, that all bacteria express their genetic information in a coordinated manner; aside from essential housekeeping genes, relatively few bacterial genes are expressed continuously. One could imagine that bacteria that would produce virulence factors constitutively (through all phases of cell growth), rather than if and when they were needed, would labor under a significant metabolic burden. As a result, this would be counter-selective compared to a more prudent organism, which was able to produce accessory factors only on an "as needed" or "just in time" basis. Therefore, it is not surprising that bacteria have evolved control systems that coordinately regulate groups of genes, such as the accessory virulence factors.[9]

Bacterial Signal Transduction

Coordinate regulation of gene expression requires that the cell possess machinery capable of detecting environmental changes. While changes in pH, temperature and carbon source often involve stimuli that can be sensed from within a cell, often the stimuli do not directly penetrate into the cytoplasm. Therefore signaling systems have evolved in virtually all cells. These signal transduction systems in bacteria often share a significant degree of structural similarities with each other even when the signals being detected or the bacteria involved are quite diverse.[10] The central elements of many of these signal transduction systems are referred to as "two component systems." In large part, two component systems consist of two proteins, usually genetically encoded in a single operon, where one of the proteins is a transmembrane "sensor" and the other is a transcription factor called a "response regulator." In general, the transmembrane protein reacts to an extracellular stimulus by binding to some specific ligand, "the signal," and undergoes autophosphorylation at a conserved histidine residue. The phosphorylated sensor then relays the phosphate to a conserved tyrosine residue on the response regulator that can, in turn, stimulate or repress target genes, most often at the level of transcription.

Expression of Virulence Factors in Culture: Dependence on the Phase of Growth

As mentioned above, expression of virulence factors is regulated in a growth phase dependent manner. Almost all of the data collected on this subject in the staphylococci and other bacteria has been obtained by the study of bacterial cells in culture, usually in a nutrient rich medium. In these studies, a typical growth curve of a strain of S. aureus grown in nutrient medium is established, which can be divided into the classic lag, log, (exponential) and stationary (post-exponential) phases of growth. However, the use of the term "stationary" for the staphylococci and other bacteria is often a misnomer. This is because while the cells in stationary phase are no longer showing an active increase in cell mass or displaying active cell division, they are still performing metabolic functions (such as producing toxic exoproteins). Table I shows a partial list of virulence factors and when they are expressed during growth in culture. In general, it has been observed that almost all of the exoproteins produced by staphylococci are produced post-exponentially.[11] Two exceptions are enterotoxin A, which is produced constitutively [throughout growth[12]] and coagulase, which is produced during logarithmic growth.[13] Conversely the cell wall associated proteins including protein A, and most proteins involved in attachment are produced during logarithmic growth rather than post-exponentially. Therefore it stands to reason that cell wall anchoring of virulence factors occurs during the process of cell wall assembly, and the enzyme(s) involved in this process (anchoring) are expressed early in growth phase, when the cell wall is being made.

TABLE I
The effect of growth phase on virulence factor production

Log Phase	Post-Exponential	Constitutive
coagulase	alpha toxin	enterotoxin A
protein A	beta hemolysin	
clumping factor	delta hemolysin	
fibronectin binding proteins	SHTs	
	(gamma hemolysin & PVL)	
fibrinogen binding protein	Exfoliative toxins A & B	
	V8 protease	
	hyaluronate lyase	
	lipase	
	capsular polysaccharide	

Shown are the effect(s) of growth phase on virulence factor expression.

Pleitropic Mutants Affecting the Production of Virulence Factors

For the staphylococci several studies have been published describing mutants which display multiple differences in the expression of exoproteins and/or virulence factors these include: *exp* mutants,[14] *agr*,[15] *sar*,[16] *lgr*,[17] *sae*.[18] Many of these have been isolated using the same strategy— transposon insertion. Each represent a classic pleitropic effect, where a presumably single transposition event gives rise to multiple phenotypic differences. It should come as no surprise that multiple loci affect the expression of *S. aureus* virulence factors, as pathogenesis is no less involved than the temporal regulation of sporulation[19] or competence[20] in *B. subtilis*, processes that are controlled by several regulatory elements.

To date, two of these loci have been cloned, sequenced and, studied in significant detail. These are the *agr* locus[15,21] and the *sar* locus.[16] In fact, these loci (*agr* and *sar*) are inextricably linked as discussed below.

The *agr* Locus

The "accessory gene regulator" (*agr*) locus was discovered as a result of multiple phenotypic differences in the expression of several virulence factors that resulted from the insertion of a single transposon, Tn551, into the chromosome of a "wild type" strain of *Staphylococcus aureus*.[15] In this mutant the production of most of the extracellular virulence factors is depressed while the cell wall associated proteins and coagulase are overexpressed. Using this mutant the *agr* locus was cloned[22] and the complete sequence determined.[23] The *agr* operon is shown in Figure 2.

The *agr* locus is organized into two divergent transcripts, referred to as RNAII and RNAIII, which are transcribed from two promoters (P2 and P3, respectively).[23,24] The RNAII transcript potentially encodes four proteins, which have been designated AgrB, AgrD, AgrC, and AgrA[24] while the RNAIII transcript contains the structural gene for the 26 amino acid peptide delta hemolysin.[25] One of the early findings concerning this locus was that RNAIII itself functioned as a regulatory molecule. It was possible to genetically inactivate delta hemolysin either by an in frame deletion[26] or by insertion of a stop codon at the beginning of the coding sequence[27] and observe either wild-type expression of virulence factors[26] or an intermediate *agr* mutant phenotype.[27]

The manner in which RNAIII regulates target genes is not yet understood. At this point, it is clear that RNAIII functions to regulate target gene expression either the level of transcription, at the level of translation, or at both. A series of studies on the role of RNAIII was undertaken by Vandenesch *et al.*,[17] in which the transcription of RNAIII was regulated by an exogenous promoter using the inducible staphylococcal beta-lactamase control system.[28] Those experiments examined the transcription of two of the principle targets of *agr* regulation: the *hla* gene encoding alpha toxin and the *spa* gene encoding protein A. Induction of RNAIII at virtually any point in the growth of a *S. aureus* culture resulted in an immediate inhibition of *spa* transcription. However, while RNAIII expression was necessary for *hla* transcription, the transcription of *hla* mRNA did not always immediately follow induction of RNAIII, but occurred at some point after the cells entered post-exponential growth. From this result Vandenesch and colleagues, concluded that there must exist at least one other "temporal factor" in addition to *agr* that is required for the expression of alpha toxin and probably other exotoxins produced by *S. aureus*. Recent work has shown that RNAIII functions as a positive effector to stimulate translation of alpha toxin mRNA.[29] This work demonstrated that RNAIII functions as an antisense RNA that base pairs with sequences on the alpha toxin mRNA upstream from the translational start and frees the ribosome binding site and start codon to allow translation of the messenger RNA molecule.

The principal role of the remainder of the *agr* locus, the RNAII transcript, is to direct transcription of RNAIII. It has been shown that transcription from P3 is dependent on each of the four Agr proteins.[24] Likewise, transcription from the P2 promoter is also dependent on the RNAII open reading frames.[24] This result suggests that RNAII expression is part of an autocatalytic feedback circuit. By virtue of their similarity with other two

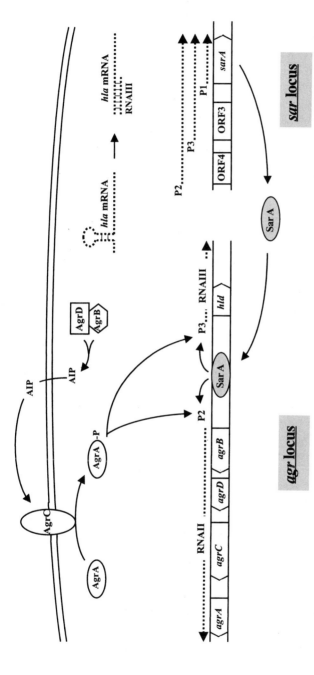

FIGURE 2. The *Staphylococcus aureus agr* and *sar* Regulatory Loci Dashed arrows (---) preceeded by "p" represent transcripts generated from various promoters. The *agr* P2-mediated RNAII transcript encodes four gene products AgrB, AgrD, AgrC and AgrA, respectively. AgrA and AgrC constitute components of a typical two component signal transduction pathway. AgrB and AgrD are thought to act in a concerted manner to produce an autoinducing peptide (AIP), which is presumed to be secreted from the cell via the activity(s) of AgrB. AIP acts as a stimulus to activate the autophosphorylating activity of the "sensor" AgrC, which in-turn, phosphorylates AgrA. In its phosphorylated state, AgrA acts as a transcriptional regulator and in combination with SarA up-regulates transcription of both RNAII and RNAIII. RNAIII subsequently down-regulates expression of virulence factor surface proteins and up-regulates expression of several exoproteins (pre-sumably most RNAIII-mediated regulation is at the transcriptional level). However, the molecular mechaniss) by which RNAIII acts as a transcriptional regulator is not yet known. In addition, RNAIII can base pair with the 5' region of *hla* mRNA, which is thought to "free" signals required for efficient mRNA translation.

component regulatory proteins Vandenesch and colleagues designed experiments which demonstrated that, the AgrC and AgrA proteins appear to be the sensor and response regulator of a two component regulatory system, as discussed above.[30] One inconsistency in this model is that attempts to demonstrate binding of any of the Agr proteins to either the P2/P3 promoter region or to target genes have only produced negative results in three different laboratories (J. Kornblum, S. Khan and S. Arvidson, unpublished results). However, it is clear that AgrC must either directly or indirectly interact with its own promoter.

Balaban and Novick[31] isolated two substances, termed RAP and RIP, that behave as regulators of exoprotein synthesis (*via* the stimulation of RNAIII production) from cultures of S. *aureus*. Characterization of the activator, RAP, revealed that it was a modified eight amino acid peptide, whose sequence is contained with the 46 amino acid *agrD* reading frame.[32] At present it is thought that AgrB functions to modify and secrete the octapeptide molecule, which in turn is the ligand for the AgrA sensory component of the *agr* signal transduction pathway. This autocrine regulation indicates that the S. *aureus agr* locus constitutes a quorum sensing regulon—detecting the presence of a critical cell mass or density, as observed in other two component regulatory systems.[33] Subsequent work has demonstrated that the specific octapeptide modification is a cyclization reaction at a cysteine residue resulting in a cyclic thiolactone.[34] Novick and colleagues have shown that all peptides that are active *in vitro* are cyclized and have gone on to show that the production of signaling cyclized thiolactone peptides is common to both coagulase positive and coagulase negative staphylococci. They have further shown that among strains of S. *aureus* no fewer than four classes of such peptides have been identified, all encoded within the same region of the corresponding *agrD* reading frames, but differing in their modification. Remarkably, some of these peptides actually interfere with rather than activate the *agr* regulon. It has been suggested that strategies which can interfere with the ability of staphylococci to appropriate regulate their expression of virulence may have therapeutic utility and understanding the biochemistry of the thiolactone regulation/interference may serve as a model in designing novel anti staphylococcal drugs.

The *sar* Locus

A second locus, identified by Cheung and colleagues, has been termed the staphylcoccal accessory regulator (*sar*) locus. This locus was identified in much the same way as the *agr* locus; a Tn917TV1 transposon insertion gave rise to a mutant displaying multiple changes in the phenotypic expression of several virulence factors.[16] The *sar* region was subsequently cloned and the sequence was determined.[35] Both sequence and blotting data demonstrated that *sar* and *agr* were indeed two distinct loci.[16] Furthermore, the double mutant, *agr, sar⁻*, was significantly more impaired in the production of virulence factors than either single mutant with both exoproteins and cell wall associated virulence factors displaying decreased expression.[36]

A map of the *sar* locus appears in Figure 2. Hybridization and mapping studies have demonstrated that there are three overlapping transcripts within the region, each of which is initiated from a distinct, independent promoter. Complementation studies in which the *sar* defect was introduced into a wild type laboratory strain demonstrated that the SarA reading frame was necessary for alpha toxin production.[37] It was also found that the *sar* locus affects alpha toxin production *via* the expression of the *agr* locus.[37] This is supported by the findings that: 1) Levels of RNAII and RNAIII, the *agr* transcripts, are markedly diminished in *sar* mutants but are partially restored in mutants complemented with the smallest of the three *sar* transcripts (*sarA*). When a *sar* mutant is complemented with sequences encompassing all three of the *sar* transcription units wild-type levels of RNAII and RNAIII are achieved. 2) Both alpha toxin and beta hemolysin levels are depressed in *sar⁻* mutants. Yet expression is restored when *agr*-RNAIII production is directed by a recombinant plasmid in trans in a *sar* mutant strain.[35] These observations indicate that RNAIII transcription is reduced in a *sar* mutant strain and the restoration of wild type levels of *agr*-RNAIII restores the ability of the cells to produce alpha toxin and beta hemolysin (and probably the other, *agr* regulated, exoproteins). Moreover, several studies have demonstrated that the SarA protein directly interacts with the *agr* locus by binding to the *agr*-P2-P3 promoter region.[38,39] In addition to its role as a transcriptional activator for the agrP2-P3 promoters, SarA also appears to independently regulate the gene encoding the collagen binding MSCRAMM, *cna*.[40]

The fact that the an *agr/sar* double mutant is more impaired in virulence factor production than either *agr* or *sar* single mutants further demonstrated that *sar* also has a role in expression of virulence factors independent of *agr*. Yet, aside for its role in transcriptional activation of the *agr* locus, it remains to be demonstrated how the *sar* locus acts as a *agr*-independent regulator of virulence factor expression.

Environmental Factors that Affect Expression of Virulence Determinants

It would be a mistake to conclude that the octapeptide-mediated regulatory system defined by *agr* is the sole regulatory element in the control of virulence factor expression, although it does appear to have a central role in the process. M.J. Betley and colleagues have demonstrated that several environmental factors affected expression of the enterotoxins and *agr*. For example it was found that the expression of enterotoxin C gene (*sec*) is regulated in response to both high NaCl concentrations (osmolarity) and the *agr* response.[41,42] In a separate study, the effect of both pH and glucose on *sec*, *hla*, and *agr* expression was examined. In that study it was observed that the *agr* transcripts, RNAII and RNAIII were poorly expressed when the pH of the culture was maintain at 6.5 or higher; therefore, *agr* expression is, to some extent, dependent on a drop in pH, which is usually observed as a culture grows. Furthermore, even at pHs that favored the expression of the *agr* transcripts (pH 5.5), the presence of glucose in the medium repressed transcription of RNAII and RNAIII.[43] The fact that expression of *agr* and, therefore, the virulence factors of *S. aureus* are subject to classic catabolite repression should come as no surprise.

Virulence of *S. aureus* Strains with Mutations in Regulatory Loci

As alluded to above, *agr* and *sar* mutants were tested in animal models of virulence in much the same way as mutants in individual virulence factors. Virtually all of the models studied, including: 1) a mouse model of arthritis,[44] 2) a rabbit model of endocarditis,[36] 3) a rabbit model of osteomyelitis,[45] and 4) a model of endophthalmitis,[46] demonstrated reduced virulence. However, while these mutant strains resulted in diminished virulence, they did not render the bacteria avirulent, an important point to consider for those who propose to target either individual virulence determinants or global regulators for antimicrobial chemotherapeutic intervention.

An interesting observation made by several investigators, but not routinely reported in the literature, is that nominally virulent strains of *S. aureus* appear to become attenuated by repeated passage *in vitro* in nutrient media. Passage of these attenuated strains through an animal sometimes restores a more virulent phenotype, but often it does not. This fact should be kept in mind by those studying virulence in these organisms.

Virulence Factors and Disease

The question now remains, how does the concerted action of the virulence determinants and their global regulators lead to staphylococcal disease? All of the in vitro and in vivo results discussed above suggest that attachment and growth are precursors to the production of most exotoxins. The fact the attachment proteins require ongoing cell wall assembly to become anchored to the cell wall is good reason for cells to produce these only during cell division and not post-exponentially. Likewise, extracellular proteins, to have an optimum effect in the immediate environment of the bacterium, would be best produced when the cells are localized and in sufficient quantity to produce enough material to have a "beneficial effect" for the bacterium. This is especially true for those exoproteins which are enzymes (e.g., hyaluronate lyase, metallo protease) or the pore-forming "invasins" (e.g., the hemolysins). Those proteins with immunomodulatory activity (enterotoxins, toxic shock syndrome toxin-1, ETA, and ETB) however, would be expected to act systemically.

This scheme suggests that sepsis due to staphylococci is not the result of a generally disseminated contamination of the bloodstream. Rather, it is the result of a focal infection in which an attached vegetation reaches a cell density sufficient to lower the local pH, deplete available nutrients, and, then, produce degratory enzymes, pore-forming invasins and immunomodulators which produce the symptoms associated with the disease.

4. CONCLUSIONS

It should be appreciated that virulence factor expression is a highly orchestrated process during both staphylococcus pathogenesis and benign colonization. As described above, the *agr* and *sar* loci play central roles in the coordinate regulation of many of these substances. In the laboratory setting these regulatory loci appear to modulate both the expression of cell wall associated proteins and exoproteins in a cell density dependent manner. It is generally accepted that these elements (*agr* and *sar*) mediate active expression of cell wall associated proteins at low cell densities; conversely, cell surface factors are subsequently down-regulated at higher cell densities. Exoproteins appear to be regulated in a *agr/sar* dependent, yet, reciprocal manner. It is reasonable that these general patterns of expression may extend into an *in vivo* (i.e., host) setting and data is now emerging that support this assumption. One can envision that early during infection it would be beneficial for a bacterial cell to produce factors that primarily allow for attachment to host tissue and evading host clearance mechanisms. Once colonization is achieved, and a critical population density is reached, quorum-sensing mechanisms may mediate the down-regulation of these factors and up-regulate factors that may be more beneficial for the organism including substances that enhance the acquisition of nutrients, such as toxins that will catabolize host tissues. Based on this scheme, it is not surprising that environmental factors such as glucose availability (as described above), also contribute to the regulation of virulence. Clearly our ability to propose roles for virulence factors and understand their regulation during infection will require both a more thorough list of virulence factors and additional *in vivo* experiments.

As described above, the *agr* locus mediated quorum-sensing mechanism is central to our current understanding of virulence factor regulation. As a result, much of the current work on staphylococcal virulence is focusing on the development of novel preventative and chemotherapeutic strategies aimed at manipulating this autoinducing regulon. It is easy to imagine that inactivation of the *agr/sar* system could lead to a novel prophylactic approach against staphylococci infections.

REFERENCES

1. Patti, J. M., *et al.*, *MSCRAMM-mediated adherence of microorganisms to host tissues. [Review] [186 refs]*. Annual Review of Microbiology, 1994. **48**: pp. 585–617.
2. Ryden, C., *et al.*, *Selective binding of bone matrix sialoprotein to Staphylococcus aureus in osteomyelitis [letter]*. Lancet, 1987. **2**(8557): p. 515.
3. Park, P. W., *et al.*, *Binding of elastin to Staphylococcus aureus.* Journal of Biological Chemistry, 1991. **266**(34): pp. 23399–406.
4. Vercellotti, G. M., *et al.*, *Extracellular matrix proteins (fibronectin, laminin, and type IV collagen) bind and aggregate bacteria.* American Journal of Pathology, 1985. **120**(1): pp. 13–21.
5. Herrmann, M., *et al.*, *Thrombospondin binds to Staphylococcus aureus and promotes staphylococcal adherence to surfaces.* Infection & Immunity, 1991. **59**(1): pp. 279–88.
6. Chhatwal, G. S., *et al.*, *Specific binding of the human S protein (vitronectin) to streptococci, Staphylococcus aureus, and Escherichia coli.* Infection & Immunity, 1987. **55**(8): pp. 1878–83.
7. Potter, K. N., *et al.*, *Staphylococcal protein A binding to VH3 encoded immunoglobulins. [Review] [55 refs]*. International Reviews of Immunology, 1997. **14**(4): pp. 291–308.
8. Bayer, A. S., *et al.*, *Hyperproduction of alpha-toxin by Staphylococcus aureus results in paradoxically reduced virulence in experimental endocarditis: a host defense role for platelet microbicidal proteins.* Infection & Immunity, 1997. **65**(11): pp. 4652–60.
9. Miller, J. F., J. J. Mekalanos, and S. Falkow, *Coordinate regulation and sensory transduction in the control of bacterial virulence. [Review] [73 refs]*. Science, 1989. **243**(4893): pp. 916–22.
10. Stock, J. B., A. J. Ninfa, and A. M. Stock, *Protein phosphorylation and regulation of adaptive responses in bacteria. [Review] [450 refs]*. Microbiological Reviews, 1989. **53**(4): pp. 450–90.
11. Arvidson, S., *Extracellular enzymes from Staphylococcus aureus.* Staphylococci and staphylococcal infections., ed. A. C. Easmon CF. Vol. 2. 1983, London: Academic Press.
12. Tremaine, M. T., D. K. Brockman, and M. J. Betley, *Staphylococcal enterotoxin A gene (sea) expression is not affected by the accessory gene regulator (agr).* Infection & Immunity, 1993. **61**(1): pp. 356–9.
13. Duthie, E., *The production of free staphylococcal coagulase.* Journal of General Microbiology, 1954. **10**: p. 427.
14. Bjorklind, A., Arvidson, S., *Mutants of Staphylococcus aureus affected in the regulation of protein exoprotein synthesis.* FEMS Microbiology Letters, 1980. **7**: p. 203.
15. Recsei, P., *et al.*, *Regulation of exoprotein gene expression in Staphylococcus aureus by agr.* Molecular & General Genetics, 1986. **202**(1): pp. 58–61.

16. Cheung, A. L., *et al.*, *Regulation of exoprotein expression in Staphylococcus aureus by a locus (sar) distinct from agr.* Proceedings of the National Academy of Sciences of the United States of America, 1992. **89**(14): pp. 6462–6.

17. Vandenesch, F., J. Kornblum, and R. P. Novick, *A temporal signal, independent of agr, is required for hla but not spa transcription in Staphylococcus aureus.* Journal of Bacteriology, 1991. **173**(20): pp. 6313–20.

18. Giraudo, A. T., *et al.*, *Characterization of a Tn925-induced mutant of Staphylococcus aureus altered in exoprotein production.* Journal of Basic Microbiology, 1994. **34**(5): pp. 317–22.

19. Hoch, J. A., *Regulation of the phosphorelay and the initiation of sporulation in Bacillus subtilis. [Review] [68 refs].* Annual Review of Microbiology, 1993. **47**: pp. 441–65.

20. Dubnau, D., *The regulation of genetic competence in Bacillus subtilis. [Review] [52 refs].* Molecular Microbiology, 1991. **5**(1): pp. 11–8.

21. Morfeldt, E., *et al.*, *Cloning of a chromosomal locus (exp) which regulates the expression of several exoprotein genes in Staphylococcus aureus.* Molecular & General Genetics, 1988. **211**(3): pp. 435–40.

22. Peng, H. L., *et al.*, *Cloning, characterization, and sequencing of an accessory gene regulator (agr) in Staphylococcus aureus.* Journal of Bacteriology, 1988. **170**(9): pp. 4365–72.

23. Kornblum, J., Kreiswirth, B., Projan, S. J., Ross, H., Novick, R. P., *Agr: a polycistronic locus regulating exoprotein synthesis in Staphylococcus aureus.* Molecular biology of the staphylococci, ed. N. RP. 1990, New York: VCH Publishers.

24. Novick, R. P., *et al.*, *The agr P2 operon: an autocatalytic sensory transduction system in Staphylococcus aureus.* Molecular & General Genetics, 1995. **248**(4): pp. 446–58.

25. Janzon, L., S. Lofdahl, and S. Arvidson, *Identification and nucleotide sequence of the delta-lysin gene, hld, adjacent to the accessory gene regulator (agr) of Staphylococcus aureus.* Molecular & General Genetics, 1989. **219**(3): pp. 480–5.

26. Novick, R. P., *et al.*, *Synthesis of staphylococcal virulence factors is controlled by a regulatory RNA molecule.* EMBO Journal, 1993. **12**(10): pp. 3967–75.

27. Janzon, L. and S. Arvidson, *The role of the delta-lysin gene (hld) in the regulation of virulence genes by the accessory gene regulator (agr) in Staphylococcus aureus.* EMBO Journal, 1990. **9**(5): pp. 1391–9.

28. Novick, R. P., *Genetic systems in staphylococci.* Methods of Enzymology, ed. J. Miller. Vol. 204. 1991, New York: Academic Press, Inc. 587–636.

29. Morfeldt, E., *et al.*, *Activation of alpha-toxin translation in Staphylococcus aureus by the trans-encoded antisense RNA, RNAIII.* EMBO Journal, 1995. **14**(18): pp. 4569–77.

30. Lina, G., *et al.*, *Transmembrane topology and histidine protein kinase activity of AgrC, the agr signal receptor in Staphylococcus aureus.* Molecular Microbiology, 1998. **28**(3): pp. 655–62.

31. Balaban, N. and R. P. Novick, *Autocrine regulation of toxin synthesis by Staphylococcus aureus.* Proceedings of the National Academy of Sciences of the United States of America, 1995. **92**(5): pp. 1619–23.

32. Ji, G., R. C. Beavis, and R.P. Novick, *Cell density control of staphylococcal virulence mediated by an octapeptide pheromone.* Proceedings of the National Academy of Sciences of the United States of America, 1995. **92**(26): pp. 12055–9.

33. Fuqua, W. C., S. C. Winans, and E. P. Greenberg, *Quorum sensing in bacteria: the LuxR-LuxI family of cell density-responsive transcriptional regulators. [Review] [87 refs].* Journal of Bacteriology, 1994. **176**(2): pp. 269–75.

34. Ji, G., R. Beavis, and R.P. Novick, *Bacterial interference caused by autoinducing peptide variants.* Science, 1997. **276**(5321): pp. 2027–30.

35. Cheung, A. L. and S. J. Projan, *Cloning and sequencing of sarA of Staphylococcus aureus, a gene required for the expression of agr.* Journal of Bacteriology, 1994. **176**(13): pp. 4168–72.

36. Cheung, A. L., *et al.*, *Diminished virulence of a sar-/agr- mutant of Staphylococcus aureus in the rabbit model of endocarditis.* Journal of Clinical Investigation, 1994. **94**(5): pp. 1815–22.

37. Cheung, A. L. and P. Ying, *Regulation of alpha- and beta-hemolysins by the sar locus of Staphylococcus aureus.* Journal of Bacteriology, 1994. **176**(3): pp. 580–5.

38. Chien, Y. T., Manna, A. C., Projan, S. J., Cheung, A. L., *SarA, a global regulator of virulence determinants in Staphylococcus aureus, binds to a conserved motif essential for sar-dependent gene regulation.* Journal of Biological Chemistry, 1999. **274**(52): pp. 37169–37176.

39. Rechtin, T. M., *et al.*, *Characterization of the SarA virulence gene regulator of Staphylococcus aureus.* Molecular Microbiology, 1999. **33**(2): pp. 307–16.

40. Blevins, J. S., *et al.*, *The Staphylococcal accessory regulator (sar) represses transcription of the Staphylococcus aureus collagen adhesin gene (cna) in an agr-independent manner.* Molecular Microbiology, 1999. **33**(2): pp. 317–26.

41. Regassa, L. B., J. L. Couch, and M. J. Betley, *Steady-state staphylococcal enterotoxin type C mRNA is affected by a product of the accessory gene regulator (agr) and by glucose.* Infection & Immunity, 1991. **59**(3): pp. 955–62.

42. Regassa, L. B. and M. J. Betley, *High sodium chloride concentrations inhibit staphylococcal enterotoxin C gene (sec) expression at the level of sec mRNA.* Infection & Immunity, 1993. **61**(4): pp. 1581–5.

43. Regassa, L. B., R. P. Novick, and M. J. Betley, *Glucose and nonmaintained pH decrease expression of the accessory gene regulator (agr) in Staphylococcus aureus.* Infection & Immunity, 1992. **60**(8): pp. 3381–8.

44. Abdelnour, A., *et al.*, *The accessory gene regulator (agr) controls Staphylococcus aureus virulence in a murine arthritis model.* Infection & Immunity, 1993. **61**(9): pp. 3879–85.

45. Gillaspy, A. F., *et al.*, *Role of the accessory gene regulator (agr) in pathogenesis of staphylococcal osteomyelitis.* Infection & Immunity, 1995. **63**(9): pp. 3373–80.

46. Booth, M. C., *et al.*, *Accessory gene regulator controls Staphylococcus aureus virulence in endophthalmitis.* Investigative Ophthalmology & Visual Science, 1995. **36**(9): pp. 1828–36.

47. Wessels, M. R., *Capsular Polysaccharide of Group A Streptococcus.* Gram-Positive Pathogens, ed. V. A. Fischetti, Novick, R. P., Ferretti, J. J., Portnay, D. A., Rood, J. I. 2000, Washington DC: ASM Press. 34–42.

48. Lowy, F. D., *Staphylococcus aureus-Eukaryotic Cell Interactions.* Gram-Positive Pathogens, ed. V. A. Fischetti, Novick, R. P., Ferretti, J. J., Portnay, D. A., Rood, J. I. 2000, Washington DC: ASM Press. 408–413.

2

Small Colony Variants of *Staphylococcus aureus*: Mechanisms for Production, Biology of Infection, and Clinical Significance

CHRISTOF von EIFF, GEORG PETERS,

and RICHARD A. PROCTOR

1. INTRODUCTION

Staphylococcus aureus has been and continue to be, a major cause of human disease, especially in the hospital setting. Indeed, it is one of the most feared pathogens because of their ability to cause overwhelming sepsis and death.[1,2] In the past staphylococci have shown a disconcerting propensity to develop resistance to antimicrobial agents. Most staphylococci are resistant to penicillin and depending on local epidemiological conditions, a significant number of isolates are resistant to methicillin, lincosamides, macrolides, aminoglycosides and fluoroquinolones.[2] Because vancomycin is the only drug with dependable activity against methicillin-resistant strains of *S. aureus*, the emergence of strains of *S. aureus* with intermediate resistance to vancomycin has heightened the fears of a pan antibiotic-resistant strain.[3] These concerns are reinforced by the existence of a number of

CHRISTOF VON EIFF and GEORG PETERS • Institute for Medical Microbiology, Westphalian Wilhelms University, Münster, Germany. RICHARD A. PROCTOR • Departments of Medicine and Medical Microbiology/Immunology, University of Wisconsin, Madison, WI 53706.

Staphylococcus aureus *Infection and Disease*, edited by Allen L. Honeyman *et al.* Kluwer Academic/Plenum Publishers, New York, 2001.

species of gram-positive cocci that are vancomycin resistant, including some strains of *S. haemolyticus* and *S. epidermidis.*

Recent studies have addressed the problem of staphylococcal anti-biotic resistance from the standpoint of classic forms of resistance, e.g., enzymatic degradation, altered penicillin-binding proteins and enhanced export.[2] However, staphylococci may have additional mechanisms for resisting therapy that extend beyond these classic mechanisms. In patients infected with susceptible organisms, some demonstrate poor clinical and bacteriologic response to standard antimicrobial regimens. Even in patients whose acute infection initially seems to respond to antimicrobial treatment, chronic relapsing disease characterized by long periods of quiescence between episodes of acute illness may occur.[1,4] Specific micro-biological factors associated with such antibiotic failures have not been fully defined, but small colony variants (SCVs) of *S. aureus* have been recovered from patients with persistent, relapsing and antibiotic-resistant infections.[5,6]

2. SCVS ARE ELECTRON TRANSPORT VARIANTS

SCV subpopulations of staphylococci have been described for many decades.[5,7–11] They represent a naturally occuring subpopulation of *S. aureus* that grow slowly on routine media, hence, their name. SCVs form mostly nonpigmented and nonhemolytic colonies and are defined by colonies about 10 times smaller than the parent strain. This small size of many clinical and laboratory SCVs on tryptic soy or Mueller-Hinton agar is often due to auxotrophy for thiamine, thymidine, menadione, or hemin.[5,7,10–12] When the medium is supplemented with these compounds (see below), SCVs grow as rapidly as the parent strains. Thiamine, mena-dione, and hemin are required for biosynthesis of electron transport chain components, while the mechanism for thymidine auxotroph formation is not likely related to that for the electron transport type SCVs. Menadione is isoprenylated to form menaquinone, the acceptor of electrons from nicotinamide adenine dinucleotide (NADH)/flavin adenine dinucleotide ($FADH_2$) in the electron transport chain. Hemin is required for the biosynthesis of cytochromes, which accept electrons from menaquinone and transports them to the ATP synthesis complex in the cell membrane. Thiamine is required for menadione biosynthesis; hence, thiamine auxotrophs are also menadione auxotrophs. Many previous reports also noted decreased respiratory activity in staphy-lococcal SCVs, which is also consistent with reduced electron transport activity.[12,13]

SCVs also demonstrate a number of other characteristics that are atypical for *S. aureus* and can be tied together by a common thread, which is alterations in electron transport. Specifically, the following findings are very likely linked to an interruption of electron transport: (i) slow growth because cell wall synthesis requires large quantities of ATP, (ii) decreased pigment formation because carotenoid biosynthesis requires electron transport, (iii) resistance to aminoglycosides as their uptake requires the large membrane potential generated by electron transport, and (iv) mannitol fermentation negative because utilization of mannitol (sugar alcohol) is decreased when electron transport is not used (Figure 1).[12–15]

3. SURVIVAL ADVANTAGES OF SCVS

Formation of *S. aureus* SCVs has important pathogenic implications. The ability to interrupt electron transport and to form a variant subpopulation affords *S. aureus* a number of survival advantages that extends beyond simply increased resistance to antibiotics. (i) *S. aureus* are phagocytized by nonprofessional phagocytes such as endothelial cells. *S. aureus* with normal phenotype produces large amounts of α-toxin that quickly lyse mammalian cells. In contrast, SCVs are ingested equally well by host cells, but they produce only small amounts of α-toxin and are able to persist within the nonprofessional phagocytes, as shown by several groups using fibroblasts, endothelial cells[11,13,15] and keratinocytes [C. von Eiff, unpublished observation]. Previous work using a site-directed mutant of *hla*, showed that this α-toxin negative mutant also persisted within endothelial cells. The intracellular position shields SCVs from host defenses and decreases exposure to antibiotics.[6,11,13,16,17] (ii) An interruption in electron transport reduces the electrochemical gradient across the bacterial membrane, resulting in decreased uptake of antimicrobial agents that require a charge differential to be active such as aminoglycosides, some lantibiotics, protamine, and some cationic bacterial proteins found in most host cells.[14,18] (iii) The very slow growth of these variants also reduces the effectiveness of cell-wall active antibiotics that are most active against rapidly growing bacteria.[12,15] (iv) Because of this slow growth, these variants may not be recovered in the clinical microbiology laboratory, a distinct advantage for the organism in our modern era. (v) Because SCVs are often relatively unstable, they can hide within the host cell, then revert to the highly virulent rapidly growing form and lyse the host cell, once the host immune response has abated and antibiotic therapy is completed. Thus, the switch of *S. aureus* into an SCV may be a potent strategy for survival against host defenses and antibiotic therapy.[6,13,15,17]

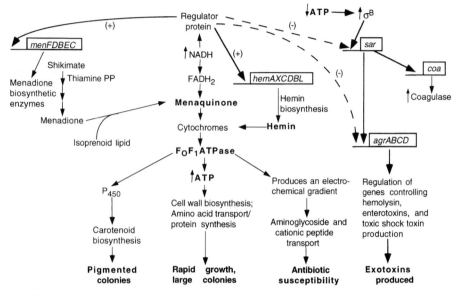

FIGURE 1. Interruption of electron transport is associated with multiple phenotypic changes in *S. aureus* that correspond to the phenotype of clinical SCVs. This model is strengthened by the observation that clinical SCVs are often auxotrophic for menadione, hemin, or thiamine, compounds involved in the biosynthesis of electron transport chain components (see also below: Characterization of a Stable Mutant in Electron Transport with SCV Phenotype). F_0F_1ATPase is the transmembrane complex that biosynthesizes ATP and creates the electrochemical gradient required for positively charged antimicrobial substances to associate with the bacterial membrane. ATP is critical for many energy-dependent activities, and decreasing levels lead to the activation of the stress sigma factor. Sigma B interacts with *sar*, one of the global regulators, which itself is reported to control *agr*, another global regulator and to positively regulate coagulase production. The *agr* operon controls the production of many toxins by *S. aureus*. Organisms among which electron transport is interrupted demonstrate reduced toxin production, despite their ability to grow >7 orders of magnitude. This suggests that some regulatory factor ("regulatory protein") may be present that down-regulates *sar* and/or *agr*. Because clinical SCVs produce only small amounts of coagulase, this suggests that the regulatory factor is at least acting upon *sar*. [Solid arrows indicate positice regulation, whereas broken arrows indicate negative regulation]. (From R. A. Proctor and G. Peters,[15] with permission of the authors and the publisher)

4. RECOVERY OF SCVS FROM PATIENTS

S. aureus SCVs were first described more than 80 years ago, yet their significance has been limited by the fact that their occurence in clinical specimen has been rarely reported.[5,15] Although *S. aureus* SCVs have been recognized for many years, connecting this phenotype to persistent and recurrent infections has only recently been appreciated.[5,6] A variant subpopulation of *S. aureus* that can hide within host cells and that is more resistant to antibiotics may help to explain the great difficulty in achieving cure for staphylococcal affections in intravascular and bone sites, even among cases for which antibiotic treatment is maintained for long periods. This ability of SCVs to persist intracellularly combined with the relatively low virulence of SCVs before they revert to the rapidly growing form help also to explain why *S. aureus* seems to be eradicated only to recur months to years later. Thus, patients were described having long disease-free intervals, the longest being 54 years.[5,12,15]

In the initial study, SCVs of *S. aureus* were cultured from five patients with unusually persistent and/or antibiotic-resistant infections.[5] All SCV strains were nonhemolytic and nonpigmented and grew very slowly on routine culture media in an ambient atmosphere. Consequently, that these phenotypic characteristics led to the initial misidentification of the organisms in the clinical microbiology laboratory. All four strains available for further studies were shown to be auxotrophs that reverted to normal colony forms in the presence of menadione, hemin, and/or CO_2 supplement. Similarly, these isolates were resistant to gentamicin, but susceptible in the presence of metabolic supplements. To evaluate clonality of infection, restriction endonuclease analysis of isolates with different colonial morphologies were performed on isolates from two patients, and this showed clonal identity of the strains, indicating phenotypic variants within individual clones. This was the first report where a model was offered that related the multiple changes in phenotypic characteristics of *S. aureus* SCVs, alterations in electron transport, and the clinical pattern of persistent and relapsing infection.[5]

The frequency of *S. aureus* SCVs among clinical isolates has not been established by prospective studies, except for the one blood culture study where stable SCVs were recovered from 1% of patients.[7] Since then, two groups of patients have been examined who have had extended exposure to antibiotics. To prospectively study patients who frequently have staphylococcal infections and receive large quantities of antibiotics, clinical specimen from cystic fibrosis (CF) patients and from patients with chronic osteomyelitis were evaluated for the presence of *S. aureus* SCVs.[10,11]

Prevalence of *S. aureus* SCVs in CF Patients

The prevalence of *S. aureus* SCVs in CF patients were determined in a 34-month prospective study including 78 patients.[11] All together; 53 patients (67.9%) harbored *S. aureus* in their respiratory specimens; of these 53, 27 (50.9%) had *S. aureus* with normal phenotype and 26 (49.1%) had normal plus SCVs, SCVs alone, or pure cultures of normal alternating with pure cultures of SCVs. In consecutive specimens from 19 of these 26 patients with recovery of these variants, SCVs were isolated over a period of 2–31 months, indicating persistence of these bacteria. Three of these patients had only SCVs and no normal *S. aureus* in their specimens. Auxotrophism for hemin could be demonstrated in 10, for menadione in 2, and for thymidine in 41 SCV strains. Double auxotrophy for thymidine plus hemin was found in 25 strains. Restriction fragments of total bacterial DNA were resolved with pulsed-field gel electrophoresis (PFGE) on specimen from 16 of 19 patients with persistent SCV colonization, and the restriction profiles of SCV and normal *S. aureus* from each patient showed clonality of the strains. In addition to the clonal SCV-normal pair, a second normal or SCV *S. aureus* strain could be isolated in five of these patients. All SCV isolates were resistant (MIC > 32) to trimethoprim-sulfamethoxazole, while the normal isolates (except one methicillin-resistant *S. aureus* strain) were trimethoprim-sulfamethoxazole-susceptible (MIC < 0.125). Of 12 SCV-normal strain pairs, 11 of 12 SCVs had higher gentamicin MICs than did their corresponding normal *S. aureus* strain.[11]

   S. aureus SCVs can be selected by antimicrobials, as shown by exposure of normal *S. aureus* to subinhibitory concentrations of gentamicin or other aminoglycosides.[16,19] In vivo, emergence of SCVs has been strongly associated with antibiotic use (for further details see below); however, SCVs may also be isolated after prolonged antibiotic-free intervals.[12,15] In the study on the prevalence of *S. aureus* SCVs in CF patients all 26 patients with SCVs had received trimethoprim-sulfamethoxazole prophylaxis, whereas only 10 of 27 patients with normal *S. aureus* received this treatment (P < .001). In addition, patients with SCVs were treated longer with trimethoprim-sulfamethoxazole (median: 23.5 months) than were patients with normal *S. aureus* (median: 18 months), but this difference did not reach significance. Also of interest, 11 of 19 patients with persistent SCV colonization received interventional aminoglycoside therapy. Notably, SCVs were isolated from patients even after extended trimethoprim-sulfamethoxazole-free intervals (3–31 months) and remained in vitro as stable SCV phenotype after primary culture and multiple passages in antibiotic-free medium. Hence, while antibiotic exposure of CF patients may contribute to SCV selection or induction, the *S. aureus* subpopulation then persist, even in the absence of selective antibiotic pressure. In addition, after transformation of *S. aureus* into an SCV, these bacteria acquire phenotypic resistance against compounds such as aminoglycosides by decreased antibiotic uptake or against antifolates by acquiring the ability to use exogenous nucleotide sources. This decreased susceptibility may then contribute to clinical persistence despite continued use of compounds such as trimethoprim-sulfamethoxazole.

In summary, the study showed for the first time that *S. aureus* SCVs are highly prevalent in respiratory secretions of CF patients, especially after long-term trimethoprim-sulfamethoxazole or interventional aminoglycoside treatment. SCVs may persist over extended periods, and thus contribute to *S. aureus* persistence in CF patients.[11]

Recovery of SCVs Following Gentamicin Bead Placement For Osteomyelitis

Gentamicin beads are used as an adjunct to debridement and antibiotic therapy for the treament of osteomyelitis. The beads slowly release the antibiotic over a period of weeks to months providing a sustained local level of drug. SCVs are more resistant to aminoglycosides (see below) and can be regularly recovered *in vitro* from cultures of normal *S. aureus* strains exposed to gentamicin.[14,16,19] In order to test whether the slow release into the local environment may be an efficient way to select for SCVs *in vivo*, bone specimens or deep tissue aspirates from patients with suspected osteomyelitis who had received gentamicin beads were carefully screened for *S. aureus* SCVs.[10] In this case-control study over an eighteen month period only patients with cultures that contained *S. aureus* were included. Patients were divided on the basis of previous placement of gentamicin beads in their bone, and their charts were reviewed. Fourteen patients were obtained on the basis of these criteria. In this study *S. aureus* SCVs were recovered from four patients, who had previously been treated with gentamicin beads. Three of these patients with SCVs had large and small colony types isolated from simultaneous or from sequential cultures which were clonal by PFGE. The SCVs were small, non-pigmented, slowly coagulase-positive, and non-hemolytic on rabbit blood agar. One SCV was a menadione and three were hemin auxotrophs. MICs for gentamicin were up to 32-fold higher for the SCVs as compared to the parent strain whereas no differences were found in susceptibilities against other antimicrobial agents. In the patients with SCVs therapy failed despite using antibiotics with *in vitro* activity against the normal parent *S. aureus*. In contrast, the other ten patients with normal *S. aureus* had no relapses of osteomyelitis occuring more than one year after primary diagnosis once active antibiotics were given for at least four weeks intravenously. Clinical evaluation showed no other major differences between the two groups. It was concluded that the recovery of *S. aureus* SCVs from patients who have been treated with gentamicin beads may be an efficient way to select for SCVs.[10] This can be demonstrated *in vitro* by exposing *S. aureus* to gentamicin and other aminoglycosides.[16,19] Selection for SCVs readily occur within 72 hours in clinical isolates of normal *S. aureus* that are exposed to gentamicin at

1 μg/ml Mueller Hinton broth. While the patient milieu is clearly more complex, parallels between the two situations are clear. To determine whether or not gentamicin beads should be used or avoided, and how often SCVs may be induced or selected by gentamicin beads will require a large prospective study because only patients that had failed gentamicin bead therapy were included in that study.

5. SCVS AND CLINICAL LABORATORY

Both, the prospective studies with CF patients and with osteomyelitis patients, strongly suggest that these pathogens must be actively sought by use of appropriate selective media and growth conditions. Furthermore, the decreased susceptibility of *S. aureus* SCVs against antimicrobials typically used for *S. aureus* prophylaxis or treatment requires the identification of these variants even in the presence of normal *S. aureus* in the specimens.

However, recovery and identification of SCVs in the microbiological laboratory can be difficult because of their fastidious growth characteristics. Considering the special phenotypic SCV characteristics, it is not surprising that most SCV isolates reported so far have been recovered from defined infectious foci, such as soft tissue abscesses or osteomyelitis, or from sterile body fluids, while in complex specimens, such as bronchial fluids, they are difficult to detect. Because of the atypical colony morphology of these variants, prerequisite for the isolation is the application of extended conventional culture and identification techniques: SCVs may be identified as nonpigmented, nonhemolytic pinpoint colonies, slow-growing after 24–72 hours' incubation on rabbit blood agar. Because SCVs and *S. aureus* with normal phenotype have the same appearance on gram staining, there is no reason to suspect a mixed culture, but the SCVs grow nine times more slowly than *S. aureus* with normal phenotype. Therefore, SCVs are rapidly overgrown and are easily missed when the normal *S. aureus* is present.[12,15,17]

Some SCVs grow more rapidly in the presence of CO_2 and on rich medium, such as Schaedler's agar which contains hemin. Hence, these SCVs can be construed to be anaerobic organisms as these conditions are often used for anaerobic blood cultures. As oxygen does not enhance growth of electron transport deficient SCVs, then their growth in an anaerobic chamber on Schaedler's agar can make the laboratory personnel believe anaerobes are present.[11,20] In addition, because of the atypical colonial morphology, the unusual biochemical reactions, and the reduced coagulase activity (often SCVs are only coagulase positive in the tube test after incubation for >18 hours), identification of SCVs as *S. aureus* is difficult.

Therefore, isolates suspicious for *S. aureus* SCVs should be confirmed as *S. aureus* by testing the species-specific *nuc* and *coa*-genes.[21]

Auxotrophy for hemin and NAD⁺ factor (Unipath, Basingstoke, UK) may be tested by using standard disks, and auxotrophy for thymidine (Fluka Chemie, Buchs, Switzerland) or menadione (Sigma Aldrich Chemie, Deisenhofen, Germany) by impregnating disks with 15 μL of thymidine or menadione at 100 μg/mL (Figure 2). To determine single auxotrophism, test isolates are inoculated on chemically defined medium (CDM) agar, impregnated disks are laid on top of the agar surface, and auxotrophism is determined as positive if a zone of normal growth surrounding the impregnated disks may be detected after 18 h of incubation. Likewise, for determination of double auxotrophy, disks may be tested on CDM agar supplemented with 100 μg of thymidine/mL, 1 μg of menadione/mL, or 1 μg of hemin/mL; for determination of triple auxotrophy, on CDM agar supplemented with 100 μg of thymidine/mL plus 1 μg of menadione/mL, 100 μg of thymidine/mL plus 1 μg of hemin/mL, or 1 μg of menadione/mL plus 1 μg of hemin/mL; and for determination of

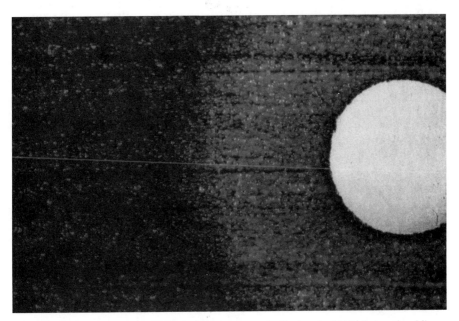

FIGURE 2. The small size of SCVs is due to auxotrophy for hemin, NAD⁺ factor, thymidine and menadione. To determine the auxotrophism, test isolates are inoculated on CDM agar with or without supplementation. Impregnated disks are laid on top of the agar surface, and auxotrophism is determined as positive if a zone of normal growth surrounding the impregnated disks may be detected after 18 h of incubation.

combined auxotrophism, on CDM agar supplemented with 100 μg of thymidine/mL, 1 μg of menadione/mL, and 1 μg of hemin/mL.

SCVs also present a challenge in terms of susceptibility testing, because the clinical isolates are often a mixed population of parent strain and SCVs. Even a small percentage (e.g., 0.1%) of normally growing organisms will rapidly replace the SCVs in liquid medium in an overnight culture because the doubling time of normal *S. aureus* is about 20 minutes, whereas SCVs double in about 180 minutes; hence, the SCVs may be overgrown to such an extent that they may not be included in the inoculum used for susceptibility testing. Furthermore, the slow growing SCVs are not always stable once they are removed from the host. Thus, results of testing by use of disk diffusion or by automated overnight methods are invalidated because the colonies may be too small to be seen on agar or detected by optical density measurements in automated systems. Consequently, testing must be performed by broth or agar dilution MIC methods.[12,15]

Even when all of the testing is properly performed, there are difficulties. *S. aureus* SCVs are not only more resistant when tested by classic methods, but they are also much more resistant to antibiotics when adherent to a biopolymer surface. In one study, during logarithmic growth phase in broth or on solid phase, i.e., adherent to a polymer surface, both parent strain with normal phenotype and SCVs were susceptible to oxacillin, vancomycin, and fleroxacin. However, two orders of magnitude more of the SCVs than the parent strain remained alive, when antibiotics were at eight times the MIC; moreover, stationary phase SCVs were much more resistant to killing with only a 10-fold reduction when in fluid phase and almost no reduction when SCVs were grown on a solid phase. Of the antibiotics tested, fleroxacin reduced adherent, stationary phase SCVs almost one $\log_{10}$, whereas the other antibiotics had essentially no effect on colony counts.[22] Thus, while *S. aureus* strains with normal phenotype show a modest decrease in susceptibility when adherent, *S. aureus* SCVs demonstrate a dramatic reduction in susceptibility once they are attached to a surface and have reached stationary phase, so that these adherent organisms have shown nearly complete resistance to the antibiotics that have been tested.[22]

6. CHARACTERIZATION OF A STABLE MUTANT IN ELECTRON TRANSPORT WITH SCV PHENOTYPE

The main characteristics of clinical SCVs are as follows: (i) isolation of the variants from patients with persistent or antibiotic resistant infectious diseases, (ii) auxotrophy of SCVs for menadione or hemin, two compounds required in the biosynthesis of electron transport chain components, menaquinone and cytochromes, respectively, and (iii) ability to persist intracellularly. Taken together, these characteristics suggested a link between electron transport defective strains and persistent infections; however, defined mutants were required to provide more definitive evidence for these connections. The strains examined so far were genetically undefined SCVs, and the clinical strains exhibit a high rate of reversion to the large colony form. In addition, genetically undefined strains might carry mutations in more than one virulence factor, especially since the clinical SCVs show multiple phenotypic changes as compared to the parent strains.

To address questions concerning possible roles of respiratory-defective *S. aureus* in the pathogenesis of staphylococcal infection, a stable mutant in electron transport was generated by interrupting *hemB* in *S. aureus*.[13] Heme is the prosthetic group of cytochromes, which plays an essential role in electron transport. The *hemB* gene is a member of the family of genes encoding enzymes of the porphyrin biosynthetic pathway; it codes for the enzyme aminolevulinic acid dehydrase, which is responsible for the conversion of delta-aminolevulinic acid to porphobilinogen. This mutant allowed us to characterize the phenotype of a genetically defined SCV of *S. aureus* and to test the hypothesis that defects in electron transport promote the development of intracellular persistence.[13]

The *S. aureus hemB* mutant showed the typical characteristics of clinical SCVs: (i) pinpoint colonies on solid agar, that are >10 fold smaller than the parent strain and slow growth of the *hemB* mutant was also observed in liquid medium (TSB or CDM). The *hemB* mutant reached stationary phase at a 10-fold lower level of total growth in comparison to the wild type. (ii) Decreased pigment formation: whitish colonies versus golden yellow colored colonies of the parent strain. (iii) Reduced hemolytic activity: the *hemB* mutant showed >90-fold reduction in percentage of lysis of rRBC compared with the parent strain 8325–4 (0.25% versus 89%). (iv) Decreased coagulase activity: in the tube coagulase test, the mutant showed a delayed coagulase reaction, being positive after 22 h incubation at 37°C whereas the parent strain was positive after 2 h. (v) Resistance to aminoglycosides: MIC for gentamicin was 16-fold higher for the mutant (MIC = 0.5 μg/ml) compared to the wild-type strain (MIC = <0.031 μg/ml) and MIC for kanamycin was 8-fold higher for the mutant (MIC = 2.0 μg/ml) compared to the wild-type strain (MIC = 0.25 μg/ml). (vi) In contrast to the parent strain and the plasmid complemented mutant, the *hemB* mutant showed biochemical characteristics that were atypical for *S. aureus*, such as reduced lactose-, turanose- and mannitol-fermentation, no nitrate reduction, and reduced N-acetyl-glucosamine utilization as analyzed in the API-systems and with conventional biochemicals. The SCV phenotype of the *hemB* mutant was essentially reversed by growing with hemin at a concentration of $1\,\mu g/ml$ or by complementation with intact *hemB*. A distinct band with a molecular mass of approximately $38\,kDa$ was observed in the protein pattern of lysostaphin cell lysates in a *hemB* complemented strain. N-terminal protein sequencing showed that this additional protein represents overproduced HemB.[13]

In order to analyze whether the *hemB* mutant produces equal amounts of extracellular and cell-associated proteins in comparison to the wild type, Western blot analyses to detect α-toxin and protein A production were performed. The Western blot analysis showed that α-toxin is produced in the parent strain, in the mutant supplemented with hemin, and in the complemented mutant. However, α-toxin was not detectable in the *hemB* mutant. Protein A was produced in the parent strain as well as in the mutant when supplemented by hemin or complemented with *hemB*. However, protein A was produced only very weak in the absence of hemin or the plasmid and was not detectable in the protein A mutant DU5875.[13]

In addition, to determine whether reduced protein levels correlated with reduced transcription, Northern blot analysis were performed to detect *spa* and *hla* transcripts. Equal amounts of RNA were isolated and used to determine the amount of *spa* (encoding protein A) and *hla* (encoding α-toxin) transcripts. In the wild type the amount of *spa* transcript was highest in the log phase (sample taken after 3 h cultivation); after 7 h cultivation no transcripts were detectable. The non-complemented *hemB* mutant exhibited no *spa* transcripts. However, if the mutant was complemented or grown with hemin, *spa* message was detectable after 7 h cultivation. Northern blot analysis of *hla* showed that transcription of *hla* was high in the early and late stationary phase, but not detectable in the log-phase. Transcription level of *hla* was high in the parent strain as well as in the plasmid complemented mutant. In the non-complemented mutant no *hla* transcript was detectable. The addition of hemin resulted only in a low level of *hla* message. Probably, *agr* and/or *sar*, the two global regulatory systems, are involved in this downregulation.[23,24] On the other hand, the export of proteins might be affected, too, because anaerobically grown *S. aureus* cells have a decreased membrane potential and showed little α-toxin production.[16] The observed lack of α-toxin production could therefore be due to downregulation and decreased secretion. Some reduction in protein synthesis could also be due to decreased energy production because protein synthesis is an energy consuming process.

Finally, in order to determine whether the *hemB* mutant could persist intracellularly within aortic bovine endothelial cells more efficiently than the parent strain *S. aureus* 8325–4, intracellular persistence assays were performed. Although hemolytic *S. aureus* strains are readily internalized by bovine endothelial cells, they efficiently lyse the endothelial cells and are thus—in contrast to SCVs—unlikely to exploit the advantages of this intracellular environment. In this model of endovascular infection higher numbers of the mutant were seen following the initial 3.5 h coincubation and a 20 min. incubation in the presence of lysostaphin compared to the parent strain and to the plasmid complemented mutant (complemented with the plasmid pCE12, tested with and without induction by xylose). Further coincubation in the continuous presence of lysostaphin revealed that >200-fold more *hemB*-mutant cells persisted intracellularly after 24 or 48 h incubation relative to the other strains tested. Supplementation of hemin reduced the intracellular persistence to the level of the parent strain[13] (Figure 3).

While the studies with clinical isolates of SCVs suggest a link between electron transport defective strains and persistent infections, the defined *hemB* mutant with the SCV phenotype provides strong additional definitive evidence for these connections. The *hemB* mutant was phagocytized by cultured endothelial cells, but did not lyse these cells, because the mutant produced very little α-toxin. The intracellular location may shield the SCVs from host defenses and antibiotics, thus providing one explanation for the difficulty in clearing *S. aureus* SCVs from host tissues.

Very recently, *S. aureus* SCVs were found to cause a persistent and antibiotic resistant mastitis in mice.[25] The investigators made a *hemB* mutant for these investigations essentially identical to that used by von Eiff *et al.*[13] This mutant invaded the epithelial cells of the mouse as well as the parent strain, but it produced a more persistent and antibiotic refractory infection. While these were defined in a murine experimental model, this clinical picture is very typical of bovine mastitis caused by *S. aureus*, which are a major problem for the dairy industry.

7. SCVS AND OTHER SPECIES

In comparison with SCVs of *S. aureus*, relatively little is known regarding infections caused by SCVs of coagulase-negative staphylococci (CoNS). There are only two well-described cases of infection due to phenotypic variants of CoNS, however strains were not characterized as slow-growing electron-transport deficient SCVs regarding their auxotrophisms.[26] Most recently, two cases of pacemaker electrode infections due to SCVs of *Staphylococcus epidermidis* and *Staphylococcus capitis*, respectively, were described.[20] In these patients isolates from blood cultures were obtained over at least a two week interval and visible growth of SCVs on subculture plates started

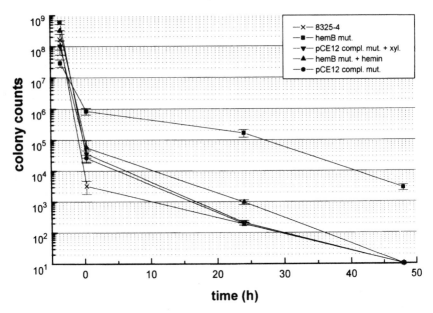

FIGURE 3. Intracellular persistence assay within cultured bovine aortic endothelial cells. Aortic bovine endothelial cell monolayers were grown to confluence. Washed bacteria were adjusted to nearly equal numbers for each strain and added to the washed monolayers. The infected monolayers were incubated for 3.5 h at 37°C in 5% CO_2 to allow adhesion and phagocytosis of the bacteria. The monolayers were then washed to remove nonattached organisms, then medium containing 10 µg of lysostaphin/ml was added, which effectively eliminated extracellular staphylococci. Incubation in the presence of lysostaphin was continued for 20 min, 24 h and 48 h. At these time points, the monolayers were washed three times to remove lysostaphin. Then sterile water was added to disrupt endothelial cells and to release intracellular organisms. Serial dilutions were made in sterile water. The number of intracellular colony-forming units (cfu) was determined by plating 100 µl aliquots on TSA in duplicate. The number of intracellular cfu at each time point was determined in duplicate or triplicate: each point represents the mean of three experiments +/– SD. (From C. von Eiff *et al.*,[13] with permission of the authors and the publisher)

only after 48–72 h incubation at 37°C yielding very small colonies. The organisms were so heterogeneous in their colonial morphology that polymicrobic infection was suspected. For most isolates biochemical testing with API Staph strips and conventional macrotube testing was not possible, except for the finding of catalase positivity, because their limited growth over 48 hours was not sufficient enough to provide positive test results in the reaction vials. Therefore, two approaches were used to identify the positive blood cultures. First, by analyzing a portion of the 16S rDNA: Sequence analysis confirmed the identity of the staphylococcal species as *S. capitis* and

S. epidermidis. Second, *Sma*I digests of the whole bacterial genome of all iso-lates analysed by PFGE, and they were found to be clonal, even though the colony morphology was very different. Thus, the isolates in both cases were proved to be from the same species and the subpopulations were also from the same clone. Analysis for auxotrophism revealed hemin dependencies for all isolated SCVs.

The two cases showed several clinical and laboratory characteristics, which are also seen with *S. aureus* SCVs infections: (i) the organisms grew very slowly and could have been easily missed, if the blood subcultures were examined for only 48 hours, particularly when normal colony forms are also present; (ii) SCVs were difficult to identify due to their slow and atypical biochemical reactions, such as reduced lactose and turanose fermentation, and/or no nitrate reduction; (iii) the presence of hetero-geneous colony forms initially suggested a mixed infection, yet all of the isolates were the same species and clonal, respectively; (iv) all SCVs isolated in these patients were hemin auxotrophs; and (v) the SCVs grew more rapidly in the presence of CO_2 and on rich medium, such as Schaedler's agar. However, in contrast to most cases reported with *S. aureus* SCVs, no differences in antibiotic susceptibilities were observed compar-ing normal phenotype and SCVs in these cases. The coagulase negative SCVs from both patients were susceptible to all antibiotics tested, includ-ing penicillins, cephalosporines, aminoglycosides, fluoroquinolones, but the testing was extended to 48–72 hours to allow sufficient growth of the controls.[20]

These cases show that SCVs of CoNS, similar to those of *S. aureus*, must be actively sought, because they grow very slowly and can easily be missed and indicate that molecular techniques may be required for identification of SCVs. We might expect to see SCVs in other genera being reported for other patients with persistent infections because a wide variety of other species are known to form SCVs, e.g., *Pseudomonas aeruginosa*, *Salmonella typhimurium*, *Shigella species*, *Brucella abortus*, *E. coli*, *Lactobacillus acidophilus*, *Serratia marcescens*, and *Neisseria gonorrhoeae*. Most SCVs from these species are characterized as respiratory deficient and/or have been described as deficient in electron transport. Aminoglycosides were recognized as having higher MICs also for some of these organisms.[6,12]

8. THERAPEUTIC IMPLICATIONS OF SCV FORMATION

Development of the SCV phenotype may not always be a clinically dis-advantageous situation. Because of their low exotoxin production, SCVs cause less tissue damage than do rapidly growing staphylococci. The presence of SCVs would be much preferable to that of a highly virulent pathogen in patients with acute bacteremia. The use of drugs that interfered with electron transport might be particularly valuable as a short-term measure if such drugs could rapidly turn off toxin production. There are currently investigations studying the effect of an electron transport inhibitor on *S. aureus*. It was found that α-toxin production and damage to cultured endothelial cells was reduced by this compound, which would represent a new class of anti-virulence factor drug (R. A. Proctor, unpublished observation).

Optimal therapy for infections due to *S. aureus* SCVs has not been defined. Reversal of the auxotrophy *in vitro* is encouraging, because reversion to the normal colony form makes these organisms more susceptible to antibiotics. In the case of menadione auxotrophs, this reversal can be easily accomplished by administering vitamin K to patients. However, whether this will prove to be of benefit remains to be determined by clinical trials. It was found, that trimethoprim-sulfamethoxazol combined with rifampin was the most active therapeutic regimen in a tissue-culture system where the SCVs were inside endothelial cells, but more research is necessary to define the optimal therapy.[12,15]

REFERENCES

1. F. A. Waldvogel, *Staphylococcus aureus* (including toxic shock syndrome), in: Principles and Practice of Infectious Diseases, G. L. Mandell, J. E. Bennett and R. Dolan, eds. pp. 1754–1777, Churchill Livingstone, New York (1995).
2. F. D. Lowy, *Staphylococcus aureus* infections, N. Engl. J. Med. 339:520–532 (1998).
3. K. Hiramatsu, N. Aritaka, H. Hanaki, S. Kawasaki, Y. Hosoda, S. Hori, Y. Fukuchi and I. Kobayashi, Dissemination in Japanese hospitals of strains of *Staphylococcus aureus* heterogeneously resistant to vancomycin, Lancet 350:1670–1673 (1997).
4. P. Korovessis, A. P. Fortis, P. Spastris and P. Droutsas, Acute osteomyelitis of the patella 50 years after a knee fusion for septic arthritis. A case report, Clin. Orthop. 272:205–207 (1991).
5. R. A. Proctor, P. van Langevelde, M. Kristjansson, J. N. Maslow and R. D. Arbeit, Persistent and relapsing infections associated with small-colony variants of *Staphylococcus aureus*, Clin. Infect. Dis. 20:95–102 (1995).
6. R. A. Proctor, J. M. Balwit and O. Vesga, Variant subpopulations of *Staphylococcus aureus* as cause of persistent and recurrent infections, Infect. Agents Dis. 3:302–312 (1994).
7. J. F. Acar, F. W. Goldstein and P. Lagrange, Human infections caused by thiamine-or menadione-requiring *Staphylococcus aureus*, J. Clin. Microbiol. 8:142–147 (1978).
8. L. L. Pelletier, M. Richardson and M. Feist, Virulent gentamicin-induced small colony variants of *Staphylococcus aureus*, J. Lab. Clin. Med. 94:324–334 (1979).
9. R. I. Wise and W. W. Spink, The influence of antibiotics on the origin of small colonies (G variants) of *Micrococcus pyogenes var aureus*, J. Clin. Invest. 33:1611–1622 (1954).

10. C. von Eiff, D. Bettin, R. A. Proctor, B. Rolauffs, N. Lindner, W. Winkelmann and G. Peters, Recovery of small colony variants of *Staphylococcus aureus* following gentamicin bead placement for osteomyelitis, Clin. Infect. Dis. 25:1250–1251 (1997).

11. B. Kahl, M. Herrmann, A. Schulze-Everding, H. G. Koch, K. Becker, E. Harms, R. A. Proctor and G. Peters, Persistent infection with small colony variant strains of *taphylococcus aureus* in patients with cystic fibrosis, J. Infect. Dis. 177:1023–1029 (1997).

12. R. A. Proctor, B. Kahl, C. von Eiff, P. E. Vaudaux, D. P. Lew and G. Peters, Staphylococcal small colony variants have novel mechanisms for antibiotic resistance, Clin. Infect. Dis. 27 (Suppl. 1):S68–S74 (1997).

13. C. von Eiff, C. Heilmann, R. A. Proctor, C. Wolz, G. Peters and F. Götz, A site-directed *Staphylococcus aureus hemB* mutant is a small colony variant which persists intracellularly, J. Bacteriol. 179:4706–4712 (1997).

14. L. A. Lewis, K. Li, M. Bharosay, M. Cannella, V. Jorgenson, R. Thomas, D. Pena, M. Velez, B. Pereira and A. Sassine, Characterization of gentamicin-resistant respiratory-deficient (*res-*) variant strains of *Staphylococcus aureus*, Microbiol. Immunol. 34:587–605 (1990).

15. R. A. Proctor and G. Peters, Small colony variants in staphylococcal infections: diagnostic and therapeutic implications, Clin. Infect. Dis. 27:419–423 (1998).

16. J. M. Balwit, P. van Langevelde, J. M. Vann and R. A. Proctor, Gentamicin-resistant menadione and hemin auxotrophic *Staphylococcus aureus* persist within cultured endothelial cells, J. Infect. Dis. 170:1033–1037 (1994).

17. O. Vesga, M. C. Groeschel, M. F. Otten, D. W. Brar, J. M. Vann and R. A. Proctor, *Staphylococcus aureus* small colony variants are induced by the endothelial cell intracellular milieu, J. Infect. Dis. 173:739–742 (1996).

18. S. P. Koo, A. S. Bayer, H. G. Sahl, R. A. Proctor and M. R. Yeaman, Staphylocidal action of thrombin-induced platelet microbicidal protein is not solely dependent on transmembrane potential, Infect. Immun. 64:1070–1074 (1996).

19. D. M. Musher, R. E. Baughn, G. B. Templeton and J. N. Minuth, Emergence of variant forms of *Staphylococcus aureus* after exposure to gentamicin and infectivity of the variants in experimental animals, J. Infect. Dis. 136:360–369 (1977).

20. C. von Eiff, P. Vaudaux, B. Kahl, D. P. Lew, A. Schmidt, G. Peters and R. A. Proctor, Blood stream infections caused by small colony variants of coagulase-negative staphylococci following pacemaker implantation, Clin. Infect. Dis. (in press).

21. O. G. Brakstad, K. Aasbakk and J. A. Maeland, Detection of *Staphylococcus aureus* by polymerase chain reaction amplification of the *nuc* gene, J. Clin. Microbiol. 30:1654–1660 (1992).

22. C. Chuard, P. Vaudaux, R. A. Proctor and D. P. Lew, Decreased susceptibility to antibiotic killing of a stable small colony variant of *Staphylococcus aureus* in fluid phase and on fibronectin-coated surfaces, J. Antimicrob. Chemother. 39:603–608 (1997).

23. J. H. Heinrichs, M. G. Bayer and A. L. Cheung, Characterization of the *sar* locus and its interaction with *agr* in *Staphylococcus aureus*, J. Bacteriol. 178:418–423 (1996).

24. J. Kornblum, B. N. Kreiswirth, S. J. Projan, H. Ross and R. P. Novick, *Agr:* A polycistronic locus regulating exoprotein synthesis in *Staphylococcus aureus*, in: Molecular biology of the staphylococci, R. P. Novick, ed., pp. 373–402, VCH Publishers, Inc., New York (1990).

25. A. Martinez, B. J. Boyll and N. E. Allen, The role of small-colony variants of *Staphylococcus aureus* in chronic bovine mastitis, Abstracts of the 99th Meeting of the American Society for Microbiology, Abstract D/B100 (1999).

26. L. M. Baddour, L. P. Barker, G. D. Christensen, J. T. Parisi and W. A. Simpson, Phenotypic variation of *Staphylococcus epidermidis* in infection of transvenous endocardial pacemaker electrodes, J. Clin. Microbiol. 28:676–679 (1990).

3

Capsule Production

CHIA Y. LEE

1. INTRODUCTION

Staphylococcus aureus produces a great number of virulence factors such as extracellular toxins, secreted enzymes and cell surface-associated antigens which are responsible for the pathogenicity of the organism. One of the cell surface-associated virulence factors is capsular polysaccharide. Most of the clinical isolates of *Staphylococcus aureus* produce capsular polysaccharides and 11 serotypes have been identified. According to colony morphology, and as discussed below, the genetic criteria and virulence properties, these capsules can also be divided into two distinct groups. Serotype 1 and 2 capsules are classified as mucoid-type capsules because strains producing these capsules are heavily encapsulated and are mucoid on solid medium. The remaining serotype 3 to 11 capsules are classified as microcapsules because strains with these capsules have a thin capsular layer and form nonmucoid colonies on solid medium. Because of the distinct mucoid appearance which are easily recognized, mucoid strains such as serotype 2 strain Smith Diffuse and serotype 1 strain M were used as the prototype in early studies of staphylococcal capsules. However, since serotypes 5 and 8 strains are clinically prevalent,[1-5] recent studies have focused on the biology of these microencapsulated nonmucoid strains. In this section, I focus on recent developments in the genetics, regulation, biosynthesis and virulence properties associated with *S. aureus* capsules. The earlier studies on mucoid-type *S. aureus* strains can be found from an excellent review by Wilkinson.[6]

CHIA Y. LEE • Department of Microbiology, Molecular Genetics and Immunology, University of Kansas Medical Center, Kansas City, KS 66160.

Staphylococcus aureus *Infection and Disease*, edited by Allen L. Honeyman *et al.* Kluwer Academic/Plenum Publishers, New York, 2001.

2. STRUCTURE OF STAPHYLOCOCCAL CAPSULES

The biochemical structures of serotypes 1, 2, 5, and 8 capsular polysaccharides have been determined and all serotypes contain hexosaminouronic acids.[6-10] The trisaccharide repeating units of type 5 and type 8 capsules are very similar. They share the same sugar composition and differ only in the linkages between the amino sugars and the position of O-acetylation. Types 1, 5 and 8 capsules also have a common sugar, N-acetylfucosamine. The repeating units of these 4 serotypes are shown below:

Type 1: →4)-α-D-GalNAcAp(1→4)-α-D-GalNAcAp(1→3)-α-D-FucNAcp(1→
       (A taurine residue is linked by an amide bond to every 4th D-GalNAcAp residue.)

Type 2: →4)-β-D-GlcNAcAp(1→4)-β-D-GlcN(N-acetylalanyl)AcAp-(1→

Type 5: →4)-3-O-Ac-β-D-ManNAcAp(1→4)-α-L-FucNAcp(1→3)-β-D-FucNAcp(1→

Type 8: →3)-4-O-Ac-β-D-ManNAcAp(1→3)-α-L-FucNAcp(1→3)-β-D-FucNAcp(1→

(Abbreviations: GalNAcA, N-acetyl-galactosaminuronic acid; FucNAc, N-acetyl-fucosamine; GlcNAcA, N-acetyl-glucosaminuronic acid; ManNAcA, N-acetyl-mannosaminuronic acid; O-Ac, O-acetyl)

3. ROLE OF STAPHYLOCOCCAL CAPSULE IN VIRULENCE

The role of mucoid-type capsules in *S. aureus* virulence has been well established. Early studies indicated that the mucoid-type capsules were important antiphagocytic virulence factors that masked C3b deposited on the bacterial cell wall thereby preventing recognition of bacterial cells by receptors on phagocytic cells.[11,12] The masking effect of the capsule is consistent with the results that the amount of capsule produced is important for virulence.[13] The virulence properties of the mucoid capsule were also confirmed by a mouse lethality study using a genetic knockout mutant derived from type 1 strain M.[14] Thus, there is little doubt that mucoid-type capsules play an important role in staphylococcal pathogenesis.

In contrast to the mucoid capsules, the role of microcapsules in virulence is controversial. An early report indicated that microcapsules conferred resistance to phagocytic killing and that antibodies to the capsules induced type-specific phagocytosis *in vitro*.[11] However, later studies showed that strains with type 5 and type 8 capsules were no more virulent than their capsule-negative mutants.[15,16] Furthermore, in a rat model of catheter-induced endocarditis, the type 5 capsule was shown to attenuate bacterial virulence and capsule-specific antibodies did not protect animals which were challenged intravenously.[17,18] On the contrary, Fattom *et al.*[19] showed that the vaccines composed of protein conjugated type 5 and type 8 capsules protected mice from a lethal dose of *S. aureus* administered intraperitoneally. This protection was also later observed by challenging the animals intraperitoneally rather than intravenously using the rat catheter-induced endocarditis model that previously failed to show protection.[20] It was suggested that the positive antibody protection results may be due to intraperitoneal challenge route which allows for a gradual generation of bacteremia and organ seeding that is perhaps more clinically relevant than the events following intravenous challenge.[19]

Most recently, by testing in different animal models, microcapsules have been directly implicated as important virulence factors in several studies. Using a mouse septic arthritis model, Nilsson *et al.*[21] showed that mice inoculated with *S. aureus* expressing a type 5 capsule had a higher frequency of arthritis and a more severe form of the disease than animals inoculated with nonencapsulated mutant strains. In addition, macrophages were less efficient in phagocytize the wild-type strains than the capsule-deficient mutants. Similarly, type 5 capsule has been shown to enhance *S. aureus* virulence in a murine bacteremia model and the virulence correlates well with resistance to phagocytosis.[22] In addition, type 5 capsule was shown to increase the ability of the organism to persist in nares in a murine nasal colonization model.[23] Thus, these recent results convincingly indicate that the microcapsules are important in staphylococcal virulence, although this conclusion is clearly dependent on the animal model of infection tested suggesting that microcapsules are disease-specific virulence factors.

4. GENETICS AND REGULATION OF THE CAPSULAR GENES

The first genetic study of staphylococcal capsule was reported by Smith *et al.*[24] who showed that the genes for capsule biosynthesis in strain Smith Diffuse were chromosomal encoded despite the high loss rate of the phenotype (1.3%). However, not until 1992 had the first cloning of the capsule genes been reported. The type 1 capsule genes (*cap1*) were first cloned by screening an *S. aureus* library for complementation of chemically-induced nonmucoid mutants derived from strain M.[25] The *cap1* locus was mapped in the G fragment of the SmaI physical map of *S. aureus* genome (Ouyang and Lee, unpublished data). Subsequent sequencing of the *cap1* locus indicates that it contains 13 tightly clustered genes, *cap1A* through *cap1M*, in a 14.6-kb region of the chromosome. Molecular characterization and mutagenesis of the *cap1* genes showed that all 13 genes were required for the type 1 capsule synthesis.[14] Northern hybridization studies indicates that all 13 genes were transcribed into a large transcript of about 14 kb in size. However, promoter mapping by reporter gene fusion and genetic complementation indicates that there are weak internal promoters within the *cap1* operon though these internal promoters are much weaker than the primary promoter located about 26 bp upstream from the ATG start codon of the first gene, *cap1A*.[26]

The primary *cap1* promoter apparently requires no upstream cis-acting element for activity as deletions upstream of the −35 region had no effect on promoter activity as measured by *xylE* reporter gene fusions.[26] These results suggest that the genes for mucoid-type capsules are constitutively expressed which is consistent with the fact that type 1 capsule expression is only modestly affected by environmental factors.[27] Nonetheless, the production of mucoid-type capsules has been shown to be unstable both *in vitro* and *in vivo*. The frequency of nonmucoid colonies arise from the mucoid strain M is 10^{-4} at 37°C and 10^{-2} to 3.8×10^{-1} at 43°C,[25] whereas the rate is 10^{-2} at 37°C or 44°C in type 2 strain Smith Diffuse.[24] Interestingly, loss of mucoid phenotype in strain M was due not to rearrangement but rather to mutations within the genes in the *cap1* locus.[28] At 37°C, the mutations occur more random than those at 43°C. Since the rate of mutation at 43°C is much higher than spontaneous mutations and that the mutations are not totally random, it is tempted to speculate that a specific system may be operating to turn off the mucoid capsule production under this condition. However, there is no apparent reason for the existence of such a system in strain M. On the other hand, switching from nonmucoid phenotype to mucoid phenotype has been observed upon animal passage. When nonmucoid mutants of strain M were injected intraperitoneally into mice, mucoid colonies were recovered from the peritoneal washings of mice that succumbed to challenge.[29] These results suggest that mucoid-type capsule may confer advantages, such as antiphagocytosis, for the bacteria in an *in vivo* environment.

Interestingly, Southern hybridization revealed that the entire *cap1* operon was specific to type 1 strains. In fact, the 14.6-kb *cap1* gene cluster is part of a discrete genetic element 33.3–35.8 kb in length.[30] In addition to the *cap1* gene cluster, the element contains a transposase-like gene and an enterotoxin-like gene near one end of the element as revealed by sequencing of the junctions between the element and the chromosome

(Ouyang and Lee, unpublished data). However, no repeated sequences were found at the junctions. It remains to be determined whether the *cap1* genes reside on a mobile genetic element.

Shortly after the *cap1* genes were cloned, cloning of *cap5* and *cap8* gene clusters was also reported. The *cap8* gene cluster was identified by screening of a genomic library of serotype 8 strain Becker with *cap1* gene probes under low-stringency conditions,[31] whereas the *cap5* gene cluster was cloned by transposon mutagenesis.[32,33] Sequencing analysis revealed that the *cap5* and *cap8* loci each contain 16 closely linked genes, *cap5(8)A* through *cap5(8)P*, transcribed in one orientation. Of the 16 genes comprising the two gene clusters, 12 are nearly identical whereas the remaining 4 genes in each gene cluster share little homology and thus are type specific.[33] The type-specific genes are located in the central region flanked by the common genes (Figure 1). In contrast, only moderate homology (61% to 71% amino acid identity) was found between *cap5(8)A-D* and respective *cap1A-D*[31,33] which apparently allowed the cloning of the *cap8* gene cluster by hybridization at low stringency.

The presence of common genes flanking type-specific genes indicates that the two *cap5* and *cap8* loci are allelic. Interestingly, these common genes are also present in strains of different capsule serotypes including serotypes 1 and 2 and in nontypeable strains suggests that all strains of *S. aureus* contain an allelic microcapsule-related locus.[31,32] However, a recent survey of bovine isolates of *S. aureus* from Argentina showed that many of these strains did not hybridize to the common genes of *cap5* and *cap8* gene clusters.[34] The fact that the mucoid type 1 strain M also contains the common genes of *cap5* and *cap8* gene clusters indicates that strain M must contain two capsule gene clusters; one specific for a mucoid type and other for a microcapsule. In fact, the second capsule locus from strain M has been cloned but not yet characterized.[31] It is interesting that both *cap5(8)* and *cap1* loci mapped closely on the same 175-kb *Sma*I-G fragment of the physical map of strain NCTC8325 (Ouyang and Lee, unpublished data).[33]

The 16 genes in the *cap8* gene cluster are transcribed by a primary promoter into a large transcript of ~17kb as revealed by Northern analysis.[35] Genetic complementation and reporter gene fusion also showed that there were numerous weak internal promoters within the *cap8* operon that are biologically active.[36] Thus, the transcriptional organization of the *cap8* locus is similar to that of the *cap1* locus in that both operons are transcribed by a primary promoter located at the beginning of the operon and that there are weak internal promoters within the operon. The difference, however, is that the *cap1* primary promoter is about 60-fold stronger than the *cap8* primary promoter in their respective genetic

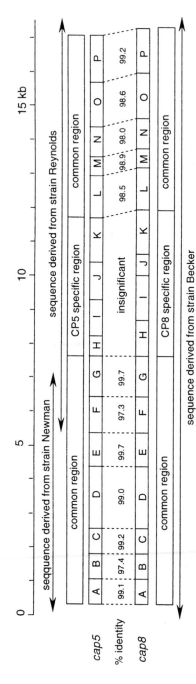

FIGURE 1. Comparison of *cap5* and *cap8* gene clusters. The *cap5* sequence is derived from strains Newman and Reynolds and the *cap8* sequence is derived from strain Becker as shown. Gene designations are shown in boxes. Percent identity indicates the amino acid identity of the deduced proteins between the two clusters. Both gene clusters are transcribed from left to right.

backgrounds.[26,35] The relative strengths of these two primary promoters may explain why the type 1 capsule is produced in a much greater amount than the type 8 capsule.

Unlike mucoid-type capsules, the production of microcapsules is influenced by environmental factors. Staphylococci grown in an iron-limited, defined medium produced 4- to 8-fold more capsule than cells grown in an iron-replete medium.[27] Similarly, cultures grown on agar plates or *in vivo* (in a rabbit endocarditis infection model) expressed >300-fold more type 8 capsule than broth-grown cultures.[27] Increased production of type 5 capsule was observed under conditions of high oxygen tension but reduced production was detected under alkaline growth conditions or in the presence of yeast extract.[37,38] In the presence of milk, increased level of capsular polysaccharide was detected from bovine mastitis isolates.[39,40] In the presence of carbon dioxide, type 5 capsule production was reduced.[41] In contrast, the effect of carbon dioxide on type 8 capsule production has been shown to be strain-dependent (Newell and Lee, unpublished data) sequence is derived from strains Newman and Reynolds and the *cap8* sequence from strain.

Recently, *agr*, a quorum-sensing global regulator that simultaneously regulates many gene products in *S. aureus*, has been shown to positively regulate the production of type 5 and type 8 capsules[42] (Luong and Lee, unpublished data). However, unlike other cell-wall associated gene products which are down-regulated by *agr* at high cell-density,[43] microcapsules are up-regulated by *agr*. This fact suggests that microcapsules may be important at a different stage of the pathogenic process compared to other cell-wall proteins. In addition to *agr*, a newly identified global regulator, *mgr*, has been shown to affect the production of type 8 capsule. However, the *mgr* negatively regulates capsule production, an effect opposite to that of *agr* (Luong and Lee, unpublished data).

In contrast to the *cap1* operon, deletion of the sequence upstream of the −35 region of the *cap8* promoter drastically reduced the promoter activity as determined by reporter gene fusions.[36] Results of deletion analysis and site-directed mutagenesis indicates that a 10-bp inverted repeat located 14 bp upstream of the −35 region of the *cap8* primary promoter is required for capsule production. A chromosomal mutation within the 10-bp repeat reduced capsule production to an undetectable level. The inverted repeat apparently serves as a protein binding site as revealed by gel mobility shift studies. These results suggest that the inverted repeat is a cis-acting binding site for a positive regulator necessary for the type 8 capsule production. In addition, gel mobility shift assay showed that yeast extract affected the regulatory protein binding to the 10-bp inverted repeat suggesting that yeast extract may affect type 8 capsule production through the putative positive regulator.[36] However, further studies are required to reveal the nature of the regulation.

5. BIOSYNTHESIS OF MICROCAPSULES

Little is known about the biosynthesis of staphylococcal capsules. However, recent cloning and sequencing of the capsule loci has allowed comparison of staphylococcal capsule genes with proteins of known functions which has led to the prediction of putative functions of most of the 16 *cap5(8)* genes.[33] The predicted functions of only a few of these genes have been confirmed by a combination of genetic and biochemical approaches. The *cap5H* gene was predicted, based on the homology to various acetyltransferases, to function as an O-acetylase which adds an O-acetyl group to the third carbon of the ManNAcA component in the trisaccharide repeating unit of type 5 capsule. This prediction was confirmed in a study which showed that the type 5 capsule produced from a mutant with a Tn*918* insertion at the *cap5H* gene lacked O-acetylation, as determined by nuclear magnetic resonance and immunological methods. Furthermore, the wild-type *cap5H* gene was shown to complement the mutant to produce O-acetylated type 5 capsule.[44] Similarly, *cap8J* is proposed to be the O-acetylation gene in the *cap8* gene cluster based on sequence comparison. The prediction was supported by the results that a monoclonal antibody specific to O-acetylated type 8 capsule failed to react with a *cap8J*-specific mutant (Sau and Lee, unpublished data). The Cap5H and Cap8J are highly dissimilar and share only a short region of homology which presumably contains the consensus motif required for acetylation. The dissimilarity is consistent with the fact that the positions of O-acetylation of ManNAcA in type 5 and type 8 capsules are different and is indicative of the substrate specificities of these enzymes.

The function of *cap5P* was elucidated initially by genetic complementation of the *E. coli rffE* gene which encodes UDP-GlcNAc-2-epimerase.[45] The *rffE* is required for converting UDP-GlcNAc to UDP-ManNAc in the biosynthesis of ManNAcA, one of the three sugar residues of the *E. coli* enterobacterial common antigen.[46] Since ManNAcA is also a component of *S. aureus* type 5 and type 8 capsules, the *cap5P* (and the nearly identical *cap8P*) gene is proposed to have function equivalent to that of the *rffE* gene. Recently, the recombinant Cap5P protein was purified and shown to have UDP-GlcNAc 2-epimerase activity in vitro confirming the previous genetic complementation.[47] Interestingly, another *cap5P* homolog with 61% identity to the *cap5P* gene is also present in the *S. aureus* chromosome. This homolog was shown to complement *E. coli rffE* mutant indicating that it is also biologically active.[47]

Similarly, *cap5O* has been shown to complement *E. coli rffD* mutant.[45] The *rffD* gene encodes UDP-ManNAc dehydrogenase which converts UDP-ManNAc to UDP-ManNAcA in the biosynthesis of *E. coli* enterobacterial common antigen.[46] The recombinant Cap5O protein has also been purified and has been demonstrated to have UDP-ManNAc dehydrogenase activity *in vitro* (J. C. Lee, personal communication). Thus, the *cap5O* (and the nearly identical *cap8O*) is a dehydrogenase which along with *cap5P* are required for synthesizing UDP-ManNAcA from UDP-GlcNAc in the type 5 capsule synthesis.

Sequence homology search shows that the *S. aureus cap8B* and cap5B genes is significantly homologous to several proteins thought to be involved in the chain-length determination of polysaccharides suggesting that *cap8B* is involved in chain length regulation.[33] In fact, a preliminary study showed that a *cap8B* mutant produced the same amount of capsule as the wild-type, but with lower molecular weight (Sau and Lee, unpublished data). This result further supports that *cap8B* is a chain length regulator.

Although only a few of the genes involved in the production of type 5 or type 8 microcapsule have been characterized by genetic or biochemical methods, in general, these results are consistent with the functional prediction based on sequence homology to known proteins. Thus, it is most likely that the other genes would function as predicted. Accordingly, a biosynthetic pathway of type 8 capsule is proposed in Figure 2. According to this proposed pathway, *cap8D, E, F, G, N, O* and *P* are amino sugar synthesis genes required for converting the precursor, UDP-D-GlcNAc, to UDP-linked D-FucNAc, L-FucNAc, and D-ManNAcA of which UDP-D-ManNAcA is further O-acetylated by the *cap8J* gene product. The three sugar monomers are then sequentially transferred by three transferases encoded by *cap8M, L* and *H* to form a repeating unit linked to a membrane-bound lipid carrier, undecaprenol phosphate, at the inner surface of the cytoplasmic membrane. The lipid-linked repeating unit is finally transported through the membrane by the *cap8I*-encoded flippase and polymerized at the outer surface by the *cap8K*-encoded polymerase. In addition, *cap8B* and possibly *cap8A* and *C* are involved in the chain-length regulation of the capsule during polymerization.

6. CONCLUSION

Molecular biology of staphylococcal capsule is still at its early stage. Recent cloning of capsule genes has opened the door for subsequent studies on genetics, regulation and pathogenesis of staphylococcal capsule at the molecular level. Although these studies have greatly advanced the knowledge of staphylococcal capsule biology, much remains to be

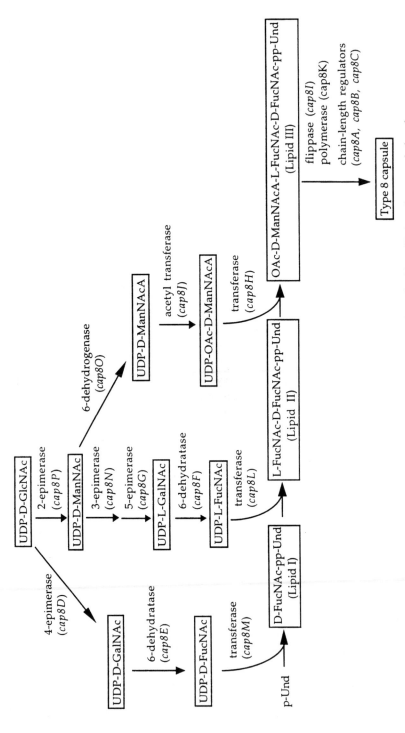

FIGURE 2. Proposed biosynthetic pathway for type 8 capsular polysaccharide. p-Und, undecaprenol phosphate.

investigated. For example, it is still unclear how capsules are synthesized and how they are regulated in response to various environmental conditions. The mechanism that microcapsules act as virulence factors has not been investigated although recent studies have established the important role of these capsules in the pathogenesis of staphylococcal diseases. Furthermore, microcapsules have recently been used as targets for vaccine development which may lead to new methods for treating *S. aureus* diseases caused by multidrug resistant strains.[48] Our understanding of the biology of capsules will be critical to the rational designing and development of a staphylococcal polysaccharide vaccine. Thus, further studies on staphylococcal capsule biology are warranted. Since the foundation for molecular studies has been laid, one should witness major advancement in staphylococcal capsule research in the near future.

ACKNOWLEDGMENTS. The author thanks J. C. Lee for communicating data prior to publication. This work was supported by NIH grant AI37027.

REFERENCES

1. Albus, A. *et al. Staphylococcus aureus* capsular types and antibody response to lung infection in patients with cystic fibrosis. *J Clin Microbiol* **26**, 2505–2509 (1988).
2. Arbeit, R. D., Karakawa, W. W., Vann, W. F. & Robbins, J. B. Predominance of two newly described capsular polysaccharide types among clinical isolates of *Staphylococcus aureus*. *Diagn Microbiol Infect Dis* **2**, 85–91 (1984).
3. Hochkeppel, H. K. *et al.* Serotyping and electron microscopy studies of *Staphylococcus aureus* clinical isolates with monoclonal antibodies to capsular polysaccharide types 5 and 8. *J Clin Microbiol* **25**, 526–530 (1987).
4. Karakawa, W. W. & Vann, W. F. Capsular polysacchrides of *S. aureus. Semin Infect Dis* **4**, 285–293 (1982).
5. Poutrel, B., Boutonnier, A., Sutra, L. & Fournier, J. M. Prevalence of capsular polysaccharide types 5 and 8 among *Staphylococcus aureus* isolates from cow, goat, and ewe milk. *J Clin Microbiol* **26**, 38–40 (1988).
6. Wilkinson, B. J. Staphylococcal capsules and slime. in *Staphylococci and staphylococcal infections* (eds. Easmon, C. S. G. & Adlam, G.) (Academic Press, New York, 1983).
7. Fournier, J. M., Vann, W. F. & Karakawa, W. W. Purification and characterization of *Staphylococcus aureus* type 8 capsular polysaccharide. *Infect Immun* **45**, 87–93 (1984).
8. Hanessian, S. & Haskell, T. H. Structural studies on staphylococcal polysaccharide. *J Biol Chem* **239**, 2758–2764 (1964).
9. Moreau, M. *et al.* Structure of the type 5 capsular polysaccharide of *Staphylococcus aureus. Carbohydr Res* **201**, 285–297 (1990).
10. Murthy, S. V., Melly, M. A., Harris, T. M., Hellerqvist, C. G. & Hash, J. H. The repeating sequence of the capsular polysaccharide of *Staphylococcus aureus* M. *Carbohydr Res* **117**, 113–123 (1983).

11. Karakawa, W. W., Sutton, A., Schneerson, R., Karpas, A. & Vann, W. F. Capsular anti-bodies induce type-specific phagocytosis of capsulated *Staphylococcus aureus* by human polymorphonuclear leukocytes. *Infect Immun* **56**, 1090–1095 (1988).
12. Peterson, P. K., Wilkinson, B. J., Kim, Y., Schmeling, D. & Quie, P. G. Influence of encapsulation on staphylococcal opsonization and phagocytosis by human polymorphonuclear leukocytes. *Infect Immun* **19**, 943–949 (1978).
13. Lee, J. C., Betley, M. J., Hopkins, C. A., Perez, N. E. & Pier, G. B. Virulence studies, in mice, of transposon-induced mutants of *Staphylococcus aureus* differing in capsule size. *J Infect Dis* **156**, 741–750 (1987).
14. Lin, W. S., Cunneen, T. & Lee, C. Y. Sequence analysis and molecular characterization of genes required for the biosynthesis of type 1 capsular polysaccharide in *Staphylococcus aureus*. *J Bacteriol* **176**, 7005–7016 (1994).
15. Albus, A., Arbeit, R. D. & Lee, J. C. Virulence of *Staphylococcus aureus* mutants altered in type 5 capsule production. *Infect Immun* **59**, 1008–1014 (1991).
16. Xu, S., Arbeit, R. D. & Lee, J. C. Phagocytic killing of encapsulated and microencapsulated *Staphylococcus aureus* by human polymorphonuclear leukocytes. *Infect Immun* **60**, 1358–1362 (1992).
17. Nemeth, J. & Lee, J. C. Antibodies to capsular polysaccharides are not protective against experimental *Staphylococcus aureus* endocarditis. *Infect Immun* **63**, 375–380 (1995).
18. Baddour, L. M. *et al. Staphylococcus aureus* microcapsule expression attenuates bacterial virulence in a rat model of experimental endocarditis. *J Infect Dis* **165**, 749–753 (1992).
19. Fattom, A. I., Sarwar, J., Ortiz, A. & Naso, R. A *Staphylococcus aureus* capsular polysaccharide (CP) vaccine and CP- specific antibodies protect mice against bacterial challenge. *Infect Immun* **64**, 1659–1665 (1996).
20. Lee, J. C., Park, J. S., Shepherd, S. E., Carey, V. & Fattom, A. Protective efficacy of antibodies to the *Staphylococcus aureus* type 5 capsular polysaccharide in a modified model of endocarditis in rats. *Infect Immun* **65**, 4146–4151 (1997).
21. Nilsson, I. M., Lee, J. C., Bremell, T., Ryden, C. & Tarkowski, A. The role of staphylococcal polysaccharide microcapsule expression in septicemia and septic arthritis. *Infect Immun* **65**, 4216–4221 (1997).
22. Thakker, M., Park, J. S., Carey, V. & Lee, J. C. *Staphylococcus aureus* serotype 5 capsular polysaccharide is antiphagocytic and enhances bacterial virulence in a murine bacteremia model. *Infect Immun* **66**, 5183–5189 (1998).
23. Kiser, K. B., Cantey-Kiser, J. M. & Lee, J. C. Development and characterization of a *Staphylococcus aureus* nasal colonization model in mice. *Infect Immun* **67**, 5001–5006 (1999).
24. Smith, R. M., Parisi, J. T., Vidal, L. & Baldwin, J. N. Nature of the genetic determinant controlling encapsulation in *Staphylococcus aureus* Smith. *Infect Immun* **17**, 231–234 (1977).
25. Lee, C. Y. Cloning of genes affecting capsule expression in *Staphylococcus aureus* strain M. *Mol Microbiol* **6**, 1515–1522 (1992).
26. Ouyang, S. & Lee, C. Y. Transcriptional analysis of type 1 capsule genes in *Staphylococcus aureus*. *Mol Microbiol* **23**, 473–482 (1997).
27. Lee, J. C., Takeda, S., Livolsi, P. J. & Paoletti, L. C. Effects of in vitro and in vivo growth conditions on expression of type 8 capsular polysaccharide by *Staphylococcus aureus*. *Infect Immun* **61**, 1853–1858 (1993).
28. Lin, W. S. & Lee, C. Y. Instability of type 1 capsule production in *Staphylococcus aureus*. *Abstracts of Annual Meeting of the American Society for Microbiology, Washington, D. C.* (1996).
29. Scott, A. C. A capsulate *Staphylococcus aureus*. *J Med Microbiol* **2**, 253–260 (1969).
30. Lee, C. Y. Association of staphylococcal type-1 capsule-encoding genes with a discrete genetic element. *Gene* **167**, 115–119 (1995).

31. Sau, S. & Lee, C. Y. Cloning of type 8 capsule genes and analysis of gene clusters for the production of different capsular polysaccharides in *Staphylococcus aureus*. *J Bacteriol* **178**, 2118–2126 (1996).

32. Lee, J. C., Xu, S., Albus, A. & Livolsi, P. J. Genetic analysis of type 5 capsular polysaccharide expression by *Staphylococcus aureus*. *J Bacteriol* **176**, 4883–4889 (1994).

33. Sau, S. *et al.* The *Staphylococcus aureus* allelic genetic loci for serotype 5 and 8 capsule expression contain the type-specific genes flanked by common genes. *Microbiology* **143**, 2395–2405 (1997).

34. Sordelli, D. O. *et al.* Capsule expression by bovine isolates of *Staphylococcus aureus* from Argentina: genetic and epidemiologic analyses. *J Clin Microbiol* **38**, 846–850 (2000).

35. Sau, S., Sun, J. & Lee, C. Y. Molecular characterization and transcriptional analysis of type 8 capsule genes in *Staphylococcus aureus*. *J Bacteriol* **179**, 1614–1621 (1997).

36. Ouyang, S., Sau, S. & Lee, C. Y. Promoter analysis of the *cap8* operon, involved in type 8 capsular polysaccharide production in *Staphylococcus aureus*. *J Bacteriol* **181**, 2492–2500 (1999).

37. Stringfellow, W. T., Dassy, B., Lieb, M. & Fournier, J. M. *Staphylococcus aureus* growth and type 5 capsular polysaccharide production in synthetic media. *Appl Environ Microbiol* **57**, 618–621 (1991).

38. Dassy, B., Stringfellow, W. T., Lieb, M. & Fournier, J. M. Production of type 5 capsular polysaccharide by *Staphylococcus aureus* grown in a semi-synthetic medium. *J Gen Microbiol* **137**, 1155–1162 (1991).

39. Sutra, L., Rainard, P. & Poutrel, B. Phagocytosis of mastitis isolates of *Staphylococcus aureus* and expression of type 5 capsular polysaccharide are influenced by growth in the presence of milk [published erratum appears in J Clin Microbiol 1990 Dec;28(12):2853]. *J Clin Microbiol* **28**, 2253–2258 (1990).

40. Mamo, W., Rozgonyi, F., Brown, A., Hjerten, S. & Wadstrom, T. Cell surface hydrophobicity and charge of *Staphylococcus aureus* and coagulase-negative staphylococci from bovine mastitis. *J Appl Bacteriol* **62**, 241–249 (1987).

41. Herbert, S. *et al.* Regulation of *Staphylococcus aureus* capsular polysaccharide type 5: CO2 inhibition *in vitro* and *in vivo*. *J Infect Dis* **176**, 431–438 (1997).

42. Dassy, B., Hogan, T., Foster, T. J. & Fournier, J. M. Involvement of the accessory gene regulator (agr) in expression of type 5 capsular polysaccharide by *Staphylococcus aureus*. *J Gen Microbiol* **139**, 1301–1306 (1993).

43. Projan, S. J. & Novick, R. P. The molecular basis of pathogenicity. in *The staphylococci in human disease* (eds. Crossley, K. B. & Archer, G. L.) (Churchill Livingstone, New York, 1997).

44. Bhasin, N. *et al.* Identification of a gene essential for O-acetylation of the *Staphylococcus aureus* type 5 capsular polysaccharide. *Mol Microbiol* **27**, 9–21 (1998).

45. Kiser, K. B. & Lee, J. C. Staphylococcus aureus cap5O and cap5P genes functionally complement mutations affecting enterobacterial common-antigen biosynthesis in Escherichia coli. *Journal of Bacteriology* **180**, 403–406 (1998).

46. Rick, P. D. & Siver, R. P. Enterobacterial common antigen and capsular polysaccharides. in *Escherichia coli and Salmonella: cellular and molecular biology* (eds. Neidhardt, F. C. *et al.*) (ASM Press, Washington, D. C., 1996).

47. Kiser, K. B., Bhasin, N., Deng, L. & Lee, J. C. *Staphylococcus aureus cap5P* encodes a UDP-N-acetylglucosamine 2-epimerase with functional redundancy. *J Bacteriol* **181**, 4818–4824 (1999).

48. Fattom, A. *et al.* Laboratory and clinical evaluation of conjugate vaccines composed of *Staphylococcus aureus* type 5 and type 8 capsular polysaccharides bound to *Pseudomonas aeruginosa* recombinant exoprotein A. *Infect Immun* **61**, 1023–1032 (1993).

4

Capsule and Vaccine Development

JEAN C. LEE

1. INTRODUCTION

Humans and rodents possess a high degree of innate immunity to infections caused by *Staphylococcus aureus*. Experimental infections are difficult to establish in animals or normal humans; they require an inoculum containing millions of organisms.[1-5] Concomitant introduction of a foreign body can reduce the infectious inoculum required to establish an infection. Individuals who abuse drugs, patients undergoing surgical procedures, those with prosthetic devices, and other immunocompromised hosts are susceptible to staphylococcal infections. *S. aureus* is the most frequently isolated bacterial pathogen in hospital-acquired infections,[6,7] and the emergence of antibiotic resistance among clinical isolates has made treatment of staphylococcal infections difficult. This scenario has sparked renewed interest in the development of a vaccine to prevent staphylococcal infections in individuals who are at high risk. Because of the safety and efficacy of other bacterial polysaccharide vaccines, studies to evaluate the vaccine potential of the *S. aureus* capsular polysaccharides have been pursued.

2. RATIONALE FOR CAPSULE AS A VACCINE TARGET

The involvement of capsular polysaccharides in the virulence of many microbial pathogens, including *Haemophilus influenzae*, *Streptococcus pneumoniae*, *Neisseria meningitidis*, and *Cryptococcus neoformans*, is well established. Encapsulated microbes are resistant to phagocytosis by leukocytes, and thus they are better suited than their nonencapsulated

JEAN C. LEE • Department of Medicine, Channing Laboratory, Brigham and Women's Hospital and Harvard Medical School, Boston, MA 02115.

Staphylococcus aureus *Infection and Disease*, edited by Allen L. Honeyman *et al.* Kluwer Academic/Plenum Publishers, New York, 2001.

counterparts to infect the blood and tissues. Because antibodies to the bacterial capsule neutralize its antiphagocytic properties, capsular polysaccharides are important targets of protective immunity.[8] Existing vaccines that confer immunity to infection by *H. influenzae*, *S. pneumoniae*, and *N. meningitidis* are composed of purified capsular polysaccharides either alone or conjugated to protein.

Similar to other invasive pathogens, *S. aureus* is also encapsulated. Although 11 putative capsular serotypes have been reported, serotypes 5 and 8 comprise the majority of strains recovered from humans.[9-12] Serotypes 1 and 2 are heavily encapsulated and produce mucoid colonies on solid medium; these types are rarely encountered among clinical isolates of *S. aureus*. The remaining serotypes, characterized by a colony morphology that is nonmucoid, are often referred to as microencapsulated because their capsules are less abundant than those produced by the serotype 1 and 2 strains. Capsular polysaccharides from only 4 of the 11 putative serotypes have been purified and chemically characterized. As shown in Figure 1, the staphylococcal capsules described to date consist of aminosugars and uronic acids. The prevalent serotype 5 and 8 strains have identical trisaccharide repeating units that differ only in the linkages between the sugars and the sites of O-acetylation on the N-acetylmannnosaminuronic acid residues.

Staphylococcal capsules have been shown to have antiphagocytic activity in vitro.[13-19] These surface-exposed polysaccharides may interfere with opsonization by antibodies to noncapsular, cell wall antigens and by C3b fragments generated by either the classical or the alternative complement pathways. Wilkinson *et al.*[20] showed that a highly encapsulated, serotype 1 *S. aureus* strain incubated with normal human serum had C3 localized on the cell wall, beneath the capsular layer. The thick capsular layer was antiphagocytic because it interfered with the recognition of cell wall-bound C3b and iC3b molecules by phagocytic cell receptors. If antibodies to the capsule were added to the bacteria, the antigen/antibody combination led

Type 1: $(\rightarrow4)$-α-D-GalNAcA-$(1\rightarrow4)$-α-D-GalNAcA-$(1\rightarrow3)$-α-D-FucNAc-$(1\rightarrow)_n$
(A taurine residue is amide-linked to every fourth D-GalNAcA residue)

Type 2: $(\rightarrow4)$-β-D-GlcNAcA-$(1\rightarrow4)$-β-D-GlcNAcA-(L-alanyl)-$(1\rightarrow)_n$

Type 5: $(\rightarrow4)$-3-*O*-Ac-β-D-ManNAcA-$(1\rightarrow4)$-α-L-FucNAc- $(1\rightarrow3)$-β-D-FucNAc-$(1\rightarrow)_n$

Type 8: $(\rightarrow3)$-4-*O*-Ac-β-D-ManNAcA-$(1\rightarrow3)$-α-FucNAc-$(1\rightarrow3)$-β-D-FucNAc-$(1\rightarrow)_n$

FIGURE 1. Structural composition of *Staphylococcus aureus* capsular polysaccharides.

to complement activation and deposition of C3 throughout the capsular layer. IgG and C3b were thus associated with the staphylococcal outer surface, and, therefore, they were available for recognition by phagocytic receptors. Studies to elucidate the interaction between complement components and the more clinically relevant capsular types 5 and 8 of *S. aureus* are in progress.

We isolated and characterized a mutant of a serotype 5 *S. aureus* strain that has a Tn*918* insertion within the *cap5H* gene.[21,22] The product of the *cap5H* gene is an O-acetyltransferase that is responsible for adding an O-acetyl group to the third carbon of the N-acetylmannosaminuronic acid residue of the type 5 capsular polysaccharide (CP5). The *cap5H* mutant, which produced wild-type levels of CP5 that was O-deacetylated, was more sensitive to complement-mediated opsonophagocytic killing than the wild-type strain.[22] The O-acetylated form of CP5 is immunodominant, and antibodies to O-acetylated CP5 are opsonic[23,24] Conflicting data exist regarding the opsonic activity of antibodies to the CP5 backbone structure.[23,25] The hypothesis that the peptidoglycan and/or teichoic acid component of the bacterial cell wall is more accessible on the bacterial surface in the absence of the O-acetyl moieties on CP5 is being tested experimentally.

3. PROTECTION AFFORDED BY CRUDE CAPSULAR PREPARATIONS

Capsular antigens were among the earliest target antigens in vaccine studies designed to protect against staphylococcal infections. Mice immunized intraperitoneally (IP) with a single dose of live or killed cells of strain Smith diffuse, a highly encapsulated serotype 2 isolate of *S. aureus*, were protected against a lethal challenge dose (10^8 CFU) of the homologous strain prepared in saline and injected IP.[26,27] Immunization with a heterologous strain (Cowan I—serotype 8) was not protective against lethality induced by the Smith diffuse strain of *S. aureus*. Moreover, immunization of mice with polysaccharide antigens extracted from cells of Smith diffuse did not protect the animals against challenge with 10^8 CFU of the homologous strain in saline.[26]

However, if the staphylococcal inoculum was mixed with 5% hog gastric mucin, the mouse lethal dose of strain Smith diffuse was reduced from 10^8 to 10^5 CFU. Under these experimental conditions, immunization with polysaccharide antigens extracted from *S. aureus* cells[26] or heat-stable culture supernatants[28] was protective against lethality induced by the homologous strain. The protection could be passively transferred to naive animals by the injection of immune serum.[26,29] However, no protection against infection by strain Smith diffuse was elicited by immunization with whole cells or culture extracts prepared from two heterologous, nonmucoid strains of *S. aureus*. Likewise, mice immunized with the Smith diffuse strain were not protected against a lethal inoculum of a heterologous *S. aureus* isolate (strain Foggie; capsular phenotype unknown).[30]

4. PURIFIED CP1 AS A PROTECTIVE IMMUNOGEN

My laboratory purified and chemically characterized capsular polysaccharide from a mucoid serotype 1 strain of *S. aureus* called SA1 mucoid.[19] The virulence of this bacterial strain for mice is indicated by its 50% lethal dose (LD_{50}) of 2.1×10^4 CFU (challenge by the IP route in saline). We immunized mice IP three times with either PBS, formalin-killed strain SA1 mucoid, or $0.1\,\mu g$ of purified type 1 capsular polysaccharide (CP1). The animals were bled before each immunization and five days after the last immunizing dose, and their serum antibody levels were evaluated by an enzyme-linked immunosorbent assay (ELISA; Figure 2).[19,31] One week after the third immunization, groups of mice were challenged IP with *S. aureus*. As shown in Figure 3, all of the mice immunized with formalin-killed bacteria survived lethal doses ranging from 2×10^5 to 5×10^6 CFU, representing 10.5 to 119 times the LD_{50} of strain SA1 mucoid. Mice immunized with CP1 were protected in a dose-dependent fashion, with 50% of the animals surviving challenge with 1.5×10^6 CFU (71 times the LD_{50}). Control mice immunized with PBS all died.

Separate groups of animals were passively immunized with normal mouse serum or immune mouse serum raised either to formalinized cells of strain SA1 mucoid or CP1. Ten of 10 mice injected with serum raised to killed *S. aureus* cells survived challenge with 1.5×10^6 CFU of SA1 mucoid. In contrast, none of 10 mice passively immunized with serum raised to CP1 survived a challenge inoculum 22 times the LD_{50} dose (6.5×10^5 CFU) for SA1 mucoid. All mice injected with normal serum died after either challenge dose. The results of these studies suggest that antibodies to CP1 are protective and that there is a correlation between capsular antibody levels and protection against lethality in mice. Active, but not passive, immunization with CP1 provided the mice with sufficient levels of CP1 antibodies to protect them against *S. aureus*—induced lethality. In a separate study, we evaluated the protection afforded by capsular antibodies in a sublethal model of *S. aureus* bacteremia and renal abscess formation. We immunized mice IP with formalin-killed cells of strain SA1 mucoid or CP1, as described above, and challenged them IV with one of three *S. aureus* strains that

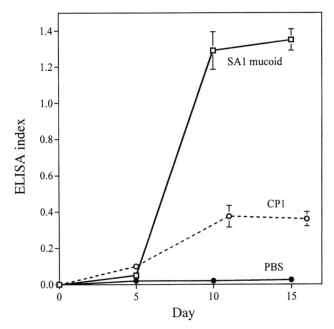

FIGURE 2. Serum antibodies to CP1 in groups of mice immunized intraperitoneally with either PBS, 10^8 CFU of formalin-killed *S. aureus* SA1 mucoid, or CP1. Arrows denote immunizations, and each point represent the mean ELISA index (±SE [bars]) of sera diluted 1:100. The ELISA index was calculated by dividing the absorbance reading of the test serum by the absorbance reading of a pool of high titered immune mouse serum (raised to killed SA1 mucoid).

varied in capsule size.[31] Quantitative cultures of blood and kidneys from the animals were performed to evaluate protection. Immunization with killed cells of the homologous strain protected mice against infection with each of the three *S. aureus* isolates.[31] Mice immunized with CP1 were protected when challenged IV with either the highly encapsulated strain SA1 mucoid or a microencapsulated serotype 1 mutant but not with an unencapsulated mutant. Protection correlated with capsular antibody levels in the immunized animals. Immunization with a heterologous strain lacking CP1 was not protective against challenge with strain SA1 mucoid. Naïve mice passively immunized with antiserum raised to strain SA1 mucoid or CP1 had significantly fewer CFU of strain SA1 mucoid in their blood and kidney samples than did mice given preimmune serum.[31]

That the staphylococcal capsule should be a major target in the search for a vaccine to prevent staphylococcal infection in humans was supported

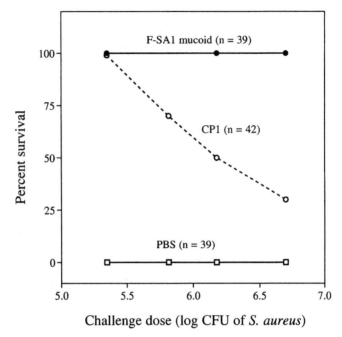

FIGURE 3. Active immunization with formalin killed cells of *S. aureus* SA1 mucoid or CP1 protects mice against lethality induced by various challenge doses of strain SA1 mucoid.

by two findings. First, the results of immunization studies with the serotype 1 and 2 strains of *S. aureus* suggested that antibodies to capsular antigens were protective. Second, antibodies specific for the capsule promoted the phagocytosis of *S. aureus* by human polymorphonuclear leukocytes in vitro.[13,16–19]

5. PROTECTION AGAINST SEROTYPE 5 AND 8 *S. AUREUS*

As noted above, highly encapsulated strains (serotypes 1 and 2) are rarely encountered among clinical isolates of *S. aureus*. Most staphylococci produce CPs that are produced in less abundance than those expressed by the highly encapsulated isolates.[32] Serotype 5 and 8 *S. aureus* strains comprise ~22% and ~53%, respectively, of clinical isolates recovered from humans.[9–12] Whether production of the serotype 5 or 8 capsules correlates with staphylococcal virulence depends upon the animal model of infection tested.[15,33,34]

Normal humans have serum antibodies to *S. aureus* cell wall components, including peptidoglycan, teichoic acid, CP5, and CP8.[35-40] However, levels of antibodies to CP5 and CP8 in normal human serum are low.[37] In an in vitro opsonophagocytic killing assay, <50% of the inoculum of a serotype 5 strain was opsonized for phagocytic killing by human polymorphonuclear leukocytes in fresh normal human serum.[15] However, if a pool of serum from humans immunized with a CP5-conjugate vaccine (see below) was added to the assay as an opsonic source, 95% of the bacterial inoculum was killed. These data suggest that the level of capsular antibodies in normal humans is not sufficient to promote efficient opsonophagocytic killing of an encapsulated *S. aureus* strain. Boosting capsular antibody levels by immunization may correlate with enhanced bacterial clearance in humans at risk for staphylococcal infections.

Several studies have evaluated the protective efficacy of antibodies to the *S. aureus* microcapsules in experimental models of staphylococcal infection. The first report evaluated the protective efficacy of capsular antibodies in a rat model of catheter-induced staphylococcal endocarditis. Rats were actively immunized with killed serotype 5 *S. aureus* cells or passively immunized with high-titer rabbit antiserum raised to whole, encapsulated bacterial cells.[41] The latter antiserum was absorbed with trypsinized cells of an unencapsulated mutant of *S. aureus* to render the serum specific for CP5. Control animals were injected with saline or passively immunized with normal rabbit serum. The rats were catheterized and then challenged IV with ~5 × 10^4 *S. aureus* cells. Protection was evaluated by quantitative cultures of blood and aortic vegetations. Despite having elevated levels of capsular antibodies, the immunized animals were susceptible to staphylococcal endocarditis, and immunized and control animals had similar numbers of bacteria in the blood and vegetations. Likewise, antibodies to teichoic acid failed to protect the animals against staphylococcal endocarditis in this study[41] and in that reported by Greenberg *et al.*[42]

6. IMMUNIZATION OF ANIMALS WITH CP5 AND CP8 CONJUGATE VACCINES

Most purified capsular polysaccharides are poor immunogens in animals and humans. The immunogenicity of polysaccharides is T cell independent, and no booster response is observed following multiple immunizations. Neither CP5 nor CP8 elicited serum antibodies when injected in mice by the subcutaneous route[37,43] (and J. Lee, unpublished observations). However, if purified polysaccharides are covalently coupled to protein carrier molecules, they gain both increased immunogenicity and T cell-dependent properties. Polysaccharide-protein conjugate vaccines elicit high levels of polysaccharide-specific antibodies, and antibody levels rise following booster doses of the vaccine. Several laboratories have synthesized conjugate vaccines consisting of *S. aureus* CP5 and CP8 covalently linked to protein.[37,44,45] These conjugates are highly immunogenic in mice and humans and induce antibodies that opsonize microencapsulated *S. aureus* for phagocytosis.[24,43] Fattom et al.[37] conjugated *S. aureus* CP5 and CP8 to nontoxic, recombinant exotoxin A from *Pseudomonas aeruginosa* (rEPA) and administered this preparation to mice. The mice developed serum antibodies to the polysaccharides after two injections; the third injection stimulated a booster response. Differences in the carrier proteins and the chemical methods utilized to couple the proteins to the polysaccharide affected the magnitude of the immune response in mice, but these variables did not affect the distribution of IgG subclasses detected in the immune serum.[46] Use of monophosphoryl lipid A as an adjuvant enhanced the immunogenicity of the conjugate vaccines and induced a shift in the IgG subclass composition toward the more opsonic IgG_{2a} and IgG_{2b} subclasses in the immunized mice.

Fattom et al.[47] tested the protective efficacy of antibodies to the CP5-rEPA conjugate vaccine in a mouse model of lethality and disseminated infection. Experimental animals were actively immunized subcutaneously with three doses of the CP5 conjugate vaccine or passively immunized with human immunoglobulin obtained from plasma donors vaccinated with the bivalent *S. aureus* CP5-/CP8-rEPA vaccine. Immunization with CP5-rEPA protected mice against lethality induced by challenging mice with 2×10^5 CFU of a serotype 5 *S. aureus* strain administered IP with 5% hog mucin. Ten days after bacterial challenge, 33 of 45 mice immunized with the conjugate survived compared with 4 of 30 mice injected with PBS. Passive immunization of mice with immune globulin resulted in a reduction in the levels of bacteremia at 6 and 24 h after IP inoculation of mice with a sublethal dose (5×10^4 CFU) of serotype 5 *S. aureus*. In addition, fewer animals given immune globulin showed metastatic infection by *S. aureus* in their livers, kidneys, and peritoneal lavage fluids (Table I).

Antibodies to the *S. aureus* CP conjugate vaccine also protected rats against infection in a modified, catheter-induced model of staphylococcal endocarditis.[24] In this study, rats were passively immunized IP with IgG purified from nonimmunized rabbits or from rabbits immunized with the bivalent CP5-/CP8-rEPA conjugate vaccine. One day later, the immunized rats were challenged IP with one of three serotype 5 *S. aureus* isolates. Bacterial challenge by the IP route resulted in a slow infusion of *S. aureus* into the blood of the catheterized rats. As shown in Table II, rats given capsular antibodies showed a significantly ($p < 0.05$) lower prevalence of

TABLE I
CP5-specific antibodies given subcutaneously protect mice against systemic infection induced by 5×10^4 CFU $S.$ $aureus$

Site	Normal IgG		Immune IgG	
	Mean CFU	Positive mice/total	Mean CFU	Positive mice/total
Peritoneal lavage fluid	0.28×10^2	7/18	7×10^1	1/20
Liver	4.03×10^2	14/18	0.37×10^1	5/20
Kidney	7.20×10^2	17/18	0.28×10^1	3/20

Adapted from Fattom *et al.*, Infect. Immun. 64:1659 (1996).

staphylococcal endocarditis (induced by each of the three strains) than rats injected with nonimmune IgG. Similarly, quantitative cultures of the blood, kidneys, and aortic valve vegetations revealed that fewer *S. aureus* cells were recovered from rats given capsule-specific IgG than from rats administered nonimmune IgG. Ongoing studies in our laboratory suggest that human antibodies to the CP5/CP8 conjugate vaccine also protect rats against endocarditis induced by two of three different serotype 8 *S. aureus* strains (unpublished).

The protection afforded by capsular antibodies elicited by the conjugate vaccine is in contrast to the lack of protection reported earlier by

TABLE II
CP5-specific antibodies given intraperitoneally protect against endocarditis in rats challenged with serotype 5 $S.$ $aureus$

Challenge strain of *S. aureus*	Log CFU/ml blood at 24 h	No. infected/total	Vegetation wt	Log CFU/g vegetation	Log CFU/g kidney
Reynolds (4×10^7 CFU)					
Normal IgG	4.31	4/4	0.012	11.0	7.33
CP-specific IgG	0.70	0/5	0	3.4	1.05
Lowenstein (6×10^7 CFU)					
Normal IgG	1.30	8/11	0.011	11.0	7.84
CP-specific IgG	0.70	4/13	0.003	3.4	4.85
VP (7×10^7 CFU)					
Normal IgG	3.93	7/9	0.009	10.2	7.20
CP-specific IgG	0.70	1/9	0	3.4	2.06

Adapted from Lee *et al.*, Infect. Immun. 65:4146 (1997).

Nemeth and Lee.[41] In that study, capsular antibodies were elicited by immunization with killed bacteria rather than by a CP-conjugate vaccine. Another difference in experimental design between the two studies was that Nemeth and Lee[41] challenged the rats with an IV bolus dose of organisms, whereas in the more recent study, the animals were challenged by the IP route of injection. Nonetheless, capsular antibodies elicited by the conjugate vaccine did not protect against endocarditis when the bacterial inoculum was delivered as a bolus dose by the IV route to rabbits[48] or rats (J. Lee, unpublished data). This finding suggests that the protective effect of capsular antibodies in the study reported by Lee et al.[24] may have been due primarily to local clearance of the bacterial cells in the peritoneal cavity, thereby preventing the staphylococci from gaining access to the bloodstream. The variable results of these vaccine studies underscore the importance of testing vaccine efficacy in multiple models of experimental S. aureus infection.

Recently, my laboratory developed a mouse model of S. aureus nasal colonization.[49] The anterior nares are the major reservoir of S. aureus in humans, and nasal carriage in a major risk factor for infection in humans, particularly in the hospital environment. Measures to reduce nasal carriage of S. aureus have proven effective in curtailing the prevalence of infection in some high-risk groups of patients. We are currently evaluating whether antibodies to S. aureus whole bacteria, capsular polysaccharides, or other staphylococcal antigens will prevent establishment of staphylococcal nasal carriage in mice. Although our studies are focused primarily on strategies of mucosal immunization, our preliminary data indicate that systemic immunization of mice with the CP5-rEPA conjugate vaccine prevents nasal colonization of mice with a serotype 5 strain of S. aureus.

7. ACTIVE IMMUNIZATION OF HUMANS WITH CP5/CP8 CONJUGATE VACCINES

Fattom and colleagues at Nabi, Inc. (Boca Raton, FL), have prepared conjugates of CP5 and CP8 linked to rEPA that are intended for commercial use. They have combined the two polysaccharide vaccines into a bivalent vaccine called StaphVAX™ that is intended for immunization of individuals at high risk for S. aureus infection.

Phase I and II Clinical Trials

The CP8- and CP5-rEPA conjugate vaccines were evaluated for safety and immunogenicity in 70 healthy adult volunteers.[37] Neither conjugate caused significant local or systemic reactions in the volunteers. The conjugate vaccine induced CP-specific antibodies of both the IgM and IgG classes. A second injection six weeks later did not have a booster effect. The authors suggest that due to low levels of prevaccination capsular antibodies in these subjects, the initial vaccination behaved more like a booster rather than a primary dose.

Nabi conducted a phase II, double-blinded, placebo-controlled clinical study of StaphVAX in ~230 chronic ambulatory peritoneal dialysis patients, individuals who are at high risk of staphylococcal disease. The patients were actively immunized with StaphVAX, and their antibody responses and infection rates were monitored. The vaccine was shown to elicit only mild local or systemic symptoms. The results of this trial indicated that the vaccine dose of 25 μg of each CP was suboptimal in these patients. Their antibody responses to the vaccine were weak, and they had infection rates similar to those of nonimmunized patients.

In subsequent phase II clinical trials, 32 volunteers with end-stage renal disease and 29 healthy controls were injected twice (6 weeks apart) with 25 μg of CP5-rEPA or the bivalent conjugate vaccine (25 μg each of CP5 and CP8 linked to rEPA). The vaccines elicited only mild local or systemic symptoms in both populations[40] (and G. Horwith, personal communication). Four weeks after the second dose of vaccine, 23 of 24 healthy volunteers and 14 of 17 patients in one study responded to the immunization with a ≥4-fold rise in preimmunization IgG and IgM antibody levels. However, the IgG and IgM levels of the patients were only ~50% of those achieved by the healthy controls at all postimmunization intervals. The monovalent and bivalent vaccines did not contain any adjuvant. Data from animal studies indicate that enhanced immunogenicity may be achieved by incorporating an adjuvant such as monophosphoryl lipid A.[46]

Phase III Clinical Trial

In 1998 a phase III clinical trial to evaluate the efficacy of StaphVAX was launched at the Kaiser Permanente Vaccine Study Center in California. This ongoing, randomized, double-blinded, placebo-controlled study is designed to assess the efficacy of StaphVAX in patients with end-stage renal disease receiving hemodialysis. Approximately 1800 patients were enrolled at the time accrual was closed in mid-1999. Half of the patients were administered a placebo, and the other half were immunized with Nabi's bivalent StaphVAX (100 μg each of CP5 and CP8 linked to rEPA). These hemodialysis patients are at high risk for staphylococcal infection, with 3 to 4 out of every 100 patients infected with *S. aureus* per year. In this clinical trial, the patients are monitored for culture-proven *S. aureus* bacteremia. Safety analyses by an interim drug safety monitoring board at 20% and 60% enrollment indicated that there were no safety issues. The study should be completed by the end of summer 2000. Because StaphVAX is the first staphylococcal vaccine to reach clinical trial, researchers and clinicians await the results with cautious optimism.

8. PASSIVE IMMUNIZATION OF HUMANS WITH CAPSULAR ANTIBODIES

Another goal of Nabi, Inc. is to immunize healthy people with StaphVAX to generate an immunoglobulin product with high levels of antibodies to *S. aureus* CP5 and CP8. Polyclonal antibodies have been purified from the plasma of healthy vaccinees. The IgG antibody generated in this fashion, referred to as StaphGAM™, is administered in passive immunization studies to patients who are at immediate risk for staphylococcal infection. The circulating half-life of such antibodies is estimated to be 14 to 21 days.[50] Twenty-nine very-low-birth-weight infants, at high risk for staphylococccal infection, were enrolled in a phase I/II safety and pharmacokinetics study conducted between 1998 and 1999 at the University of Texas. Subjects, stratified by weight (501–1000 g and 1001–1500 g) were administered two injections of AltaStaph two weeks apart. Three dosages (500, 750, and 1000 µg/kg) of AltaStaph were administered, assessing the safety of each dosage prior to escalating to the next dosage level. The results indicated that all of the dosages were well tolerated. Additional trials with AltaStaph are planned to test its efficacy as a prophylactic agent to prevent bacteremia. In addition, Nabi hopes to evaluate the therapeutic effect of AltaStaph an as an adjunct to antibiotics in patients with documented *S. aureus* infection (G. Horwith, personal communication).

9. POLY-N-SUCCINYL β-1 → 6 GLUCOSAMINE (PNSG)

Recently, a previously unrecognized, surface-associated polysaccharide was identified on *S. aureus* strains isolated from either humans or ruminants.[51] This polysaccharide, composed of PNSG, is structurally identical to the capsular polysaccharide adhesin produced by *Staphylococcus epidermidis*.[52] PNSG is also similar in structure to the polysaccharide intercellular adhesin that is present both in *S. aureus* and in several other species of staphylococci.[53] Few strains of *S. aureus* express PNSG in vitro, but the polysaccharide could be detected by serologic methods on organisms recovered from infections. The protective efficacy of immunization with PNSG was evaluated in a murine model of renal abscess formation. Mice that were immunized with three 100-µg doses of PNSG (five to six days apart) before bacterial challenge showed significant reductions in the CFU of *S. aureus* per gram of kidney compared with mice immunized with an irrelevant polysaccharide. Mice that were passively immunized with rabbit antibodies to PNSG before IV challenge with *S. aureus* and again 18 h after challenge were also protected against renal infection, and they showed lower lethality than animals injected with antiserum to an irrelevant polysaccharide. Because PNSG is also elaborated by many isolates of coagulase-negative staphylococci, a PNSG vaccine might target both coagulase-positive and coagulase-negative staphylococci. Previous studies showed that PNSG was effective in laboratory animals as a vaccine against infections caused by coagulase-negative staphylococci.[54,55]

10. CAPSULAR VACCINES AGAINST BOVINE MASTITIS

In addition to its importance for humans, *S. aureus* is also a major veterinary pathogen. Many attempts have been made to produce an effective *S. aureus* vaccine to control mastitis in ruminants. Bovine mastitis is the most economically important disease of dairy cattle in the United States, and *S. aureus* is a major cause of this infection. In the absence of an efficacious vaccine, culling of infected animals or treatment with antibiotics is indicated. However, the bacteriologic cure rate for infected, lactating cows treated with antibiotics is <30%.

Watson reported in 1978 that immunization with a live *S. aureus* vaccine provided better protection for the mammary gland than did a vaccine of killed staphylococci that were grown *in vitro*.[56] Furthermore, *S. aureus* cultivated *in vivo* (within a dialysis sac implanted for 48 h in the peritoneal cavity of a sheep) produced an antigen that was not detectable in conventional broth cultures grown *in vitro*.[57] Watson named this extracellular substance a "pseudocapsule" and reported that production of this material conferred on the staphylococci an increased resistance to phagocytosis. *In vivo* growth conditions were simulated by growing *S. aureus* in nutrient broth with 10% sterile ovine milk whey; these in vitro conditions were permissive for expression of the pseudocapsule.[58] Immunization of sheep with killed staphylococci grown in the presence of milk whey resulted in high concentrations of circulating IgG_2 antibodies directed against surface antigens of staphylococci grown *in vivo*. Antibodies to the pseudocapsular antigens were opsonic in an *in vitro* opsonophagocytic assay.[59] Furthermore, ewes immunized with the killed vaccine showed a substantial degree of resistance to experimental staphylococcal mastitis.[58] A field trial involving five commercial dairy herds in Australia was conducted to test the efficacy of the killed vaccine. Vaccinates had 45–52% fewer cases of *S. aureus*-related clinical mastitis and 25% fewer intramammary infections than controls.[60] To determine the influence of Watson's vaccine on the immunologic status of nonlactating animals, Nickerson *et al.*[61] immunized cows in the United States. Following challenge by intramammary infusion with a heterologous *S. aureus* strain, 92% of the control cows developed intramammary staphylococcal infection compared with 36% and 60% of the animals vaccinated intramuscularly and in the supramammary lymph node, respectively.

Although the pseudocapsule has been visualized by transmission electron microscopy,[62] Watson and coworkers have not reported the purification of the pseudocapsular material. The chemical composition of the pseudocapsule remains undisclosed, and its relationship to the staphylococcal capsular polysaccharides has not been reported. My laboratory has shown that CP8 production is enhanced in the presence of milk whey (unpublished data). However, the preferential expression of the pseudocapsule in vivo suggests that it may be related to PNSG.

In more recent studies, Gilbert *et al.*[44] immunized six dairy cows subcutaneously with purified CP5 or a CP5-ovalbumin conjugate in Freund's incomplete adjuvant. Whereas purified CP5 did not induce a humoral response in the cows, the conjugate vaccine elicited a CP5 antibody response that was primarily of the IgG_2 subclass. A booster injection given 3 months later resulted in a rapid rise in antibody titer. Whether systemic immunization of cows with a CP5- or CP8-based conjugate vaccine would protect against bovine mastitis is unknown. Systemic immunization of formalin-killed, serotype 5 *S. aureus* cells elicited higher titers of serum antibodies to CP5 than did immunization with a CP5-human serum albumin conjugate vaccine (T. Tollersrud, personal communication). Although whole cell preparations are not suitable for use as human vaccines, such preparations might be of use in veterinary vaccines.

11. PROSPECTS FOR THE FUTURE

New strategies are needed to combat infections caused by antibiotic-resistant strains of *S. aureus*. Because of the complexity of staphylococcal infections and the myriad of virulence factors produced by this organism, it is not apparent that antibodies to a single antigen will protect a susceptible host. The ideal vaccine against *S. aureus* would induce antibodies to prevent bacterial adherence, promote opsonophagocytic killing by leukocytes, and neutralize toxic exoproteins produced by the bacterium. The results of animal studies suggest that antibodies to CP5 and CP8 have a positive impact on reducing experimental staphylococcal infections. Nonetheless, the results of ongoing clinical trials of CP5-/CP8-rEPA in humans will provide the ultimate test of vaccine efficacy. The data available at present support the inclusion of CP5 and CP8 antigens in a multicomponent staphylococcal vaccine for humans. As basic research studies on the pathogenesis of staphylococcal infections unravel the secrets of this complex bacterial pathogen, we will move closer to the design of an effective *S. aureus* vaccine.

ACKNOWLEDGMENTS. This work was supported by Public Health Service grants AI-29040 AND AI-44136 from the National Institute of Allergy and Infectious Diseases. I thank all the members of my laboratory over the years for their contributions to this work.

REFERENCES

1. R. H. Gorrill. The establishment of staphylococcal abscesses in the mouse kidney. *Br J Exp Pathol.* 39: 203 (1958).
2. T. M. Donnelly, and D. M. Stark. Susceptibility of laboratory rats, hamsters, and mice to wound infection with *Staphylococcus aureus. Am J Vet Res.* 46: 2634 (1985).
3. G. Singh, R. R. Marples, and A. M. Kligman. Experimental *Staphylococcus aureus* infections in humans. *J Invest Dermatol.* 57: 149 (1971).
4. J. J. Hoogeterp, H. Mattie, A. M. Krul, and R. van Furth. The efficacy of rifampicin against *Staphylococcus aureus* in vitro and in an experimental infection in normal and granulocytopenic mice. *Scand J Infect Dis.* 20: 649 (1988).
5. S. R. Sharar, R. K. Winn, C. E. Murry, J. M. Harlan, and C. L. Rice. A CD18 monoclonal antibody increases the incidence and severity of subcutaneous abscess formation after high-dose *Staphylococcus aureus* injection in rabbits. *Surgery.* 110: 213 (1991).
6. F. D. Lowy. Medical progress: *Staphylococcus aureus* infections. *N Engl J Med.* 339: 520 (1998).
7. G. L. Archer. *Staphylococcus aureus:* A well-armed pathogen. *Clin Infect Dis.* 26: 1179 (1998).
8. J. B. Robbins, S. R, W. B. Egan, W. Vann, and D. Liu. Virulence properties of bacterial capsular polysaccharides-unanswered questions, in *The Molecular Basis of Microbial Pathogenicity.* H. Smith, J. Skehel, M. Turner, eds. Verlag Chemie GmbH, Weinheim, (1980).
9. D. Sompolinsky, Z. Samra, W. W. Karakawa, W. F. Vann, R. Schneerson, and Z. Malik. Encapsulation and capsular types in isolates of *Staphylococcus aureus* from different sources and relationship to phage types. *J Clin Microbiol.* 22: 828 (1985).
10. H. K. Hochkeppel, D. G. Braun, W. Vischer, A. Imm, S. Sutter, U. Staeubli, and R. Guggenheim. Serotyping and electron microscopy studies of *Staphylococcus aureus* clinical isolates with monoclonal antibodies to capsular polysaccharide types 5 and 8. *J Clin Microbiol.* 25: 526 (1987).

11. W. W. Karakawa, and W. F. Vann. Capsular polysaccharides of *Staphylococcus aureus*. *Semin Infect Dis.* 4: 285 (1982).

12. R. D. Arbeit, W. W. Karakawa, W. F. Vann, and J. B. Robbins. Predominance of two newly described capsular polysaccharide types among clinical isolates of *Staphylococcus aureus*. *Diagn Microbiol Infect Dis.* 2: 85 (1984).

13. W. W. Karakawa, A. Sutton, R. Schneerson, A. Karpas, and W. F. Vann. Capsular antibodies induce type-specific phagocytosis of capsulated *Staphylococcus aureus* by human polymorphonuclear leukocytes. *Infect Immun.* 56: 1090 (1988).

14. P. Peterson, B. Wilkinson, Y. Kim, Schmeling, and P. Quie. Influence of encapsulation on staphylococcal opsonization and phagocytosis by human polymorphonuclear leukocytes. *Infect Immun.* 19: 943 (1978).

15. M. Thakker, J.-S. Park, V. Carey, and J. C. Lee. *Staphylococcus aureus* serotype 5 capsular polysaccharide is antiphagocytic and enhances bacterial virulence in a murine bacteremia model. *Infect Immun.* 66: 5183 (1998).

16. M. Melly, L. Duke, D.-F. Liau, and J. Hash. Biological properties of the encapsulated *Staphylococcus aureus* M. *Infect Immun.* 10: 389 (1974).

17. B. J. Wilkinson, P. K. Peterson, and P. G. Quie. Cryptic peptidoglycan and the antiphagocytic effect of the *Staphylococcus aureus* capsule: model for the antiphagocytic effect of bacterial cell surface polymers. *Infect Immun.* 23: 502 (1979).

18. S. Xu, R. D. Arbeit, and J. C. Lee. Phagocytic killing of encapsulated and microencapsulated *Staphylococcus aureus* by human polymorphonuclear leukocytes. *Infect Immun.* 60: 1358 (1992).

19. J. C. Lee, F. Michon, N. E. Perez, C. A. Hopkins, and G. B. Pier. Chemical characterization and immunogenicity of capsular polysaccharide isolated from mucoid *Staphylococcus aureus*. *Infect Immun.* 55: 2191 (1987).

20. B. J. Wilkinson, S. P. Sisson, Y. Kim, and P. K. Peterson. Localization of the third component of complement on the cell wall of encapsulated *Staphylococcus aureus* M: implications for the mechanism of resistance to phagocytosis. *Infect Immun.* 26: 1159 (1979).

21. A. Albus, R. D. Arbeit, and J. C. Lee. Virulence of *Staphylococcus aureus* mutants altered in type 5 capsule production. *Infect Immun.* 59: 1008 (1991).

22. N. Bhasin, A. Albus, F. Michon, P. J. Livolsi, J.-S. Park, and J. C. Lee. Identification of a gene essential for O-acetylation of the *Staphylococcus aureus* type 5 capsular polysaccharide. *Mol Microbiol.* 27: 9 (1998).

23. A. I. Fattom, J. Sarwar, L. Basham, S. Ennifar, and R. Naso. Antigenic determinants of *Staphylococcus aureus* type 5 and type 8 capsular polysaccharide vaccines. *Infect Immun.* 66: 4588 (1998).

24. J. C. Lee, J.-S. Park, S. E. Shepherd, V. Carey, and A. Fattom. Protective efficacy of antibodies to the *Staphylococcus aureus* type 5 capsular polysaccharide in a modified model of endocarditis in rats. *Infect Immun.* 65: 4146 (1997).

25. M. Propst, S. Stewart, J. C. Lee, S. Fuller, and G. S. Bixler. Opsonophagocytosis of *Staphylococcus aureus* type 5: involvement of the O-acetyl moiety on the capsular polysaccharide, in: *Abstract of the 98th General Meeting of the American Society for Microbiology*. E-47 (1998).

26. R. D. Ekstedt. Studies on immunity to staphylococcal infection in mice. II. Effect of immunization with fractions of *Staphylococcus aureus* prepared by physical and chemical methods. *J Infect Dis.* 112: 152 (1963).

27. R. Ekstedt. Studies on immunity to staphylococcal infection in mice. I. Effect of dosage, viability, and interval between immunization and challenge on resistance to infection following injection of whole cell vaccines. *J Infect Dis.* 112: 143 (1963).

28. S. Fisher. A heat stable protective staphylococcal antigen. *Aust J Exp Biol.* 38: 479 (1960).
29. M. Fisher, H. Devlin, and A. Erlandson. A new staphylococcal antigen. Its preparation and immunizing activity against experimental infections. *Nature.* 199: 1074 (1963).
30. R. Ekstedt. Studies on immunity to staphylococcal infection in mice. IV. The role of specific and nonspecific immunity. *J Infect Dis.* 116: 514 (1966).
31. J. C. Lee, N. E. Perez, C. A. Hopkins, and G. B. Pier. Purified capsular polysaccharide-induced immunity to *Staphylococcus aureus* infection. *J Infect Dis.* 157: 723 (1988).
32. B. J. Wilkinson. Staphylococcal capsules and slime, in: *Staphylococci and Staphylococcal Infections.* C. Easmon, C. Adlam, eds. Vol 2. Academic Press, London, 1983.
33. I.-M. Nilsson, J. C. Lee, T. Bremell, C. Ryden, and A. Tarkowski. The role of staphylococcal polysaccharide microcapsule expression in septicemia and septic arthritis. *Infect Immun.* 65: 4216 (1997).
34. L. M. Baddour, C. Lowrance, A. Albus, J. H. Lowrance, S. K. Anderson, and J. C. Lee. *Staphylococcus aureus* microcapsule expression attenuates bacterial virulence in a rat model of experimental endocarditis. *J Infect Dis.* 165: 749 (1992).
35. B. Christensson, A. Boutonnier, U. Rydiing, and J. M. Fournier. Diagnosing *Staphylococcus aureus* endocarditis by detecting antibodies against *S. aureus* capsular polysaccharide type 5 and 8. *J Infect Dis.* 163: 530 (1991).
36. A. Albus, J. M. Fournier, C. Wolz, A. Boutonnier, M. Ranke, N. Hoiby, and H. Hochkeppel. *Staphylococcus aureus* capsular types and antibody response to lung infection in patients with cystic fibrosis. *J Clin Microbiol.* 26: 2505 (1988).
37. A. Fattom, S. R., D. C. Watson, W. W. Karakawa, D. Fitzgerald, I. Pastan, and X. Li. Laboratory and clinical evaluation of conjugate vaccines composed of *Staphylococcus aureus* type 5 and type 8 capsular polysaccharides bound to *Pseudomonas aeruginosa* recombinant exoprotein A. *Infect Immun.* 61: 1023 (1993).
38. H. Verbrugh, R. Peters, M. Rozenberg-Arska, P. Peterson, and J. Verhoef. Antibodies to cell wall peptidoglycan of *Staphylococcus aureus* in patients with serious staphylococcal infections. *J Infect Dis.* 144: 1 (1981).
39. H. I. Wergeland, L. R. Haaheim, O. B. Natas, F. Wesenberg, and P. Oeding. Antibodies to staphylococcal peptidoglycan and its peptide epitopes, teichoic acid, and lipoteichoic acid in sera from blood donors and patients with staphylococcal infections. *J Clin Microbiol.* 27: 1286 (1989).
40. P. G. Welch, A. Fattom, J. Moore, R. Schneerson, J. Shiloach, D. A. Bryla, and X. R. Li. Safety and immunogenicity of *Staphylococcus aureus* type 5 capsular polysaccharide-*Pseudomonas aeruginosa* recombinant exoprotein a conjugate vaccine in patients on hemodialysis. *J Amer Soc Nephrol.* 7: 247 (1996).
41. J. Nemeth, and J. C. Lee. Antibodies to capsular polysaccharides are not protective against experimental *Staphylococcus aureus* endocarditis. *Infect Immun.* 63: 375 (1995).
42. D. P. Greenberg, J. I. Ward, and A. S. Bayer. Influence of *Staphylococcus aureus* antibody on experimental endocarditis in rabbits. *Infect Immun.* 55: 3030 (1987).
43. A. Fattom, R. Schneerson, S. C. Szu, W. F. Vann, J. Shiloach, W. W. Karakawa, and J. B. Robbins. Synthesis and immunologic properties in mice of vaccines composed of *Staphylococcus aureus* type 5 and type 8 capsular polysaccharides conjugated to *Pseudomonas aeruginosa* exotoxin A. *Infect Immun.* 58: 2367 (1990).
44. F. B. Gilbert, B. Poutrel, and L. Sutra. Immunogenicity in cows of *Staphylococcus aureus* type 5 capsular polysaccharide-ovalbumin conjugate. *Vaccine.* 12: 369 (1994).
45. L. Reynaud-Rondier, A. Voiland, and G. Michel. Conjugation of capsular polysaccharide to a-hemolysin from *Staphylococcus aureus* as a glycoprotein antigen. *FEMS Microbiol Lett.* 76: 193 (1991).
46. A. Fattom, X. Li, Y. H. Cho, A. Burns, A. Hawwari, S. E. Shepherd, and R. Coughlin. Effect

of conjugation methodology, carrier protein, and adjuvants on the immune response to *Staphylococcus aureus* capsular polysaccharides. *Vaccine.* 13: 1288 (1995).

47. A. I. Fattom, J. Sarwar, A. Ortiz, and R. Naso. A *Staphylococcus aureus* capsular polysaccharide (CP) vaccine and CP-specific antibodies protect mice against bacterial challenge. *Infect Immun.* 64: 1659 (1996).

48. A. S. Bayer, M. Ing, E. Kim, M. R. Yeaman, S. Shepherd, R. Naso, and A. Fattom. Role of anticapsular IgG in modifying the course of experimental *Staphylococcus aureus* endocarditis, in *Abstracts of the 36th International Conference on Antimicrobial Agents and Chemotherapy.* American Society for Microbiology, G096 (1996).

49. K. B. Kiser, J. M. Cantey-Kiser, and J. C. Lee. Development and characterization of a *Staphylococcus aureus* nasal colonization model in mice. *Infect Immun.* 67: 5001 (1999).

50. R. Naso, and A. Fattom. Polysaccharide conjugate vaccines for the prevention of grampositive bacterial infections. *Adv Exp Med Biol.* 397: 133 (1996).

51. D. McKenney, K. L. Pouliot, Y. Wang, V. Murthy, M. Ulrich, G. Doring, J. C. Lee, D. A. Goldmann, and G. B. Pier. Broadly protective vaccine for *Staphylococcus aureus* based on an in vivo-expressed antigen. *Science.* 284: 1523 (1999).

52. D. McKenney, J. Hubner, E. Muller, Y. Wang, D. A. Goldmann, and G. B. Pier. The *ica* locus of *Staphylococcus epidermidis* encodes production of the capsular polysaccharide/adhesin. *Infect Immun.* 66: 4711 (1998).

53. S. E. Cramton, C. Gerke, N. F. Schnell, W. W. Nichols, and F. Gotz. The intercellular adhesion (*ica*) locus is present in *Staphylococcus aureus* and is required for biofilm formation. *Infect Immun.* 67: 5427 (1999).

54. S. Takeda, G. B. Pier, Y. Kojima, M. Tojo, E. Muller, T. Tosteson, and D. A. Goldmann. Protection against endocarditis due to *Staphylococcus epidermidis* by immunization with capsular polysaccharide/adhesin. *Circulation.* 84: 2539 (1991).

55. Y. Kojima, M. Tojo, D. A. Goldmann, T. D. Tosteson, and G. B. Pier. Antibody to the capsular polysaccharide/adhesin protects rabbits against catheter related bacteremia due to coagulase-negative staphylococci. *J Infect Dis.* 162: 435 (1990).

56. D. L. Watson, and C. G. Lee. Immunity to experimental staphylococcal mastitis—comparison of live and killed vaccines. *Aust Vet J.* 54: 374 (1978).

57. D. L. Watson. Virulence of *Staphylococcus aureus* grown in vitro or in vivo. *Res Vet Sci.* 32: 311 (1982).

58. D. L. Watson. Vaccination against experimental staphylococcal mastitis in ewes. *Res Vet Sci.* 45: 16 (1988).

59. D. L. Watson. Ovine opsonins for *Staphylococcus aureus* cell wall and pseudocapsule. *Res Vet Sci.* 46: 89 (1989).

60. D. L. Watson, and C. L. Schwartzkoff. A field trial to test the efficacy of a staphylococcal mastitis vaccine in commercial dairies in Australia. *Proc International Symp on Bovine Mastitis.* Indianapolis, 73 (1990).

61. S. C. Nickerson, W. E. Owens, and R. L. Boddie. Effect of a *Staphylococcus aureus* bacterin on serum antibody, new infection, and mammary histology in nonlactating dairy cows. *J Dairy Sci.* 76: 1290 (1993).

62. D. L. Watson. Expression of a pseudocapsule by *Staphylococcus aureus:* influence of cultural conditions and relevance to mastitis. *Res Vet Sci.* 47: 152 (1989).

5

Superantigen Activation of Macrophages

STEPHEN K. CHAPES,[1] ALBION D. WRIGHT[1], and ALISON A. BEHARKA[1,2]

1. STAPHYLOCOCCAL SUPERANTIGENS

Staphylococcus aureus is a Gram-positive bacterium that can secrete over 30 distinct extracellular proteins.[1] Many of these contribute to the pathogenicity of the organism.[2] Staphylococcal exoproteins are broadly characterized as epidermolytic toxins (ETA and ETB), the enterotoxin family of toxins which includes SEA, SEB, SEC 1, 2 and 3, SED, SEE, SEG, SEH, SEI and SEJ as well as streptococcal pyrogenic exotoxin A, toxic shock syndrome toxin-1 (TSST-1) and membrane-damaging toxins (α, β, δ, γ toxins and others). Coagulase and staphylokinase also are important extracellular secretion products of staphylococci.[1,3–5]

The enterotoxins are a group of closely related molecules, known to cause "food poisoning" and toxic shock[6] and they have some homology to streptococcal pyrogenic toxins.[7,8] They have been categorized into several groups based on their similarities.[1,4,9] Enterotoxins A and E have 81% sequence homology and have been grouped together.[1,9] In this same classification scheme, SED is grouped with SEA and SEE.[5] However, others have listed it separately[4] with (approximately 55% amino acid [AA] homology to SEA and SEE). SEJ shares 78% sequence homology to SEA and 64% similarity with SED when conservative amino acid substitutions are included.[5] SEC and SEB are in a third distinct group (66% AA homology between SEB and SEC; approximately 31% AA homology between SEB/SEC and

STEPHEN K. CHAPES and ALBION D. WRIGHT • Division of Biology, Kansas State University, Manhattan, KS 66506. ALISON A. BEHARKA • Division of Biology, Kansas State University, and Department of Veterans Affairs, Division of Infectious Disease, University of Iowa, Iowa City, IA 52246.

Staphylococcus aureus Infection and Disease, edited by Allen L. Honeyman *et al.* Kluwer Academic/Plenum Publishers, New York, 2001.

SEA/SEE) and SEG is in a fourth group (28% AA homology to SEA/SEE and approximately 44% AA homology to SEB/SEC). Two distinct enterotoxins have been designated SEH and they are antigenically distinct from the other enterotoxins.[10] The toxins range in size from 26–29.6 kDa, have a conserved pair of cysteines that form a disulfide loop, and have isoelectric points ranging from 7.0–8.6.[3] Thus, there is significant diversity as well as similarity between the enterotoxins.

2. WHAT ARE SUPERANTIGENS?

Many of the secreted proteins of *Staphylococcus aureus* were recognized for their "mitogenic" properties in 1975.[11,12] However, we have learned most of what we know about the immunological impact of these molecules within the last 10 years.[13,14] In particular, several groups investigated how these bacterial products affected T cells. Now referred to as "superantigens", staphylococcal exoproteins stimulate specific T cell subpopulations based on their interaction with the variable region of the T cell receptor β chain.[15,16] It was originally believed that T cell stimulation by superantigens required antigen presenting cells[17] but the presentation of the superantigen was not major histocompatibility complex (MHC)-haplotype restricted.[18] Studies by our group and others suggest that T cells may be activated when superantigen is bound by immunoglobulin in the absence of accessory cells or MHC II molecules.[19,20] Under these circumstances, activation was greatly reduced and the activated T cell subpopulations were more limited. Some superantigens can activate the same T cell subpopulations (e.g. $V_\beta 8.3$) even in the absence of MHC II. However, it is not known whether this is true of all superantigens.[21]

3. MACROPHAGE-SUPERANTIGEN INTERACTIONS

Macrophages also are activated by superantigens. Ikejima *et al.*,[22] soon followed by Parsonnet *et al.*[23,24] found that human mononuclear phagocytes secreted IL-1 in response to toxic shock syndrome toxin-1. Other studies, including our own, demonstrated that TSST-1, the enterotoxins and the exfoliative toxins activated human, rat and mouse macrophages.[25–28] In addition, macrophages and monocytes can be induced to produce tumor necrosis factor-α[27–29] (TNFα), nitric oxide,[27,28,30] interleukin-6,[27] granulocyte monocyte colony stimulating factor[31] and IL-10 (See Table I). Furthermore, in the presence of interferon-γ (IFN-γ) these toxins can induce

TABLE I
Summary of exotoxin activation of MHC II +/+ (C57BL/6J) and MHC II −/− (C2D) murine peritoneal macrophages

Treatment[1]	Secretion by C2D cells (MHC II −/−)				Secretion by B6 cells (MHC II +/+)			
	TNF (U/ml)	IL-6 (pg/ml)	IL-10 (pg/ml)	NO$_2^-$ (µM)	TNF (U/ml)	IL-6 (pg/ml)	IL-10 (pg/ml)	NO$_2^-$ (µM)
SEB	9 ± 2	1153 ± 322	84 ± 8	<3	7 ± 3	1132 ± 362	84 ± 84	<3
SEC	7 ± 5	1660 ± 190	58 ± 19	<3	15 ± 6	2468 ± 668	220 ± 149	10 ± 3
SEE	11 ± 3	1377 ± 591	312 ± 63	<3	24 ± 7	5642 ± 400	138 ± 46	12 ± 3
LPS − PMB	49 ± 5	1797 ± 164	706 ± 128	10 ± 2	53 ± 9	2783 ± 544	412 ± 53	29 ± 9
LPS + PMB	6 ± 3	535 ± 37	ND[3]	ND[3]	11 ± 3	854 ± 143	ND	ND

[1]Adherent peritoneal macrophages were stimulated with medium ± 10 ug/ml of each enterotoxin (A, B, Cl or E) and 10 ug/ml polymyxin B (PMB) or 12.5 ug/ml E. coli 055:B5 lipopolysaccharide ± 10 ug/ml PMB. Cells were stimulated with each agonist for 18 hours.

[2]Mean of at least three independent experiments ± SEM.

[3]Not Determined (ND).

macrophages to become cytolytic.[27,28] Clearly, superantigens directly stimulate macrophages.

Staphylococcal superantigens are pathogenic. Their ability to cause "food poisoning", toxic shock syndrome, and scalded skin syndrome have been appreciated for some time[1,6] even though more recent claims about their ability to cause symptoms related to autoimmune disease, Kawasaki syndrome and others is more controversial.[32-39] Moreover, there is not unanimity about the contributions of macrophages to the various physiological and pathological manifestations. It is clear that engagement of cellular MHC II molecules induces signal transduction and cellular activation.[40-48] Therefore, macrophage activation can occur when superantigens directly engage MHC II. Alternatively, T cells make IFN-γ which can be used to stimulate macrophages.[49-51] Even so, many have found the T cell as the major leukocyte contributor to superantigen-induced pathologies. Studies using nude mice[52] or cyclosporin-treated mice[53] demonstrated that SEB-induced weight loss or shock were ameliorated in the absence of T cells. Koesling *et al.*[54] found that mice depleted of splenic macrophages had relatively normal splenic V$\beta8^+$ T cell responses and only slightly delayed CD4$^+$, V$\beta8^+$ T cell responses after SEB treatment. SEA-induced T cell responses were also reported as normal in these studies. These data, along with several mutagenesis studies correlating the inability of mutant superantigens SEA, SEB and TSST-1 to activate T cells with the absence of pathogenesis[55-57] confirm that the T cell response is important to bacterial superantigen-mediated pathogenesis. Nevertheless, there is considerable data to suggest that other leukocytes contribute to pathogenesis. For example, Alber *et al.*,[58] using anti-idiotypic antibodies and carboxymethylation of SEB histidine residues, separated the T cell response from the ability to cause emetic responses. Similarly, Harris *et al.*[59] created SEA and SEB mutants that dissociated emetic responses from T cell activation. Macrophages from C3H/HeJ mice do not respond well to staphylococcal superantigens[27] but the T cells respond normally *in vitro* and *in vivo.*[60] Furthermore, enterotoxin was significantly less toxic to D-galactosamine-sensitized C3H/HeJ mice (3/14 died, 21%) compared to similarly sensitized C3HeB/FeJ mice (11/11 died, 100%). Macrophages from C3HeB/FeJ mice and other mouse strains respond well to staphylococcal superantigens by secreting several cytokines[27,61] (See Table I for a summary). Therefore, there is a strong correlation between macrophage function and pathogenesis.

Our group has shown that T cells are not necessary for superantigen activation of murine macrophages *in vitro.*[61,62] Human monokines can also be elicited by superantigens in the absence of T cells.[63] However, a more realistic situation *in vivo* should reflect the presence of both T cells and macrophages. Indeed, human peripheral blood cells produce both monokines and lymphokines when stimulated with superantigens.[64] In the murine system, the production of TNFα was required for pathogenesis. Its optimal production required the presence of both macrophages and T cells.[65,66] Bright *et al.* found that binding of SEB to MHC II induced macrophages to produce IL-12, a molecule necessary for the induction of a Th1 response and many autoimmune diseases.[67] Without doubt, macrophages contribute to superantigen-mediated pathogenesis. They can be activated directly to help activate T cells and they can respond to the cytokines secreted by superantigen-activated T cells.

4. MACROPHAGES HAVE DISPARATE RESPONSES TO STAPHYLOCOCCAL SUPERANTIGENS

We have spent several years examining how macrophages are activated by staphylococcal superantigens. Macrophages respond within 30 seconds of exposure to several superantigens including SEA and SEB.[62] By 1 hour, subtle differences can be detected amongst macrophages stimulated by various superantigens.[68] For example, SEB (10 μg/ml) did not induce the phosphorylation (as detected in macrophage lysates run in O'Farrell gels[69]) of any macrophage proteins compared to unstimulated macrophage controls (Figure 1). In contrast, macrophages incubated with SEA expressed 6 unique phosphoproteins not expressed by macrophages incubated in medium alone or by macrophages activated by LPS, SEB or ETA (66 kDa, pI 5.5; 65 kDa, pI 5.5; 60 kDa, pI 5.5; 56 kDa, pI 9.0; 53 kDa, and 46 kDa, pI 5.0; Figure 1, labeled as A–F, respectively). In the same pH range, ETA (and ETB, not shown) induced the phosphorylation of a unique 43 kDa protein with a pI of 6.1 (Figure 1, labeled as G). In addition, SEA induced the phosphorylation of a 60 kDa protein in the 8.2–9.5 pH range (pI 9.0; Figure 2, labeled as H). ETA (and ETB, not shown) also induced the 60 kDa phosphoprotein that was seen after SEA stimulation. Moreover, in the same pH range, ETA (and ETB not shown) induced two additional phosphoproteins with 60 kDa molecular weights and pIs of 8.4 and 8.8 respectively (Figure 2, Labeled as I and J). The exfoliative toxins also induced a 12 kDa phosphoprotein with a pI of 6.1 that was not induced by SEA or SEB (Figure 3, labeled as K).

The dramatic differences in the induced macrophage phosphoproteins after SEA and SEB treatment translate into a distinct difference in the cytokines that are subsequently secreted. Whereas, SEA and SEB both stimulated IL-6 efficiently (See Table I), SEA but not SEB stimulated the transcription and eventual secretion of TNFα.[27,62] Macrophages stimulated

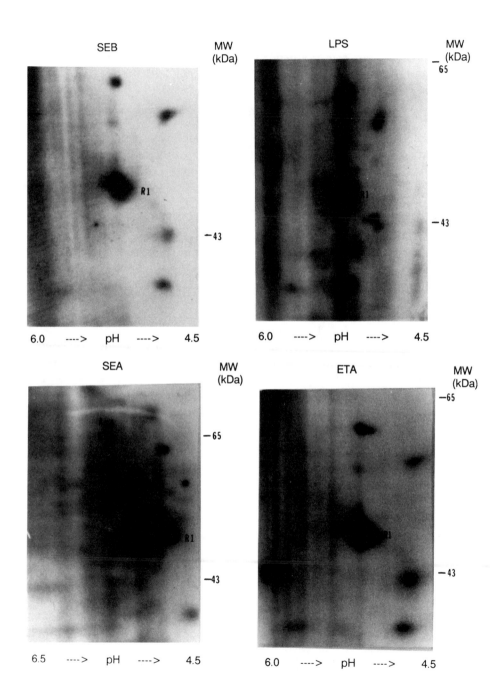

with SEB and IFN-γ did secrete TNFα[62] which suggested to us that multiple signals or costimulation are necessary for superantigen induction of the TNFα response. Indeed, receptor interactions by SEA and SEB determine the outcome of the macrophage response (See below) and recent data confirm that similar outcomes occur after the ligation and cross-linking of MHC II on T cells.[70]

5. THE MHC II HAS TWO DISTINCT SUPERANTIGEN BINDING EPITOPES THAT REGULATE MACROPHAGE RESPONSES

After it was established that superantigens bind MHC II.[71–74] Russell et al.,[75] Karp et al.[76] and Kappler and Marrack and colleagues[77,78] demonstrated that SEA bound to both helices of the MHC II molecule. Others further defined the SEA-MHC II interaction. Zinc is an important element involved in the interaction of SEA, SEE and other superantigens with the MHC II molecule,[79–84] however, other toxins like SEB did not exhibit Zn^{++}-dependent binding.[15,79] Based on competition assays with human[74,85] and mouse[86,87] leukocytes, SEA appeared to have at least one unique and one common binding site with SEB on cell surfaces. The SEA-MHC II interaction was also distinct from the SEB-MHC II complex in that SEA binding was affected by peptides bound in the peptide-binding groove[88] similarly to the observations made using TSST-1.[89,90] SEB does not appear to interact with the MHC II peptide binding groove.[91] Several groups have complemented these observations with exciting data which indicates that the amino terminal end of SEA has a low affinity binding site for the α chain of MHC II and a zinc-dependent, medium affinity binding site in the carboxy end, that binds to the β chain of the MHC II molecule.[79–82] Their

----

FIGURE 1. Two-dimensional gel electrophoretic analysis of superantigen-induced macrophage phosphoproteins with pIs between 4.5 and 6.0. ^{32}Pi-equilibrated macrophages (1 hr.) were stimulated for 1 hr. with 10 μg/ml of SEA, SEB, or ETA or 12.5 μg LPS. Macrophages were solubilized and analyzed by isoelectric focusing followed by SDS polyacrylamide gel electrophoresis. Differences between phosphoproteins with pIs between 4.5 and 6.0 are compared in this experiment. The phosphoprotein labeled R1 is provided to aid orientation. SEA induces 6 unique phosphoproteins of 66 kDa (labelled as A), 65 kDa (labeled as B), 60 kDa (labeled as C), 56 kDa (labeled as D) 53 kDa (labeled as E) and 45 kDa (labeled as F) with pI's of 5.5, 5.5, 5.5, 5.4 and 5.0 respectively. These phosphoproteins are not induced in response to SEB. The phosphoproteins detected after SEB stimulation are shown and are the same as when cells are incubated in medium alone. Phosphoproteins not specifically labeled are phosphoproteins not unique to SEA treatment (e.g. also induced by LPS). The phosphoprotein labeled as G is induced specifically in response to the exfoliative toxins, ETA and ETB (ETB gel not shown).

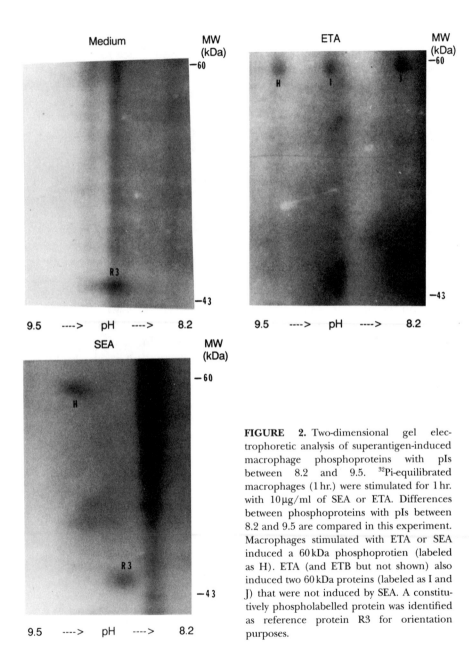

FIGURE 2. Two-dimensional gel electrophoretic analysis of superantigen-induced macrophage phosphoproteins with pIs between 8.2 and 9.5. ^{32}Pi-equilibrated macrophages (1 hr.) were stimulated for 1 hr. with 10 μg/ml of SEA or ETA. Differences between phosphoproteins with pIs between 8.2 and 9.5 are compared in this experiment. Macrophages stimulated with ETA or SEA induced a 60 kDa phosphoprotien (labeled as H). ETA (and ETB but not shown) also induced two 60 kDa proteins (labeled as I and J) that were not induced by SEA. A constitutively phospholabelled protein was identified as reference protein R3 for orientation purposes.

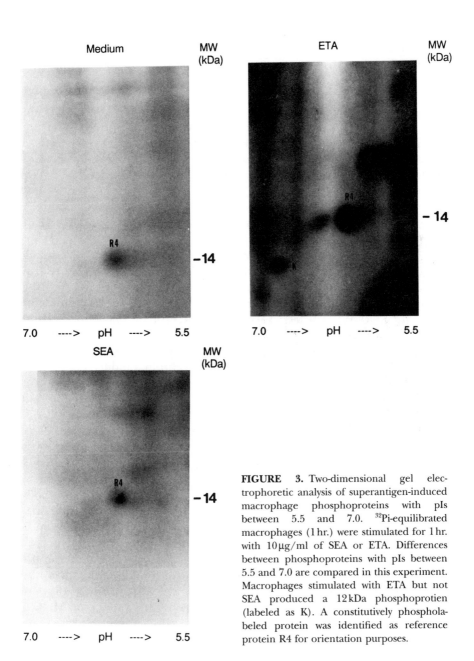

FIGURE 3. Two-dimensional gel electrophoretic analysis of superantigen-induced macrophage phosphoproteins with pIs between 5.5 and 7.0. ^{32}Pi-equilibrated macrophages (1 hr.) were stimulated for 1 hr. with 10 μg/ml of SEA or ETA. Differences between phosphoproteins with pIs between 5.5 and 7.0 are compared in this experiment. Macrophages stimulated with ETA but not SEA produced a 12 kDa phosphoprotien (labeled as K). A constitutively phospholabeled protein was identified as reference protein R4 for orientation purposes.

observations would be consistent with early studies that found that the amino terminus[92–95] and the carboxyl terminus[94,96] of the SEA molecule were involved in MHC II binding. Moreover, the two MHC II SEA binding sites would allow for cross-linking of MHC II molecules on the macrophage plasma membrane.[80] Indeed, this cross-linking process appears responsible for the potent SEA-induced macrophage response. When SEA is mutagenized so that the SEA binding site (amino acid 227) in the MHC II β chain or in the MHC II α chain (amino acid 47) is disrupted, the ability of human macrophage-like cells to transcribe TNFα is ameliorated.[97] Therefore, because SEB lacks a Zn^{++} binding domain it does not bind the β-chain of MHC II[81,82,91] and it cannot cross-link MHC II molecules.

6. THE LOW AFFINITY SUPERANTIGEN EPITOPES CONTROL IL-6

In spite of the fact that SEB lacks a Zn^{++} binding domain, its binding to the MHC II α-chain causes immediate changes in macrophage F-actin concentration.[62] However, as pointed out earlier, the failure to bind the MHC II β chain does have subsequent consequences. The magnitude of the cytokine response is less (Table I) and the proteins phosphorylated in response to SEA are not phosphorylated in response to SEB (Figure 1). Nevertheless, IL-6 is secreted. This proposed MHC IIα-chain-dependent response appears analogous to another low affinity binding epitope for SEA and SEB that we first detected on wild-type macrophages[62] and later defined using macrophages from MHC II[−/−] mice.[87,98] SEA and SEB bind H-2D[b].[98] SEA and SEC1 bind to H-2K[k] and H-2D[k].[99] We have recently discovered that SEA also binds to HLA-A2 with a K_d of approximately 1.4×10^{-6} M. The binding of SEA or SEB to MHC II[−/−] macrophages induces relatively poor TNFα responses. The IL-6 response, in contrast, is comparable to wild-type mouse macrophages[87] (See Table I). It is clear that there is a biologically active superantigen binding epitope on MHC I. Antibody specific for H-2D[b] significantly inhibited the IL-6 response *in vitro,* SEA-induced septic shock *in vivo*[98] and exfoliation *in vivo.*[100] SEA is also significantly less toxic in the absence of MHC I *in vivo.*[101] Therefore, MHC I is a superantigen-binding receptor and is biologically active. In addition, the superantigen-induced IL-6 response is controlled differently than the TNFα response. Because of these observations with MHC I, we also propose that IL-6 is induced by engagement of the low affinity epitope on MHC II in the absence of receptor crosslinking.

We propose a receptor paradigm that encompasses all superantigen interactions with macrophages. Specifically, three superantigen receptor epitopes can be found on macrophages each capable of signaling a cellular response. Two of these epitopes are on the MHC II molecule and one is found on MHC I. We further propose that one of the MHC II epitopes (the MHC IIα chain) and the MHC I epitope are low affinity receptors responsible for signaling the macrophage IL-6 response. The medium affinity receptor epitope on MHC II is dependent on cationic Zn and works in concert with the low affinity MHC II epitope to produce a high affinity interaction to induce more pronounced macrophage cytokine responses. The inability of T cells that lack the MHC IIβ chain binding site for SEA to produce IFN-γ or phosphorylate proteins[70] supports this proposal.

7. SUPERANTIGEN-MEDIATED MHC I RECEPTOR CROSS-LINKING ENHANCES MACROPHAGE ACTIVATION

Houlden *et al.*[102] demonstrated that antibody binding to MHC I molecules stimulated cellular proliferation. MHC I molecule engagement induces protein phosphorylation and up regulation of co-stimulatory molecules.[103] Indeed, engaging murine H-2D^b with monoclonal antibody has the ability to induce macrophage secretion of TNFα and IL-6[104] (Also see Figure 4). Because MHC I could function as a signal transducing receptor on murine macrophages, we addressed the mechanism of how superantigens function to activate cells through the MHC I receptor.[104] We found that directly cross-linking MHC I, by using SEA bound to MHC I and anti-SEA antibody or cross-linking biotinylated SEA with avidin, dramatically increased TNFα or IL-6 secretion by MHC II$^{-/-}$ macrophages[104] (Also see Figure 5). In many ways, this experiment could represent what occurs in normal physiological systems. That is, many individuals have antibody titers against staphylococcal toxins. Therefore, crosslinking the toxins that have bound to cells expressing MHC I is a realistic process because all nucleated cells express MHC I and the toxin concentrations that stimulate cells can be produced during *Staphylococcus aureus* infection.

What remains unresolved are questions about the interactions between MHC I and MHC II receptor epitopes. Engaging the low affinity epitope on MHC I or MHC II alone is sufficient to induce macrophage responses and pathogenicity. We know this because macrophages from either wild-type mice respond by making IL-6 in response to SEB, and MHC II$^{-/-}$ mouse macrophages respond by making relatively normal concentrations of IL-6 in response to staphylococcal superantigens even though the TNFα responses are significantly reduced and because the absence or blocking of either MHC I or MHC II affects pathogenicity *in vivo*.[98,100,101] However, it is not known if there are any synergistic, cooperative or inhibitory effects between MHC I and MHC II. For example, differences in the ways these molecules regulate IL-10 production may impact the kinds of host responses that are induced.[64,105] The fact that SEA does

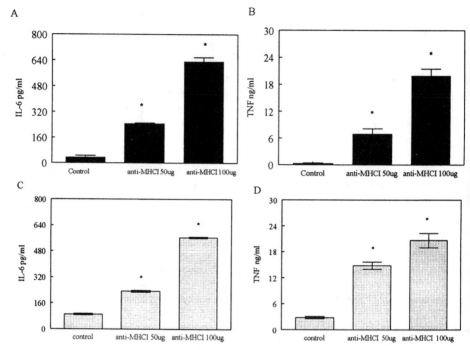

FIGURE 4. Incubation of C2D (Panels A and B) or C57BL/6J (Panels C and D) macrophages with anti-MHC I antibody induces the secretion of TNFα (Panels B and D) and IL-6 (Panels A and C). Peritoneal macrophages were stimulated for 18 hours with medium alone or cross-linked with anti-D^b-specific monoclonal antibody (IgM isotype, HB36, American Type Culture Collection) at 50 or 100μg concentrations. Cytokine determinations were done using bio-assays previously described by our group.[27,87] *indicates a statistically significant difference compared to control using a Student's *t* test, p < 0.05.

not similarly activate B cells with different allelic forms of MHC II[48] also suggest more complex interactions may occur between MHC II and other surface molecules, one of which could be MHC I. Therefore, several interesting questions about receptor interactions remain to be resolved.

8. CONTRIBUTION OF MACROPHAGE-RESPONSE GENES IN SUPERANTIGEN PATHOGENESIS

Macrophages can secrete at least 80 defined products in response to various agonists, cytokines and microorganisms.[106,107] Although we are beginning to appreciate some of the genes that control these processes, we

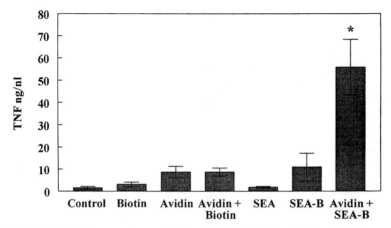

FIGURE 5. MHC II$^{-/-}$ macrophages incubated with biotinylated-SEA and avidin secrete TNFα. C2D mouse macrophages were incubated with 10 μg of biotinylated SEA for 2 hours on ice. Cells were subsequently incubated with avidin for 18 hours at 37°C to complete cross linking. TNFα was quantitated by bioassay.[27,87]

still have a lot to learn, especially about how various genes interact. To address this issue, our group has developed a series of recombinant mice which express combinations of functional and nonfunctional alleles of three macrophage response genes: the *Lps* gene, the *Nramp* gene and the genes of the MHC II complex, A_α and A_β. The development of these recombinant mice provided us a novel model system to determine how these genes and gene combinations impact superantigen pathogenesis. Before describing some of those experiments we will give some background on these genes.

The *Lps* gene is located on the murine 4th chromosome. The gene has recently been identified as a *Tlr4*-like gene.[108–111] Its expression has been characterized by cells and animals that are sensitive to the stimulatory effects of Gram-negative bacterial endotoxin or lipopolysaccharide (LPS). The *Lps*^{n} designation or allele was assigned to animals that were sensitive to the effects of LPS and the *Lps*^{d} designation was assigned to animals resistant to LPS.[112] It is not clear how mutations in the *Lps* gene impact macrophage function, however, signal transduction through the MyD88 pathway[113] and/or other pathways appears to be impacted.[114–117]

The natural resistance associated macrophage protein-1 (*Nramp1*) gene has been closely associated with macrophage function. Natural resistance to several intracellular pathogens like *Salmonella*, *Mycobacteria* or *Leishmania* was noted many years ago and was mapped to chromosome

1.[118-120] The construction of *Nramp1* gene knock-out mice with the same sensitive phenotype to intracellular infections established *Ity, Bcg* or *Lsh* genes as the same gene.[121,122] A guanine to adenine mutation in nucleotide position 596 causes a glycine to aspartic acid substitution in a transmembrane domain of the *Nramp*-gene product.[123,124] The molecule has been associated with late lysosomal granules in macrophages and not with plasma or nuclear membranes.[125] The molecule serves a role as a transport protein which modifies the phagolysosome to allow killing of phagocytosed bacteria.[125] Specifically, mice with defective *Nramp1* alleles fail to fuse late endosomes with phagosomes in the presence of viable bacteria and have diminished numbers of ATP-dependent H^+ pumps with which to acidify the vacuole.[126] In addition, other defects have been associated with defective *Nramp1* alleles. For example, macrophages from *Nramp*-sensitive mice produce less superoxide and nitric oxide than wild-type (resistant) mice, iron transport is disrupted and cytokine RNA stability may be reduced in "sensitive" animals.[127-129]

The major histocompatibility complex is a group of well defined genes located on the mouse 17th and human 6th chromosomes which control T cell responsiveness. The crystal structures of both MHC I and MHC II molecules[130,131] reveal the elegant way these molecules engage peptides and how MHC II polymorphism regulates immune responsiveness.[132-134] As discussed above, these molecules also bind superantigens which leads to both T cell and macrophage activation.

Because $Lps^{d/d}$, MHC II[+/+](C3H/HeJ) mice were significantly more resistant to superantigen-induced death[60] and $Lps^{n/n}$, MHC II[-/-] (C2D) mice were susceptible,[98] we used recombinant $Lps^{d/d}$, MHC II[-/-] mice[135] to determine whether a functional *Lps* gene was required for pathogenesis in the absence of MHC II molecules. In this system, mice were challenged (i.p.) with 20 mg of D-galactosamine, 2 ng of LPS and 100 μg of SEB as was described previously.[60,98] C3H/HeJ mice were not killed by 2 ng of LPS or 100 μg of SEB. Moreover, when SEB and LPS were administered together only about a quarter of the mice died (Table II). C2D mice were more sensitive to LPS and SEB when each was administered individually, however, the majority of mice survived unless SEB and LPS were injected together when 100% of the C2D mice died. Recombinant mice that are $Lps^{d/d}$, MHC II[-/-] were not susceptible to SEB induced death (Table II). $Lps^{d/d}$, MHC II[-/-] mice survived after SEB and LPS challenge regardless of whether they carried the C3H/HeJ mouse, *Nramp*[r/r] genotype, the C2D mouse *Nramp*[s/s] genotype or were heterozygous for *Nramp*. These data support the hypothesis that MHC II molecules are not necessary for the effects of SEB pathogenesis. Indeed, by blocking MHC I molecules we have inhibited

TABLE II
Contribution of Macrophage-Response Genes to Superantigen Pathogenesis

Mouse Strain[1]	Genotype[2]	LPS[3]	SEB[3]	#Surviving Mice/total[4]	% Surviving Mice
C3H/HeJ	MHC II$^{+/+}$, $Lps^{d/d}$, $Nramp^{r/r}$	+	−	7/7	100
C3H/HeJ	MHC II$^{+/+}$, $Lps^{d/d}$, $Nramp^{r/r}$	−	+	3/3	100
C3H/HeJ	MHC II$^{+/+}$, $Lps^{d/d}$, $Nramp^{r/r}$	+	+	17/23	74
C2D	MHC II$^{-/-}$, $Lps^{n/n}$, $Nramp^{s/s}$	+	−	16/23	70
C2D	MHC II$^{-/-}$, $Lps^{n/n}$, $Nramp^{s/s}$	−	+	14/15	93
C2D	MHC II$^{-/-}$, $Lps^{n/n}$, $Nramp^{s/s}$	+	+	0/29	0
C2D × C3H/HeJ	MHC II$^{-/-}$, $Lps^{d/d}$, $Nramp^{s/s}$	+	+	8/8	100
C2D × C3H/HeJ	MHC II$^{-/-}$, $Lps^{d/d}$, $Nramp^{s/s}$	+	+	8/8	100
C2D × C3H/HeJ	MHC II$^{-/-}$, $Lps^{d/d}$, $Nramp^{r/r}$	+	+	8/8	100

[1]C3H/HeJ mice were crossed with C2D (MHC II$^{-/-}$), mice and selected for the absence of MHC II and $Lps^{d/d}$ alleles in the F$_2$ and subsequent generations as described[135].
[2]C3H × HeJ mice (MHC II$^{-/-}$, $Lps^{d/d}$) were selected for heterozygosity, or homozygosity at the $Nramp$ gene as described[135].
[3]Mice were injected i.p. with 20 mg/D-galactosamine simultaneously with 2 ng LPS ± 100 ug SEB as described[60].
[4]Numbers represent survivors 4 days after challenge.

superantigen-mediated effects in the absence of MHC II.[98,100] In addition, the Lps ($Tlr4$) gene is important for the manifestations of staphylococcal superantigen pathogenesis in the presence or absence of MHC II. These data also suggest that at least some of the signal transduction processes activated by engaging MHC I and MHC II molecules are similar or have some necessary common component. Interestingly, the $Nramp$ gene did not play a role in superantigen pathogenesis. This is consistent with other studies where $Nramp^{s/s}$ and $Nramp^{r/r}$ mice could both be killed by staphylococcal superantigens.[53]

The impact of the Lps gene on superantigen-mediated pathogenesis suggests a role for macrophages in this process. We investigated macrophage function of the recombinant mice *in vitro* to examine their role in host superantigen responses. In this experiment, we assessed peritoneal macrophage contributions to the activation of C3H/HeJ T cells by a mixture of two superantigens, SEA and SEB. C3H/HeJ T cells were used to standardize the responding T cell population and eliminate differences amongst the various recombinant mouse T cell subpopulations. T cell activation was assessed by the production of IL-2. As summarized in Table III, T cells not incubated with macrophages did not produce IL-2. In contrast, macrophages from C3HeB/FeJ and C3H/HeJ mice activated T cells to

TABLE III
Superantigens activate T cells in the Presence of MHC II$^{-/-}$ Macrophages

Macrophage[1]	Genotype[2,3]	IL-2 (U/ml)[3]	% Wild-type
C3Heb/FeJ	MHC II$^{+/+}$, $Lps^{n/n}$, $Nramp^{r/r}$	30 ± 1	—
C3H/HeJ	MHC II$^{+/+}$, $Lps^{d/d}$, $Nramp^{r/r}$	29 ± 2	97
FeJxC2D(R)	MHC II$^{-/-}$, $Lps^{n/n}$, $Nramp^{r/r}$	40 ± 1	133
FeJxC2D(S)	MHC II$^{-/-}$, $Lps^{n/n}$, $Nramp^{s/s}$	11 ± 0	37
HeJxC2D(R)	MHC II$^{-/-}$, $Lps^{d/d}$, $Nramp^{r/r}$	22 ± 0	73
HeJxC2D(S)	MHC II$^{-/-}$, $Lps^{d/d}$, $Nramp^{s/s}$	16 ± 1	53
None	T cells from C3H/HeJ	0 ± 0	0

[1]C3H/HeJ or C3HeB/FeJ mice were crossed with MHC II$^{-/-}$, C2D mice and selected for the presence or absence of desired MHC II and *Lps* alleles in the F$_2$ and subsequent generations as described[135].
[2]Recombinant mice were selected for Homozygous $Nramp^{r/r}$ or $Nramp^{s/s}$ alleles as described[135].
[3]Nylon wool purified C3H/HeJ splenic T cells were incubated for 6 days with peritoneal macrophage harvested from recombinant mice. Cultures were pulsed with 10 ug/ml of SEA and SEB. On day 4, cultures were pulsed with 10 u/ml human IL-2. Murine IL-2 was detected using a capture ELISA using mouse-specific anti-IL-2 antibodies as was described previously[60].

produce 29–30 units/ml IL-2. The null-expression of MHC II did not diminish the ability of macrophages to support T cell activation. T cells incubated with FeJ x C2D macrophages[136] (MHC II$^{-/-}$, $Lps^{n/n}$) secreted the most IL-2 of all the experimental groups.

The absence of MHC II and a functional *Lps* gene impacted the production of IL-2 by only approximately 25%. This slightly diminished IL-2 response did not correlate with the reduced susceptibility of HeJ x C2D mice to SEB-induced death. Furthermore, in contrast to our lethality studies where there were no differences in animals with $Nramp^{s/s}$ and $Nramp^{r/r}$ genotypes, macrophages carrying the $Nramp^{r/r}$ allele stimulated T cells significantly better than macrophages from mice carrying the $Nramp^{s/s}$ allele (Table III). Therefore, pathogenesis did not correlate with T cell activation. It is not clear how *Nramp* functions to allow better T cell stimulation, however, because of its previous impact on RNA stability, signal transduction and secretion,[128] there are many potential mechanisms that could be impacted by these allelic differences. Nevertheless, these data support the hypothesis that T cells can be activated by superantigens in the absence of functional MHC II and *Lps* genes. Moreover, these data strongly support the hypothesis that macrophages help regulate the host response to superantigens with the macrophage response gene, *Lps* (*Tlr4*), playing an important role.

9. CONCLUSION

Superantigens are molecules that powerfully stimulate the immune system. Activation has severe consequences on host physiological responses and can be lethal. We have provided evidence that macrophages play a role in these responses. Superantigens induce changes in macrophages within 30 seconds of ligand-receptor contact. Macrophages have disparate responses to various staphylococcal superantigens and these can be clearly distinguished by 1 hour after exposure. At least three distinct receptor epitopes can be documented for superantigens. These epitopes are present on MHC I and MHC II molecules. Moreover, crosslinking of these epitopes appears to be an important step in the induction of robust macrophages responses. Lastly, the host response to superantigens appears to be strongly impacted by the macrophage response gene, *Lps* (*Tlr4*) and other macrophage response genes *Nramp* and MHC II also appear to impact the ability of macrophages to regulate the T cell response to staphylococcal superantigens.

ACKNOWLEDGMENTS. We would like to thank Ms. Connie Carlson, Ms. Jennifer Ewert, Dr. Dorothy Feese, Dr. Allan Forsman, Ms. Angela Herpich-Matthews and Dr. John Iandolo for their help with various aspects of our work. Our studies have been supported past and present by the American Heart Association, grants KS-GS-94-33 and KS-GS-97-02; the Army Research and Development Command, grant DAMD-17-89-Z-9039; the National Aeronautics and Space Administration, grants NAGW-1197, NAGW-2328, NAG2-1274 and the NASA Kansas EPSCoR Program; the National Cancer Institute, grant CA09418; the United States Department of Agriculture Animal Health Funds Section 1433, Grant 4-81895; the Kansas Agriculture Experiment Station and the Kansas Health Foundation. This is Kansas Agriculture Experiment Station Publication number 00-21-B.

REFERENCES

1. Iandolo, J. J. Genetic analysis of extracellular toxins of *Staphylococcus aureus*. *Annu. Rev. Microbiol.* 43, 375 (1989).
2. Tao, M., H. Yamashita, K. Watanabe and T. Nagatake. Possible virulence factors of *Staphylococcus aureus* in a mouse septic model. *FEMS Immunology* 23, 135 (1999).
3. Johnson, H., J. Russell and C. Pontzer. Staphylococcal enterotoxin microbial superantigens. *FASEB J.* 5, 2706 (1991).
4. Betley, M., D. Borst and L. Regassa. in *Biological significance of superantigens* (ed. B. Fleischer) p. 1 (Karger, Basel, 1992).

5. Zhang, S., J. J. Iandolo and G. C. Stewart. The enterotoxin D plasmid of Staphylococcus aureus encodes a second enterotoxin determinant (sej). *FEMS Microbiol. Lett.* 168, 227 (1998).

6. Bergdoll, M. in *Food bourne infections and intoxications* (eds. H. Riemann & F. L. Bryan) pp. 444 (Academic Press, New York, 1979).

7. Leonard, B., P. Lee, M. Jenkins and P. Schlievert. Cell and receptor requirements for *Streptococcal pyrogenic* exotoxinT cell mitogenicity. *Infect. Immun.* 59, 1210 (1991).

8. Abe, R., J. Forrester, F. Nakahara, J. Lafferty, B. Kotzin and D. Leung. Selective stimulation of human T cells with streptococcal erythrogenic toxins A and B. *J. Immunol.* 146, 3747 (1991).

9. Bayles, K. and J. Iandolo. Genetic and molecular analysis of the gene encoding staphylococcal enterotoxin D. *J. Bacteriol.* 171, 4799 (1989).

10. Su, Y. C. and A. C. L. Wong. Identification and purification of a new staphylococcal enterotoxin , J. *Applied and Environmental Microbiology* 61, 1438 (1995).

11. Warren, J., D. Leatherman and J. Metzger. Evidence for cell-receptor activity in lymphocyte stimulation by staphylococcal enterotoxin. *J. Immunol.* 115, 49 (1975).

12. Smith, B. and H. Johnson. The effect of staphylococcal enterotoxins on the primary *in vitro* immune response. *J. Immunol.* 115, 575 (1975).

13. Leung, D. Y. M., B. T. Huber and P. M. Schlievert (eds.) *Superantigens: Molecular Biology, Immunology, and Relevance to Human Disease* (Marcel Dekker, Inc., New York, 1997).

14. Thibodeau, J. and R.-P. Sekaly (eds.) *Bacterial Superantigens: Structure, Function and Therapeutic Potential* (Springe-Verlag, Heidelberg, 1995).

15. Papageorgiou, A. C., H. S. Tranter and K. R. Acharya. Crystal structure of microbial surperantigen staphylococcal enterotoxin B at 1.5A resolution: implications for superantigen recognition by MHC class II molecules and T-cell receptors. *J. Mol. Biol.* 277, 61 (1998).

16. Papageorgiou, A. C., C. M. Collins, D. M. Gutman, J. B. Kline, S. M. O'Brien, H. S. Tranter and K. R. Acharya. Structural basis for the recognition of superantigen streptococcal pyrogenic exotoxin A (SpeA1) by MHC class II molecules and T-cell receptors. *EMBO J.* 18, 9 (1999).

17. Carlsson, R., H. Fischer and H. Sjogren. Binding of staphlyococcal enterotoxin A to accessory cells is a requirement for its ability to activate human T cells. *J. Immunol.* 140, 2484 (1988).

18. Fleischer, B. and H. Schrezenmeier. T cell stimulation by staphylococcal enterotoxins. Clonally variable response and requirement for major histocompatibility complex class II molecules on accessory or target cells. *J. Exp. Med.* 167, 1697 (1988).

19. Chapes, S., S. Hoynowski, K. Woods, J. Armstrong, A. Beharka and J. Iandolo. Staphylococcus-mediated T cell activation and spontaneous natural killer cell activity in the absence of major histocompatibility complex class II molecules. *Infect. Immun.* 61, 4013 (1993).

20. Hamad, A. R., A. Herman, P. Marrack and J. Kappler. Monoclonal antibodies defining functional sites on the toxin superantigen staphylococcal enterotoxin B. *J. Exp. Med.* 180, 615 (1994).

21. Rovira, P., M. Buckle, J. P. Abastado, W. J. Peumans and P. Truffa-Bachi. Major histocompatibility class I molecules present *Urtica dioica* agglutinin, a superantigen of vegetal origin, to T lymphocytes. *Eur. J. Immunol.* 29, 1571 (1999).

22. Ikejima, T., C. Dinarello, D. Gill and S. Wolff. Induction of human interleukin-1 by a product of *Staphylococcus aureus* associated with toxic shock syndrome. *J. Clin. Invest.* 73, 1312 (1984).

23. Parsonnet, J., R. Hickman, D. Eardley and G. Pier. Induction of human interleukin-1 by toxic-shock-syndrome toxin-1. *J. Infect. Dis.* 151, 514 (1985).

24. Parsonnet, J., Z. Gillis and G. Pier. Induction of interleukin-1 by strains of *Staphylococcus aureus* from patients with nonmenstrual toxic shock syndrome. *J. Infect. Dis.* 154, 55 (1986).

25. Beezhold, D., G. Best, P. Bonventre and M. Thompson. Synergistic induction of interleukin-1 by endotoxin and toxic shock syndrome toxin-1 using rat macrophages. *Infect. Immun.* 55, 2865 (1987).

26. Fast, D., P. Schlievert and R. Nelson. Toxic shock syndrome-associated staphlococcal and streptococcal pyrogneic toxins are potent inducers of tumor necrosis factor. *Infect. Immun.* 57, 291 (1989).

27. Fleming, S. D., J. J. Iandolo and S. K. Chapes. Murine macrophage activation by staphylococcal exotoxins. *Infect. Immun.* 59, 4049 (1991).

28. Fast, D., B. Shannon, M. Herriott, M. Kennedy, J. Rummage and R. Leu. Staphylococcal exotoxins stimulate nitric oxide-dependent murine macrophage tumoricidal activity. *Infect. Immun.* 59, 2987 (1990).

29. Trede, N., R. Geha and T. Chatila. Transcriptional activation of IL-1β and tumor necrosis factor genes by MHC class II ligands. *J. Immunol.* 146, 2310 (1991).

30. Isobe, K. I. and L. Nakashima. Feedback suppression of staphylococcal enterotoxin-stimulated T-lymphocyte proliferation by macrophages through inductive nitric oxide synthesis. *Infect. Immun.* 60, 4832 (1992).

31. Bratton, D. L., K. R. May, J. M. Kailey, D. E. Doherty and D. Y. Leung. Staphylococcal toxic shock syndrome toxin-1 inhibits monocyte apoptosis. *J. Allergy Clin. Immunol.* 103, 895 (1999).

32. Mancia, L., J. Wahlstrom, B. Schiller, L. Chini, G. Elinder, P. D'Argenio, D. Gigliotti, H. Wigzell, P. Rossi and J. Grunewald. Characterization of the T-cell receptor V-beta repertoire in Kawasaki disease. *Scand. J. Immunol.* 48, 443 (1998).

33. Soos, J. M., J. Schiffenbauer, B. A. Torres and H. M. Johnson. Superantigens as virulence factors in autoimmunity and immunodeficiency diseases. *Medical Hypotheses* 48, 253 (1997).

34. Fischer, P., M. M. Uttenreuther-Fischer and G. Gaedicke. Superantigens in the aetiology of Kawasaki disease. *Lancet.* 348, 202 (1996).

35. Lueng, D. Y. M. Superantigens related to Kawasaki syndrome. *Springer Seminars in Immunopath.* 17, 385 (1996).

36. Inocencio, J. and R. Hirsch. The role of T cells in Kawasaki disease. *Critical Reviews in Immunol.* 15, 349 (1995).

37. Curtis, N., R. Zheng, J. Lamb and M. Levin. Evidence for a superantigen mediated process in Kawasaki disease. *Arch. Dis. in Childhood* 72, 308 (1995).

38. Rowley, A. H. and T. S. Stanford. Letter to the editor-reply. *Pediatric Res.* 43, 291 (1998).

39. Choi, I.-H., Y.-J. Chwae, W.-S. Shim, D.-S. Kim, D.-H. Kwon, J.-D. Kim and S.-J. Kim. Clonal expansion of CD8⁺ T cells in Kawasaki disease. *J. Immunol.* 159, 481 (1997).

40. St-Pierre, Y., N. Nabavi, Z. Ghogawala, L. Glimcher and T. Watts. A fuctional role for signal transduction via the cytoplasmic domains of MHC class II proteins. *J. Immunol.* 143, 808 (1989).

41. Fuleihan, R., W. Mourad, R. Geha and T. Chatila. Engagement of MHC-Class II molecules by staphylococcal exotoxins delivers a comitogenic signal to human B cells. *J. Immunol.* 146, 1661 (1991).

42. Chen, Z., J. McGuire, K. Leach and J. Cambier. Transmembrane signaling through B cell MHC class II molecules: Anti-Ia antibodies induce protein kinase C translocation to the nuclear fraction. *J. Immunol.* 138, 2345 (1987).

43. Mooney, N., C. Grillot-Courvalin, C. Hivroz, L. Y. Ju and D. Charron. Early biochemical events after MHC class II-mediated signaling on human B lymphocytes. *J. Immunol.* 145, 2070 (1990).

44. Chatila, T. and R. Geha. Signal transduction by microbial superantigens via MHC class II molecules. *Immunol. Rev.* 131, 43 (1993).

45. Morio, T., R. Geha and T. Chatila. Engagement of MHC class II molecules by staphylococcal superantigens activates src-type protein tyrosine kinases. *Eur. J. Immunol.* 24, 651 (1994).

46. Matsuyama, S., Y. Koide and T. Yoshida. HLA class II molecule-mediated signal transduction mechanism responsible for the expression of interleukin-1β and tumor necrosis factor-α genes induced by a staphylococcal superantigen. *Eur. J. Immunol.* 23, 3194 (1993).

47. Mourad, W., K. Mehindate, T. Schall and S. McColl. Engagement of major histocompatibility complex class II molecules by superantigens induces inflammatory cytokine gene expression in human rheumatoid fibroblast-like synoviocytes. *J. Exp. Med.* 175, 613 (1992).

48. Guo, W., W. Mourad, D. Charron and R. Al-Daccak. Ligation of MHC class II molecules differentially upregulates TNFβ gene expression in B cell lines of different MHC class II haplotypes. *Hum. Immunol.* 60, 312 (1999).

49. Ruco, L. and M. Meltzer. Macrophage activation for tumor cytotoxicity: development of macrophage cytotoxic activity requires completion of a sequence of short-lived intermediary reactions. *J. Immunol.* 121, 2035 (1978).

50. Pace, J., S. Russell, B. Torres, H. Johnson and P. Gray. Recombinant mouse gamma interferon induces the priming step in macrophage activation for tumor cell killing. *J. Immunol.* 130, 2011 (1983).

51. Boehm, U., T. Klamp, M. Groot and J. C. Howard. in *Annual Review of Immunology* (eds. W. E. Paul, C. G. Fathman & H. Metzger) pp. 749 (Annual Reviews Inc., Palo Alto, 1997).

52. Marrack, P., M. Blackman, E. Kushnir and J. Kappler. The toxicity of staphylococcal enterotoxin B in mice is mediated by Tcells. *J. Exp. Med.* 171, 455 (1990).

53. Miethke, T., C. Wahl, K. Heeg, B. Echtenacher, P. Krammer and H. Wagner. T cell-mediated lethal shock triggered in mice by the superantigen Staphylococcal Enterotoxin B: Critical role of tumor necrosis factor. *J. Exp. Med.* 175, 91 (1992).

54. Koesling, M., O. Rott and B. Fleischer. Macrophages are dispensable for superantigen-mediated stimulation and anergy induction of peripheral T cell *in vivo*. *Cell. Immunol.* 157, 29 (1994).

55. Bonventre, P., H. Heeg, C. Edwards III and C. Cullen. A mutation at histidine residue 135 of toxic shock syndrome toxin yields an immunogenic protein with minimal toxicity. *Infect. Immun.* 63, 509 (1995).

56. Hoffman, M., M. Tremaine, J. Mansfield and M. Betley. Biochemical and mutational analysis of the histidine residues of staphylococcal enterotoxin A. *Infect. Immun.* 64, 885 (1996).

57. Woody, M. A., T. Krakauer, R. G. Ulrich and B. G. Stiles. Differential immune responses to staphylococcal enterotoxin B mutations in a hydrophobic loop dominating the interface with major histocompatibility complex class II receptors. *J. Infectious Diseases* 177, 1013 (1998).

58. Alber, G., D. Hammer and B. Fleischer. Relationship between enterotoxic- and T lymphocyte-stimulating activity. *J. Immunol.* 144, 4501 (1990).

59. Harris, T., D. Grossman, J. Kappler, P. Marrack, R. Rich and M. Betley. Lack of complete correlation between emetic and T-cell-stimulatory activities of staphylococcal enterotoxins. *Infet. Immun.* 61, 3175 (1993).

60. Chapes, S. K. and A. A. Beharka. Lipopolysaccharide is required for the lethal effects of enterotoxin B after D-galactosamine sensitization. *J. Endotoxin Res.* 2, 263 (1995).

61. Beharka, A. A., J. W. Armstrong and S. K. Chapes. Macrophage cell lines derived from major histocompatibility complex II-negative mice. *In Vitro Cell. Dev. Biol.* 34, 499 (1998).
62. Chapes, S. K., A. Beharka, M. Hart, M. Smeltzer and J. J. Iandolo. Differential RNA regulation by staphylococcal enterotoxins A and B in murine macrophages. *J. Leukoc. Biol.* 55, 523 (1994).
63. Kotb, M., H. Ohnishi, G. Majumdar, S. Hackett, A. Bryant, G. Higgins and D. Stevens. Temporal relationship of cytokine release by peripheral blood mononuclear cells stimulated by the streptococcal superantigen pep M5. *Infect. Immun.* 61, 1194 (1993).
64. Rink, L., J. Luhm, M. Koester and H. Kirchner. Induction of a cytokine network by superantigens with parallel TH1 and TH2 stimulation. *J. Interferon and Cytokine Res.* 16, 41 (1996).
65. See, R., W. Kum, A. Chang, S. Goh and A. Chow. Induction of tumor necrosis factor and interleukin-1 by purified staphylococcal toxic shock syndrome toxin 1 requires the presence of both monocytes and T lymphocytes. *Infect. Immun.* 60, 2612 (1992).
66. Grossman, D., J. Lamphear, J. Mollick, M. Betley and R. Rich. Dual roles for class II major histocompatibility complex molecules in staphylococcal enterotoxin-induced cytokine production and *in vivo* toxicity. *Infect. Immun.* 60, 5190 (1992).
67. Bright, J. J., Z. Xin and S. Sriram. Superantigens augment antigen-specific Th1 responses by inducing IL-12 production in macrophages. *J. Leukoc. Biol.* 65, 665 (1999).
68. Beharka, A. A., J. Iandolo and S. K. Chapes. Description of protein kinase activation in murine macrophages by *Staphylococcus aureus* superantigens. *J. Leukoc. Biol.* Supplement 1994, 22 (1994).
69. O'Farrell, P. High resolution two-dimensional electrophoresis of proteins. *J. Biol. Chem.* 250, 4007 (1975).
70. Nielsen, M. B., N. Odum, J. Gerwien, A. Svejgaard, K. Bendtzen, S. Bregentholt, C. Ropke, C. Geisler, M. Dohlsten and K. Kaltoft. Staphylococcal enterotoxin-A directly stimulates signal transduction and interferon-gamma production in psoriatic T-cell lines. *Tissue Antigens* 52, 530 (1998).
71. Mollick, J., R. Cook and R. Rich. Class II MHC molecules are specific receptors for staphylococcus enterotoxin A. *Science* 244, 817 (1989).
72. Scholl, P., A. Diez, W. Mourad, J. Parsonnet, R. Geha and T. Chatila. Toxic shock syndrome toxin 1 binds to major histocompatibility complex class II molecules. *Proc. Natl. Acad. Sci. USA* 86, 4210 (1989).
73. Herrmann, T., R. Accolla and H. MacDonald. Different staphylococcal enterotoxins bind preferentially to distinct major histocompatibility complex class II isotypes. *Eur. J. Immunol.* 19, 2171 (1989).
74. Fraser, J. High-affinity binding of staphylococcal enterotoxins A and B to HLA-DR. *Nature* 339, 221 (1989).
75. Russell, J., C. Pontzer and H. Johnson. Both alpha-helices along the major histocompatibility complex binding cleft are required for staphylococcal enterotoxin A function. *Proc. Natl. Acad. Sci. USA* 88, 7228 (1991).
76. Karp, D. and E. Long. Identification of HLA-DR1 β chain residues critical for binding Staphylococcal enterotoxins A and E. *J. Exp. Med.* 175, 415 (1992).
77. Herman, A., N. Labrecque, J. Thibodeau, P. Marrack, J. Kappler and R. P. Sekaly. Identification of the staphylococcal enterotoxin A superantigen binding site in the $\alpha 1$ domain of the human histocompatibility antigen HLA-DR. *Proc. Natl. Acad. Sci. USA* 88, 9954 (1991).
78. Dellabona, P., J. Peccoud, J. Kappler, P. Marrack, C. Benoist and D. Mathis. Superantigens interact with MHC class II molecules outside of the antigen groove. *Cell* 62, 1115 (1990).

79. Fraser, J., R. Urban, J. Strominger and H. Robinson. Zinc regulates the function of two superantigens. *Proc. Natl. Acad. Sci. USA* 89, 5507 (1992).

80. Hudson, K., R. Tiedemann, R. Urban, S. Lowe, J. Strominger and J. Fraser. Staphylococcal enterotoxin A has two cooperative binding sites on major histocompatibility complex class II. *J. Exp. Med.* 182, 711 (1995).

81. Abrahmsen, L., M. Dohlsten, S. Segren, P. Bjork, E. Jonsson and T. Kalland. Characterization of two distinct MHC class II binding sites in the superantigen staphylococcal enterotoxin A. *EMBO J.* 14, 2978 (1995).

82. Schad, E., I. Zaitseva, V. Zaitsev, M. Dohlsten, T. Kalland, P. Schlievert, D. Ohlendorf and L. Svensson. Crystal structure of the superantigen staphylococcal enterotoxin type A. *EMBO J.* 14, 3292 (1995).

83. Papageorgiou, A., K. Acharya, R. Shapiro, E. Passalacqua, R. Brehm and H. Tranter. Crystal structure of the superantigen enterotoxin C2 from *Staphylococcus aureus* reveals a zinc-binding site. *Structure* 3, 769 (1995).

84. Schad, E. M., A. C. Papageorgiou, L. A. Svensson and K. R. Archarya. A structural and functional comparison of staphylococcal enterotoxins A and C2 reveals remarkable similarity and dissimilarity. *J. Mol. Biol.* 269, 270 (1997).

85. Chintagumpala, M., J. Mollick and R. Rich. Staphylococcal toxins bind to different sites on HLA-DR. *J. Immunol.* 147, 3876 (1991).

86. Buxser, S., P. Bonventre and D. Archer. Specific receptor binding of staphylococcal enterotoxins by murinesplenic lymphocytes. *Infect. Immun.* 33, 827 (1981).

87. Beharka, A. A., J. Armstrong, J. J. Iandolo and S. K. Chapes. Binding and activation of major histocompatibility complex class II-deficient macrophages by staphylococcal exotoxins. *Infect. Immun.* 62, 3907 (1994).

88. Dowd, J., R. Jenkins and D. R. Karp. Inhibition of antigen-specific T cell activation by staphylococcal enterotoxins. *J. Immunol.* 154, 1024 (1995).

89. Kim, J., R. Urban, J. Strominger and D. Wiley. Toxic shock syndrome toxin-1 complexed with a class II major histocompatibility molecule HLA-DR1. *Science* 266, 1870 (1994).

90. Thibodeau, J., I. Cloutier, P. Lavoie, N. Labrecque, W. Mourad, T. Jardetzky and R. Sekaly. Subsets of HLA-DR1 molecules defined by SEB and TSST-1 binding. *Science* 266, 1874 (1994).

91. Jardetzky, T., J. Brown, J. Gorga, L. Stern, R. Urban, Y.-I. Chi, C. Stauffacher, J. Strominger and D. Wiley. Three-dimensional structure of a human class II histocompatibility molecule complexed with superantigen. *Nature* 368, 711 (1994).

92. Pontzer, C., J. Russell and H. Johnson. Localization of an immune functional site on staphylococcal enterotoxin A using the synthetic peptide approach. *J. Immunol.* 143, 280 (1989).

93. Griggs, N., C. Pontzer, M. Jarpe and H. Johnson. Mapping of multiple binding domains of the superantigen staphylococcal enterotoxin A for HLA. *J. Immunol.* 148, 2516 (1992).

94. Mollick, J., R. McMasters, D. Grossman and R. Rich. Localization of a site on bacterial superantigens that determines T cell receptor β chain specificity. *J. Exp. Med.* 177, 283 (1993).

95. Harris, T. and M. Betley. Biological activities of staphylococcal enterotoxin type A mutants with N-terminal substitutions. *Infect. Immun.* 63, 2133 (1995).

96. Hedlund, G., M. Dohlsten, T. Herrmann, G. Buell, P. Lando, S. Segren, J. Schrimsher, H. Macdonald, H. Sjogren and T. Kalland. A recombinant C-terminal fragment of staphylococcal enterotoxin A binds to human MHC class II products but does not activate T cells. *J. Immunol.* 147, 4082 (1991).

97. Mehindate, K., J. Thibodeau, M. Dohlsten, T. Kalland, R.-P. Sekaly and W. Mourad. Cross-linking of major histocompatibility complex class II molecules by staphylococcal

enterotoxin A superantigen is a requirement for inflammatory cytokine gene expression. *J. Exp. Med.* 182, 1573 (1995).

98. Beharka, A. A., J. J. Iandolo and S. K. Chapes. Staphylococcal enterotoxins bind H-2D^b molecules on macrophages. *Proc. Natl. Acad. Sci. USA.* 92, 6294 (1995).

99. Chapes, S. K. and A. R. Herpich. Complex high affinity interactions occur between MHC I and superantigens. *J. Leukoc. Biol.* 64, 587 (1998).

100. Iandolo, J. J. and S. K. Chapes. in *Superantigens: Relevance to Human Disease and Basic Biology* (eds. D. Leung, B. Huber & P. Schlievert) p. 231 (Marcel Dekker, Inc., New York, 1996).

101. Stiles, B. G., S. Bavari, T. Krakauer and R. G. Ulrich. Toxicity of staphylococcal enterotoxins potentiated by lipopolysaccharide: Major histocompatibility complex class II molecules dependency and cytokine release. *Infect. Immun.* 61, 5333 (1993).

102. Houlden, B., S. Widacki and J. Bluestone. Signal transduction through class I MHC by a monoclonal antibody that detects multiple murine and human class I molecules. *J. Immunol.* 146, 425 (1991).

103. Bregenholt, S., M. Ropke, S. Skov and M. H. Claesson. Ligation of MHC class I molecules on peripheral blood T lymphocytes induces new phenotypes and functions. *J. Immunol.* 157, 993 (1996).

104. Wright, A. D. and S. K. Chapes. Staphylococcal enterotoxin A bound to MHC class I requires cross linking for the induction of TNF-α. Submitted for Publication (1999).

105. Hasko, G., L. Virag, G. Egnaczyk, A. L. Salzman and C. Szabo. The crucial role of IL-10 in the suppression of the immunological response in mice exposed to staphylococcal enterotoxin B. *Eur. J. Immunol.* 28, 1417 (1998).

106. Adams, D. and T. Hamilton. The cell biology of macrophage activation. *Ann. Rev. Immunol.* 2, 283 (1984).

107. Unanue, E. The regulation of lymphocyte functions by the macrophage. *Immunol. Rev.* 40, 227 (1978).

108. Du, X., P. Thompson, E. K. L. Chan, J. Ledesma, B. Roe, S. Clifton, S. N. Vogel and B. Beutler. Genetic and physical mapping of the lps locus: identification of the toll-4 receptor as a candidate gene in the critical region. *Blood Cells Mol. Dis.* 24, 340 (1998).

109. Hoshino, K., O. Takeuchi, T. Kawai, H. Sanjo, T. Ogawa, Y. Takeda, K. Takeda and S. Akira. Cutting Edge: Toll-Like Receptor 4 (TLR4)-Deficient Mice Are Hyporesponsive to Lipopolysaccharide: Evidence for *TLR4* as the *Lps* Gene Product. *J. Immunol.* 162, 3749 (1999).

110. Poltorak, A. *et al.* Defective LPS signaling in C3H/HeJ and C57BL/10ScCr mice: mutations in *Tlr4* gene. *Science* 282, 2085 (1998).

111. Qureshi, S. T., L. Larivi#re, G. Leveque, S. Clermont, K. J. Moore, P. Gros and D. Malo. Endotoxin-tolerant Mice Have Mutations in Toll-like Receptor 4 (Tlr4). *J. Exp. Med.* 189, 615 (1999).

112. Watson, J., M. Largen and K. McAdam. Genetic control of endotoxic responses in mice. *J. Exp. Med.* 147, 39 (1978).

113. Muzio, M., G. Natoli, S. Saccani, M. Levrero and A. Mantovani. The human toll signaling pathway: divergence of nuclear factor kappa B and JNK/SAPK activation upstream of tumor necrosis factor receptor-associated factor 6 (TRAF6). *J. Exp. Med.* 187, 2097 (1998).

114. Vogel, S. N. and D. Fertsch. Macrophages from endotoxin-hyporesponsive (*Lps^d*) C3H/HeJ mice are permissive for vesicular stomatitis virus because of reduced levels of endogenous interferon: possible mechanism for natural resistance to virus infection. *J. Virol.* 61, 812 (1987).

115. Barber, S., P.-Y. Perera and S. N. Vogel. Defective ceramide response in C3H/HeJ (*Lps*^d) macrophages. *J. Immunol.* 155, 2303 (1995).
116. Thieblemont, N. and S. D. Wright. Mice genetically hyporesponsive to lipopolysaccharide (LPS) exhibit a defect in endocytic uptake of LPS and ceramide. *J. Exp. Med.* 185, 2095 (1997).
117. Kraatz, J., L. Clair, J. L. Rodriguez and M. A. West. *In vitro* macrophage endotoxin tolerance: defective *In vitro* macrophage map kinase signal transduction after LPS treatment is not present in macrophages from C3H/HeJ endotoxin resistant mice. *Shock* 11, 58 (1999).
118. Plant, J. and A. Glynn. Genetics of resistance to infection with *Salmonella typhimurium* in mice. *J. Infect. Dis.* 133, 72 (1976).
119. Plant, J. and A. Glynn. Locating *Salmonella* resistance gene on mouse chromosome 1. *Clin. Exp. Immunol.* 37, 1 (1979).
120. Bradley, D. Genetic control of *Leishmania* populations within the host. II. Genetic control of acute susceptibility of mice to *L. donovani* infection. *Clin. Exp. Immunol.* 30, 130 (1977).
121. Vidal, S., P. Gros and E. Skamene. Natural resistance to infection with intracellular parasites: molecular genetics identifies *Nramp1* as the *Bcg/Ity/Lsh* locus. *J. Leukoc. Biol.* 58, 382 (1995).
122. Vidal, S., M. Tremblay, G. Govoni, S. Gauthier, G. Sebastiani, D. Malo, E. Skamene, M. Olivier, S. Jothy and P. Gros. The *Ity/Lsh/Bcg* locus: natural resistance to infection with intracellular parasites is abrogated by disruption of the *Nramp1* gene. *J. Exp. Med.* 182, 655 (1995).
123. Gruenheid, S., M. Cellier, S. Vidal and P. Gros. Identification and characterization of a second mouse *Nramp* gene. *Genomics* 25, 514 (1995).
124. Vidal, S. M., D. Malo, K. Vogan, E. Skamene and P. Gros. Natural resistance to infection with intracellular parasites: isolation of a candidate for *Bcg*. *Cell* 73, 469 (1993).
125. Gruenheid, S., E. Pinner, M. Desjardins and P. Gros. Natural resistance to infection with intracellular pathogens: the *Nramp1* protein is recruited to the membrane of the phagosome. *J. Exp. Med.* 185, 717 (1997).
126. Hackam, D. J., O. D. Rotstein, W.-J. Zhang, S. Gruenheid, P. Gros and S. Grinstein. Host resistance to intracellular infection: Mutation of natural resistance-associated macrophage protein 1 (Nramp 1) impairs phagosomal acidification. *J. Exp. Med.* 188, 351 (1998).
127. Blackwell, J., T. Roach, S. Atkinson, J. Ajioka, C. Barton and M. A. Shaw. Genetic regulation of macrophage priming activation: The *Lsh* gene story. *Immunol. Lett.* 30, 241 (1991).
128. Blackwell, J. M. and S. Searle. Genetic regulation of macrophage activation: understanding the function of Nramp1 (=Ity/Lsh/Bcg). *Immunol. Lett.* 65, 73 (1999).
129. Kuhn, D. E., B. D. Baker, W. P. Lafuse and B. S. Zwilling. Differential Iron Transport into phagosomes isolated from RAW264.7 macrophage cell lines transfected with Nramp1^{Gly169} or Nramp1^{Asp169}. *J. Leukoc. Biol.* 66, 113 (1999).
130. Bjorkman, P., M. Saper, B. Samraoui, W. Bennett, J. Strominger and D. Wiley. Structure of the human class I histocompatibility antigen, HLA-A2. *Nature* 329, 506 (1987).
131. Brown, J., T. Jardetzky, J. Gorga, L. Stern, R. Urban, J. Strominger and D. Wiley. Three-dimensional structure of the human class II histocompatibility antigen HLA-DR1. *Nature* 364, 33 (1993).
132. Fremont, D. H., W. A. Hendrickson, P. Marrack and J. Kappler. Structures of an MHC Class II molecule with covalently bound single peptides. *Science* 272, 1001 (1996).

133. Fremont, D. H., M. Matsumura, E. A. Stura, P. A. Peterson and I. A. Wilson. Crystal structures of two viral peptides in complex with murine MHC class I H-2K^b. *Science* 257, 919 (1992).

134. Matsumura, M., D. H. Fremont, P. A. Peterson and I. A. Wilson. Emerging principles for the recognition of peptide antigens by MHC class I molecules. *Science* 257, 927 (1992).

135. Wright, A. D. and S. K. Chapes. LPS sensitivity in recombinant mice lacking functional alleles at MHC II, *Lps*, and *Nramp1* Genes. Submitted for Publication (1999).

136. Wright, A. D. and S. K. Chapes. Macrophages defective for *Nramp1*, *Lps* and MHC II suppress IFN-γ production. Submitted for Publication (1999).

6

Toxin Production

JEREMY M. YARWOOD and PATRICK M. SCHLIEVERT

1. INTRODUCTION

Staphylococci have developed a highly regulated system of toxin production that researchers are only beginning to understand. These toxin control systems respond to a wide range of environmental conditions, from catabolite and oxygen concentrations to bacterial cell density. Understanding the mechanisms of toxin regulation and production and how these systems might be manipulated to prevent toxin production will greatly enhance our ability to control staphylococcal infections. Furthermore, elucidating environmental conditions that promote toxin production by staphylococci may explain why specific toxins are associated with certain disease conditions and why not all patients that carry toxin-producing strains experience staphylococcal diseases.

This chapter will review the available data concerning the production of the exotoxins by *Staphylococcus aureus*. These toxins include toxic shock syndrome toxin-1 (TSST-1), staphylococcal enterotoxins A through D (SEA, SEB, SEC, SED), exfoliative toxins A and B (ETA, ETB), α-, β-, δ-, and γ-hemolysins, and Panton-Valentine leukocidin (PVL). Although additional enterotoxins have been identified (SEE, SEG, SEH, SEI, SEJ), relatively little is known regarding their regulation, and existing data indicate that the number of clinical isolates producing these toxins and associated with serious infection is relatively small. Very few coagulase-negative staphylococci have been demonstrated to produce enterotoxins. In addition, no significant differences between the regulation of toxin production in coagulase-negative staphylococci and *S. aureus* have been found. For these reasons, this chapter will address toxin production primarily by *S. aureus*.

JEREMY M. YARWOOD and PATRICK M. SCHLIEVERT • Department of Microbiology, University of Minnesota Medical School, Minneapolis, MN 55455.

Staphylococcus aureus *Infection and Disease*, edited by Allen L. Honeyman *et al.* Kluwer Academic/Plenum Publishers, New York, 2001.

2. TOXIN PRODUCTION PROFILES AND DISEASE ASSOCIATION

For reasons that are not entirely clear, certain staphylococcal toxins are rarely produced together by the same clinical isolate, while other toxins are consistently produced together. TSST-1 and SEB, for instance, are rarely, if ever, produced by the same toxic shock syndrome (TSS) isolates, an observation also true for SEB and SEC. TSST-1 and SEA, however, are often produced together, as are TSST-1 and SEC. Recent examination of 12 *S. aureus* clinical isolates (nine from cases of TSS and 3 from staphylococcal scarlet fever patients) that had previously tested negative for TSST-1, SEA-SEE, and SEH, found that all were positive for both SEG and SEI, suggesting that these toxins are genetically linked and occasionally cause serious disease.[1] Complete analysis of the genetic elements carrying these toxins will likely elucidate the nature of toxin associations or exclusions. Current hypotheses include exclusion factors encoded by the mobile genetic elements carrying the genes or exclusive insertion sites for the genetic elements.

The production of toxins can vary significantly with staphylococcal genotype. In a survey of 4,088 *S. aureus* clinical isolates obtained from a university clinic and community hospitals in Frankfurt, Germany, 5% were found to be methicillin resistant *S. aureus* (MRSA).[2] The MRSA could be grouped by macrorestriction analysis into 26 different genotypes which strongly correlated with the toxin production profiles of the isolates. One genotype, containing 60 isolates, produced none of the enterotoxins (SEA-D) nor TSST-1, while members of other genotypic groups consistently produced one or two particular toxins.

Isolates from patients with particular staphylococcal diseases often show a skewed toxin production profile compared to isolates from patients with a different staphylococcal disease. Almost all isolates from patients with menstrual TSS produce TSST-1, for example, while only 50 to 60% of isolates from nonmenstrual cases of TSS are TSST-1 positive. Nearly all of the remaining isolates from nonmenstrual TSS cases produce SEB and SEC. SEA can be associated with septicemia and food poisoning, and is also associated with approximately 75% of menstrual TSS isolates and 40% of non-menstrual isolates. Strains isolated from various body sites may also exhibit skewed toxin production profiles. *S. aureus* isolates from blood cultures, for instance, were found to produce SED in significantly larger amounts and at higher frequencies than did isolates from other body sites.[3] Part of the reason for associations between toxins and disease may lie in the environmental conditions encountered by staphylococci in various body sites. Conditions not conducive to toxin production may prevent certain strains from colonizing particular body sites. Toxin production profiles do not necessarily vary among patients groups, however. Among 300 *S. aureus* strains isolated from wound swabs of patients in treatment centers near Manchester, England, 50 (17%) produced TSST-1, with no significant difference in toxin production between isolates from hospital inpatients, outpatients and burn units.[4]

There exists conflicting opinion on whether or not toxin production profiles vary significantly between methicillin-resistant *S. aureus* (MRSA) and methicillin-sensitive *S. aureus* (MSSA). Schmitz *et al.*[5] examined 181 MRSA and 100 MSSA isolates from different patients and stated that they were unable to find a statistically significant difference in the abilities of the MRSA and MSSA isolates to produce toxin. Overall, 51% of the MRSA and 40% of the MSSA produced enterotoxin or TSST-1. Their data do show, however, a tendency for MRSA to produce SEA at higher frequencies than the MSSA (24% vs. 14%, respectively), while MSSA produced SEC at significantly higher frequencies than did the MRSA (20% vs. 0.6%, respectively). A comparison of the findings by Wichelhaus *et al.*[2] and Lehn *et al.*[3] also reveals differences between toxin production by MRSA and MSSA. Wichelhaus *et al.* demonstrated that, of 26 MRSA genotypes, 23% produced enterotoxin A, 23% enterotoxin B, and 8% toxic shock syndrome toxin 1 (TSST-1). None were found to produce enterotoxin C or D. In contrast, Lehn *et al.* found that among 183 clinical isolates (not necessarily MRSA), 20.2% of the isolates produced SEA, 7.7% SEB, 5.5% SEC, 3.3% SED, and 13.7% TSST-1. Toxins most often found together were TSST-1 with SEA, and SEA with SED. Overall, 40% produced one or more toxins, similar to the findings of Wichelhaus *et al.* (38% producing one or more toxins). In contrast to these studies, it is our experience that nearly all MRSA isolates associated with nonmenstrual TSS make SEB or SEC and not TSST-1 or SEA. Therefore, while toxin production profiles do seem to vary with the susceptibility of *S. aureus* to methicillin, conclusions regarding how these profiles vary must take into account both the geographical origin and disease association of the isolates.

Some association of hemolysin production profiles with specific disease conditions may also be found. Of 15 *S. aureus* isolates from patients with TSS, all (15/15) produced α-hemolysin, 10 of 15 produced γ-hemolysin, while none produced δ-hemolysin.[6] A similar hemolysin production profile was found in 10 non-TSS associated isolates, except that while only 2 of the 15 TSS isolates produced α-hemolysin, 9 of the 10 non-TSS isolates produced this toxin. Notably, all of the TSS isolates had the α-hemolysin gene (*hla*), despite the fact that only 2 produced the toxin *in vitro*. This agrees with the results of Christennson and Hedstrom,[7] who found that strains producing TSST-1 rarely produce α-hemolysin, and α-hemolysin production by *S. aureus* septicemia strains is less frequent. In a survey of 139 clinical *S. aureus* isolates for Panton-Valentine leukocidin (PVL), 8 (5.8%) were found that produced the toxin.[8] All 8 isolates were from injured superficial soft tissues and were not associated with severe infection.

Production of identical toxins may also vary significantly from strain to strain. A comparison of TSST-1 production by several TSS isolates revealed that one produced 15–20 μg TSST-1/ml, whereas the remainder made only 3 μg/ml.[10] Furthermore, ovine isolates positive for TSST-O (a variant of TSST-1) may make less than 0.3 μg/ml. In a study of *seb* cloned from 3 wild-type strains, each with identical upstream promoter regions, all three produced equal amounts of *seb* mRNA and extracellular SEB when cloned into the same strain (reviewed by Betley *et al.*[9]). In their parental strains, however, these *seb* genes produced significantly different amounts of SEB, indicating that host factors present in the parental strains are responsible for variation in SEB production among the isolates. Concentrations of RNAIII, the effector molecule of the accessory gene regulator (*agr*) locus, correlated with the levels of *seb* mRNA, suggesting that one of the host factors responsible for the variation in toxin production might be the *agr* regulatory system. Variation in α-hemolysin production among *S. aureus* strains can also be explained by variation in the level of RNAIII transcript concentrations between strains.[11] Other host factors besides *agr* likely play a role in variation in toxin production, however. The variation in *sea* mRNA levels and SEA production between two *S. aureus* strains could be partially attributed to the *sea*-containing phages. When the *sea*-containing phage from each strain was used to lysogenize an *sea⁻* strain, the lysogen with the phage from the first parental strain produced 2- to 4-fold less SEA than the lysogen with the phage from the second parental strain.[9]

3. REGULATION AND CONTROL OF TOXIN PRODUCTION

The global regulators of virulence factors, including the accessory gene regulator (*agr*) and the staphylococcal accessory regulator (*sar*), discussed more thoroughly in the chapter entitled "Global regulators", play key roles in the regulation of toxin production[9,12] (Figure 1). Several studies have demonstrated that increased RNAIII, the effector RNA molecule encoded by the *agr* locus, leads to increased levels of toxins under *agr* regulation. Indeed, *agr⁻* strains produce significantly less toxin than do their *agr⁺* counterparts. Furthermore, levels of RNAIII are markedly decreased in *sar* mutants, and production of toxins is impaired. *Agr/sar* double mutants produce even less toxin than either the *agr* or *sar* single mutants. Available evidence suggests that SarA, the protein encoded by *sar* operon,

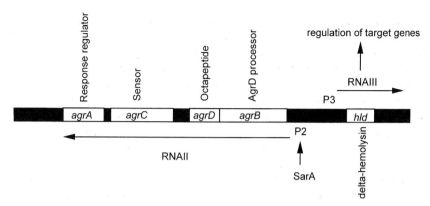

FIGURE 1. The *agr* locus from *Staphylococcus aureus.* P2 and P3 are the promoters for the RNAII and RNAIII transcripts, respectively, which are divergently transcribed. The proposed functions for *agr*A-D and *hld* are indicated. Figure adapted from Projan and Novick.[12]

interacts directly with the *agr* locus by binding to the *agr*-P2 promoter, thus regulating transcription of RNAIII. As will become evident in this review, however, additional systems that control toxin production remain uncharacterized. In particular, those systems that respond to environmental conditions, such as oxygen concentrations or the presence of catabolites, may operate independently of the *agr* and *sar* systems and likely mediate a complex network of regulatory signals.

Translational vs. Transcriptional Control

The majority of studies that have examined regulation of toxin production have found that variance in toxin mRNA correlates directly with extracellular toxin levels, indicating that regulation of toxin production occurs primarily at the level of transcription. Regassa *et al.,*[13] for instance, showed that the dramatic increase of SEC following postexponential growth of *S. aureus* FRI1230 correlated with a peak in the level of *sec* mRNA. The addition of glucose to the culture not only reduced the amount of extracellular SEC, but also the amount of *sec* mRNA. This suggests that catabolite repression of toxin synthesis, as with other environmental conditions, occurs at the transcriptional level. The *agr* effect itself is likely at the level of steady-state mRNA.[14] Transcriptional regulation of *seb, sec, sed, tst, eta,* and *hla* by *agr* likely occurs via the action of the RNAIII molecule encoded by the *agr* locus that is thought to bind to the promoter region of these toxin gene operons.[12,15] Thus, variation in toxin gene transcription (and toxin production) often reflects changes in the level of RNAIII transcript. Induction of RNAIII does not necessarily result in immediate production of toxin mRNA, however. Vandenesch et al.[16] showed that a "temporal factor", in addition to RNAIII, was required for expression of hla after entry into postexponential growth.

While mRNA levels may strongly correlate with extracellular toxin concentrations, strain-specific translational or protein export controls may affect the amount of toxin exported by the cell relative to the amount of toxin mRNA present. Regassa et al.[13] observed a 16-fold difference in extracellular SEC concentrations between two SEC producing strains, while only a two- to three-fold difference in steady-state sec mRNA under the same growth conditions. One S. aureus isolate with high RNAIII levels was shown to produce high levels of α-hemolysin, even though it had low levels of hla mRNA. This observation may be explained by the fact that this strain lacked extracellular proteases, which may act on α-hemolysin as well as other proteins.[11]

Temporal Regulation

As illustrated in Figure 2 and reviewed by Projan and Novick,[12] numerous studies of virulence factor production by S. aureus in batch cultures have shown that most exoproteins produced by staphylococci, including exotoxins, are produced only in the postexponential phase of bacterial growth. Cell-wall associated virulence factors, such as protein A, are instead produced during logarithmic growth. Exceptions to the postexponential "rule" include coagulase, which is produced during logarithmic growth, and SEA, which is produced constitutively. The agr regulatory system appears to play an essential role in this temporal regulation of toxin production. SEA, which is produced throughout growth, is not under agr control, while TSST-1, SEB, SEC, SED, ETA, ETB and the hemolysins, which are under agr control, are produced postexponentially. Vandenesch et al.[16] showed that induction of RNAIII expression, via an inducible β-lactamase control system, inhibited spa transcription immediately and, together with a temporal factor, induced expression of hla after the cells entered postexponential growth. In theory, production of exotoxins during postexponential growth may facilitate the spread of a S. aureus infection when large bacterial cell populations have exhausted nutrient supplies in local infection sites.

Environmental Conditions

The ability of staphylococci to sense and respond to environmental conditions facilitates their infection of conducive sites in the human patient, as well as their growth in food products. While toxin producing

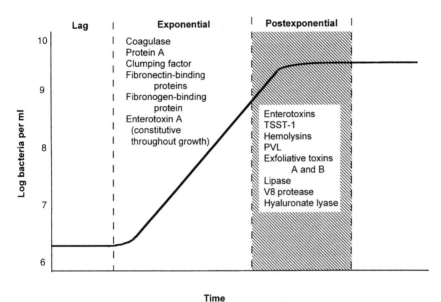

FIGURE 2. Effect of growth phase on virulence factor production by staphylococci in an idealized flask culture. In general, the synthesis of surface proteins occurs during exponential growth, while production of exotoxins takes place during the postexponential phase. Abbreviations: TSST-1, toxic shock syndrome toxin-1; PVL, Panton-Valentine leukocidin.

strains of *S. aureus* may colonize a non-menstruating female patient with no clinical symptoms, the neutral pH and elevated protein, carbon dioxide and oxygen levels associated with the use of certain tampons during menstruation stimulates the production of TSST-1 by *S. aureus*, causing TSS. Manipulating these responses to environmental conditions to control staphylococcal toxin production and infection has the potential to be a very effective therapeutic approach. Environmental conditions also greatly affect the ability of staphylococci to produce toxins while colonizing foods. One *S. aureus* strain, for example, produces significantly more SEB than SEA in batch culture. Yet in pasta dough and Manchego-type cheese, SEB production by the same strain is undetectable while SEA is made in significant amounts (reviewed by Betley *et al.*[9]). This example also highlights the challenge of attempting to replicate natural environments or host conditions in the laboratory when evaluating toxin production by staphylococci.

The sensing mechanisms employed by *S. aureus* in responding to environmental conditions are generally unknown. One area of great interest is the two-component systems ubiquitous throughout the prokaryotic world (Figure 3). These systems enable the organism to sense and respond to changes in environmental conditions, even when the stimuli do not penetrate the cytoplasm. Two-component systems consist of a transmembrane sensor (also known as a histidine kinase) and a cytoplasmic response regulator. The sensor may bind to a specific ligand or alter its conformation in the presence of specific chemical species. This signal event results in autophosphorylation of a conserved histidine residue on the cytoplasmic side of the sensor. The phosphate group is then transferred to an asparagine residue on the response regulator, which in turn stimulates or represses target genes at the transcriptional level. Since environmental conditions have been repeatedly shown to affect toxin production,[17] these two-component systems may play a key role in staphylococcal virulence. AgrA and AgrC, discussed more thoroughly in the chapter "Global regulators", provide an example of a sensor and response regulator pair, respectively (Figure 1). The *agrD* gene encodes a protein cleaved to make an octapeptide that is exported outside of the cell and likely functions as the ligand for AgrC, which in turn phosphorylates AgrA. AgrA likely binds within the *agr* promoter region, increasing RNAIII transcription and, thus, toxin gene transcription. This resembles a quorum-sensing mechanism in which toxin

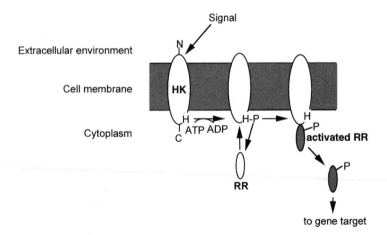

FIGURE 3. Two-component regulatory systems. In response to a stimulus at the N-terminal domain (N), the histidine kinase (HK) autophosphorylates at the histidine residue. The response regulator (RR) associates with the C-terminus (C) of the histidine kinase, and the phosphoryl group (P) is transferred to the response regulator. The activated response regulator disassociates from the histidine kinase and affects gene transcription of its target.

production is not initiated until a sufficient cell density has achieved, and would explain why toxin production occurs only after entry into the post-exponential growth phase. A possible advantage of this system is that *S. aureus* produces toxins only when a sufficient number of bacteria are present to have a sufficient effect on the host immune response, perhaps by preventing migration of polymorphonuclear (PMN) cells into the area of infection.[18] Alternatively, this system may simply signal *S. aureus* that cell populations are exhausting local nutrient sources and toxin synthesis is initiated to assist in the spread of the infection.

Several studies point to a link between alterations in DNA topology induced by signals such as osmolarity, anaerobiosis and the presence of certain catabolites, and expression of virulence genes by pathogenic bacteria (reviewed by Dorman[19]). Indeed, the suppression of *eta* in *S. aureus* by the presence of osmolytes is relieved when supercoiling is inhibited using a DNA gyrase inhibitor.[20] The osmolyte suppression of *tst*, however, occurs independently of DNA supercoiling.[21]

Alternative sigma factor σ^B has been characterized in response to environmental stress and starvation-survival, and a role for σ^B in the regulation of virulence determinant production in response to environmental conditions has been proposed.[22] Deora and Misra[23] showed that a purified σ^B protein interacts with core RNA polymerase to bind to the *sarC* promoter. Kullik and Fuchs[24] found that lipase production was significantly increased in a *sigB* deletion mutant as compared to the parent strain. The deletion mutant was also transiently more resistant to hydrogen peroxide activity, suggesting that σ^B may be a negative regulator of both lipase and at least one of the staphylococcal catalases. Examination of a mutant *S. aureus* strain with an insertionally inactivated *sigB*, however, failed to find a major role for σ^B in the production of SarA, the transcription of *hla* and *spa*, the production of lipase, DNase, protease and α- and β-hemolysins, or pathogenicity in a mouse subcutaneous abscess model.[22] Chan *et al.* did find, however, that in a *sar* mutant *sigB* transcription was reduced during the stationary phase of growth. This suggests a possible role for SarA in the *S. aureus* stress response. Given the limited amount of research in this area, a role for σ^B in enterotoxin gene transcription under appropriate environmental conditions cannot be ruled out. A role for SarA in environmental signal transduction, including the response to aeration stimuli, has been suggested;[25] the evidence remains inconclusive, however.

Catabolite Repression

Numerous labs have found that sufficient concentrations of catabolites such as glucose, galactose, sucrose, glycerol and maltose, inhibit production of toxins, including TSST-1, SEA, SEB and SEC, hemolysins and lipase (reviewed by Betley et al.[9]). Agr contributes to the catabolite repression effect under conditions in which pH is not controlled. In these cultures, dramatic decreases in RNAII, the gene transcript encoding AgrA-D, and RNAIII levels are observed as pH drops, resulting in significant reduction of hla and sec expression. This suppression effect is not only due to the pH drop that normally accompanies glucose metabolism, however. When pH is controlled, the concentrations of RNAIII are unaffected, yet hla and sec expression are significantly reduced, though not to the extent seen in strains with active agr systems. Furthermore, glucose-mediated suppression of sec expression is still observed in strains with an insertionally inactivated agr. As with other environmental condition-mediated responses, this suggests an as yet uncharacterized regulatory system responsible for catabolite suppression. The addition of glucose to the growth medium results in not only decreased extracellular SEC, but also decreased amounts of steady-state sec mRNA, suggesting that glucose repression of toxin synthesis occurs at the transcriptional level.[13] The suppression effect is not due to increased osmotic pressure, as the addition of NaCl does not decrease the extracellular SEC concentrations. It has been shown that an intact phosphoenolpyruvate phosphotransferase system is necessary to demonstrate glucose repression of toxin production in S. aureus, but the mechanism of repression remains unknown.[26]

Chan and Foster[21] examined the repression of hla, tst and spa expression by sucrose and confirmed that the suppression did not necessarily involve the agr regulatory system. The presence of sucrose did, however, reduce production of SarA. This suggests that sucrose regulation of toxin gene expression is mediated via additional mechanisms than for osmolyte regulation, which does not affect SarA production.

Osmolyte Regulation

S. aureus is a remarkably osmotolerant organism, an attribute that likely facilitates its growth on skin and in a number of foods and subsequent causation of staphylococcal food poisoning. Numerous labs have examined osmolyte repression of staphylococcal toxins (reviewed by Regassa and Betley[28]). Interestingly, only those toxin genes that are under agr control are also osmolyte regulated (i.e., tst, seb, sec, eta, hla, spa), yet an intact agr system is not required for osmolyte-mediated repression of toxin production. Production of SEB and SEC is much more sensitive to high osmolarity than SEA production. Variance in SEA production correlates with increased or decreased growth, while SEB and SEC production is repressed by high osmolyte concentrations even when correcting for decreased growth. Furthermore, the repression of *sec* by high-osmotic-strength (1.2 M NaCl) growth media occurs at the level of mRNA.[28] The salt repression of *sec* in a *agr⁻* derivative of the wild-type strain (FRI1230) was identical to that observed in the parent, however, indicating that repression of *sec* expression occurs independently of *agr*. The nature of the ion also appears to alter its effect on toxin production. *Hla* expression, also repressed by the presence of osmolytes, is more sensitive to potassium ions than sodium ions, and glutamate ions more than chloride ions. It also appears that osmolyte regulation of *hla*, and presumably other toxins, is not due to increased intracellular concentrations of potassium or glutamate ions.[29]

Chan and Foster[21] examined the suppression of *hla*, *tst* and *spa* expression by NaCl (1 M) using reporter gene fusions and found that the presence of NaCl in the growth medium significantly reduced the expression of both the toxins and surface protein genes. It was also confirmed that *agr* was not involved in the salt repression. In addition, SarA production was relatively unaffected by the presence of the osmolyte, suggesting that additional mechanisms are involved in the osmolyte regulation of virulence determinant production. NaCl-mediated suppression of *tst* expression was not reversed by the addition of novobiocin, an inhibitor of DNA gyrase. Unlike the expression of *eta*,[20] therefore, *tst* expression does not appear to be sensitive to the presence of NaCl via DNA-supercoiling.

Temperature

While it might be expected that optimal toxin production by pathogenic *S. aureus* would occur at normal body temperature (37°C), a number of studies have shown that this is not necessarily the case. Although significantly more toxin is made at 37°C than at 30°C or lower,[30] optimal production of α-hemolysin and TSST-1 occurs at 40–42°C.[29,31] Interestingly, one strain showed a growth-phase dependent *hla* regulation influenced by temperature.[29] At 37°C, induction of *hla* occurred in the late exponential phase of growth, while at 42°C, induction occurred as early as the mid-exponential phase. Furthermore, induction of *hla* transcription at 42°C was not coupled with higher concentrations of *agr* RNAIII, suggesting a partially *agr*-independent temperature regulation mechanism. It has been proposed that a higher ratio of active RNAIII to inactive RNAIII may be obtained following growth at 42°C versus 37°C, leading to increased translation of *hla* mRNA.[32] It is also likely that the regulation of toxin production by temperature is at least partially mediated by staphylococcal enzymes whose optimal activity occurs at temperatures likely to be encountered during colonization of food products or the human.

Minimum temperatures at which toxins are produced are primarily of concern for the food industry. A number of studies, reviewed by Schmitt et al.,[33] establish the lower temperature limit for detectable SE production at 15°C after incubation for seven days. The number of isolates producing detectable amounts of SE at temperatures less than 18°C, however, are relatively rare. It has been possible to detect enterotoxin formation at 10°C only after extended storage (2–4 months). Temperature limits vary widely from strain to strain. Examination of 77 S. aureus strains isolated from different foods revealed that the lower and upper temperature limits for detectable enterotoxin production after seven days ranged from 14 to 38°C and 35 to 44°C, respectively.[33] Lower and upper temperature limits for production of heat stable nuclease were between 6.5 and 12.5°C and 39.5 to 48.5°C, respectively.

pH

Several studies have examined the affect of pH on toxin production (reviewed by Regassa and Betley[27] and Dinges et al.[34]) and determined that optimal expression of TSST-1, SEB, SEC, SED, as well as the hemolysins, occurs within a pH range of 6.5 to 8. Todd et al.[31] showed that material removed from focal infections had a nearly neutral pH, and that optimal expression of TSST-1 occurred at pH 7.0 in batch cultures. A necessary condition for toxin production by S. aureus during TSS is the neutral pH of menstrual blood flow, vastly different from the pH 4 of the vagina when menstruation is not occurring. TSST-1 production by S. aureus is significantly inhibited in the presence of the Today contraceptive sponge, likely due to the acidic pH maintained by the sponge's citric acid-sodium citrate buffering system.[35]

Optimal expression of sec also occurs at pH 7.0.[27] Optimal expression coincides with maximum RNAIII levels at pH 7.0, while RNAIII levels are undetectable at pH 8.0 or above. Furthermore, sec expression is reduced in alkaline pH in S. aureus FRI1230, but not in its agr⁻ derivative, suggesting that the agr system mediates the effect of pH on toxin expression.

Irradiation

The effect of low-dose irradiation on growth and toxin production by S. aureus in foods has also been examined.[36] Irradiation does not appear to affect toxin production directly, but rather significantly reduces the number of viable bacteria. The reduction in cell number delays the time required for S. aureus populations to reach critical cell densities necessary to initiate toxin production (presumably mediated by S. aureus quorum-sensing mechanisms). Toxin production is initiated in both irradiated and non-irradiated food samples once *S. aureus* cell densities reach approximately 10^7 cfu/gram.

Mixed Culture

Enterotoxin production by *S. aureus* in mixed cultures is unlikely unless the staphylococci outnumber the other contaminating organisms.[37] While staphylococci can grow to sufficient numbers to produce enterotoxin in laboratory medium in the presence of equal numbers of other organisms, this is not the case in food products. As much as 3 to $4 \log_{10}$ greater inoculum sizes (vs. competing organisms) are required for staphylococci to produced detectable enterotoxin in meat media. The reason for this inhibition by competing organisms is not entirely clear and is not simply due to preventing *S. aureus* populations from reaching densities required for induction of toxin production. Even when cell densities reached 5×10^9 CFU/ml, SEA production is not observed when competing cell populations are sufficiently high.

Oxygen and Carbon Dioxide

Most of the research into oxygen regulation of toxin production has used TSST-1 as the representative toxin. Our lab proposed in the early 1980's that the introduction of oxygen into the vaginal environment by the insertion of a tampon was a critical factor in the production of TSST-1 by *S. aureus* during TSS. Since then, studies have examined the role of aerobic conditions in toxin production.[58] In general, anaerobic conditions suppress TSST-1 production, while mildly aerobic conditions enhance toxin production. Excess aeration, in the absence of carbon dioxide, suppresses toxin production. The oxygen response is greatly modified in the presence of carbon dioxide, however. Not only does the presence of carbon dioxide greatly enhance toxin production (by up to ten-fold in batch culture), but alleviates the suppression effect of excess aeration (up to 21% oxygen [v/v], or atmospheric levels).

Optimum TSST-1 production occurs *in vivo* and *in vitro* in aerobic conditions with 5–7% CO_2, pH 7.0 and high levels of protein.[31] Todd *et al.* showed that materials from infected focal lesions are consistent with these conditions, which are also associated with tampon use during menstruation. The vaginal pH rises from approximately 4 to around 7 during menstruation and menstrual blood flow provides both protein and elevated carbon dioxide levels. The vaginal environment is normally anaerobic but insertion of a tampon increases the oxygen tension in the vaginal environmental to nearly atmospheric conditions while reducing carbon dioxide levels to less than 1% [v/v].[38] While the vaginal oxygen levels remain elevated for at least 8 hours, however, carbon dioxide levels quickly recover from atmospheric to nearly normal *in vivo* levels (5–7% [v/v]) within a half hour. This implies that staphylococci colonizing the vagina will encounter elevated oxygen and carbon dioxide conditions concurrently, an optimal environment for TSST-1 production.

Other toxins, such as α-hemolysin, β-hemolysin, and γ-hemolysin have also been shown to require the presence of oxygen and are strongly enhanced in the presence of carbon dioxide (reviewed by Dinges *et al.*[34]). Furthermore, the effect of oxygen and carbon dioxide on regulation of α-toxin production occurs on a transcriptional level,[29] which is likely the case for other toxins, as well.

Ions

Early epidemiological studies pointed out a link between high-absorbency tampons and TSS.[39] Kass *et al.*[40] proposed that binding of magnesium to tampons created a magnesium-limiting growth environment for *S. aureus* and that this condition stimulated TSST-1 production. Examination by our lab, however, showed that while magnesium was necessary for growth and toxin production, increasing magnesium concentrations above those necessary for growth did not inhibit toxin production.[41] We propose that the apparent stimulation of toxin production by limiting magnesium concentrations occurs as a result of a longer lag period and delayed growth of staphylococci in these conditions.[42] When TSST-1 production on a per-cell basis is measured at equivalent stages of growth between cultures containing various magnesium concentrations, TSST-1 production is equivalent, provided enough magnesium is present to sustain growth of the organism. Interestingly, Sarafian and Morse[43] observed that magnesium had no effect on toxin production under anaerobic conditions, while it appeared to inhibit TSST-1 production at concentrations above 0.4 mM in aerobic conditions. The effect of oxygen on the response of *S. aureus* to magnesium may have contributed to the disparities in data between the different laboratories investigating the magnesium effect. Recent work by Chan and Foster[21] found that addition of $MgCl_2$ to batch cultures resulted in a two-fold decrease of *tst* expression (measured using a *tst::lacZ* fusion strain), while addition of $CaCl_2$ or $FeSO_4$ reduced β-galactosidase activity of the *tst::lacZ* fusion to 50% and 70%, respectively, of that in control flasks. In summary, while several labs have found some effect on toxin production by the presence of divalent cations, it remains to be seen whether this phenomenon is an artifact of variable growth conditions or is a truly significant, independent regulatory mechanism of toxin production.

Solid Surfaces

As mentioned earlier, epidemiological studies pointed out a link between high-absorbency tampons and TSS,[39] an association whose cause has not been conclusively determined. Studies performed in several labs showed that tampon composition of commercially available tampons has little effect on toxin production. Both the Schlievert[44] and Parsonnet[45] labs found that TSST-1 production by *S. aureus* on cotton tampons was no less than in cultures using cotton/rayon mixtures. Furthermore, the presence of the tampon itself does not enhance toxin production when compared with cultures in which no tampon was present, provided that the effect of the introduction of oxygen by the tampon is negated by shaking the cultures.[45] Tampons with a larger volume or higher absorbency do stimulate both bacterial growth and toxin production in still cultures, possibly due to the introduction of more oxygen into the culture environment by these products.

It has been our experience that *S. aureus* produces significantly more TSST-1 (ten-fold or more) on a per-cell basis when cultivated in a thin film on a layer of polyethylene mesh than in a batch culture (Yarwood, J. M., and Schlievert, P. M. J. Clin. Microbiol. Submitted). We have also observed significant production of TSST-1 by *S. aureus* when grown on occlusive wound dressings, except those that contain chitosan, on which TSST-1 production is almost completely suppressed. These observations are supported by the work of Ohlsen *et al.*[29] who found that the expression of an *hla::lacZ* fusion was slightly induced after cultivation on solid medium. This may reflect the adaptation of staphylococci to growth on a variety of tissues, including mucosal surfaces, as well as wound dressings and tampons.

Topical Agents and Antibiotics

A number of topical agents and antibiotics have been shown to affect the amount of toxin produced by *S. aureus* clinical isolates, properties that may influence the outcome of antistaphylococcal chemotherapy. The clinical severity of staphylococcal disease is usually toxin mediated, rather than a response to an overwhelming bacterial infection. Immediate inhibition of exotoxin production, therefore, is critical in controlling disease progression. Treatment of patients with antibiotics to which the staphylococci are resistant and that stimulate toxin production may negatively effect the outcome of the infection, while use of agents that inhibit toxin production may be a useful tool in controlling staphylococcal infection.

A number of β-lactam based antibiotics, as well as fluoroquinolones, have been shown to stimulate toxin production. The expression of a hla::lacZ fusion was strongly induced in the presence of β-lactam antibiotics, and, to a lesser extent, fluoroquinolones.[46] Penicillin and methicillin have also been shown to increase hemolytic activity of S. aureus by as much as 8- to 16-fold.[47] Nafcillin stimulates the hemolytic activity of both nafcillin-sensitive and nafcillin–resistant isolates.[48] Likewise, methicillin enhances Hla production by both methicillin sensitive S. aureus (MSSA) and methicillin resistant S. aureus (MRSA).[46] In addition, sterile broth filtrates of cultures grown in the presence of nafcillin are more rapidly lethal when injected intraperitoneally in mice than are filtrates of the same strain grown in the absence of nafcillin.[48] While isolates grown in the presence of nafcillin produce more α-hemolysin mRNA than do nafcillin-free cultures, agr RNAIII levels are comparable, suggesting that the effect of nafcillin on α-hemolysin production is not entirely attributable to agr.

Exposure of strains to tunicamycin (also a β-lactam antibiotic) results in up to a 100% increase in TSST-1 concentrations in growth media.[49] Dickgiesser et al. proposed that the increase was not due to increased toxin production but an uncontrolled release of TSST-1 through the damaged cell wall. It is difficult to imagine, however, that S. aureus retains enough TSST-1 intracellularly to account for a nearly two-fold increase of TSST-1 in the growth medium upon damage of the cell wall. It is instead likely that the presence of the β-lactam antibiotic affects toxin production at the level of transcription or translation. The data suggest that the induction of toxin gene expression by β-lactams may depend on specific interactions of the antibiotic agents with penicillin-binding proteins. The data also raise the possibility that use of β-lactams to combat infections of β-lactam resistant S. aureus may only enhance the virulence of the organism by stimulating toxin production.

Macrolides and aminoglycosides, on the other hand, appear to be particularly effective inhibitors of toxin production, at least in vitro. Subinhibitory (insufficient to affect bacterial growth) concentrations of clindamycin, erythromycin, lincomycin, kanamycin and tetracycline are all capable of partially or completely inhibiting TSST-1 production without significant change in bacterial count.[49] Subinhibitory concentrations of clindamycin, erythromycin and several aminoglycosides almost completely repressed the expression of a hla::lacZ fusion in S. aureus.[46] (Glycopeptide antibiotics were found to have no effect on hla expression.[46]) Interestingly, clindamycin, which is thought to interfere with protein synthesis by staphylococci, fails to inhibit growth of *S. aureus* strain MN8, despite completely suppressing TSST-1 production.[10] This suggests that either *S. aureus* has ribosomes that are dedicated to toxin production or that clindamycin has an additional mechanism of toxin suppression besides inhibiting protein synthesis.

Because some agents effectively inhibit toxin production both during logarithmic and static growth, but are ineffective in reducing bacterial cell numbers of some strains,[10] effective antibiotic regimens may combine both a toxin inhibitor as well as a potent bacteriocidal agent. Langevelde *et al.*[50] found that the combination of a β-lactam antibiotic (flucloxacillin) and an aminoglycoside agent (gentamicin) effectively reduced bacterial cell numbers as well as inhibited toxin production.

Edwards-Jones and Foster[4] examined the effect of sub-lethal concentrations of five topical antimicrobial compounds on toxin production by 55 TSST-1 producing *S. aureus* clinical isolates. They reported that stabilized hydrogen peroxide cream and chlorhexidine gluconate/cetrimide solution increased toxin production in some strains while inhibiting toxin production in others. Povidone iodine, frequently used on burns, did not affect toxin production by most strains. Silver sulphadiazine cream, also routinely used for burn treatment, caused significantly increased toxin production in 45% of the strains, while mupirocin ointment caused a significant decrease in toxin production in 47% of the strains (the remainder of the isolates were not affected by the silver sulphadiazine cream or mupirocin ointment). The mechanism by which these agents affect toxin production can only be speculated. The sulphadiazine moiety appears to affect membrane permeability and thus may affect toxin export. Silver ions can act as intercalating agents and distort the shape of DNA, possibly affecting *tst* transcription. Mupirocin acts at the level of translation by inhibition of protein synthesis, a property which may affect TSST-1 mRNA translation in some strains.

Cerulenin, an antibiotic that stops fatty-acid synthesis, was shown to inhibit secretion of α-hemolysin by *S. aureus*.[51] At the concentrations used, cerulenin did not affect cell growth or protein synthesis, but did reduce lipid synthesis by 50%. It has been speculated that the amphipathic structure of many exotoxins and their high affinity for both cell membranes and lipid-containing structures facilitates their translocation across the plasma membrane. Cerulenin may alter the properties of the membrane, thus interfering with either the interaction of a membrane-bound docking protein with the toxin or the actual transport of the toxin across the membrane. However, the precursor form of α-hemolysin fails to accumulate in bacterial cells in the presence of cerulenin, suggesting that inhibition by cerulenin may occur at an earlier stage of toxin synthesis.

Glycerol monolaurate (GML), a common surfactant, has been shown to inhibit both growth and production of toxins by *S. aureus*, including TSST-1, ETA and hemolysin.[52] GML also inhibits hemolysin production by *S. hominis*. Concentrations of GML above 100 ug/ml in dialyzed beef heart media inhibit both growth and toxin production by *S. aureus* strains from patients with TSS or scalded skin syndrome (SSS). Concentrations of GML below those necessary to inhibit growth, however, continue to inhibit elaboration of α-hemolysin, TSST-1, SEA, and ETA. GML also inhibits TSST-1 production *in vivo*, as confirmed using a rabbit model of tampon associated TSS.[53] Although lipase is partially inhibited by GML, some lipase is made and released, eventually degrading GML in the medium. This release of lipase suggests that exoprotein secretion is not blocked by the compound. GML also does not inhibit the production of *agr* transcripts RNAII or RNAIII.[54] However, the presence of GML does appear to inhibit TSST-1 and α-hemolysin at the level of transcription. GML also blocks the induction of β-lactamase, but not its constitutive synthesis. GML likely acts, therefore, by interfering with signal transduction in a regulatory mechanism independent of *agr*. This hypothesis is consistent with the nature of GML, as its strongly hydrophobic nature makes it likely that any biological effect would be due to association of GML with the bacterial cell membrane rather than an interaction between GML and an intracellular process. Other surfactant-type agents have been investigated in regard to their effect on toxin, including Standamul, which inhibits TSST-1 production at concentrations below those necessary for growth inhibition,[55] and Pluronic L92, which appears to amplify TSST-1 production above that in untreated controls.[56] We have also observed that occlusive wound dressings containing chitosan, a polyglucosamine purified from crab shells, are highly inhibitory to TSST-1 production. Wound dressings lacking chitosan have no effect on toxin production as compared to controls with no wound dressing.

The use of subinhibitory concentrations of topical agents and antibiotics elicits some controversy. Potential disadvantages to these type of treatments include favoring the development of mutants resistant to antibiotics by exposing them to concentrations of antibiotics insufficient to destroy the organism. Also, the effect of some treatments may be difficult to predict, with some agents stimulating toxin production by some strains, while inhibiting it in others.

It has become apparent, however, that treatment with antibiotics in concentrations sufficient to destroy an infecting organism may also destroy non-pathogenic members of the normal human microflora. This allows possible recolonization of the patient with antibiotic-resistant or other deleterious microorganisms. Some consensus exists that antimicrobial chemotherapy should instead focus on preventing the actual agents of the disease (in this case, the staphylococcal toxins) while leaving the natural microflora intact. Judicious use of agents such as those discussed in this chapter, or other emerging inhibitors of toxin production, may allow the control of staphylococcal infection with minimum impact on the patient. Certain individuals who have recurring TSS despite antibiotic therapy, for example, may respond well to treatment with low levels of toxin-inhibiting antibiotics at the time of menses, thus preventing TSS even in the presence of *tst⁺ S. aureus*. The use of topical agents that have been shown to only decrease the amount of toxin production, if affecting production at all (e.g., mupirocin), appears to have only beneficial potential effects. Finally, drug combinations that both inhibit growth of and toxin production by *S. aureus* may be the most effective means of controlling staphylococcal infection.

4. TOXIN PROCESSING AND SECRETION

The mechanism by which toxins are secreted from the cell has not been closely examined in the staphylococci. Similarities between the signal sequences of the staphylococcal toxins with those in other bacteria suggest a secretion system homologous to the Sec system in *Escherichia coli* and its homolog in *Bacillus subtilis* (reviewed by White[57]). These signal peptides, located near the N-terminus of the toxins, target the toxins to translocation systems located in the membrane of the cell, perhaps in the presence of a chaperone protein. According to the current model, once attached to the membrane-bound translocase, the N-terminus of the signal peptide remains on the cytoplasmic side of the membrane, while the carboxy-terminal of the peptide "flips" into the lipid bilayer. During this "flipping" movement, the protein (in this case, the toxin) enters a channel formed by the translocase. The rest of the protein is then translocated through the channel driven by energy derived from ATP binding to the translocation proteins and subsequent hydrolysis. Once the protein has been secreted through the translocase channel, membrane associated proteases cleave the signal peptide and release the protein into the extracellular environment. The hydrophilic nature of many exoproteins likely facilitates their export across the cell membrane as well.

ACKNOWLEDGMENTS. We gratefully acknowledge John McCormick for his thoughtful review of the manuscript.

REFERENCES

1. Jarraud, S. *et al.* Involvement of enterotoxins G and I in staphylococcal toxic shock syndrome and staphylococcal scarlet fever. *J Clin Microbiol* **37**, 2446–9 (1999).
2. Wichelhaus, T. A., Schulze, J., Hunfeld, K. P., Schafer, V. and Brade, V. Clonal heterogeneity, distribution, and pathogenicity of methicillin-resistant *Staphylococcus aureus*. *Eur J Clin Microbiol Infect Dis* **16**, 893–7 (1997).
3. Lehn, N., Schaller, E., Wagner, H. and Kronke, M. Frequency of toxic shock syndrome toxin- and enterotoxin-producing clinical isolates of *Staphylococcus aureus*. *Eur J Clin Microbiol Infect Dis* **14**, 43–6 (1995).
4. Edwards-Jones, V. and Foster, H. A. The effect of topical antimicrobial agents on the production of toxic shock syndrome toxin-1. *J Med Microbiol* **41**, 408–13 (1994).
5. Schmitz, F. J. *et al.* Enterotoxin and toxic shock syndrome toxin-1 production of methicillin-resistant and methicillin-sensitive *Staphylococcus aureus* strains. *Eur J Epidemiol* **13**, 699–708 (1997).
6. Clyne, M., De Azavedo, J., Carlson, E. and Arbuthnott, J. Production of gamma-hemolysin and lack of production of alpha-hemolysin by *Staphylococcus aureus* strains associated with toxic shock syndrome. *J Clin Microbiol* **26**, 535–9 (1988).
7. Christensson, B. and Hedstrom, S. A. Biochemical and biological properties of *Staphylococcus aureus* septicemia strains in relation to clinical characteristics. *Scand J Infect Dis* **18**, 297–303 (1986).
8. Finck-Barbancon, V., Prevost, G. and Piemont, Y. Improved purification of leukocidin from *Staphylococcus aureus* and toxin distribution among hospital strains. *Res Microbiol* **142**, 75–85 (1991).
9. Betley, M. J., Borst, D. W. and Regassa, L. B. Staphylococcal enterotoxins, toxic shock syndrome toxin and streptococcal pyrogenic exotoxins: a comparative study of their molecular biology. *Chem Immunol* **55**, 1–35 (1992).
10. Schlievert, P. M. and Kelly, J. A. Clindamycin-induced suppression of toxic-shock syndrome–associated exotoxin production. *J Infect Dis* **149**, 471 (1984).
11. Li, S., Arvidson, S. and Mollby, R. Variation in the *agr*-dependent expression of alpha-toxin and protein A among clinical isolates of *Staphylococcus aureus* from patients with septicemia. *FEMS Microbiol Lett* **152**, 155–61 (1997).
12. Projan, S. J. and Novick, R. P. The molecular basis of pathogenicity. in *The Staphylococci in Human Disease* (eds. Crossley, K. B. and Archer, G. L.) 55–81 (Churchill Livingstone Inc., New York, 1997).
13. Regassa, L. B., Couch, J. L. and Betley, M. J. Steady-state staphylococcal enterotoxin type C mRNA is affected by a product of the accessory gene regulator (*agr*) and by glucose. *Infect Immun* **59**, 955–62 (1991).
14. Gaskill, M. E. and Khan, S. A. Regulation of the enterotoxin B gene in *Staphylococcus aureus*. *J Biol Chem* **263**, 6276–80 (1988).
15. Recsei, P. *et al.* Regulation of exoprotein gene expression in *Staphylococcus aureus* by *agr*. *Mol Gen Genet* **202**, 58–61 (1986).
16. Vandenesch, F., Kornblum, J. and Novick, R. P. A temporal signal, independent of *agr*, is required for *hla* but not *spa* transcription in *Staphylococcus aureus*. *J Bacteriol* **173**, 6313–20 (1991).
17. Miller, J. F., Mekalanos, J. J. and Falkow, S. Coordinate regulation and sensory transduction in the control of bacterial virulence. *Science* **243**, 916–22 (1989).
18. Fast, D. J., Schlievert, P. M. and Nelson, R. D. Nonpurulent response to toxic shock syndrome toxin 1-producing *Staphylococcus aureus*. Relationship to toxin-stimulated production of tumor necrosis factor. *J Immunol* **140**, 949–53 (1988).

19. Dorman, C. J. DNA supercoiling and environmental regulation of gene expression in pathogenic bacteria. *Infect Immun* **59**, 745–9 (1991).

20. Sheehan, B. J., Foster, T. J., Dorman, C. J., Park, S. and Stewart, G. S. Osmotic and growth-phase dependent regulation of the *eta* gene of *Staphylococcus aureus*: a role for DNA supercoiling. *Mol Gen Genet* **232**, 49–57 (1992).

21. Chan, P. F. and Foster, S. J. The role of environmental factors in the regulation of virulence-determinant expression in *Staphylococcus aureus* 8325–4. *Microbiology* **144**, 2469–79 (1998).

22. Chan, P. F., Foster, S. J., Ingham, E. and Clements, M. O. The *Staphylococcus aureus* alternative sigma factor sigmaB controls the environmental stress response but not starvation survival or pathogenicity in a mouse abscess model. *J Bacteriol* **180**, 6082–9 (1998).

23. Deora, R., Tseng, T. and Misra, T. K. Alternative transcription factor sigmaB of *Staphylococcus aureus*: characterization and role in transcription of the global regulatory locus *sar*. *J Bacteriol* **179**, 6355–9 (1997).

24. Kullik, I., Giachino, P. and Fuchs, T. Deletion of the alternative sigma factor sigmaB in *Staphylococcus aureus* reveals its function as a global regulator of virulence genes. *J Bacteriol* **180**, 4814–20 (1998).

25. Chan, P. F. and Foster, S. J. Role of SarA in virulence determinant production and environmental signal transduction in *Staphylococcus aureus*. *J Bacteriol* **180**, 6232–41 (1998).

26. Smith, J. L., Bencivengo, M. M., Buchanan, R. L. and Kunsch, C. A. Enterotoxin A production in *Staphylococcus aureus*: inhibition by glucose. *Arch Microbiol* **144**, 131–6 (1986).

27. Regassa, L. B. and Betley, M. J. Alkaline pH decreases expression of the accessory gene regulator (*agr*) in *Staphylococcus aureus*. *J Bacteriol* **174**, 5095–100 (1992).

28. Regassa, L. B. and Betley, M. J. High sodium chloride concentrations inhibit staphylococcal enterotoxin C gene (*sec*) expression at the level of sec mRNA. *Infect Immun* **61**, 1581–5 (1993).

29. Ohlsen, K., Koller, K. P. and Hacker, J. Analysis of expression of the alpha-toxin gene (*hla*) of *Staphylococcus aureus* by using a chromosomally encoded *hla::lacZ* gene fusion. *Infect Immun* **65**, 3606–14 (1997).

30. Schlievert, P. M. and Blomster, D. A. Production of staphylococcal pyrogenic exotoxin type C: influence of physical and chemical factors. *J Infect Dis* **147**, 236–42 (1983).

31. Todd, J. K., Todd, B. H., Franco-Buff, A., Smith, C. M. and Lawellin, D. W. Influence of focal growth conditions on the pathogenesis of toxic shock syndrome. *J Infect Dis* **155**, 673–81 (1987).

32. Morfeldt, E., Taylor, D., von Gabain, A. and Arvidson, S. Activation of alpha-toxin translation in *Staphylococcus aureus* by the trans-encoded antisense RNA, RNAIII. *EMBO J* **14**, 4569–77 (1995).

33. Schmitt, M., Schuler-Schmid, U. and Schmidt-Lorenz, W. Temperature limits of growth, TNase and enterotoxin production of *Staphylococcus aureus* strains isolated from foods. *Int J Food Microbiol* **11**, 1–19 (1990).

34. Dinges, M. M., Orwin, P. M. and Schlievert, P. M. Exotoxins of *Staphylococcus aureus*. *Clin Microbiol Rev*. Submitted. (2000).

35. Remington, K. M., Buller, R. S. and Kelly, J. R. Effect of the Today contraceptive sponge on growth and toxic shock syndrome toxin-1 production by *Staphylococcus aureus*. *Obstet Gynecol* **69**, 563–9 (1987).

36. Grant, I. R., Nixon, C. R. and Patterson, M. F. Effect of low-dose irradiation on growth of and toxin production by *Staphylococcus aureus* and *Bacillus cereus* in roast beef and gravy. *Int J Food Microbiol* **18**, 25–36 (1993).

37. Noleto, A. L., Malburg Junior, L. M. and Bergdoll, M. S. Production of staphylococcal enterotoxin in mixed cultures. *Appl Environ Microbiol* **53**, 2271–4 (1987).

38. Wagner, G., Bohr, L., Wagner, P. and Petersen, L. N. Tampon-induced changes in vaginal oxygen and carbon dioxide tensions. *Am J Obstet Gynecol* **148**, 147–50 (1984).

39. Berkley, S. F., Hightower, A. W., Broome, C. V. and Reingold, A. L. The relationship of tampon characteristics to menstrual toxic shock syndrome. *Jama* **258**, 917–20 (1987).

40. Kass, E. H., Kendrick, M. I., Tsai, Y. C. and Parsonnet, J. Interaction of magnesium ion, oxygen tension, and temperature in the production of toxic-shock-syndrome toxin-1 by *Staphylococcus aureus*. *J Infect Dis* **155**, 812–5 (1987).

41. Schlievert, P. M. Effect of magnesium on production of toxic-shock-syndrome toxin-1 by *Staphylococcus aureus*. *J Infect Dis* **152**, 618–20 (1985).

42. Kass, E. H., Schlievert, P. M., Parsonnet, J. and Mills, J. T. Effect of magnesium on production of toxic-shock-syndrome toxin-1: a collaborative study. *J Infect Dis* **158**, 44–51 (1988).

43. Sarafian, S. K. and Morse, S. A. Environmental factors affecting toxic shock syndrome toxin-1 (TSST-1) synthesis. *J Med Microbiol* **24**, 75–81 (1987).

44. Schlievert, P. M. Comparison of cotton and cotton/rayon tampons for effect on production of toxic shock syndrome toxin. *J Infect Dis* **172**, 1112–4 (1995).

45. Parsonnet, J., Modern, P. A. and Giacobbe, K. D. Effect of tampon composition on production of toxic shock syndrome toxin-1 by *Staphylococcus aureus* in vitro. *J Infect Dis* **173**, 98–103 (1996).

46. Ohlsen, K. *et al.* Effects of subinhibitory concentrations of antibiotics on alpha-toxin (*hla*) gene expression of methicillin-sensitive and methicillin-resistant *Staphylococcus aureus* isolates. *Antimicrob Agents Chemother* **42**, 2817–23 (1998).

47. Hallander, H. O., Laurell, G. and Lofstrom, G. Stimulation of staphylococcal haemolysin production by low concentrations of penicillin. *Acta Pathol Microbiol Scand* **68**, 142–8 (1966).

48. Kernodle, D. S. *et al.* Growth of *Staphylococcus aureus* with nafcillin in vitro induces alpha-toxin production and increases the lethal activity of sterile broth filtrates in a murine model. *J Infect Dis* **172**, 410–9 (1995).

49. Dickgiesser, N. and Wallach, U. Toxic shock syndrome toxin-1 (TSST-1): influence of its production by subinhibitory antibiotic concentrations. *Infection* **15**, 351–3 (1987).

50. van Langevelde, P., van Dissel, J. T., Meurs, C. J., Renz, J. and Groeneveld, P. H. Combination of flucloxacillin and gentamicin inhibits toxic shock syndrome toxin 1 production by *Staphylococcus aureus* in both logarithmic and stationary phases of growth. *Antimicrob Agents Chemother* **41**, 1682–5 (1997).

51. Saleh, F. A. and Freer, J. H. Inhibition of secretion of staphylococcal alpha toxin by cerulenin. *J Med Microbiol* **18**, 205–16 (1984).

52. Schlievert, P. M., Deringer, J. R., Kim, M. H., Projan, S. J. and Novick, R. P. Effect of glycerol monolaurate on bacterial growth and toxin production. *Antimicrob Agents Chemother* **36**, 626–31 (1992).

53. Melish, M., Fukunaga, C. and Murata, S. Efficacy of glycerol monolaurate (GML) in a vaginal tampon model for TSS. in *European conference on toxic shock syndrome* (eds. Arbuthnott, J. and Furman, B.) (The Royal Society of Medicine Press, London, England, 1998).

54. Projan, S. J., Brown-Skrobot, S., Schlievert, P. M., Vandenesch, F. and Novick, R. P. Glycerol monolaurate inhibits the production of beta-lactamase, toxic shock toxin-1, and other staphylococcal exoproteins by interfering with signal transduction. *J Bacteriol* **176**, 4204–9 (1994).

55. Schlievert, P. M., Blomster, D. A. and Kelly, J. A. Toxic shock syndrome *Staphylococcus aureus*: effect of tampons on toxic shock syndrome toxin 1 production. *Obstet Gynecol* **64**, 666–71 (1984).

56. Melish, M., Fukunaga, C. and Murata, S. Effect of glycerol monolaurate (GML) and pluronic L92 (PL92) on illness and TSST-1 production in a subcutaneous depot model for TSS. in *European conference on toxic shock syndrome* (eds. Arbuthnott, J. and Furman, B.) (The Royal Society of Medicine Press, London, England, 1998).

57. White, D. *The Physiology and Biochemistry of Prokaryotes* (Oxford University Press, New York, 1995).

58. Yarwood, J. M. and Schlievert, P. M. Oxygen and carbon dioxide regulation of toxic shock syndrome toxin 1 production by Staphylococcus aureus MN8. *J Clin Microbiol* **38**(5): 1797–1803, 2000.

7

Staphylococcal Enterotoxins

SHUPING ZHANG and GEORGE C. STEWART

1. STAPHYLOCOCCAL FOOD POISONING

Staphylococcus aureus is a common cause of confirmed bacterial food borne disease in the United States.[1] After an incubation period of 30 minutes to 8 hours, consumption of staphylococcal contaminated foods results in symptoms of vomiting, diarrhea, and abdominal cramping.[2] The disease is an intoxication, not an infection, which accounts for the short incubation time prior to the onset of symptoms. The protein toxin responsible, the enterotoxin, is produced by *S. aureus* during growth on the contaminated food. A toxin dose of less than one microgram in contaminated food will elicit symptoms of food poisoning. This toxin level is reached when the bacterial population exceeds 10^5 per gram.[3] Foods often incriminated in staphylococcal food poisoning include meat (especially ham), poultry and egg products, casseroles, bakery products, and milk and dairy products. Implicated foods are often those that require considerable handling during preparation and are kept at slightly elevated temperatures after preparation. The bacteria replicate in the food and elaborate one or more enterotoxins. The halotolerance of the bacteria and the relative heat resistance of the enterotoxin contribute to prevalence of the disease. Food handlers are the usual source of the bacterial contamination and the majority of these have no obvious lesions.[2] Human strains of *S. aureus* are more likely produce enterotoxin than are animal associated strains. However, recent reports have indicated that a significant percentage of bovine and ovine mastitis isolates (28–88%) produce one or more enterotoxins.[4-7] However, substantial geographical variation has been found as isolates from certain geographical locations have not yet been found to produce enterotoxin.[6] The epidemiology of staphylococcal food poisoning is thus

SHUPING ZHANG and GEORGE C. STEWART • Department of Diagnostic Medicine / Pathobiology, College of Veterinary Medicine, Kansas State University, Manhattan, KS 66506.

Staphylococcus aureus *Infection and Disease*, edited by Allen L. Honeyman *et al.* Kluwer Academic/Plenum Publishers, New York, 2001.

very different from that caused by *Salmonella, Campylobacter,* or *Escherichia coli* where the animal or a product from the animal is the usual source of the contamination.

2. ENTEROTOXINS

The virulence factors producing the foodborne illness are enterotoxins. Staphylococcal enterotoxins are secreted proteins with molecular weights of approximately 28,000 (Table I). The enterotoxins are resistant to proteolytic digestion with trypsin, chymotrypsin, pepsin, rennin, and papain and are relatively heat resistant. In crude preparations of toxin, boiling of the sample for 30 minutes is inadequate to completely inactivate the enterotoxin.[8] The enterotoxins have the property of inducing emesis and gastroenteritis upon oral administration to primates. Recent studies have also shown that emesis can be induced in ferrets,[9] shrew mice,[10] and actinomycin D-primed mice.[11] Thus nonprimate animal models of enterotoxigenicity may be available to researchers. To date, a number of enterotoxins have been identified which are distinguished serologically. These are designated staphylococcal enterotoxin A (SEA) through J (SEJ).[12-22] Minor sequence variants of SEC have also been reported.[20] A toxin which is a sequence variant of SEG, Seg$_v$, has been identified.[23] Toxic shock syndrome

TABLE I
Size of Staphylococcal Enterotoxins

| Toxin | Number of Amino Acid Residues | | |
	Precursor form	Mature form	Mol. Wt. (Mature Form)
SEA	257	233	27,100
SEB	266	239	28,366
SEC1	266	239	27,496
SEC2	266	239	27,531
SEC3	266	239	27,563
SED	258	228	26,360
SEE	257	230	26,425
SEG	258	233	27,043
SEH	241	218	25,210
SEI	242	218	24,928
SEJ	268	244	28,460

toxin-1 (TSST-1) was once referred to as enterotoxin F.[23,24] Characterization of TSST-1 revealed that this toxin shared many biological activities with enterotoxins, but did not cause emesis. Thus there is no SEF. Additional enterotoxin-like sequences have been identified in *S. aureus*. An enterotoxin-like pseudogene, *sezA* has also been reported.[25] This determinant is transcribed but is not translated because it lacks an initiation codon. An enterotoxin homolog, labeled SE-TS in Table II, was identified within the 15.2 kb toxic shock syndrome toxin mobile pathogenicity island.[26] Nucleotide sequence analysis revealed that the *sei* determinant is flanked by open reading frames that resemble enterotoxin genes. The orf downstream of *sei* contains a frameshift mutation, and thus no functional product is produced. A gene product was not detected for the orf upstream of *sei*. Enterotoxin related sequences, but not an intact open reading frame, was also found flanking *seg*. Thus it is likely that additional staphylococcal enterotoxin determinants will be discovered as additional producing strains are examined and more complete genome sequences become available.

The known enterotoxin genes share 26–97% amino acid sequence identity (Table II). These toxins can be grouped into three families based on sequence relatedness. These are the SEA-SEH family, the SEB-SEC-SED, and the SEI-SE-tsi family (Figure 1). The sequence variants of SEC and SEG belong to the respective prototype families. Among the known enterotoxins, SEA is the serotype most commonly associated with food poisoning episodes.[2]

3. ENTEROTOXIN MODE OF ACTION

The typical symptoms associated with staphylococcal food poisoning are vomiting with or without diarrhea and abdominal cramping. In severe cases, patients may experience fever and shock. Enteritis resulting from food poisoning in humans was initially studied by Palmer.[27] Thereafter, many animals including cats, dogs, monkeys, rabbits, chinchillas, rats, and mice have been used to study the pathologic feature of staphylococcal food poisoning. Some early studies showed that injection of enterotoxins induced symptoms in cats similar to those seen in food poisoning cases and repeated daily injection of enterotoxins caused moderate to severe jejunitis in cats and kittens.[28] Severe gastroenteritis was produced in dogs by intrajejunal instillation of crude staphylococcal filtrates.[29] Vomiting, diarrhea, shock, and acute gastroenteritis marked by regional edema, hypermenia, mucosal exudation, muscular irritation, and destruction of intestinal villi

TABLE II

Percent amino acid sequence identity between precursor forms of staphylococcal enterotoxins

	SEA	SEB	SEC1	SEC2	SEC3	SED	SEE	SEG	SEGv	SEH	SEI	SEJ	SE-TSI
SEA	100	33	30	31	31	50	83	27	27	37	39	64	31
SEB		100	68	67	69	35	32	44	44	33	31	33	30
SEC1			100	97	94	31	29	41	41	27	26	30	26
SEC2				100	96	31	30	42	42	27	28	31	27
SEC3					100	32	29	42	42	26	27	30	26
SED						100	52	26	28	35	33	51	33
SEE							100	27	26	35	35	63	32
SEG								100	97	34	28	29	28
SEGv									100	34	28	30	28
SEH										100	33	35	28
SEI											100	34	67
SEJ												100	33
SE-TSI													100

Sequence comparison was performed with program BLASTP. Sequences were obtained from GenBank. SE-TSI refers to the enterotoxin gene sequence identified in the toxic shock sydrome toxin pathogenicity island (see reference 26). The SEGv sequence variant is described in reference 23.

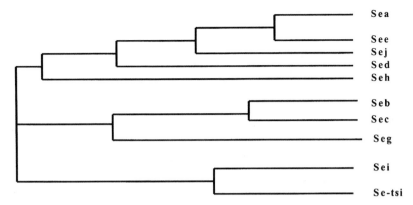

FIGURE 1. Staphylococcal Enterotoxin Families. Phylogenetic tree was built using the neighbor joining method of Saitou and Nei.[104] The SEC subtypes are included with SEC and SEGv is included with SEG.

were observed 2 to 3 hours after receiving one or two large doses of enterotoxin. Lymphoid hyperplasia was observed after repeated instillation of enterotoxin filtrates. Monkeys have been proven to be the most susceptible laboratory animals to enterotoxins.

Vomiting and diarrhea occurred 2 to 8 hours after oral administration of enterotoxins, though some animals did not develop symptoms until 16 hours after feeding of toxins.[30] Acute gastroenteritis was well developed by 2 hours, reached a maximum at 4 to 8 hours, and rapidly regressed after 12 to 72 hours. The lesions found in small intestine were characterized by epithelial damage, villus distension, and crypt lengthening. Electron microscopy revealed mitochondrial alterations in villus and crypt epithelial cells, as well as in diverse cells of the jejunal mucosa.[31] Though emetic response and the severity of tissue destruction correlated well, vomiting and intestinal lesions did not always occur at the same time. For instance, after repeated daily feeding of enterotoxins, monkeys became refractory to emesis, but intestinal lesions were still observable.[30] It was suggested that specific receptors for enterotoxins were located within the gastrointestinal tract, and the sensory stimulus reached the vomiting center *via* vagus and sympathetic nerves.[32,33] However, such receptors have not been identified. Studies with human kidney proximal tubular cells have identified a neutral glycosphingolipid as a putative receptor for enterotoxin.[34] This study may provide clues as to the nature of the receptor on intestinal epithelial cells.

4. A ROSE BY ANY OTHER NAME—PYROGENIC TOXIN SUPERANTIGENS

Naming toxins is a tricky business. They are usually assigned a name based upon their most obvious activity. The a hemolysin of *S. aureus*, the toxin responsible for the zone of complete hemolysin around a colony on a sheep blood agar plate, was renamed α toxin when it became known that its contribution to virulence was its effects on other cell types rather than the lysis of red blood cells. The enterotoxins were named because of their role in food poisoning, but their role in staphylococcal virulence is much different. The enterotoxins can induce profound immune system responses by stimulating T cells with particular $V\beta$ elements. The fraction of responding T cells can be orders of magnitude greater than that evoked by conventional antigens. Accordingly, they are termed "superantigens".[35] The enterotoxins are functionally bivalent T cell mitogens that bind simultaneously to MHC II molecule on antigen presenting cells and the variable region of the β chain ($V\beta$) of the T cell receptor (TCR).[36] Consequently, a large amount of proinflammatory cytokines, including tumor necrosis factor a (TNFα), interferon gamma (INF-γ), and interleukins-1 and 2 (IL-1 and 2) are produced and which can cause clinical symptoms that include f ever, hypotension, and shock.[37–40]

These superantigens bind to the $V\beta$ chain of the TCR regardless of the composition of the variable regions. A given type of superantigen can bind to all of the T cells bearing a particular $V\beta$ chain. For example, SEA exhibits binding specificity for murine $V\beta1$, 3, 11, and 12, while SEB shows affinity for murine $V\beta3$, 7, 8.1, 8.2, 8.3, and 11.[41,42] SEA has also been shown to bind to the MHC class I molecule and produce a cytokine response, although with a lower efficiency than the response seen with cells bearing MHC II.[43]

The pharmacological properties of the enterotoxins are thus similar to those of toxic shock syndrome toxin 1 (TSST-1) of *S. aureus*. TSST-1, SEA, SEB, SEC, and SED have been shown to fold into highly similar three dimensional structures.[44–49] In addition, the biological properties of the enterotoxins and the amino acid sequences are highly similar to those of the pyrogenic exotoxins of *Streptococcus pyogenes*.[50] These toxins, the enterotoxins, TSST-1 and the streptococcal pyrogenic exotoxins, have been grouped as the pyrogenic toxin superantigens (PTSAgs). Of the PTSAgs, only the enterotoxins are emetic. Superantigenicity and emesis have been shown to result from distinct regions of the staphylococcal enterotoxins.[51,52] Carboxymethylated SEA and SEB did not induce vomiting in monkeys, but carboxymethylated SEB was still able to stimulate T cell activation.[51,52] To further assess the correlation between emesis and T cell activation, SEA and SEB mutants have been constructed and analyzed by Betley and co-workers.[53] These mutants were divided into the following three groups: one group of the mutants failed to induce murine T cell proliferation *in vitro*, but caused emesis in monkeys; the second group of mutants were able to stimulate murine T cells, but did not induce emesis; the third group of mutants showed reduced ability to induce T cell proliferation and emesis. To identify the sequences responsible for emesis, mutant forms of SEC have been generated.[54] An SEC1 mutant with a cysteine to alanine substitution is not emetic. Based on these data, the investigators has proposed that the disulfide bond contributes to a conformation that causes emesis in primates. However, the disulfide loop is not essential for emesis. SEI has only one cysteine residue, but still retains the ability to induce vomiting in monkeys.[18]

Blood composition changes resulting from administration of enterotoxins, providing *in vivo* evidence for their role as superantigens, have been reported. Leucocytosis of a few hours duration occurred within 30 minutes after feeding of SEA, SEB, or SEC to monkeys.[55] Besides causing food poisoning, enterotoxins are also associated with menstrual and non-menstrual staphylococcal toxic shock syndrome which is characterized by rapid onset of fever, hypotension, rash, and multiple organ failure. Enterotoxin (SEA to SEE, SEG and SEI) producing strains have been found in patients with nonmenstrual TSS which is usually secondary to *S. aureus* infection.[56–59] Histopathological examination of fatal TSS cases revealed aseptic inflammatory lesions in multiple organs and changes in abdominal lymphoid tissue.[60,61] These pathological changes are observable in rabbits receiving large doses of enterotoxins.[58] Intoxication in monkeys following intragastric administration of SEB was shown to correlate with elevated plasma levels of acharidonic acid cascade metabolites.[62] Cysteinyl leukotrienes, such as leukotriene E_4, have also been implicated as mediators of SEB intoxication.[63] It has not yet been determined if these compounds play a direct role in the intoxication process or are produced indirectly, as a consequence of the intoxication.

Enterotoxins may have other action sites located within gastrointestinal tract as suggested by some early experiments. However, *in vitro* studies have produced conflicting results. Enterotoxins SEA and SEB did not damage the integrity of cultured Henle 407 human intestinal cells as measured by leakage of cytoplasmic constituents, amino acid transport, and macromolecular synthesis.[64] However, SEB was shown to have a direct effect on the barrier function of endothelial cells.[65] The damage induced by SEB was prevented using inhibitors of protein tyrosine kinases. The pathogenic effect of enterotoxins on the gastrointestinal tract could also result from production of cytokines by local immune cells, such as macrophages, mast cells, and other MHC II bearing cells lining the gut, and /or T cells located in this area. In this regard, one study has shown that SEB, through its effect to expand T cell populations (see below) gives rise to T cells which induce apoptosis in syngeneic intestinal epithelial cells.[66] The autoreactive activity of the T cells was suppressed by the addition of IL-10. The authors suggest that the bacterial toxin has the potential to abrogate self tolerance by stimulating autoreactive T cells which are cytolytic to the target cells.

5. ENTEROTOXIN ROLE IN STAPHYLOCOCCAL DISEASES

Clinical isolates of *S. aureus* frequently produce one or more enterotoxins.[67] Enterotoxin production has been associated with clinical isolates from patients suffering from toxic shock syndrome, staphylococcal scarlet fever, recalcitrant erythematous desquamating disorder, and arthritis, and in some cases enterotoxin producing strains have been shown to cause these diseases in experimental animals.[56–59,67,68] Co-production of SEA with TSST-1 has been shown to enhance TSST-1 mediated mortality in a murine model of lethal shock.[69] Immunization of mice with a recombinant SEA which was devoid of superantigenic properties was shown to provide protection against sepsis caused by an SEA-producing *S. aureus* strain.[70] These disease conditions arise, at least in part, from an inappropriate hyperexpression of cytokines as a consequence of the superantigenicity of these toxins. The enterotoxin superantigens are not only activators of T cells, but also are potent inducers of T cell tolerance. In mouse studies, enterotoxin exposure induced massive expansion of the T cells reactive to the corresponding superantigen in lymphoid tissues.[71] The elevated percentage of the superantigen-reactive T cells, however, declined rapidly to control-like levels within 2–3 days. Neither $CD4^+$ nor $CD8^+$ T cells remaining in the lymphoid tissues exhibited either proliferation or lymphokine production in response to restimulation with the same superantigen *in vitro*.[71–73] Thus anergy induction accompanied superantigen exposure. Apoptotic cell death seems to be involved in the decline of the superantigen-reactive T cells arising from priming with enterotoxin *in vivo*.[74–78] Implantation of an osmotic pump containing human recombinant IL-2 prolonged the expanded states of the polyclonally expanded Vβ3+ and Vβ11+ cells in SEA-injected mice,[79] suggesting that IL-2 deprivation may be involved in the apoptotic elimination of the expanded T cell population. SEE stimulation of murine splenic T cells *in vitro* differed from *in vivo* exposure in that memory state was induced in the resultant $CD4^+$ T cell blasts rather than the tolerence.[73] However, the anergic state was induced in the resultant $CD8^+$ T cell blasts.

Enterotoxin-induced T cell depletion is suspected to play a role in other staphylococcal diseases. Infection with enterotoxin producing staphylococci has been implicated in aggravation of atopic dermatitis through this mechanism.[80] Enterotoxin production thus appears to be an important virulence tool in the arsenal of S. aureus. These PTSAgs disrupt normal immune function and therefore may promote persistence of the bacteria in the infected host.

6. NATURE OF THE GENETIC ELEMENTS ENCODING THE ENTEROTOXINS

The best genetically characterized strain of S. aureus is 8325, a phage group III clinical strain isolated more than 40 years ago. This strain, as well as many other animal and human isolates, does not produce an enterotoxin. This provides an indication that enterotoxins are not typical chromosomal genes in this species. S. aureus can be envisioned as having a modular genome.[81] In addition to its "standard" chromosome, it can contain a variable number of mobile genetic elements that include transposons, temperate and defective bacteriophage, plasmids, pathogenicity island(s), and foreign DNA inserts of uncharacterized type. It is through acquisition of these genetic modules that a strain becomes able to produce one or more enterotoxin.

Genetic studies revealed that the sea determinant mapped to a location in the staphylococcal chromosome between the purB110 and ilv-129 markers.[82] However, not all SEA-producing strains carry the sea determinant at this site in the chromosome. The purB- ilv site corresponds to the attachment site for a temperate phage and the sea structural gene is carried on this prophage.[83] The sea-containing phage comprise a family of related, but not identical, phage as evidenced by differences in physical maps. The actual prophage integration site is within the hlb locus, encoding the sphingomyelinase known as β-toxin. The sea-containing phage are referred to as double coverting, or triple converting phage.[84] Strains acquiring this prophage lose the capacity to produce β-toxin due to insertional inactivation of hlb by the integration of the prophage. Doubling converting phage thus lose β-toxin synthesis simultaneously with acquisition of production of SEA. Triply converting phage carry sak, the gene for staphylokinase, along with sea and, therefore lysogens produce both SEA and staphylokinase while losing β-toxin production.

The sezA pseudogene is carried on a temperate phage which can be induced by exposure of the lysogens to ultraviolet light.[25] The gene encoding SEE was also identified on UV-inducible phage which share sequence homology with *sea* containing phage.[85] Because the UV-induced *see* containing phage were not able to form plaques on various *S. aureus* strains tested, it was suggested that the *see* containing phage may be defective. The *sed* and *sej* determinants are carried on a 27.6 kb penicillinase-type plasmid in *S. aureus*.[21,86] The determinants are oriented in opposite directions and the open reading frames are separated by an 895 bp intergenic sequence. Physical mapping of 21 independent *sed* encoding plasmids indicated that *sej* is always coresident.[21,86,87] Thus SED producing staphylococci also produce SEJ. The *seh* determinant as well as the *sec* family of enterotoxins (with the one exception listed below) are found in the chromosome of the respective enterotoxin-producing strains, but the nature of the genetic element on which they reside, bacteriophage, transposon, integrated plasmid, etc., has not been elucidated.[17,87,88] The *seg* and *sei* enterotoxin genes have been shown to be present together and genetically linked in strains which produce these enterotoxins.[18,59,89] Their co-inheritance would suggest that these determinants are part of a discrete mobile genetic element.

Southern hybridization analysis of the chromosomal DNA from both *seb+* and *seb–* strains demonstrated that the gene determinant for SEB resides on a discrete genetic element with a minimum size of 26.8 kb.[90] The SEB element gene contains at least 24.5 kb of DNA upstream of *seb* and 1.5 kb downstream of this enterotoxin determinant. Some enterotoxin B negative strains lack the entire *seb* element, whereas other *seb*-negative strains contain the flanking regions but not the structural gene for SEB. It has been postulated that the latter strains are a result of imprecise excision of an *seb* element.[90] What then is the nature of the element that carries *seb*? To date, no viable phage has been induced by UV-irradiation of *seb+* strains, which makes it less likely that *seb* is encoded as part of a prophage. The size of *seb* element is larger than known staphylococcal transposons. It is likely that the *seb* element is part of an integrated plasmid or, perhaps, a pathogenicity island analogous to the toxic shock syndrome toxin encoding island. There is one report of a plasmid location for the *seb* determinant.[91] A 56.2 kb plasmid, referred to as pZA10, encoding β-lactamase and heavy metal resistance was identified from an enterotoxigenic clinical isolate. The physical map of pZA10 and subsequent co-transformation analysis indicated that *seb*, *sec*, *bla*, and metallic ion resistance genes were linked and associated with a 18.1 kb *Sal* I fragment. Elimination of pZA10 resulted in a loss of SEB production. The plasmid was physically and segregationally unstable. Chromosomal integration of pZA10 was observed. These observations may provide support for the *seb* element being the remnant of an integrated plasmid. Lastly, an enterotoxin-like gene has been identified embedded in the toxic shock syndrome toxin-1 pathogenicity island.[26]

7. EXPRESSION AND REGULATION OF ENTEROTOXIN GENES

The expression of enterotoxins varies among serological types. SEA and SEJ are produced in an apparently unregulated fashion during the exponential phase of growth.[21,92,93] However, as much as an eight-fold difference in the amount of SEA produced can be attributed to the specific *sea*-harboring temperate phage present.[87] In contrast, SEB, SEC, and SED are maximally produced during the transition from exponential to stationary phase of growth.[86,92,94] In addition to differences in the kinetics of expression, the amount of toxin synthesized also varies widely. SEA, SED, SEE, and SEJ are often produced at concentrations less than 5 µg/ ml of culture supernatant, whereas SEB and SEC are produced in larger quantities, usually on the order of 100 µg/ml of culture supernatant.[95] Production of a given enterotoxin may also vary with the host background. For instance, S6, DU4916, and COL produce 375, 50, and 12 µg /ml of SEB, respectively.[96,97] Strains isolated from clinical cases produce higher amount of SEC (≥25 µg/ml) than food strains and animal strains.[20] Most of the bovine and ovine isolates produce less than 5 µg/ml of SEC. Similar information concerning SEH, SEG, and SEI expression levels are not yet available.

The postexponential growth phase stimulation of *seb, sec,* and *sed* expression is a characteristic of many staphylococcal extracellular virulence factors which are under the control of *agr* regulation. The *agr*-associated regulation of enterotoxin gene expression has been examined by Iandolo, Betley, a Khan and their coworkers.[21,86,96–99] Their experiments demonstrated that loss of *agr* signal transduction system resulted in substantial reductions of enterotoxin protein and mRNA production. The reductions in mRNA levels were 4-fold for *seb,* 5.5-fold for *sed,* and 2–3 fold for *sec.* The reduction in enterotoxin protein production was more dramatic. For example, the amount of SEC was reduced 16 to32-fold as revealed by western blot analysis.[98] The mechanism by which RNAIII regulates the expression of enterotoxin genes is currently unknown. The levels of staphylococcal enterotoxin B (SEB) produced by various naturally occurring toxogenic strains of *S. aureus* are highly variable. The *seb* determinants from a high-producer strain, S6, and from DU4916 and COL (medium-and low-level toxin-producer strains, respectively) showed that their open reading frame upstream sequences are identical.[97] The *seb* determinants from these three strains, when cloned into a strain 8325 genetic background, each were expressed to the same extent. RNAIII, the regulatory species of the *agr* system, was shown by Northern blot analysis to vary in an identical fashion as *seb* RNA levels in strains S6, DU4916, and COL. These results suggest that differences in the *agr* system are responsible for the differential enterotoxin production by many naturally occurring strains.

In addition to *agr* and *sar* systems, the expression of enterotoxin genes is also affected by glucose concentration in culture medium. Several early studies suggested that addition of glucose to culture medium resulted in decreased production of SEA, SEB, SEC and other exoproteins. Because these early experiments were carried out without a strictly controlled glucose concentration and pH, it was not known whether the glucose effect was due to a catabolite repression mechanism or is a result of the decreased pH resulting from metabolism of the glucose. Regassa *et al.* were able to demonstrate that repression of *sec* expression by glucose occurred even when the culture pH was maintained at 6.5.[98] Furthermore, the glucose effect was shown to be independent of a functional *agr* system. Smith *et al.* found that the sugar-related repression of SEA production was dependent upon an intact phosphotransferase system, even if the repressing sugar was not transported into the bacterial cell by this pathway.[100]

To understand the transcription regulation, it is essential to characterize the promoter for a target gene, identify the *cis*-regulatory sequence(s), and study the interaction between the potential regulatory species and the *cis* sequence. The promoter for *sea*, a non-*agr*-regulated enterotoxin gene, has been characterized by primer extension in conjunction with deletion mutagenesis.[101] The transcription start site (+1) of *sea* was located at 87±1 upstream to the translation start site. A region from −35 to +11 was identified to be sufficient for *sea* transcription. Within this region, two sequences (5'TAGACA3' and 5'TAATAT3', separated by 18 bp) closely resembling *E. coli* −35 and −10 promoter elements, were identified. Deletion of either sequence element resulted in diminished production of SEA. Comparison of the promoter sequences for *sea* isolated from strains FRI100 and FRI722 indicated that two mutations, $-28_{A/G}$ and $+3_{T/C}$, occurred in strain FRI722 and are responsible for the 20-fold increase in SEA expression by this strain.[102,103]

The promoters for the *agr*-regulated enterotoxin genes have not, for the most part, been well characterized. The transcription start site for *seb* was determined by S1 nuclease protection assays and localized at 42 ± 1 bases upstream of the translation start site. Sequence analysis revealed a putative −10 element (5'TATATT3'), located 8 bases upstream of +1 and a −35 element (5'TTGAAT3') separated by 18 nucleotides from the Pribnow Box sequence. Deletion mutagenesis analysis indicated that a region from

−93 to +1 was sufficient for *seb* transcription.[99] When the deletion extended to base position −59, the production of SEB was dramatically reduced which suggested that a DNA sequence located between −93 and −59 was required for *seb* transcription. There are repeat sequences present upstream of the *seb* promoter and it has been postulated that these sequences may be important for *agr* regulation. However, this hypothesis has not yet been tested experimentally.

For *sed*, S1 nuclease protection and primer extension studies mapped the transcription start site to a position 265 nucleotides upstream from the translation start site.[21,86] The presence of a −10 sequence (5′TATAAT3′) was found 5 bases upstream of +1. A poor −35 sequence (ATGAAA) was identified. To further study enterotoxin gene expression and *agr*-associated regulation, deletion and site-specific mutagenesis was carried out on the *sed* promoter.[21] A 51 bp sequence, extending from −34 to +17 contained full *sed* agr-regulated promoter activity. DNA sequences downstream of the start site of transcription (+1 to +17) were required for promoter function. The downstream sequences could be replaced by sequences from another enterotoxin gene (*seb*), but not by sequences from the staphylococcal lactose operon. When the −35 element was altered to match the consensus TTGACA sequence, promoter strength increased and the requirement for the downstream (+1 to +17) sequence was eliminated.

The organization of the enterotoxin gene promoters with regard to required elements for expression and critical *agr*-associated regulatory sequences differs between the *seb* and *sed* determinants (Figure 2). The *seb* promoter requires sequences upstream of the −35 element for expression and there is no requirement for sequences beyond the start site of transcription for promoter activity. Conversely, sequences upstream of the −35 element are not involved in *sed* promoter activity or regulation by the *agr* system. Thus the regulatory organization of these two enterotoxin

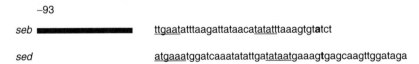

FIGURE 2. The promoter region sequences of the *seb* and *sed* enterotoxin genes. The −35 and −10 promoter elements are underlined and the nucleotide position corresponding to the start site of transcription is in bold. The *sed* sequence is the minimal promoter fragment containing full promoter activity and control sequences for regulation by the *agr* system. The *seb* promoter contains a sequence located between −93 and −58 which is required for promoter activity.[99] The sequence from −93 to +4 possess full promoter strength and is subject to *agr* control. The *seb* sequence is taken from reference 99.

```
                 192              179  247    241
            auguuacuuucauu  uucaacc
            ::.:::::::::::.:  :::::::
  atgaaatggatcaaatatattgatataatgaaagtgagcaagttggatagattgcggc
  tactttacctagtttatataactatattactttcactcgttcaacctatctaacgccg
  ::::::::                    ::: :.:::::::
    aaauggau                     aaaauuagcaagu
   124      131                 259          271
            ::::: :::::
            aaauagauuga
            436         442
```

FIGURE 3. The DNA sequence of the *sed* promoter is shown with the −35 and −10 promoter elements underlined. Aligned with the DNA sequences are sequence segments from RNAIII. The numbers refer to base positions in the RNAIII molecule. Double dots signify positions of complementary base pairs and single dots indicate G-U pairs. The alignments are meant as examples of possible alignments but do not represent all of the possible alignments.

determinants are very different. There are additionally no obvious sequence matches in the promoters of the two enterotoxin genes (other than the Pribnow box sequences) which might be candidates for the *agr* system *cis* elements. However, it may not be reasonable to expect that the enterotoxin genes would all interact with the *agr* system in the same manner. The enterotoxin genes have all been introduced into *S. aureus* on different types of genetic elements (bacteriophage, plasmid, pathogenicity island) and the degree of influence of the *agr* system on transcription of the enterotoxin genes also varies markedly. Therefore, the enterotoxin genes may have evolved regulatory sites for *agr* control in an independent fashion and there may not be one overall method for enterotoxin gene regulation by this global regulatory system. There are sequences within the RNAIII molecule which are identical or complementary to sequences within the *sed* promoter element and interactions between the promoter and this regulatory RNA species may be involved in *agr* control of SED expression (Figure 3). Whether the RNAIII regulatory molecule of the *agr* system interacts directly or indirectly with the enterotoxin gene promoters is not yet known and is the subject of current investigations in our laboratory.

REFERENCES

1. Bean, N. H., Goulding, J. S., Loa, C., and Angula, F. J., Surveillance for foodborne-disease outbreaks-United States, 1988–1992, Morb. Mortal. W. Rep. 45 (SS-5), 1 (1996).
2. Holmberg, S. D. and Blake, P. A., Staphylococcal food poisoning in the United States. New facts and old misconceptions, JAMA 251:487 (1984).

3. Food and Drug Administration, 1998, *Staphylococcus aureus*, in: Foodborne Pathogenic Microorganisms and Natural Toxins Handbook (Bad Bug Book), URL: http://vm.cfsan.fda.gov/~mow/intro.html, (1998).

4. Adesiyun, A. A., Characteristics of *Staphylococcus aureus* strains isolated from bovine mastitic milk: bacteriophage and antimicrobial agent susceptibility, and enerotoxigenicity, Zentralbl Veterinarmed [B] 42:129 (1995).

5. Kenny, K., Reiser, R. F., Bastida-Corcuera, F. D., and Norcross, N. L., Production of enterotoxins and toxic shock syndrome by bovine mammary isolates of *Staphylococcus aureus*, J. Clin. Microbiol. 31:706 (1993).

6. Lee, S. U., Quesnell, M., Fox, L. K., Yoon, J. W., Park, Y. H., Davis, W. C., Falk, D., Deobald, C. F., and Bohach, G. A., Characterization of staphylococcal bovine mastitis isolates using the polymerase chain reaction, J. Food Prot. 61:1384 (1998).

7. Orden, J. A., Cid, D., Blanco, M. E., Ruiz Santa Quiteria, J. A., Gomez-Lucia, E., and de la Fuente, R., Enterotoxin and toxic shock syndrome toxin-one production by staphylococci isolated from mastitis in sheep, APMIS 100:132 (1992).

8. Bergdoll, M. S., Enterotoxins, in: Staphylococci and Staphylococcal Infections vol. 2, C.S.F. Easmon and C. Adlum, eds, Academic Press, London (1983).

9. Wright, A., Andrews, P. L., and Titball, R. W., Induction of emetic, pyrexic, and behavioral effects of *Staphylococcus aureus* enterotoxin B in the ferret, Infect. Immun. 68:2386 (2000).10. Hu, D. L., Omoe, K., Shimura, H., Ono, K., Sugii, S., and Shinagawa, K., Emesis in the shrew mouse (*Suncus murinus*) induced by peroral and intraperitoneal administration of staphylococcal enterotoxin A, J. Food Prot. 62:1350 (1999).

11. Chen, J., Y.-J., Qiao, Y, Komisar, J. L., Baze, W. B., Hsu, I.-C., and Tseng, J., Increased susceptibility to staphylococcal enterotoxin B intoxication in mice primed with actinomycin D, Infect. Immun. 62:4626 (1994).

12. Casman, E. P., Further serological studies of staphylococcal enterotoxin, J. Bacteriol. 79:849 (1960).

13. Bergdoll, M. S., Surgalla, M. J., and Dack, G. M., Staphylococcal enterotoxin. Identification of a specific precipitating antibody with enterotoxin-neutralizing property, J. Immunol. 83:334 (1959).

14. Borja, C. R. and Bergdoll, M. S., Purification and partial characterization of enterotoxin C produced by *Staphylococcus aureus* strain 137, Biochem. 6:1467 (1967).

15. Casman, E. P., Bennett, R. W., Dorsey, A. E., and Isa, J. A., Identification of a fourth staphylococcal enterotoxin, enterotoxin D, J. Bacteriol. 94:1875 (1967).

16. Bergdoll, M. S., Borja, C. R., Robbins, R. N., and Weiss, K. F., Identification of enterotoxin E, Infect. Immun. 4:593 (1971).

17. Ren, K., Bannan, J. D., Pancholi, V., Cheung, A. L., Robins, J. C., Fishette, V. A., and Zabriskie, J. B., Charcterization and biological properties of a new staphylococcal exotoxin, J. Exp. Med. 180:1675 (1994).

18. Muson, S. H., Tremaine, M. T., Betley, M. J., and Welch, R. A., Identification and characterization of staphylococcal enterotoxin type G and I from *Staphylococcus aureus*, Infect. Immun. 66:337 (1998).

19. Bergdoll, M. S., Borja, C. R., and Avena, R. M., Identification of new enterotoxin as enterotoxin C, J. Bacteriol. 90:1481 (1965).

20. Marr, J. C., Lyon, J. D., Robberson, J. R., Lupher, M., Davis, W. C., and Bohach, G. A., Characterization of novel type C staphylococcal enterotoxins: biological and evolutionary implications, Infect. Immun. 61:4254 (1993).

21. Zhang, S., Iandolo, J. J., and Stewart, G. C., The enterotoxin D plasmid of *Staphylococcus aureus* encodes a second enterotoxin determinant (*sej*), FEMS Microbiol. Lett. 168:227 (1998).

22. Abe, J., Ito, Y., Onimaru, M., Kohsaka, T., and Takeda, T., Characterization and distribution of a new enterotoxin-related superantigen produced by *Staphylococcus aureus*, Microbiol. Immunol. 44:79 (2000).

23. Bergdoll M. S., Crass, B. A., Reiser, R. F., Robbins, R. N., and Davis, J. P., A new staphylococcal enterotoxin, enterotoxin F, associated with toxic-shock-syndrome *Staphylococcus aureus* isolates. Lancet 9:1017 (1991).

24. Bergdoll, M. S., Crass, B. A., Reiser, R. F., Robbins, R. N., Lee, A. C., Chesney, P. J., Davis, J. P., Vergeront, J. M., and Wand, P. J., An enterotoxin-like protein in *Staphylococcus aureus* strains from patients with toxic shock syndrome, Ann. Intern. Med. 96(6 Pt 2):969 (1982).

25. Soltis, M. T., Mekalanos, J. J., and Betley, M. J., Identification of a bacteriophage containing a silent staphylococcal variant enterotoxin gene (*sezA*), Infect. Immun. 58:1614 (1990).

26. Lindsay, J. A., Ruzin, A., Ross, H. F., Kurepina, N., and Novick, R. P., The gene for toxic shock toxin is carried by a family of mobile pathogenicity islands in *Staphylococcus aureus*, Mol. Microbiol. 29:527 (1998).7. Palmer, E. D., The morphologic consequences of acute exogenous (staphylococcic) gastroenteritis of the gastric mucosa, Gastroenterol.19:462 (1951).

28. Tan, T. L., Drake, C. T., Jacobson, M. J., and Prohaska, J. V., The experimental development of pseudomembranous enterocolitis. Surg. Gynec. Obst. 108:415 (1959).

29. Warren, S. E., Jacobson, M., Mirany, J., and Prodaska, J. V., Acute and chronic enterotoxin enteritis. J. Exp. Med. 120:561 (1964).

30. Kent, T. H., Staphylococcal enterotoxin gastroenteritis in rhesus monkeys, Am. J. Pathol. 48:387 (1966).

31. Merrill, T. G., Sprinz, H., 1968. The effect of staphylococcal enterotoxin on the fine structure of the monkey jejunum, Lab. Invest. 18:114 (1968).

32. Sugiyama, H., and Hayama, T., Comparative resistance of vagotomized monkeys to intravenous vs. intragastric staphylococcal enterotoxin challenges, Proc. Soc. Exp. Biol. Med. 115:243 (1964).

33. Sugiyama, H. and Hayama, T., Abdominal viscera as site of emetic action for staphylococcal enterotoxin in monkeys. J. Infect. Dis. 115:243 (1965).

34. Chatterjee, S. and Jett, M., Glycosphingolipids: the putative receptor for *Staphylococcus aureus* enterotoxin-B in human kidney proximal tubular cells. Mol. Cell. Biochem. 113:25 (1992).

35. Marrack, P. and Kappler, J., The staphylococcal enterotoxins and their relatives, Science 248, 705 (1990).

36. Fraser, J. D., High-affinity binding of staphylococcal enterotoxins A and B to HLA-DR, Nature 339:221 (1989).

37. Hoiden, I., Cardell, S., and Moller, G., Commitment to lymphokine profile during primary in vitro stimulation. Scand. J. Immunol. 38:515 (1993).

38. Fast, D. J., Schlievert, P. M., and Nelson, R. D., Toxic shock syndrome-associated staphylococcal and streptococal pyrogenic toxins are potent inducers of tumor necrosis factor production, Infect. Immun. 57:291 (1989).

39. Huang, W. T., Lin, M. T., Won, S. J., Staphylococcal enterotoxin A-induced fever is associated with increased circulating levels of cytokines in rabbits, Infect. Immun. 65:2656 (1997).

40. Takimoto, H., Yoshikai, Y., Kishihara, K., Matsuzaki, G., Kuga, H., Otani, T., Nomoto, K., Stimulation of all T cells bearing V beta 1, V beta 3, V beta 11 and V beta 12 by staphylococcal enterotoxin A. Eur. J. Immunol. 20:617 (1990).

41. Baudet, V., Hurez, V., Lapeyre, C., Kaveri, S. V., and Kazatchkine, M. D., Intravenous immunoglobulin (IVIg) modulates the expansion of V beta 3+ and V beta 17+ T cells induced by staphylococcal enterotoxin B superantigen in vitro. Scand J. Immunol. 43:277 (1996).

42. Schad, E., Zaitseva, I., Zaitsev, V., Dohlsten, M., Kalland, T., Schlievert, P., Ohlendorf, D., and Svensson, L., Crystal structure of the superantigen staphylococcal enterotoxin type A. EMBO. J. 14:3292 (1995).

43. Wright, A. D. and Chapes, S. K., Cross-linking staphylococcal enterotoxin A bound to major histocompatibility complex class I is required for TNF-alpha secretion, Cell. Immunol. 197:129 (1999).44. Hoffmann, M. L., Jablonski, L. M., Crum, K. K., Hackett, S. P., Chi, Y. I., Stauffacher, C. V., Stevens, D. L., and Bohach, G. A., Predictions of T-cell receptor and major histocompatibility complex binding sites on staphylococcal enterotoxin C_1, Infect. Immun. 62:3396 (1994).

45. Papageorgiou, A. C., Acharya, K. R., Shapiro, R., Passalacqua, R., Brehm, R. D., and H. S. Tranter, Crystal structure of the superantigen enterotoxin C2 from *Staphylococcus aureus* reveals a zinc-binding site, Structure 3:769 (1995).

46. Prasad, G. S., Earhart, C. A., Murray, D. L., Novick, R. P., Schlievert, P. M., and Ohlendorf, D. H., Structure of toxic shock syndrome toxin-1, Biochem. 32:13761 (1993).

47. Schad, E. M., Zaitseva, I., Zaitsev, V. N., Dohlsten, M., Kalland, T., Schlievert, P. M., Ohlendorf, D. H., and Svensson, L. A., Crystal structure of the superantigen staphylococcal enterotoxin type A, EMBO J. 14:3292 (1995).

48. Sundström, M., Abrahmsén, L., Antonsson, P., Mehindate, K., Mourad, W., and Dohlsten, M., The crystal structure of staphylococcal enterotoxin type D reveals Zn^{2+}-mediated homodimerization, EMBO J. 15:6832 (1996).

49. Swaminathan, S., Furey, W., Pletcher, J., and Sax, M., Crystal structure of staphylococcal enterotoxin B, a superantigen, Nature 359:801 (1992).

50. Dinges, M. M., Orwin, P. M., and Schlievert, P. M., Exotoxins of *Staphylococcus aureus*, Clin. Microbiol. Rev. 13:16 (2000).

51. Reck B., Scheuber, P. H., Londong, W., Sailer-Kramer, B., Bartsch, K., Hammer, D. K., Protection against the staphylococcal enterotoxin-induced intestinal disorder in the monkey by anti-idiotypic antibodies, Proc. Natl. Acad. Sci. USA 85:3170 (1988).

52. Stelma, G. N., Jr. and Bergdoll, M. S., Inactivation of staphylococcal enterotoxin A by chemical modification. Biochem. Biophys. Res. 105:121 (1982).

53. Harris, T. O., Grossman, D., Kappler, J. W., Marrack, P., Rich, R. R., and Betley, M. J., Lack of complete correlation between emetic and T-cell stimulatory activities of staphylococcal enterotoxins. Infect. Immun. 61:3175 (1993).

54. Hovde, C. J., Marr, J. C., Hoffmann, M. L., Hackett, S. P., Chi, Y.-i., Crum, K. K., Stevens, D. L., Stauffacher, C. V., and Bohach, G. A., Investigation of the role of the disulphide bond in the activity and structure of staphylococcal enterotoxin C_1, Mol. Microbiol. 13:897 (1994).

55. Sugiyama, H. and McKissic Jr., E. M., Leukocytotic response in monkeys challenged with staphylococcal enterotoxin. J. Bacteriol. 92:349 (1966).

56. Garbe, P. L., Arko, R. J., Reingold, A. L., Graves, L. M., Hayes, P. S., Hightower, A. W., Chandler, F. W., and Broome, C. V., *Staphylococcus aureus* isolates from patients with nonmenstrual toxic shock syndrome. Evidence for additional toxins. JAMA 253:2538 (1985).

57. Kain, K. C., Schulzer, M., and Chow, A. W., Clinical spectrum of nonmenstrual toxic shock syndrome (TSS): comparison with menstrual TSS by multivariate discriminant analyses. Clin. Infect. Dis. 16:100 (1993).

58. McCollister, B. D., Kreiswirth, B. N., Novick, R. P., and Schlievert, P. M., Production of toxic shock syndrome-like illness in rabbits by *Staphylococcus aureus* D4508: association with enterotoxin A, Infec. Immun. 58:2067 (1990).

59. Jarraud, S., Cozon, G., Vandenesch, F., Bes, M., Etienne, J., and Lina, G., Involvement of enterotoxins G and I in staphylococcal toxic shock syndrome and staphylococcal scarlet fever, J. Clin. Microbiol. 37:2446 (1999).0. Larkin S. M., Williams, D. N., Osterholm, M. T., Tofte, R. W., and Posalaky, Z., Toxic shock syndrome: clinical, laboratory, and pathologic findings in nine fatal cases. Ann. Intern. Med. 96:858 (1982).

61. Paris, A. L., Harwardt, L. A., Blum, D., Schmid, G. P., and Shands, K. N., Pathologic findings in twelve fetal cases of toxic shock syndrome. Ann. Intern. Med. 96. 852 (1982).

62. Jett, M., Brinkley, W., Neill, R., Gemski, P., and Hunt, R., *Staphylococcus aureus* enterotoxin B challenge of monkeys: correlation of plasma levels of arachidonic acid cascade products with occurrence of illness, Infect. Immun. 58:3494 (1990).

63. Scheuber, P. H., Golecki, J. R., Kickhofen, B., Scheel, D., Beck, G., and Hammer, D. K., Cysteinyl leukotrienes as mediators of staphylococcal enterotoxin B in the monkey, Eur. J. Clin. Investig. 17:455 (1987).

64. Buxser, S. and Bonventre, P. F., Staphylococcal enterotoxins fail to disrupt membrane integrity or synthetic function of Henle 407 intestinal cells. Infect. Immun. 31:929 (1981).

65. Campbell, W. N., Fitzpatrick, M., Ding, X., Jett, M., Gemski, P., and Goldblum, S. E., SEB is cytotoxic and alters EC barrier function through protein tyrosine phosphorylation in vitro, Am. J. Physiol. 273:L31 (1997).

66. Ito, K., Takaishi, H., Yin, Y., Song, F., Denning, T. L., and Ernst, P. B., Staphylococcal enterotoxin B stimulates expansion of autoreactive T cells that induce apoptosis in intestinal epithelial cells: regulation of autoreactive responses by IL-10, J. Immunol. 164:2994 (2000).

67. Tsen, H. Y., Yu, G. K., Wang, K. C., Wang, S. J., Chang, M. Y., and Lin, L. Y., Comparison of the enterotoxigenic types, toxic shock syndrome toxin I (TSST-1) strains and antibiotic susceptibilities for enterotoxigenic *Staphylococcus aureus* strains isolated from food and clinical samples, Food Microbiol. 15:33 (1998).

68. Bremell, T. and Tarkowski, A., Preferential induction of septic arthritis and mortality by superantigen-producing staphylococci, Infect. Immun. 63:4185 (1995).

69. De Boer, M. L., Kum, W. W. S., Pang, L. T. Y., and Chow, A. W., Co-production of staphylococcal enterotoxin A with toxic shock syndrome toxin-1 (TSST-1) enhances TSST-1 mediated mortality in a D-galactosamine sensitized mouse model of lethal shock, Microb. Path. 27:61 (1999).

70. Nilsson, I.-M., Verdrengh, M., Ulrich, R. G., Bavari, S., and Tarkowski, A., Protection against *Staphylococcus aureus* sepsis by vaccination with recombinant staphylococcal enterotoxin A devoid of superantigenicity, J. Infec. Dis. 180:1370 (1999).

71. Kawabe, Y. and Ochi, A., Selective anergy of $V\beta8^+$, $CD4^+$ T cells in *Staphylococcus* enterotoxin B-primed mice, J. Exp. Med. 172:1065 (1990).

72. Rellahan, B. L., Jones, L. A., Kruisbeek, A. M., Fry, A. M., and Matis, L. A., *In vivo* induction of anergy in peripheral $V\beta8^+$ T Cells by staphylococcal enterotoxin B, J. Exp. Med. 172:1091 (1990).

73. Yan, X.-J., Li, X.-Y., Imanishi, K., Kumazawa, Y., and Uchiyama, T., Study of activation of murine cells with bacterial superantigens. *In vivo* induction of enhanced responses in $CD4^+$ T cells and anergy in $CD8^+$ T cells, J. Immunol. 150:3873 (1993).

74. Kawabe, Y. and Ochi, A., Programmed cell death and extrathymic reduction of $V\beta8^+$ $CD4^+$ T cells in mice tolerant to *Staphylococcus aureus* enterotoxin B, Nature 349:245 (1991).

75. Renno, T., Hahne, M., and MacDonald, H. R., Proliferation is a prerequisite for bacterial superantigen-induced T cell apoptosis *in vivo*, J. Exp. Med. 181:2283 (1995).76.
Renno T., Attinger, A., Locatelli, S., Bakker, T., Vacheron, S., and MacDonald, H. R., Cutting edge: apoptosis of superantigen-activated T cells occurs preferentially after a discrete number of cell divisions *in vivo*, J. Immunol. 162:6312 (1999).

77. Vabulas, R., Bittlingmaier, R., Heeg, K., Wagner, H., and Miethke, T., Rapid clearance of the bacterial superantigen staphylococcal enterotoxin B *in vivo*, Infect. Immun. 64:4567 (1996).

78. Aroeira, L. S., Moreno, M. C., and Martinez, C., *In vivo* activation of T-cell induction into the primed phenotype and programmed cell death by staphylococcal enterotoxin B, Scand. J. Immunol. 43:545 (1996).

79. Kuroda, K., Yagi, J., Imanishi, K., Yan, X. J., Li, X. Y., Fujimaki, W., Kato, H., Miyoshi-Akiyama, T., Kumazawa, Y., Abe, H., and Uchiyama, T., Implantation of IL-2-containing osmotic pump prolongs the survival of superantigen-reactive T cells expanded in mice injected with bacterial superantigen, J. Immunol. 157:1422 (1996).

80. Yoshino, T., Asada, H., Sano, S., Nakamura, T., Itami, S., Tamura, M., and Yoshikawa, K., Impaired responses of peripheral blood mononuclear cells to staphylococcal superantigen in patients with severe atopic dermatitis: a role of T cell apoptosis, J. Invest. Dermatol. 114:281 (2000).

81. Iandolo, J. J., Bannantine, J. P., and Stewart, G. C., Genetic and physical map of the chromosome of *Staphylococcus aureus*, in: The Staphylococci in Human Disease, K. B. Crossley and G. L. Archer, eds., Churchill Livingstone, New York (1997).

82. Mallonee, D. H., Glatz, B. A., and Pattee, P. A., Chromosomal mapping of a gene affecting enterotoxin A production in *Staphylococcus aureus*, Appl Environ. Microbiol. 43:397 (1982).

83. Betley, M. J. and Mekalanos, J. J., Staphylococcal enterotoxin A is encoded by phage, Science 229:185 (1985).

84. Coleman, D. C., Sullivan, D. J., Russell, R. J., Arbuthnott, J. P., Carey, B. F., and Pomeroy, H. M., *Staphylococcus aureus* bacteriophages mediating the simultaneous lysogenic conversion of β-lysin, staphylokinase and enterotoxin A: molecular mechanism of triple conversion, J. Gen. Microbiol. 135:1679 (1989).

85. Couch, J. L., Soltis, M. T., and Betley, M. J., Cloning and nucleotide sequence of the type E staphylococcal enterotoxin gene, J. Bacteriol. 170:2954 (1988).

86. Bayles, K. W. and Iandolo, J. J., Genetic and molecular analyses of the gene encoding staphylococcal enterotoxin D, J. Bacteriol. 171:4799 (1989).

87. Betley, M. J., Borst, D. W., and Regassa, L. B., Staphylococcal enterotoxins, toxic shock syndrome toxin and streptococcal pyrogenic exotoxins: a comparative study of their molecular biology, Chem. Immunol. 55:1 (1992).

88. Bohach, G. A. and Schlievert, P. A., Expression of staphylococcal enterotoxin C_1 in *Escherichia coli*, Infec. Immun. 55:428 (1987).

89. Monday S. R. and Bohach, G. A., Use of multiplex PCR to detect classical and newly described pyrogenic toxin genes in staphylococcal isolates, J. Clin. Microbiol. 37:3411 (1999).

90. Johns, Jr., M. B. and Khan, S. A., Staphylococcal enterotoxin B gene is associated with a discrete genetic element, J. Bacteriol. 170:4033 (1988).

91. Altboum, Z., Hertman, I., and Sarid, S., Penicillinase plasmid-linked genetic determinants for enterotoxin B and C_1 production in *Staphylococcus aureus*. Infect. Immun. 47:514 (1985).

92. Bergdoll, M. S., Czop, J. K., and Gould, S. S., Enterotoxin synthesis by the staphylococci, Ann. NY Acad. Sci. 236:307 (1974).

93. Noleto, A. L. and Bergdoll, M. S., Production of enterotoxin by a *Staphylococcus aureus* strain that produces three identifiable enterotoxins, J. Food. Prot. 45:1096 (1982).

94. Otero, A., Garcia, M. L., Garcia, M. C., Moreno, B., and Bergdoll, M. S., Production of staphylococcal enterotoxins C_1 and C_2 and thermonuclease throughout the growth cycle, Appl. Environ. Microbiol. 56:555 (1990).

95. Bergdoll, M. S., Staphylococcal intoxications, in Foodborne Infections and Intoxications, H. Riemann and F. L. Bryan, eds, Academic Press, New York (1979).

96. Gaskill, M. E., and Khan, S. A., Regulation of the enterotoxin B gene in *Staphylococcus aureus*, J. Biol. Chem. 263:6276 (1988).

97. Compagnone-Post, P., Malyankar, U., and Khan, S. A., Role of host factors in the regulation of the enterotoxin B gene, J. Bacteriol. 173:1827 (1991).

98. Regassa, L. B., Couch, J. L., and Betley, M. J., Steady-state staphylococcal enterotoxin type C mRNA is affected by a product of the accessory gene regulator (*agr*) and by glucose, Infect. Immun. 59:955 (1991).

99. Mahmood, R. and Khan, S. A., Role of upstream sequences in the expression of the staphylococcal enterotoxin B gene. J. Biol. Chem. 15:4652 (1990).

100. Smith, J. L., Bencivengo, M. M., and Kunsch, C. A., Enterotoxin A synthesis in *Staphylococcus aureus*: inhibition by glycerol and maltose, J. Gen. Microbiol. 132:3375 (1986).

101. Borst, D. W. and Betley, M. J., Promoter analysis of the staphylococcal enterotoxin A gene, J. Biol. Chem. 269:1883 (1994).

102. Friedman, M. E. and Howard, M. B., 1971. Induction of mutants of *Staphylococcus aureus* 100 with increased ability to produce enterotoxin A, J. Bacteriol. 106:289 (1971).

103. Borst, D. W. and Betley, M. J., Mutations in the promoter spacer region and early transcribed region increase expression of staphylococcal enterotoxin A, Infect. Immun. 61:5421 (1993).

104. Saitou, N. and Nei, M., The neighbor-joining method: a new method for reconstructing phlogenetic trees, Mol. Biol. Evol.06 (1987).

8

Staphylococcal Extracellular/Surface Enzymatic Activity

VIJAYKUMAR PANCHOLI

1. INTRODUCTION

During the bacterium-host cell interaction, bacterial surface proteins play a key role in the pathogenesis of disease. These proteins expressed in various sizes and shape on the bacterial surface sequentially engage with complimentary receptors on target cells. These early events play a primary role in the bacterial adherence, colonization and internalization. Once the initial niche has been established, bacteria may use their extracellular armamentarium to gain access to the tissue either by subverting host defense mechanisms, therapeutic regimes, host cellular signaling systems, by employing molecular mimicry, or by using a brutal force of their ability to digest the target tissue. In this regard, staphylococci, like many other pathogenic gram-positive cocci such as pneumococci and streptococci, are the perfect example to assign the role of some or all of these mechanisms in the causation of a variety of diseases they cause. With the recent emergence of methicillin resistant staphylococci (MRSA), staphylococcal infections in general has remained a major health concerns whether they are minor infections such as pustules or furuncles, or serious and often fatal infections, such as endocarditis, osteomyelitis, and septic shock syndrome. The surface of staphylococci, like streptococci are decorated with an array of variety of proteins. In addition, staphylococci secrete a variety of proteins many of them are in fact enzymes of a variety of nature. This chapter reviews this extracellular armamentarium of enzymes to elucidate

VIJAYKUMAR PANCHOLI • Bacterial Pathogenesis and Immunology, The Rockefeller University, New York, NY 10021.

Staphylococcus aureus *Infection and Disease*, edited by Allen L. Honeyman *et al.* Kluwer Academic/Plenum Publishers, New York, 2001.

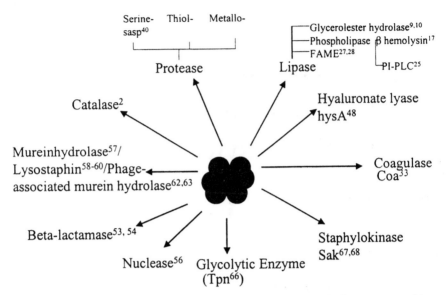

FIGURE 1. Innate Extracellular/Surface enzymatic activity. Schematic diagram summarizing the staphylococcal extracellular/surface enzymatic activity. Numbers in superscript indicate the reference number.

pathogenicity of staphylococci. Staphylococci also possess property to acquire and binds to host protease enzymes and use this property to their own advantage for invading the tissue where they may have made an initial niche. Accordingly, staphylococcal surface enzymatic activity is broadly classified into two categories. Conceptually, these two major categories are: (1) Innate surface enzyme activity (2) Acquired surface enzyme activity. (Figures 1 and 2).

2. INNATE SURFACE ENZYME ACTIVITY

Staphylococci secrete number of enzymes which catalyzed their reactions using both specific and non specific substrates that include specific cellular protein, carbohydrate or lipid. Although their biochemical properties may allow them to classify in a special category, their actual role in infection process remain speculative. It is a fact that staphylococci are not a designated pathogen since whoever harbors this organism at the mucosal surface or the skin may not necessarily always contract disease. In normal circumstances, the mucous membrane and the skin are the efficient barrier

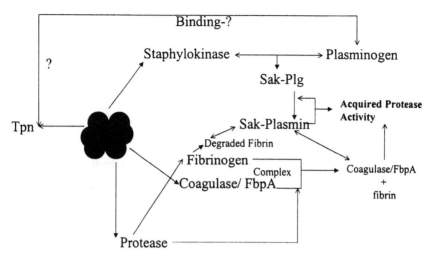

FIGURE 2. Acquired enzymatic activity. Schematic diagram summarizing different pathways by which staphylococci can acquired plasminogen which may then converted into plasmin by staphylokinase or other plasminogen activators. Plasmin then imparts its serine protease activity. Some of the proposed pathways may need experimental validation as described in the text.

for staphylococcal infection, however, once there is a breach in these barriers due to trauma or surgery, initial niche of staphylococci is established. It is at this time such secretory products may allow staphylococci to survive longer and secrete sufficient amount of some of these secretory product which may cause deleterious effect. Thus, in the context of infection, some or combination of these secretory enzymes may serve as virulence factors. Earlier studies have clearly shown clinical isolates display significant variations from strain to strain in the type and amount of such enzyme activities and suggested that the cause of staphylococcal infection is multifactorial. This notion has been confirmed by several recent genetic studies in which individual or more then one putative virulent genes were either deleted or replaced with their defective isogenic counter part rendering staphylococci still pathogenic. On the basis of the proven potential virulence property, the surface enzyme activity in this category is further divided into two categories: (A) enzyme activity with potential virulence property. (B) Enzyme activity with no known virulence property. The latter category, however, has been used for diagnosis purpose and at times used as diagnostic markers to designate the clinical strain with potential virulence property. Thus in category (A) catalase, coagulase, lipase, protease, hyaluronidase, β-lactamase are included, while in category (B) lysostaphin, nuclease, phosphatase, are included (Figure 1).

Catalase

All staphylococci have capacity to convert hydrogen peroxide into non-toxic H_2O and O_2, however, quantitative analysis of Gelosa[1] indicated that coagulase positive staphylococci produced higher levels of catalase and coagulase negative staphylococci produced lower levels or catalase. He suggested, therefore, that the catalase assay may be include as one of the biochemical tests of pathogenicity. Several earlier studies[2,3] have shown that staphylococcal catalase activity is closely related to oxygen content of the culture, thus any compound which reduces oxygen tension is likely serve as an inducer of catalase activity. Kovac's study[2] also showed that catalase when attached to the membrane of staphylococcal cell remains unfolded and hence remain in an inactive form but when the enzyme is induced and detached from the membrane, it unfolds and becomes an extremely active hydrogen peroxide-decomposing agent.[3] Since oxygen-free poly-morphonuclear neutrophils (PMN) cannot kill *S. aureus* normally, the usual mechanisms for PMN bactericidal activity probably involve hydrogen peroxide or superoxide. Mandell[4] demonstrated good correlation between staphylococcal catalase activity and mouse lethality but no correlation between staphylococcal superoxide dismutase activity and mouse lethality. Similarly, exogenous catalase increased the virulence of low-catalase staphylococci, but exogenous superoxide did not alter the virulence of staphylococcal strains.[4] These findings thus concluded that staphylococcal catalase protects intraphagocytic microbes by destroying hydrogen peroxide produced by the phagocyte. Thus, catalase may be a significant staphylococcal virulence factor.

Lipase

Staphylococci produce several lipid hydrolyzing enzymes. Biochemically this group of enzymes are glycerol ester hydolases. This lipolysis is depended on three enzymes classified as lipase, esterases, and phosphatidase.[5] According to the study of Elek,[6] almost all human staphylococci are lipolytic in nature.

Glycerol Ester Hydrolases

These enzymes belong to a family of serine esterases and in principle there are two major types of glycerol ester hydrolases depending on their ability to degrade water-insoluble long chain triacylglycerols or water soluble short chain glycerol ester.[7,8] The class of enzymes that belongs to the former category is the true ester hydrolases and are less common in comparison with those belong to the latter category. While both the types of enzymes are produced by S. aureus and have an apparent molecular mass of 44–45 kDa, their corresponding gene product measure around 75 kDa, suggesting these are synthesized as preproenzymes. The gene encoding true glycerol hydrolases is denoted as *geh*.[9] The pH optima of the corresponding enzymes product is around 8.5. Since the activity of more common but less true glycerol hydrolases was seen on butyryl ester, the gene encoding this enzyme was recently denoted as *beh*.[10] In contrast to the previous category this enzymes show best activity at pH 6.5. Cheung *et al*.[11] have shown that expression of these enzymes are up and down regulated by global regulator *agr* and *sar* respectively, however, it is not yet known which lipase enzymes are regulated by these global regulators.

The role of this enzymes is not fully understood in staphylococcal pathogenicity, although the study of Rollof and Normak[12] suggest that staphylococcal lipase may serve as a virulence factor by virtue of their ability to impair neutrophil functions. Since these enzymes are present in almost all the staphylococcal species, it is likely that it is the less common true glycerol ester hydrolase may have a role in staphylococcal virulence or at best they may be playing a role in bacterial nutrition.

Phospholipases

Staphylococci produce two phospholipases: (i) β-Hemolysin as sphingomyelinase and (ii) Phosphoinositol specific phospholipase C (PI-PLC).

Staphylococcal β-Hemolysin

It is well known for its hot-cold lysis of red blood cells,[13,14] is a neutral sphingomyelinase[15] and its production is more associated with animal isolates (>80%) then with human isolates (10–45%).[16] The molecular mass of staphylococcal β-toxin is 33.7 kDa and is encoded by a gene, *hlb*[17] which carries an attachment site for serological group F converting phages.[18] In the lysogenic stage the *hlb* gene is disrupted by a prophage integration.[18] Although the structural studies on this enzyme has not been carried out, this protein is related to sphingomyelinase of *Bacillus cereus*, exhibiting 58% identity at the amino acid level and to a similar extent with that of *Leptospira interrogans*.[19] The degree of sensitivity of staphylococcal sphingomyelinase activity which converts sphingomyelin into phosphorylcholine and ceramide, depends on the membrane sphingomyelin content of the erythrocytes. Accordingly, staphylococcal shpingomyelinase activity is species dependent with maximum activity with sheep, cow and goat erythrocytes, intermediate activity with human erythrocytes and almost no activity with murine or canine erythrocytes.[14] The purified staphylococcal β-toxin is up to 150 fold less toxic compared to α-toxin.[13]

Since free ceramide plays an important role in the intracellular signal transduction process that ultimately leads to apoptosis, it is reasonable to believe that the enzymatic activity of this toxin may play a role in cellular signaling process and causation of cell apoptosis. Although Jarvis et al.[20] recently showed that staphylococcal β-toxin induces apoptosis of certain cell lines possibly through sphingomyelin pathway, the role of ceramide in β toxin-mediated apoptosis of monocytes was found to be questionable.[21] The latter study, however, attributed selective killing of monocytes by beta toxin to its stimulatory activity on IL-1β, IL6 receptor and soluble CD14.

PI-PLC

Acts on membrane associated inositol phospholipids. Although this protein is known to be secreted in the culture supernatant since 1965,[22] its importance was recognized[23] with the advent of the knowledge of a new class of eukaryotic proteins which are anchored to membrane through a novel glycan-phosphoinositol lipid anchor (GPI-anchor).[24] PI-PLC has been cloned, sequenced, and its biochemical properties have been characterized in detail.[25] The *plc* gene encodes a mature protein with a molecular mass of 34,107 Da with a high specificity for PI at pH 5.5. Although it is not a cysteine-containing enzyme, its inhibition pattern match more with that of sulphydryl-enzyme.

This enzyme is now extensively used in the release and the extraction of eukaryotic GPI-anchored surface proteins many of which serve as adhesion molecules, receptors for intracellular cell signaling.[24] Inositol phospholipid plays an important role as an mediator of many signaling events.[26] In view of these facts, it is likely that staphylococcal PI-PLC may play an important role in the disease process.

Fatty Acid Modifying Enzyme (FAME)

FAME is found in the culture supernatant of both *S. aureus* as well as *S. epidermidis* strains.[27] It is an extracellular enzyme that inactivates bactericidal saturated fatty acid by esterifying them at pH optima of 5.5 to cholesterol.[28] However, its activity is inhibited by unsaturated di-triglyceride. Like many other extracellular products, FAME is also up- and down-regulated by the global regulator Agr and Sar.[29] Chemberlin[30] recently found a low molecular weight (<3000 kDa) non-proteinecious activator from the culture supernatant of S. aureus and S. epidermidis which induces FAME production. The activator from S. aureus induces production of FAME not only in S. aureus but also in S. epidemidis. In contrast, a similar activator from S. epidermidis induces FAME production only in S. epidermidis. The nature of this activator is, however, not known.

FAME may serve as a staphylococcal virulent factor since it can esterify large quantity of bactericidal long chain fatty acid present in staphylococcal abscesses and inactivate them, allowing them to survive longer or at best may serve as an scavenging enzyme for nutrition purpose.

Coagulase

Coagulase activity of staphylococci on human plasma has been taken as the main criterion to differentiate S. aureus from S. epidermidis although some S. aureus strains do show coagulase negative pattern as a result of transcriptional or post transcriptional defects.[31] Coagulase binds to prothrombin and nonproteiolytically converts it into staphylothrombin complex which then converts soluble fibrinogen to fibrin.[32] Coagulase which is encoded by the gene coa,[33] is distinct from other fibrinogen binding staphylococcal clumping factor(fbpA),[34] since it does not possess a classical gram-positive hexapeptide surface sorting signal, LPXTG[35,36] and acts only on soluble and not solid-phase fibrinogen. On the basis of neutralization test, S. aureus strains have been divided into 8 serotypes. The type specificity of these serotypes is located in the N-terminal variable region which span upto 270 amino acid residues. This region is also responsible for the binding to prothrombin. The C-terminal region which contains 5–8 repeats each of 27 amino acid residues is more constant and is responsible for the binding to fibrinogen. In contrast to many other secretory enzymes, the expression of staphylococcal coagulase is negatively regulated by agr.[37] Other then a fact that staphylococcal has an ability to bind prothrombin and converts into enzymatically active thrombin to cause coagulation of serum, there is no direct evidence that shows that coagulase may serve as a virulence factor, since isogenic coagulase producing and coagulase non-producing strains show no difference in their relative virulence.[38]

Proteases

Most strains of S. aureus produce protease enzymes. They are divided in to three major categories (1) Serine protease (2) thiol/cysteine protease (3) metaloprotease.

Serine Protease

Staphylococcal serine protease or V8-protease is a Glu-specific enzyme and widely used for the site-specific fragmentation of proteins before the internal amino acid sequencing. While the amino acid sequence comparison of V8-protease depicts only up to 20–25 % sequence identity with other similar Glu-specific enzymes isolated from different micro-organisms, the catalytic domain consisting of a triad of His-51, Asp-93, and Ser-168 and its flanking regions are well conserved.[39,40] V8-protease is encoded by the gene, *sasp*.[40] It is also conspicuously presented with a tripep-tide repeats, Pro-Asn/Asp-Asn up to 19 times, the function of which is not known.[40]

Since V8-protease can cleave and inactivate IgG, and α_1-proteinase inhibitor, it is proposed that this activity may impair host defense by blocking the antibodies or by inactivating granulocytes defensins.[41] Further, its proteolytic activity on important host proteins may cause tissue destruc-tion and enhance bacterial invasiveness.[42] Since many nonpathogenic bacteria also produce similar enzymes, it is likely that the primary function of this enzyme may simply be to serve as an scavenger in order to provide the bacterium useful low molecular weight nutrient. Its limited pro-teolytic activity as alone may not necessarily play a role in staphylococcal virulence.

Thiol Protease

Potempa *et al.*,[43] reported a 13 kDa cysteine protease from the culture supernatant of *S. aureus.* This enzyme shows strong activity against elastin. Its gene sequence is not known. It is likely that there are two more thiol-protease are expressed in the staphylococcal culture supernatant. None of these enzymes are biochemically well characterized or sequenced.[44]

Metallolprotease

The second most characterized staphylococcal protease enzyme is aureolysisn or Protease III.[45] The molecular mass of this enzyme is 33 kDa. It is a calcium-binding and zinc-dependent enzyme. The former activity imparts stability to the enzyme while the latter activity requires for the catalytic activity. While the crystal structure of this enzyme is available at 1.7 A resolution, the corresponding gene for this enzyme has not been identified.[45] According to Drapeau,[46] the function of this enzyme is likely to convert V8 protease zymogen to its enzymatically active form. The structurally similar metalloprotease produced by *S. epidermidis* has elastase activity.[47] This activity and others point to the fact that metalloprotease may have a role in digestion of extracellular matrix and connective tissue.

Hyaluronate Lyase

Staphylococcal hyaluronidase and hyaluronate lyase enzymes digest hyaluronic acid which is uniformly present in the extracellular matrix of vertebrates in the form of a linear polysaccharide. The latter is composed of repeating subunits of D-glucuronic acid (1-β-3)N-acetyl-D-glucosamine(1-β-4). Staphylococcal hyaluronate lyase degrades hyaluronic acid into disaccharides that contain glucuronosyl residues. The molecular mass of this enzyme is 92 kDa and is encoded by the *hysA* gene.[48] Its amino acid sequence shows 35% identity (including the conserved catalytic His-479 amino acid residue) with those of group B streptococcal and pneumococcal hyaluronate lyases which have been considered as their important virulence factors.[49] Thus, although genetic and biochemical characterization of this enzyme is not well explored, it is likely that staphylococcal hyaluronate lyase may participate in promoting spread through degradation of the tissue, and thus play an important role in staphylococcal pathogenesis. Unlike other staphylococcal enzymes, the production of this enzyme is not regulated by *agr* since it is produced only during the bacterial exponential phase of growth.[50]

β-Lactamase

Staphylococcal extracellular β-lactamases contains 257 amino acids with a molecular mass of 28.8 kDa an and hydrolyze the β-lactam ring of penicillin and convert it into its inactive form, thus rendering staphylococci resistant to penicillin.[51,52] β-lactamases are found either bound to the membrane or released in the medium. From the detailed structural analyses, β-lactamases are seemed to behave like trypsin like serine proteases. In principal, they catalyse the splitting of the lactam amide bond of β-lactams with the help of a serine-ester linked acyl intermediate.

Acylation   deacylation

E + penicillin<---------->EP---------->EP*---------->E + penicilloic acid

(Acylated)

From the crystal structure, the active center of β-lactamase enzyme which participates in the hydrolysis of β-lactam antibiotics, involves four motifs with amino acid sequence S(70)TSK(73), S(130)DN(132), E(166)IELN(170), K(234)SG(236).[53,54] Serine residue-70 is involved in the acylation. Glu-166 is involved in both acylation and deacylation reaction, since in solution form, Glu-166 remains in direct contact and can serve as a base for acylation and can be used in the activation of water molecule required for the deacylation process.[55] Impact of the presence of this enzyme in staphylococcal drug resistance and in drug treatment is enormous is separately treated in this book in two different chapters and hence not elaborated in this chapter (see Chapters 3 and 4 in this volume).

Nuclease

S. aureus, *S. hyicus*, and *S. intermedius* produce a thermostable nuclease (Tnase, Snase or Nuclease A) that is used on a both single- or doble-stranded DNA and RNA for taxonomic purposes.[56] In the presence of calcium, it hydrolyses DNA/or RNA at 5′ end of the phosphodieaster bond into 3′phosphomononucleotide hence it is in fact a phosphodieasterase with both exo and endo nuclease activity. The molecular mass of this enzyme (149 amino acid) is 16.8 kDa.[56] Its role in staphylococcal pathogenesis is not clear.

Murein Hydrolases/Lysostaphin/Phage-coded Murein Hydrolases

The group of enzymes that play a crucial role in the physiological growth of cell wall are called the murein hydrolases. These activities have been summarized and reviewed recently.[57] They are grouped according to their enzymatic activities. Muramidase or N-Acetylmuramidase acts on MurNac(β1-4)GlcNac. Glucosaminidase or N-acetylglucosiminidase acts on GlcNAc(β1-4)MurNAc.

Amidase cleave amide bond between D-lactyl group of MurNAc and amide group of D-Ala. Lysostaphin is produced by *S. simulans* and is a bacterial zinc metalloproteinase.[58] Park *et al.*[59] have shown that it has specific affinity for elastin and degrades elastin which is distinct from its glycyl-glycine endopeptidase activity that cleaves pentaglycine cross bridge of staphylococcal peptidoglycan.[58] The N-terminal sequence Ala-Ala-Thr-His-Glu is involved in the elastin degradation. Lysostaphin is synthesized as a preproenzyme. The proenzyme/prolysostaphin is 5 fold less active than the mature lysostaphin. Once the N-terminal repeat region is cleaved by staphylococcal thiolprotease, the mature lysostaphin cleaves the pentaglycine bridge of the *S. aureus* peptidoglycan much more efficiently.[60] Mature lysostaphin does not act effciently on *S. simulans* because of the incorporation of serine residue into the cell wall cross-bridge.[60] In other words, incorporation of serine into the peptidoglycan cross bridge that renders *S. simulans* immune to the lysostaphin action, is a reminiscent of bacteriocin action which acts on a competing bacteria in a mixed culture. The enzyme that incorporates serine in the wall is called lysostaphin inhibitory factor (LIF) and is encoded by the gene *lif*.[60] Baba and Schneewind[61] have shown that cell wall degrading activity of lystaphin activity lies in the c-terminal region which along with some specific but unknown factor(s), recognizes species-specific peptidocglycan for its action.

The phage encoded murein hydrolases were identified due to the induction of lysogenic phages at the end of logarithmic phase of culture. S. aureus ϕ11 expresses a murein hydrolase (Lyt A) which lacks an N-terminal signal peptide but has C-terminal targetting signal for the wall similar to that of lysostaphin and N-terminal domain that codes for both its D-Ala-Gly endopeptidase and amidase activity.[62] Borchardt *et al*.[63] analyzed a downstream region to the *lytA* gene which encodes a protein with sequence homology to the holins (lysis protein) of bacteriophages of gram-negative bacteria. Navarre and Schneewind[36] suggested that phage-encoded murein hydrolases are released from the cytoplasm of gram-positive bacteria only after the disruption of cytoplasmic membrane caused by holin like lysis protein.

Glycolytic Enzyme

After the discovery of the presence of two glycolytic enzymes, glyceraldehyde-3-phosphate dehydrogenase[64] and α-enolase[65] on the surface of group A streptococci, there has been a several reports describing the presence of glycolytic enzymes in other organisms including staphylococci.[65] Modun and William[66] identified a 42 kDa transferrin binding protein (Tpn) on the surface of S. *aureus* and S. *epidermidis* to be glycerldehyde-3-phosphate dehydrogenase. Staphylococcal GAPDH was, however, not detected on the surface or in the cell wall extract of S. *saprophyticus* and S. *warneri*.[66] Intact S. *aureus* and S. *epidermidis*, like group A streptococci, exhibit GAPDH activity by catalyzing the conversion of glycerladehyde-3-phosphate to 1,3-diphosphoglycerate. Transferrin binding protein is involved in the acquisition of transferrin-bound iron. The ability of staphylococcal GAPDH to bind human transferrin could be one of the multifunction nature of GAPDH molecule in general and may be similar as in the case of streptococcal GAPDH(SDH). The direct role of this protein in staphylococcal pathogenesis is still unclear.

3. ACQUIRED SURFACE ENZYMATIC ACTIVITY

In this category, surface/extracellular proteins that are presented on the surface of bacteria, may not necessarily behave as an enzyme, however, by virtue of having specific binding sites for an host enzyme, they acquire enzymatic activity from their environment. The most notable example of this *de novo* enzymatic activity is through the acquisition of plasminogen/plasmin by the bacterium from the host plasma. Plasminogen is an inactive glycoprotein. In the presence of specific activators, plasminogen is cleaved into a potent serine protease, plasmin. Thus, by acquiring plasminogen/plasmin system, certain pathogen may display protease activity which may be advantageous for their dissemination in the host tissue (Figure 2).

Staphylokinase

Staphylokinase, a 163-amino acid protein (mature protein 136 amino acid) produced by certain strains of *S. aureus*, is a potent plasminogen activator.[67] It is encoded by the gene, *sak*.[68] Staphylokinase (SAK) is produced by lysogenic strains that carry certain prophage. There are three naturally occurring staphylokinase variants with minor differences in their primary structures.[69] SAK is not an enzyme by itself but forms a stoichiomatric complex with plasmin in a ratio of 1:1 which in turn activates other plasminogen molecules. SAK itself has much lower affinity for native plasminogen than for plasmin. However, it binds strongly to plasminogen which is bound to partially degraded fibrin. The mechanism of SAK-mediated activation of plasminogen is reviewed recently.[70] Compared to a similar plasminogen activation by streptokinase, the major difference in the SAK-mediated thrombolysis lies in the fact that it is more fibrin-specific. When streptokinase is added to human plasma containing fibrin clot, it makes complex with plasminogen found at the fibrin clot surface as well as in solution. This complex then becomes the potent activator of other plasminogen molecule and resistant to all proteinase inhibitor such as α_2-antiplasmin. SAK on the other hand, when added to human plasma containing fibrin clot, reacts poorly with free plasminogen but react with high affinity with traces of plasmin at the clot surface resulting into SAK-plasmin complex which in turn activates plasminogen to plasmin at the clot surface. The bound form of SAK-plasmin complex and plasmin at the clot surface are protected by from inhibition by α_2-antiplasmin, however, the complex and plasmin liberated from the clot in the plasma are rapidly (100 fold faster) inactivated by α_2-antiplasmin. Thus, unlike streptokinase, staphylokinase can be used as a potent, uniquely fibrin-selective thrombolytic agent which does not allow excessive liberation of plasmin and confines its activity only where it is needed without being inactivated. However, its use has remained limited because most patients develop high titre of neutralizing antibodies against SAK within 2 weeks of its first introduction in the plasma.[70]

4. GLYCERALDEHYDE-3-PHOSPHATE DEHYDROGENASE (GAPDH)

Staphylococcus aureus isolates have been reported to express surface plasmin(ogen) binding protein. Staphylococcal strain containing the *sak* gene, can acquire plasminogen from plasma or serum and show surface protease activity.[71,72] In a similar study, Kuusella and Sakesela[73] have shown that staphylococci are capable of binding and activating cell surface bound Lys-plasminogen, although this study did not identify the bacterial receptor involved in the binding of plasminogen. Staphylococcal transferrin binding protein (TPN), which was identified as GAPDH, may serve as plasmin(ogen) binding receptor as a structurally similar molecule, Plr [plasmin binding receptor[74] or streptococcal surface dehydrogenase-SDH[64]] was also identified as a strong plasminogen binding receptor on the surface of streptococci. However, in the light of two recent reports which indicated that the streptococcal GAPDH does not not contribute to the overall plasminogen binding activity of group A streptococci,[65,75] it seems unlikely that staphylococcal TPN really functions as plasminogen binding protein on the surface of staphylococci.

Fibrinogen Binding Protein

As mentioned before, mechanism of staphylokinase-mediated activation of plasminogen is fibrin specific, it is likely that many fibrinogen binding proteins may secondarily acquire plasminogen, once they bind to fibrinogen or its partially digested form, fibrin.[71] Based on this, Boyle and Lottenberg[76] extended their model of plasminogen activation by streptokinase and showed that by using purified fibrinogen, streptokinase and plasminogen, group A streptococci can acquire enzymatic activity in a multistep process. Although such a multistep-plasminogen activation mediated by initial binding of fibrinogen to a specific staphylococcal receptor has not been described clearly, it is very likely that some or all of the fibrinogen binding proteins such as clumping factor,[33] fibrinogen binding protein (fbpA)[34] may play a critical role in plasminogen activation on the surface of staphylococci. However, at this time, this hypothesis demands experimental validations.

REFERENCES

1. L. Gelosa, Catalase contents of Staphylococci. *G. Batt. Virol. Immun.* 54:391 (1961).
2. E. Kovacs, and H. H. Mazarean, Investigation of the action mechanism and induction of catalase in the culture of *Staphylococcus aureus*. *Enzymologia.* 30:19 (1966).

3. V. M. Amin, and N. F. Olson, Influence of catalase activity on resistance of coagulase positive staphylococci to hydrogen peroxide. *Appl. Microbiol.* 16:267 (1968).

4. G. L. Mandell, Catalase, superoxide dismutase, and virulence of *Staphylococus aureus. In vitro* and *In vivo* studies with emphasis on staphylococcal-leukocyte interaction. *J. Clin. Invest.* 55:556 (1975).

5. G. T. Stewart, The lipases and pigments of staphylococci. *Ann. N.Y. Acad. Sci.* 128:132 (1965).

6. S. D. Elek, *Staphylococcus pyogenes and its relation to diseases.* E. S. Livingstone, London (1959).

7. J. Kotting, H. Eibl, and F. J. Fehrenbach, Substrate specificity of *Staphylococcus aureus,* (TEN5) lipase withisomeric oleyl-sn-glycerol esters as substrate. *Chem. Phys. Lipids* 47:117 (1988).

8. J.-W. Simons, H. Adams, R. C. Cox, N. Dekker, F. Gotz, A. J. Slotboom, and H. M. Verheij, The lipase from *Staphylococcus aureus:* expression in *Escherichia coli,* large-scale purification and comparison of substrate specificity to *Staphylococcus hyicus* lipase. *Eur. J. Biochem.* 242:760 (1996).

9. C. Y. Lee, and J. J. Iandolo, Lysogenic conversion of staphylococcus lipase is caused by insertion of the bacteriophage L54a genome into the lipase structural gene. *J. Bacteriol.* 166:385 (1986).

10. K. Nikoleit, R. Rosenstein, H. M. Verheij, and M. Gotz, Comparative biochemical and molecular analysis of the *Staphylococcus hyicus, Staphylococcus aureus* and hybrid lipase. *Eur. J. Biochem.* 228:732 (1995).

11. A. L. Cheung, J. M. Koomey, C. A. Butler, S. J. Projan, and V. A. Fischetti, Regulation of exoprotein expression in *Staphylococcus aureus* by a locus (*sar*) distinct from agr. *Proc. Nat. Acad. Sci. USA* 89:6462 (1992).

12. J. Rollof, and S. Normak, *In vivo* processing of *Staphylococcus aureus* lipase. *J. Bacteriol.* 174:1844 (1992).

13. G. M. Wiseman, Some characteristics of the beta hemolysin of *Staphylococcus aureus. J. Pathol. Bacteriol.* 89:187 (1965).

14. G. M. Wiseman, The nature of staphylococcal beta-hemolysin. II Effect on mammalian cells. *Can J. Microbiol.* 14:179 (1968).

15. T. Wadstrom, and R. Mollby, Studies on extracellular proteins from *Staphylococcus aureus.* VII. Studies on beta-hemolysin. *Biochem. Biophys. Acta.* 242:308 (1972).

16. S. D. Elek, and E. Levy, Distribution of hemolysins in pathogenic and nonpathogenic staphylococci. *J. Pathol. Bacteriol.* 62:541 (1950).

17. S. J. Projan, J. Kornblum, B. Kreiswirth, S. L. Moghazeh, W. Eisner, and R. P. Novick, Nucleotide sequence: the β-hemolysin gene of *Staphylococcus aureus. Nucleic Acid. Res.* 17:3305 (1989).

18. D. C. Coleman, J. P. Arbuthnott, H. M. Pomeroy, and T. H. Birkbeck, Cloning and expression in *Escherichia coli* and *Staphylococcus aureus* of the beta-lysin determinant from *Staphylococcus aureus:* evidence that bacteriophage conversion of beta hemolysin activity is caused by insertional inactivation of beta-lysin determinant. *Microb. Pathog.* 1:549 (1986).

19. T. Tomita, Y. Ueda, H. Tamura, R. Taguchi, and H. Ikezawa, The role of acidic amino acid residues in catalytic and adsorptive sites of *Bacillus cereus* shingomyelinase. *Biochim. Biophys. Acta.* 1203:85 (1993).

20. W. D. Jarvis, R. N. Kolesnick, F. A. Fornari, R. S. Traylor, D. A. Gerwitz, and S. Grant, Induction of apoptotic DNA damage and cell death by activation of the sphingomyelinase pathway. *Proc. Natl. Acad. Sci. U.S.A.* 91:73 (1994).

21. I. Walev, U. Weller, S. Strauch, T. Foster, and S. Bhakdi, Selective killing of human monocytes and cytokine release provoked by sphinomyelinase (beta toxin) of *Staphylococcus aureus. Infect. Immun.* 64:2974 (1996).

22. H. M. Doery, B. J. Magnusson, J. Gulasekharam, and J. E. Pearson, The properties of phospholipase enzymes in staphylococcal toxins. *J. Gen. Microbiol.* 40:283 (1965).
23. M. B. Marques, P. F. Weller, J. Parsonnet, B. J. Ransil, and A. Nicholson-Weller, Phosphatidyl-inositol specific phospholipase C, a possible virulence factor for Staphylococcus aureus. *J. Clin. Microbiol.* 27:2451 (1987).
24. M. A. Ferguson, and A. F. Williams, Cell-surface anchoring of proteins via glycosylphosphatidylinositol structures. *Annu. Rev. Biochem.* 57:285 (1988).
25. S. Daugherty, and M. G. Low, Cloning, expression, and mutagenesis of phosphatidylinositol-specific phospholipase C from *Staphylococcus aureus*: a potential staphylococcal virulence factor. *Infect. Immun.* 61:5078 (1993).
26. W. D. Singer, H. A. Brown, and P. C. Sternweis, Regulation of eukaryotic phosphatidylinositol-specific phospholipase C and phospholipase D. *Annu. Rev. Biochem.* 66:475 (1997).
27. J. P. Long, J. Hart, W. Albers, and F. A. Kapral, The production of fatty acid modifying enzyme (FAME) and lipase by various staphylococcal species. *J. Med. Microbiol.* 37:232 (1992).
28. J. E. Mortensen, T. R. Shryock, and F. A. Kapral, Modification of bactericidal fatty acid s by an enzyme of *Staphylococcus aureus*. *J. Med. Microbiol.* 36:293 (1992).
29. N. R. Chamberlain, and B. Imanoel, Genetic regulation of fatty acid modifying enzyme from Staphylococcus aureus. *J. Med. Microbiol.* 44:125 (1996).
30. N. R. Chamberlain, Identification and partial characterization of an extracellular activator of fatty acid modifying enzyme (FAME) expression in *Staphylococcus epidermidis* *J. Med. Microbiol.* 46:693 (1997).
31. F. Vandenesch, C. Lebeau, M. Bes, D. McDEvitt, T. Greenland, R. P. Novick, and J. Etienne, Coagulase deficiency in clinical isolates of *Staphylococcus aureus* involves both transcriptional and posttranscriptional defects. *J. Med. Microbiol.* 40:344 (1994).
32. S. Kawabata, T. Morita, S. Iwanaga, and H. Igarashi, Enzymatic proerties of staphylothrombin, an active molecule complex formed between staphylocoagulase and human prothrombin. *J. Biochem.* 98:1603 (1985).
33. P. Phonimdaeng, M. O'Reilly, P. Nowlan, A. J. Brame, and T. J. Foster, The coagulase of *Staphylococcus aureus* 8325–4. Sequence analysis and virulence of site specific coagulase deficient mutants. *Mol. Microbiol.* 4:393 (1990).
34. A. L. Cheung, S. J. Projan, R. E. Edelstein, and V. A. Fischetti, Cloning expression, and nucleotide sequence of a *Staphylococus aureus* gene (fbpA) encoding a fibrinogen-binding protein. *Infect. Immun.* 63:1914 (1995).
35. V. A. Fischetti, V. Pancholi, and O. Schneewind, Conservation of a hexapeptide sequence in the anchor region of surface proteins from Gram-positive cocci. *Mol. Microbiol.* 4:1603 (1990).
36. W. W. Navarre, and O. Schneewind, Surface proteins of Gram-positive bacteria and mechanisms of their targetting to the cell wall envelope. *Microbiol. Mol. Biol. Rev.* 63:174 (1999).
37. C. Lebeau, F. Vandenesch, T. Greenland, R. P. Novick, and J. Etiene, Coagulase expression in *Staphylococcus aureus* is positively and negatively modulated by an agr-dependent mechanism. *J. Bacteriol.* 176:5534 (1994).
38. L. M. Baddour, M. M. Tayidi, E. Walker, D. McDevitt, and T. J. Foster, Virulence of coagulase-deficient mutants of *Staphylococcus aureus* in experimental endocarditis. *J. Med. Microbiol.* 41:259 (1994).
39. G. H. Drapeau, The primary structure of staphylococal protease. *Can. J. Biochem.* 56:534 (1978).
40. C. Carmona, and G. L. Gray, Nucleotide sequence of the serine protease gene of *Staphylococcus aureus*, Strain V8. *Nucleic. Acids. Res.* 15:6757 (1987).

41. M. E. Selsted, Y. Q. Tang, W. L. Morris, P. A. McGuire, M. J. Novotny, W. Smith, A. H. Henschen, and J. S. Cullor, Purification, primary structures, and antibacterial activities of beta-defensins, a new family of antimicrobial peptides from bovine neutrophils. *J. Biol. Chem.* 9:6641 (1993).

42. J. D. Goguen, N. P. Hoe, and Y. V. Subrahmanyam, Proteases and bacterial virulence, a view from the trenches. *Infect. Agent Dis.* 4:47 (1995).

43. J. Potempa, A. Dubin, G. Korzus, and J. Travis, Degradation of elastin by cysteine proteinase from *Staphylococcus aureus. J. Biol. Chem.* 261:14330 (1988).

44. S. Arvidson, Extracellular enzymes. In: *Gram positive pathogen.* V. A. Fischetti, R. P. Novick, J. Ferreti, D. Portnoy, J. Rood, ASM Publication. Washington D.C. p. 379 (2000).

45. A. Banbula, J. Potempa, J. Travis, C. Fernandes-Catalan, K. Mann, R. Huber, W. Bode, and F. J. Medrano, Amino acid sequence and three dimensional structure of *Staphylococcus aureus* metalloproteinase at 1.72 A resolution. *Structure* 6:1185 (1998).

46. G. R. Drapeau, Role of metalloprotease in activation of the precursor of staphylococcal protease. *J. Bacteriol.* 136:607 (1978).

47. P. Teufel, and F. Gotz (1993) Characterization of an extracellular metalloprotease with elastase activity from *Staphylococcus epidermidis. J. Bacteriol.* 175:4218 (1993).

48. A. M. Farrell, D. Taylor, and K. T. Holland, Cloning, nucleotide sequence determination and expression of the *Staphylococcus aureus* hyaluronate lyase gene. *FEMS Microbiol. Lett.* 130:81 (1995).

49. B. S. Steiner, S. Romero-Steiner, D. Cruce, and R. George, Cloning and sequencing of the hyaluronate lyase gene from *Propionibacterium acnes. Can. J. Microbiol.* 43:315 (1997).

50. D. Taylor, and K. T. Holland, Differential regulation of toxic shock syndrome toxin-1 and hyaluronate lyase production by *Staphylococcus aureus. Zentalbl. Bakteriol. Mikrobiol. Hyg. Suppl.* 21:209 (1991).

51. J.-M. Frere, Beta-lactamases and bacterial resistance to antibiotics. *Mol. Microbiol.* 16:385 (1995).

52. D. J. Zygmunt, C. W. Stratton, and D. S. Kernodle, Characterization of four β-lactamases produced by *Staphylococcus aureus. Antimicrob. Agents Chemother.* 36:440 (1992).

53. R. P. Ambler, A. F. W. Coulson, J. M. Frere, J. M. Ghuysen, B. Joris, M. Forsman, R. C. Levesque, G. Tiraby, and S. G. Waley, Standard numbering scheme for the class A beta-lactamases. *Biochem. J.* 276:269 (1991).

54. O. Herzberg, Refined crystal structure of β-lactamase from *Staphylococcus aureus* PC1 at 2.0 A resolution. *J. Mol. Biol.* 217:701 (1991).

55. R. M. Gibson, H. Christensen, and S. G. Waley, Site directed mutagenesis of β-lactamase I. Single and double mutants of Glu-166 and Lys-73. *Bichem. J.* 272:613 (1990).

56. O. Chesneau, and N. El Solh, Primary structure and biological features of a thermostable nuclease isolated from *Staphylococcus hyicus. Gene.* 145:41 (1994).

57. G. D. Shockman, and J.-V. Holtje, Microbial peptidoglycan (murein) hydrolases. p. 131. In J.-M. Ghusen and R. Hakenbeck *Bacterial cell wall.* Elsevier Science BV, Amsterdam, Netherland. (1994).

58. C. A. Schindler, and V. T. Schuhardt, Lysostaphin: a new bacteriolytic agent for the staphylococcus *Proc. Natl. Acad. Sci. U.S.A.* 51:414 (1964).

59. P. W. Park, R. M. Senior, G. L. Griffin, T. J. Broekelmann, M. S. Mudd, and R. P. Mecham Binding and degradation of elastin by the staphylolytic enzyme lysostaphin. *Int. J. Biochem. Cell Biol.* 2:139 (1995).

60. G. Thumm, and F. Gotz, Studies on prolysostaphin processing and characterization of the lysostaphin immunity factor (lif) of *Staphylococcus simulans* biovar. *Staphylolyticus. Mol. Microbiol.* 23:1251 (1997).

61. T. Baba, and O. Schneewind, Target cell specificity of a bacteriocin molecule: a C-terminal signal directs lysostaphin to the cell wall of *Staphylococcus aureus. EMBO J.* 15:4789 (1996).
62. X. Wang, N. Mani, P. A. Patter, B. J. Wilkinson, and R. K. Jayaswal, Analysis of peptidoglycan hydrolase gene from *Staphylococcus aureus* NCTC 8325. *J. Bacteriol.* 174:6303 (1992).
63. S. A. Borchardt, A. V. Babvah, and R. K. Jayswal, Sequence analysis of the region downstream from a peptidoglycan hydrolase-encoding gene from *Staphylococcus aureus* NCTC 8325. *Gene.* 137:253 (1993).
64. V. Pancholi, and V. A. Fischetti, A major surface protein on group A streptococci is a Glycerladehyde-3-phosphate dehydrogenase with multiple binding activity. *J. Exp. Med.* 176:415 (1992).
65. V. Pancholi, and V. A. Fischetti, α-Enolase, a novel strong plasmin(ogen) binding protein on the surface of pathogenic streptococci. *J. Biol. Chem.* 273:14503 (1998).
66. B. Modun, and P. William, The staphylococcal transferrin-binding protein is a cell wall glycerladehyde-3-phosphate dehydrogenase. *Infect. Immun.* 67:1086 (1999).
67. C. H. Lack, Staphylokinase: An activator of plasma protease. *Nature.* 161:559 (1948).
68. T. Sako, and N. Tsuchida, Nucleotide sequence of the staphylokinase gene from *Staphylococcus aureus. Nucleic Acid. Res.* 11:7679 (1983).
69. A. Gase, E. Birch-Hirschfeld, K. H. Guhrs, M. Hartmann, S. Vetterman, G. Damaschun, H. Damaschun, K. Gast, R. Misselwitz, and D. Zirwer, The thermostability of natural variants of bacterial plasminogen-activator staphylokinase. *Eur. J. Biochem.* 1:303 (1994).
70. D. Collen, Staphylokinase: a potent uniquely fibrin-selective thrombolytic agent *Nat. Med.* 4:279 (1998).
71. V. Sakharov, H. R. Lijnen, and D. C. Rijken, Interaction between staphylokinase, plasmin(ogen), and fibrin. Staphylokinase discriminates between free plasminogen and plasminogen bound to partially degraded fibrin. *J. Biol. Chem.* 271:27912 (1996).
72. R. B. Christner, and M. D. P. Boyle, Role of staphylokinase in the acquisition of plasmin(ogen)-dependent enzymatic activity by staphylococci. *J. Infect. Dis.* 173:104 (1996).
73. P. Kuusela, and O. Saksela, Binding and activation of plasminogen at the surface of *Staphylococcus aureus.* increase in affinity after conversion to the Lys form of the ligand. *Eur. J. Biochem.* 193:759 (1990).
74. R. Lottenberg, C. C. Broder, M. D. P. Boyle, S. J. Kain, B. L. Schroeder, and R. Curtis III, Cloning, sequence anlysis, and expression in *Escherichia coli* of a streptococcal plasmin receptor. *J. Bacteriol.* 174:5204 (1992).
75. S. B. Winram, and R. Lottenberg, Site-directed mutagenesis of streptococcal plasmin receptor protein (Plr) identifies the C-terminal Lys[334] as essential for plasmin binding, but mutation of the *plr* gene does not reduce plasmin binding to group a streptococci. *Microbiology* 144:2025 (1998).
76. M. D. P. Boyle, and R. Lottenberg, Plasminogen activation by invasive human pathogen. *Thromb. Haemost.* 77:1 (1997).

9

Surface Protein Anchoring and Display in Staphylococci

HUNG TON-THAT, SARKIS K. MAZMANIAN, GWEN LIU, and OLAF SCHNEEWIND

1. INTRODUCTION

Staphylococci, Gram-positive microorganism that colonize the human skin and nares, account for more than 80% of all suppurative infections in hospitals.[1] Staphylococcus aureus is the causative agent of a variety of human diseases ranging from minor wound infections to septicemia, osteomyelitis, endocarditis, and septic shock.[1] Treatment of nosocomial infections caused by *S. aureus* is challenging because of the emergence of strains that are resistant to all known antibiotics.[2,3] Several other Gram-positive pathogens, including *Staphylococcus epidermidis*, *Streptococcus pneumoniae* and *Enterococcus faecalis*, have also developed resistance mechanisms to many, if not all, known antibiotics.[4] Thus, the identification of novel targets for anti-bacterial therapy is urgently needed.[5] The cell wall sorting mechanism described below may present such a target as surface proteins play an important role during infection, providing for the attachment of bacteria to host tissues and the escape of invading pathogens from the immune system.

2. STAPHYLOCOCCAL SURFACE PROTEINS

Figure 1 and Table I list the known surface proteins of *S. aureus* that can be grouped according to their ligands, i.e., proteins in the human

HUNG TON-THAT, SARKIS K. MAZMANIAN, GWEN LIU, and OLAF SCHNEEWIND • Department of Microbiology and Immunology, UCLA School of Medicine, University of California, Los Angeles, Los Angeles, CA 90095.

Staphylococcus aureus *Infection and Disease*, edited by Allen L. Honeyman *et al.* Kluwer Academic/Plenum Publishers, New York, 2001.

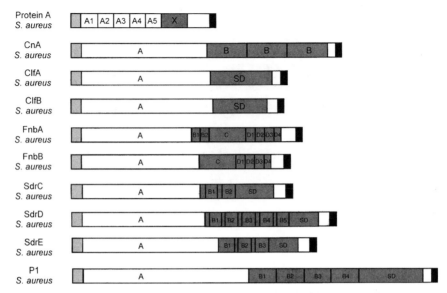

FIGURE 1. Domain organization of *S. aureus* surface proteins. All surface proteins harbor an N-terminal signal peptide (shaded box) and a C-terminal sorting signal (black box). The N-terminal domains of mature surface proteins are comprised of repeat domains (A, B, C or D) that display various ligand binding activities (see text for detail). A proline rich region (white box) upstream of the cell wall sorting signal is thought to span the peptidoglycan layer of the cell wall envelope. Some surface protein harbor extensive repeats at the C-terminal end, for example the serine (S) asparatate (D) repeats or the region X of protein A. See text for details. The figure has been modified after Foster and Höök.[6]

TABLE I
Staphylococcal surface proteins

Surface Protein	Size (aa)	Cell Wall Repeat	Ligand	References
Spa	454	KEDNNKPG	IgG	(110)
CnA	1185	ETTSISGEKVWDD	Collagen	(73)
ClfA	933	SD	Fibrinogen	(59)
ClfB	913	SD	Fibrinogen	(69)
FnbA	1018	TPPTPEVPSEPET	Fibronectin	(88)
FnbB	940	TPPTPEVPSEPET	Fibronectin	(69)
P1	1637	SD(A)	unknown	GI4185564
SdrC	947	SD	Fibrinogen?	(42)
SdrD	1315	SD	Fibrinogen?	(42)
SdrE	1166	SD	Fibrinogen?	(42)

blood or the extra-cellular matrix.[6] Protein A (Spa) was the first surface protein to be identified in *S. aureus* due to its property of binding immunoglobulins.[7,8] Five N-terminal repeat domains of protein A promote binding to the Fc portion of immunoglobulins.[9] Region X, the C-terminal domain of protein A, is divided into two subdomains.[10] Region Xr is composed 13 tandem repeats of the peptide sequence KEDNNKPG and is followed by region Xc, a sequence that is rich in proline residues.[10] During infection, protein A binding to immunoglobulins is thought to camouflage bacteria and allow their escape from opsono-phagocytosis.[11,12]

Several staphylococcal surface proteins bind to extracellular matrix components such as collagen, fibrinogen and fibronectin. Two fibronectin binding proteins, FnbA and FnbB, are expressed simultaneously during staphylococcal growth.[13–16] Three repeat domains, named D1-3, of FnbA and FnbB bind to the N-terminal domain of fibronectin, at a site that is distinct from the RGD domain of this extra-cellular matrix protein.[17–19] Thus, staphylococcal binding to fibronectin can be viewed as a molecular bridge between bacteria and integrins,[20] receptor molecules that are displayed on the surface of epithelial or immune cells.[21] Staphylococcal FnbA and FnbB are thought to provide for bacterial attachment to host tissues[17] as well as for the invasion of microbes into epithelial cells.[22] It seems likely that the N-terminal A, B and C domains of FnbA and FnbB also play a role in bacteria host interactions, however specific ligands for these domains have not yet been characterized. The collagen adhesin Cna has been identified in *S. aureus* strains that were isolated from osteomyelitis and septic arthritis cases.[23,24] Staphylococcal adhesion to collagen within bone and cartilage tissue is thought to be an important aspect for the pathogenesis of these infections.[20,25] Nevertheless, *S. aureus* strains isolated from wound, skin or blood borne infections may not express Cna surface protein.[26,27]

The clumping factor ClfA is necessary for the binding of stationary phase staphylococci to fibrinogen.[28] The N-terminal A domain of ClfA binds to the γ-chain of fibrinogen.[29,30] The C-terminal serine-aspartate (SD) repeat region functions as a tether between the surface exposed A domain and the cell wall anchor structure.[31] By using DNA probes encoding the SD repeat region, Foster and colleagues identified 4 additional surface proteins in the staphylococcal genome: ClfB, SdrC, SdrD and SdrE.[32,33] The A domain of ClfB interacts with fibrinogen α- and β-chains, but not with the γ-chain.[32] During exponential growth both clumping factors, ClfA and ClfB, contribute to staphylococcal fibrinogen binding.[32] However, only ClfA, but not ClfB, is found on the surface of stationary phase staphylococci. The SdrC, SdrD and SdrE proteins are similar to ClfA and ClfB and composed of an N-terminal A domain and a C-terminal SD repeat region.[33,34] What distinguishes these proteins from ClfA and ClfB, is the insertion of a B repeat region immediately downstream of the A domain.[34] Each B repeat folds into a structure containing several low affinity calcium binding sites as well as an EF hand fold for high affinity binding to calcium.[34] Although it is clear that the B regions promote binding to calcium, the role of this activity during infection has not yet been established. Another staphylococcal surface protein containing an SD repeat region, P1, has been identified by genome sequence analysis. The role of P1 as a ligand for eukaryotic proteins or during bacterial pathogenesis is unknown. Binding of staphylococci to fibrinogen may serve several functions. Once within the blood stream, bacteria are generally phagocytosed and killed by the reticuloendothelial system.[35] Adherence to small fibrin deposits within vascular and endocardic lesions may allow staphylococci to avoid transport via the blood stream and exposure to macrophages.[35] Further, the deposition of fibrin on the bacterial surface may physically shield staphylococci from phagocytosis. In contrast to *S. aureus*, *S. epidermidis* has been thought to not bind to fibrinogen. This concept may have to be reconsidered due to the recent observation that *S. epidermidis* express a fibrinogen binding protein (clumping factor) on their surface.[36]

3. CELL WALL ANCHORED PROTEIN A

The structure and assembly of protein A in the cell wall envelope have been extensively characterized.[37] The predicted amino acid sequence of protein A (Spa) revealed the presence of an N-terminal signal peptide, which is absent from the mature cell wall anchored polypeptide.[38-40] The N-terminal domain, containing five IgG binding repeats (A1-5), is exposed on the bacterial surface.[9] Each repeat unit is a small globular protein built of three parallel helices arranged in a triangular array. The repeats bind to the first two helices of Fc that are attached to segments of CH2 and CH3 of the immunoglobulin fold.[41] The C-terminal region X presumably forms an elongated, largely unstructured thread that weaves through the peptidoglycan layer of the cell wall envelope.[10] Incubation of staphylococci with thermolysin removes the N-terminal A domains and part of region X, thereby generating a C-terminal peptide fragment that is protected from further proteolytic cleavage by the cell wall envelope.[10] As all protease protected fragments display the same size, protein A must be linked to the cell wall in a manner preserving a uniform distance between the cell surface and the C-terminal anchor structure. This result favors a model of longitudinal growth of the bacterial cell wall. An alternative model, proposing vectorial growth of the cell wall like the bark of an aging tree, can be dismissed as surface proteins would be positioned at various positions within the cell wall envelope.[42] Purified cell wall sacculi of staphylococci contain linked protein A molecules.[43] Extraction with detergent, organic solvents or acids can not solubilize protein A from the murein sacculus.[43] Digestion of the peptidoglycan with lysostaphin, a glycyl-glycine endopeptidase that cleaves the crossbridges, or muramidase, which cuts the glycan stands of the cell wall, released protein A from the cell wall.[37] Lysostaphin and muramidase-released protein A species differ in mass, indicating that the C-terminal end of the polypeptide must be linked to the cell wall envelope.[37]

4. THE CELL WALL SORTING REACTION

A model for the mechanism of protein A anchoring to the cell wall of S. aureus is displayed in Figure 2. Two topogenic signals, the N-terminal signal peptide and the C-terminal cell wall sorting signal, are required for the cell wall anchoring of protein A.[44] The 35-residue C-terminal sorting signal consists of an LPETG sequence motif, followed by a hydrophobic domain and a positively charged tail.[45] After synthesis in the cytoplasm, the protein A precursor is first initiated into the secretory pathway (Sec) of S. aureus and the N-terminal signal peptide is removed by signal peptidase. The C-terminal hydrophobic domain and the positively charged tail retain protein A within the secretory pathway,[45] thereby permitting cleavage of the polypeptide between the threonine (T) and the glycine (G) of the LPETG motif.[46] The liberated carboxyl group of threonine subsequently forms an amide bond with the amino group of the pentaglycine crossbridge, thereby tethering the C-terminal end of protein A to the cell wall envelope.[47] This amide bond exchange reaction is catalyzed by sortase, a transpeptidase that is located in the cytoplasmic membrane of S. aureus.[48] Sortase presumably uses precursor molecules of two pathways as substrates for the sorting reaction: surface protein precursor and the peptidoglycan precursor, lipid II.[49] The product of the sorting reaction, surface protein linked to lipid II,[49] is thought to be incorporated into the cell wall by the transglycosylase and transpeptidase activities of the cell wall synthesis machinery (penicillin binding proteins)[50,51] (Figure 2).

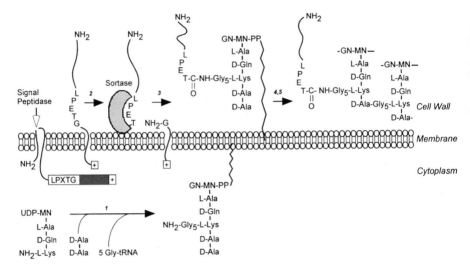

FIGURE 2. Model for the sorting of surface proteins to the staphylococcal cell wall. Surface proteins are synthesized as precursors in the bacterial cytoplasm bearing an N-terminal signal peptide and a Ct-terminal sorting signal (P1 precursor). The sorting signal is comprised of an LPXTG sequence motif, followed by a hydrophobic domain (black box) and tail of positively charged residues (boxed +). Following cleavage of the N-terminal signal peptide, the hydrophobic domain and charged tail of the P2 precursor retain surface proteins in the secretory pathway. The P2 precursor is substrate for cleavage by sortase, a membrane anchored transpeptidase, thereby generating an acyl enzyme intermediate and the cleaved sorting signal. The acyl enzyme intermediate, a thioester bond between the thiol of sortase and he carboxyl of threonine at the C-terminal end of surface proteins, is resolved by the nucleophilic attack of the amino group of the pentaglycine crossbridge. Presumably, the lipid II precursor serves as a peptidoglycan substrate for the sorting reaction. Cell wall synthesis begins in the bacterial cytoplasm via the assembly of nucleotide linked wall peptides. After the precursor is transferred to undecaprenylpyrophosphate, the lipid II molecules are translocated across the cytoplasmic membrane. Surface proteins linked to lipid II may be incorporated into the cell wall envelope by the transglycosylation and transpeptidation reactions to generate mature cell wall anchored surface protein.

5. SORTING SIGNALS AND SURFACE PROTEINS

Cell wall sorting signals have been found at the predicted C-terminus of all *S. aureus* surface proteins: Spa, FnbA, FnbB, ClfA, ClfB, SdrC, SdrD, SdrE, Cna and P1[6](Table II). The LPXTG motif is conserved in all of these signals, however there is considerable variation is sequence and amino acid composition of the hydrophobic domain and charged tail.[42] The protein A sorting signal has been altered by various deletion or point mutations.[44] Truncation of the C-terminal positively charged tail caused protein A to be

TABLE II
Staphylococcal surface proteins containing sorting signals

Protein	Sorting signals	Ref.
Spa	**LPETG**EENPFIGTTVFGGLSLALGAALLAGRRREL	(110)
Cna	**LPKTG**MKIITSWITWVFIGILGLYLILRKRFNS	(73)
ClfA	**LPDTG**SEDEANTSLIWGLLASIGSLLLFRRKKENKDKK	(59)
ClfB	**LPETG**DKSENTNATLFGAMMALLGSLLLFRKRKQDHKEKA	(69)
FnbA	**LPETG**GEESTNKGMLFGGLFSILGLALLRRNKKNHKA	(88)
FnbB	**LPETG**GEESTNNGMLFGGLFSILGLALLRRNKKNHKA	(40)
P1	**LPDTG**NDAQNNGTLFGSLFAALGGLFLVGRRRKNKNNEEK	GI4185564
SdrC	**LPETG**SENNNSNNGTLFGGLFAALGSLLSFGRRKKQNK	(42)
SdrD	**LPETG**NENSGSNNATLFGGLFAALGSLLLFGRRKKQNK	(42)
SdrE	**LPETG**SENNGSNNATLFGGLFAALGSLLLFGRRKKQNK	(42)
Fbe	**LPDTG**ANEDYGSKGTLLGTLFAGLGALLLGKRRKNRKNKN	(70)

secreted into the extracellular medium.[44] All further truncations, including the hydrophobic domain and the LPXTG motif, displayed the same phenotype.[44] Deletion of the LPXTG motif alone caused a different phenotype.[44] The protein A mutant was found missorted in the cytoplasm, the membrane and the cell wall compartment and was not linked to the cell wall peptidoglycan. Point mutations replacing the proline (P) of the LPXTG motif with asparagine (N) resulted in a similar phenotype, whereas replacement of the threonine (T) with either alanine (A) or serine (S) had no effect on the sorting reaction. These results are consistent with observed sequence variations in the LPXTG motif of more than 100 surface proteins from many different Gram-positive bacteria. While the threonine (T) is sometimes replaced with either serine or alanine, the three other residues are absolutely conserved.[42] In *S. aureus* sorting signals, the position X of the LPXTG motif is typically a negatively charged residue. The one exception to this rule is the sorting signal of Cna, which is not functional when transplanted onto the C-terminus of reporter proteins and tested in *S. aureus* strain 8325-4 or derivaties.[45] Three arginines within the positively charged tail of the protein A sorting signal are required to retain the polypeptide from the secretory pathway for subsequent cleavage by sortase at the LPXTG motif.[45] As arginines can be replaced with lysine residues, it is likely that the retention signal is composed of positive charges rather than signaling via the recognition of specific amino acid residues. Further, the positive charges must be properly spaced downstream of the LPXTG motif in order for cell wall anchoring to occur. Shortening of the spacing between the LPXTG motif and the positive charges caused protein A mutants to be secreted into the extracellular medium. An increase in the spacing of sorting signals resulted in impaired bacterial growth and viability.[45] The hydrophobic domain of sorting signals does generally not seem to function as a membrane anchor. Removal of the LPXTG motif caused missorting of protein A mutants but failed to stably insert polypeptides into the cytoplasmic membrane.[45]

Do cell wall sorting signals promote anchoring of all polypeptides that are initiated into the secretory pathway? To address this question, the protein A sorting signal was fused to the C-terminus of enterotoxin B (Seb) and staphylococcal β-lactamase (BlaZ). Enterotoxin B is exported by a type I signal peptide, cleaved by signal peptidase and secreted into the extra-cellular medium.[52,53] Fusion of the protein A sorting signal to the C-terminus of Seb caused cell wall sorting of the hybrid protein.[45] β-lactamase is synthesized as a precursor bearing an N-terminal type II signal peptide.[54] Following export, approximately half of all β-lactamase is cleaved by signal peptidase II and thioether lipid modified at its N-terminal cysteine. This modification directs mature BlaZ to the cytoplasmic membrane.[55] The remainder of the polypeptide is cleaved by signal peptidase seven residues downstream of the cysteine and the cleaved polypeptide is secreted into the extra-cellular medium.[55] Fusion of the protein A sorting signal to the C-terminus of β-lactamase generated two species: cell wall anchored BlaZ with and without an N-terminal lipid modification.[55] These results suggest that fusion of the sorting signal to any polypeptide bearing an N-terminal signal peptide results in cell wall sorting of the hybrid protein.

Lysostaphin, a bacteriocin that is secreted into the extracellular medium of *S. simulans* biovar *staphylolyticus* cultures,[56,57] is synthesized as a pre-pro enzyme and exported via its N-terminal signal peptide. Following secretion of the pro-enzyme, 13 N-terminal repeat domains are cleaved by a cysteine protease.[58,59] Mature lysostaphin is targeted to the envelope of *S. aureus* cells.[60] By virtue of its glycyl-glycine endopeptidase activity, lysostaphin digests the peptidoglycan and causes osmotic lysis of staphylococci.[56,59] Bacteriocin targeting to the cell wall of *S. aureus* requires a targeting signal that is located at the C-terminal end of lysostaphin.[60] The targeting signal is not required for enzymatic activity. However, without this signal lysostaphin cannot distinguish between host (*S. simulans*) and target cells (*S. aureus*). Expression of lysostaphin in *S. aureus* did not result in secretion of the polypeptide into the extra-cellular medium.[60] Instead, the bacteriocin was found targeted to the cell wall envelope. Fusion of the protein A sorting signal to the C-terminus of the targeting signal did not result in cell wall linked polypeptides. In contrast, fusion of the targeting signal to the C-terminal end of the sorting signal did not interfere with cell wall anchoring.[60] We do not know how the targeting signal interferes with the function of cell wall sorting signals. Perhaps the targeting signal sequesters the polypeptide in a manner that prevents recognition of the LPXTG motif by sortase.

6. DISPLAY OF PROTEINS ON THE STAPHYLOCOCCAL SURFACE

Several laboratories have developed expression systems that allow the display of recombinant proteins on the surface of staphylococci or other Gram-positive bacteria.[61–63] Typically, these systems allow insertion of coding sequence into the scaffold of a cell wall anchored surface protein. To determine the site for optimal expression and surface display, Strauss and Gotz varied the length of the cell wall spanning domain of FnbA.[64] Decreasing the wall spanning domain beyond a critical length (90 residues) abolished surface display, without interfering with the cell wall anchoring of the recombinant polypeptides.[64] Thus, this experiments further supports the notion that surface proteins are anchored at a uniform distance between the surface and the cell wall anchor structure. Similar results were obtained for the cell wall spanning domain of the clumping factor ClfA, i.e. the serine-aspartate repeat region.[31] The protein A scaffold has been engineered to accept immunoglobulin domains.[65] In this manner, bacteria can be manipulated to represent an immunologically reactive particle. Another application for the engineered display of surface proteins is the manufacturing of recombinant live vaccines.[62,63]

7. THE PEPTIDOGLYCAN SUBSTRATE OF THE SORTING REACTION

Genetic analysis of staphylococcal methicillin resistance has provided insights into the synthesis of peptidoglycan crossbrigdes.[66] Staphylococcal strains expressing the penicillin binding protein PBP2a (PBP2') are resistant to most β-lactam antibiotics including methicillin.[67,68] Genetic screens designed to identify elements that are also necessary for methicillin resistance yielded mutations in approximately ten different *fem* (*aux*) genes.[69–71] Some of these genes are involved in the synthesis of the pentaglycine crossbridge,[72–75] or the amidation of D-iso-glutamyl within the wall peptide.[76,77] Staphylococcal strains harboring mutations in the *femA*, *femB*, or *femX* gene synthesize altered cell wall crossbridges with either three glycine *femB*, one glycine *femA*, or a combination of no or one glycine.[78] The latter phenotype has been reported for a mutant with a combination of a *femA* mutation and a second one leading to a partial non-funtional *FemX* (Fmhb) protein.[78,79] Biochemical studies on the synthesis of staphylococcal peptidoglycan revealed that the pentaglycine crossbridge is synthesized via modification of the lipid II precursor (undecaprenylpyrophosphate-MurNAc(-L-Ala-D-iGln-L-Lys-D-Ala-D-Ala)-(β1-4)-GlcNAc).[80–82] Thus, it seems likely that *FemA*, *FemB*, and the recently identified FmhB[79] catalyze the addition of glycine to the ε-amino group of L-lysine to generate the pentaglycine crossbridge of lipid II.

If the sorting reaction utilized the lipid II molecule as a precursor, an alteration of the pentaglycine crossbridge, may interfere with the anchoring of staphylococcal surface proteins. An experimental scheme was developed that allowed measurement of the cleavage of surface protein precursor and the characterization of the cell wall anchored surface proteins in *fem* mutant staphylococci.[83] *S. aureus* strains carrying mutations in the *fem* genes displayed a decreased rate of precursor cleavage as compared to the wild-type strains, suggesting that the altered crossbridges slowed the anchoring of surface proteins.[83] Analysis of the cell wall anchor structures showed that surface proteins could be linked to mono-, tri-, or pentaglycine as well as tetra-glycine-monoserine crossbridges but not to the ε-amino group of lysine in neuropeptides.[83] These results suggest that the sorting mechanism requires specific peptidoglycan substrates to catalyze the amide bond exchange mechanism.

8. SORTASE AND THE SORTING REACTION

To identify genes that act in the cell wall sorting pathway, one thousand temperature-sensitive *S. aureus* mutants were screened with a pulse-labeling assay for a defect in cleaving protein A.[48] A mutant strain was identified, transformed with a plasmid library of chromosomal DNA and screened for restoration of this defect. One gene, *srtA* (staphylococcal surface protein sorting A), complemented the defect. The *srtA* gene specifies a 206 amino acid polypeptide with an N-terminal hydrophobic domain that functions as a signal peptide/membrane anchor domain[48] (Figure 3). Preliminary results suggest that SrtA is assembled in the membrane envelope as a type II membrane protein with its N-terminus in the cytoplasm and the C-terminal end positioned in the cell wall. Knockout mutations of *srtA* were constructed by allelic replacement of *srtA* with the *ermC* gene.[84] The mutant *srtA⁻:ermC* allele could be transduced into various *S. aureus* strains, thereby abolishing the expression of SrtA. *SrtA⁻* mutant strains were defective in cleaving the sorting signals of protein A, fibronectin binding

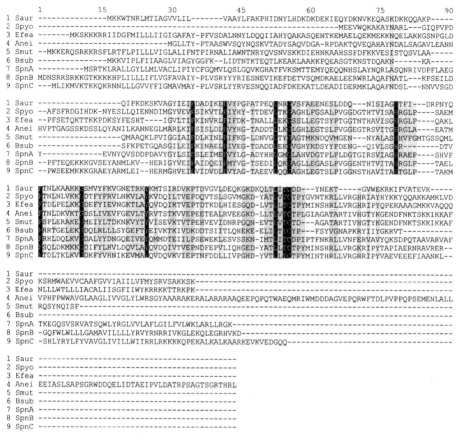

FIGURE 3. The *srtA* gene is conserved in Gram-positive bacteria. The sequence alignment compares the predicted primary structure of the SrtA protein (Sortase) with that of homologous sequences identified by database searches. Note the conservation of a single cysteine residue as well as its surrounding sequence. The databases used were for (1) *S. aureus*, (2) *S. pyogenes*, (3) *E. faecalis*, (4) *A. naeslundii* (Genbank),[118] (5) *S. mutans*, (6) *B. subtilis*, and (7–9) *S. pneumoniae*. The Institute for Genomic Research (TIGR), personal communication.

protein (FnbA and FnbB) and clumping factor (ClfA) at the LPXTG motif.[84] The surface protein precursor species are not linked to the cell wall but can be found in the cytoplasm and the membrane of *srtA*⁻ mutant staphylococci. Neither the protein secretion pathway nor the retention of surface proteins lacking an LPXTG motif within the secretion pathway were affected by knockout mutations of the *srtA* gene. Thus, *srtA* is absolutely necessary for the cell wall anchoring of all surface proteins bearing a

C-terminal sorting signal,[84] suggesting that *srtA* encodes the transpeptidase sortase.

Sortase may catalyze a transpeptidation reaction by forming an acyl-enzyme intermediate with the carboxyl group of threonine at the C-terminal end of cleaved surface proteins.[85] Acyl-enzyme intermediates involve either an active site hydroxyl or thiol group, leading to the formation of an ester or thioester bond between the enzyme and its substrate.[85] In a second reaction, the acyl enzyme is resolved by the nucleophilic attack of the free amino group of the pentaglycine cross-bridge.[85] If sortase formed an acyl-enzyme containing thioester, the addition of the strong nucleophile hydroxylamine should release surface proteins into the extracellular medium. Lipmann first showed that hydroxylaminolysis led to the formation of substrate hydroxamate and the regeneration of enzyme thiol.[86] This prediction was tested and the addition hydroxylamine to staphylococcal cultures indeed caused the release of surface protein hydroxamate into the extracellular medium.[85] Hydroxylaminolysis of surface proteins expressed by S. *aureus* required the single cysteine residue of sortase, suggesting that the thiol may function as the active site nucleophile during the transpeptidation reaction.[85] This hypothesis is supported by the observation that the staphylococcal sorting reaction can be inhibited with methanethiosulfonates, compounds that react very quickly with free thiol.[49] Slower reacting sulfhydryl reagents (iodoacetate, iodoacetamide and N-ethylamleimide) have no effect on the sorting reaction.[49] The formation of sortase acyl-enzyme intermediates presumably prevents access of these reagents to the active site thiol.[85]

Staphylococcal extracts, purified SrtA and purified SrtA$_{\Delta N}$, a mutant enzyme in which the N-terminal hydrophobic domain has been replaced with an affinity tag, all catalyze the slow hydrolysis of peptides bearing an LPXTG motif[85] (Figure 4). Cleavage is specific for substrates bearing an LPXTG motif, as peptides with a scrambled motif are not cleaved. The addition of hydroxylamine to purified sortase increased the rate of peptide cleavage. To determine the in vitro cleavage site of sortase, LPXTG substrate peptides were incubated with or without SrtA$_{\Delta N}$ and reaction products were analyzed by rpHPLC and mass spectrometry. Hydrolysis occurred between the threonine (T) and the glycine (G) of the LPXTG motif.[87] To test whether sortase catalyzed a transpeptidation reaction in the presence of its physiological nucleophile, i.e. the amino group of glycine. SrtA$_{\Delta N}$ was incubated with LPXTG peptides and NH$_2$-Gly$_3$. Analysis of the reaction products revealed the presence of transpeptidation (LPXTGG) but not of hydrolysis products (LPXT).[87] Thus, sortase preferred the amino group of the peptidoglycan substrate as a nucleophile to accept the carboxyl of threonine at the C-terminal end of surface protein. Further, these data

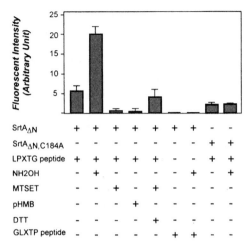

SrtA$_{\Delta N}$	+	+	+	+	+	+	+	-	-
SrtA$_{\Delta N,C184A}$	-	-	-	-	-	-	-	+	+
LPXTG peptide	+	+	+	+	+	-	-	+	+
NH2OH	-	+	-	-	-	-	+	-	+
MTSET	-	-	+	-	+	-	-	-	-
pHMB	-	-	-	+	-	-	-	-	-
DTT	-	-	-	-	+	-	-	-	-
GLXTP peptide	-	-	-	-	-	+	+	-	-

FIGURE 4. Sortase cleaves LPXTG motif bearing peptides *in vitro*. Purified SrtA$_{\Delta N}$ was incubated with the LPXTG peptide (DABCYL-QAGLETPEE-EDANS) and cleavage monitored as an increase in fluorescence. The reaction was inhibited by the addition of methanethiosulfonate (MTSET) or organic mercurial (pHMB), while the addition of 0.2 M NH$_2$OH accelerated cleavage. MTSET-treated SrtA$_{\Delta N}$ could be rescued by incubation with 10 mM DTT. The peptide DABCYL-QAGLETPEE-EDANS (GLXTP) served as a control for cleavage specificity of purified SrtA$_{\Delta N}$. Purified SrtA$_{\Delta N,C184A}$ contains a replacement of cysteine 184 with alanine. When incubated with LPXTG peptide, SrtA$_{\Delta N,C184A}$ caused only a small increase in fluorescence, which may be due to the binding of substrate to the mutant enzyme. The addition of NH$_2$OH to SrtA$_{\Delta N,C184A}$ did not generate an increase in fluorescence, indicating that no cleavage of LPXTG peptide occurred.

suggest that sortase is necessary and sufficient to catalyze the cell wall anchoring reaction of surface proteins at the LPXTG motif.

9. TRANSPEPTIDATION REACTIONS: SORTASE, PENICILLIN BINDING PROTEINS AND TRANSAMIDASE

The cell wall sorting reaction is an amide bond exchange reaction and can be viewed as two distinct reactions. First, the nucleophilic attack of the enzyme thiol results in the formation of an acyl-enzyme thioester intermediate and in the transfer of one proton to the amino group of glycine at the N-terminus of the cleaved sorting signal.[85] Second, the thioester enzyme intermediate is resolved by the nucelophilic attack of the amino group of the pentaglycine crossbridge of the peptidoglycan precursor lipid II.[85] The observation that hydroxylamine releases acyl-enzyme intermediates as surface protein with a C-terminal hydroxamate into the extra-cellular medium of staphylococci suggests that under physiological conditions, the specificity of the sorting reaction is determined by the availability of nucleophiles.[85] As the cell wall of *S. aureus* contains only one type of amino group, i.e. the amino of the peptidoglycan crossbridge,[88] the C-terminus of all anchored surface proteins is tethered to pentaglycine.

The crosslinking of peptidoglycan strands during bacterial cell wall synthesis proceeds by a similar amide bond exchange mechanism.[89] The lipid II precursor contains a five residue peptide, L-Ala-D-iGlu-L-Lys-D-Ala-D-Ala, which is tethered to the disaccharide MurNac-(β1-4)-GlcNac[90] via an amide bond between the amino of L-Ala and the carboxyl of the lactyl moiety within MurNac.[91] To synthesize bacterial peptidoglycan, high molecular weight transpeptidases first polymerize the glycan strands via a transglycosylation reaction, which is fueled by the hydrolysis of the phosphodiester bonds within the lipid II precursor.[92] The same group of enzymes catalyzes the crosslinking of nascent peptidoglycan strands. The terminal amide bond of the wall peptide is cleaved, causing the formation of an acyl enzyme intermediate with the carboxyl of D-Ala at position four.[93] The acyl-enzyme intermediate is resolved by the nucleophilic attack of the amino group within pentaglycine crossbridges.[94] This transpeptidation reaction, but not the one catalyzed by sortase, is inhibited by penicillin and other β-lactam antibiotics. After cleavage of the antibiotic and the formation of an acyl-enzyme, the inhibitors occupy the active site in a manner that cannot be released by the nucleophilic attack of either water or the pentaglycine crossbridges.[92] Transpeptidases (penicillin binding proteins) use an active site hydroxyl (serine) to cleave wall peptides between D-alanyl-D-alanine.[95-97] Nevertheless, the acyl-enzyme of penicillin binding proteins can also be released by the addition of hydroxylamine.[96,97]

Surface proteins of yeast, protozoa and mammalian cells are inserted into the plasma membrane via a C-terminal glycosylphosphatidylinositol (GPI) modification.[98] For example, the protozoan pathogen *Trypanosoma brucei* assembles a surface coat composed of variable surface glycoproteins (VSG) that undergo continuous antigenic variation and must be shed at regular intervals from the plasma membrane.[99] Surface protein assembly involves C-terminal GPI modification.[100] During antigenic variation, *T. brucei* are thought to express a phospholipase that cleaves the GPI moiety,[101] thereby shedding VSG proteins into the medium and allowing assembly of a new, antigenically distinct VSG coat.[102] VSG precursors contain an N-terminal signal peptide and a C-terminal hydrophobic segment.[103,104] The

N-terminal signal peptide initiates the precursor into the secretory pathway. After VSG translocation into the lumen of the endoplasmic reticulum, the C-terminal hydrophobic domain anchors the polypeptide in the membrane.[102] Membrane insertion is followed by cleavage of the polypeptide and concomittant attachment of the GPI moiety.[98,105] The overall reaction can be viewed as an amide bond exchange reaction, during which an enzyme named transamidase cleaves the polypeptide at a designated site[106,107] to form an acyl-enzyme intermediate.[102] The amino of ethanolamine within GPI anchors presumably performs the nucleophilic attack to resolve the enzyme intermediate, thereby generating GPI modified proteins that are transported to the plasma membrane.[98] GPI anchoring is thought to occur by a universal mechanism in all eukaryotic organisms.[98,108]

A search for yeast mutants defective in GPI synthesis and protein modification[109,110] identified two proteins, GAA1 and GPI-8, that are absolutely essential for the attachment of GPI to protein.[111,112] The addition of strong nucleophiles, hydroxylamine or hydrazine, to a mammalian *in vitro* protein translocation and GPI modification reaction results in the formation of cleaved precursor lacking the C-terminal hydrophobic domain.[113] Presumably, these nucleophiles released an acyl-enzyme intermediate between surface protein and transamidase. Hydroxylaminolysis is dependent on functional GPI-8, as extracts prepared from mammalian cells lacking GPI-8 fail to release a processed precursor.[114] While these results suggest that GPI-8 functions as a transamidase to attach GPI anchors to surface proteins, the role of GAA1 still remains to be characterized.

10. CELL WALL SORTING IN OTHER GRAM-POSITIVE BACTERIA

Surface proteins with C-terminal sorting signals have been identified sin almost all Gram-positive bacteria.[42] Furthermore, sortase is conserved is the genomes of all Gram-positive bacteria that have been sequenced to date: *Actinomyces naeslundi, Bacillus subtilis, Enterococcus faecalis, Streptococcus mutans, Streptococcus pneumoniae,* and *Streptococcus pyogenes*[48] (Figure 3). As the substrates for the sorting reaction, i.e. the LPXTG motif and the amino group of peptidoglycan crossbridges, as well as the enzymatic machinery are conserved, it seems likely that cell wall sorting occurs by a universal mechanism in Gram-positive bacteria.[42] For example, *Actinomyces naeslundi* elaborate fimbriae that are composed of fimbrial subunits bearing C-terminal sorting signals with an LPXTG motif.[115] Fimbrial assembly is reported to be dependent an actinomycetal sortase homolog.[116] Furthermore, characterization of the cell wall anchor structure of surface proteins in *L. monocytogenes* revealed that surface protein anchoring occurs by a mechanism that is identical to that described for *S. aureus*.[117]

11. CONCLUSIONS

As sortase and the cell wall anchoring of surface adhesins are universal in Gram-positive bacteria, compounds that interfere with sortase function may be useful for the treatment of human infections. Sortase inhibitors should act as antiinfective agents that disrupt the display of surface proteins of Gram-positive microorganisms. As non-pathogenic microbes can be rapidly cleared by the immune system, immunocompetent individuals that have been infected with Gram-positive pathogens should benefit from the use of sortase inhibitors. Furthermore, the sorting reaction may be useful for the design of microorganisms that are engineered to perform immunological or biotechnological functions or can be used as vaccine delivery vehicles. All these applications require a rigorous and detailed understanding of the cell wall sorting mechanism. The recent description of in vivo and in vitro assays for the sorting reaction as well as the identification of sortase should help to further our understanding of this mechanism. The biochemical characterization of sortase, its sorting substrates, intermediate and final products are the most important questions that need to be addressed in the future.

ACKNOWLEDGMENTS. H.T.T. acknowledges support from the Predoctoral Training Program in Microbial Pathogenesis at UCLA (AI07323). S.K.M. was supported by the Predoctoral Training Program in Genetic Mechanisms at UCLA (T32GM07104). Work in O.S.'s laboratory is supported by a grant from the NIH-NIAID, Infectious Disease Branch AI33987.

REFERENCES

1. Lowy, F. D. *Staphylococcus aureus* infections. *New Engl. J. Med.* **339**, 520–532 (1998).
2. Hiramatsu, K. *et al.* Dissemination in Japanese hospitals of strains of *Staphylococcus aureus* heterogeneously resistant to vancomycin. *Lancet* **350**, 1670–1673 (1997).
3. Sieradzki, K., Roberts, R. B., Haber, S. W. & Tomasz, A. The development of vancomycin resistance in a patient with methicillin-resistant *Staphylococcus aureus* infection. *New Engl. J. Med.* **340**, 517–523 (1999).
4. Gold, H. S. & Moellering, R. C. Antimicrobial-drug resistance. *New Engl. J. Med.* **335**, 1445–1453 (1996).
5. Neu, H. C. The crisis in antibiotic resistance. *Science* **257**, 1064–1073 (1992).

6. Foster, T. J. & Höök, M. Surface protein adhesins of *Staphylococcus aureus*. *Trends Microbiol.* **6**, 484–488 (1998).

7. Jensen, K. A normally occuring staphylococcus antibody in human serum. *Acta Path. Microbiol. Scandin.* **44**, 421–428 (1958).

8. Forsgren, A. Protein A from *Staphylococcus aureus*. VI. Reaction with subunits from guinea pig gamma-1- and gamma-2-globulin. *J. Immunol.* **100**, 927–930 (1968).

9. Sjödahl, J. Repetitive sequences in protein A from *Staphylococcus aureus*. Arrangement of five regions within the protein, four being highly homologous and Fc-binding. *Eur. J. Biochem.* **73**, 343–351 (1977).

10. Guss, B. *et al.* Region X, the-cell-wall-attachment part of staphylococcal protein A. *Eur. J. Biochem.* **138**, 413–420 (1984).

11. Jonsson, P., Lindberg, M., Haraldsson, I. & Wadstrom, T. Virulence of *Staphylococcus aureus* in a mouse mastitis model: studies of hemolysin, coagulase, and protein A as possible virulence determinants with protoplast fusion and gene cloning. *Infect. Immun.* **49**, 765–769 (1985).

12. Patel, A. H., Nowlan, P., Weavers, E. D. & Foster, T. Virulence of protein A-deficient and alpha-toxin-deficient mutants of *Staphylococcus aureus* isolated by allele replacement. *Infect. Immun.* **55**, 3103–3110 (1987).

13. Flock, J. I. *et al.* Cloning and expression of the gene for a fibronectin-binding protein from *Staphylococcus aureus*. *EMBO J.* **6**, 2351–2357 (1987).

14. Signas, C. *et al.* Nucleotide sequence of the gene for a fibronectin-binding protein from *Staphylococcus aureus*: use of this peptide sequence in the synthesis of biologically active peptides. *Proc. Natl. Acad. Sci. USA* **86**, 699–703 (1989).

15. Jönsson, K., Signäs, C., Müller, H. P. & Lindberg, M. Two different genes encode fibronectin binding proteins in *Staphylococcus aureus*. The complete nucleotide sequence and characterization of the second gene. *Eur. J. Biochem.* **202**, 1041–1048 (1991).

16. Greene, C. *et al.* Adhesion properties of mutants of *Staphylococcus aureus* defective in fibronectin-binding proteins and studies on the expression of fnb genes. *Mol. Microbiol.* **17**, 1143–1152 (1995).

17. Sottile, J., Schwarzbauer, J., Selegue, J. & Mosher, D. F. Five type I modules of fibronectin form a functional unit that binds to fibroblasts and *Staphylococcus aureus*. *J. Biol. Chem.* **266**, 12840–12843 (1991).

18. McGavin, M. J., Raucci, G., Gurusiddappa, S. & Höök, M. Fibronectin binding determinants of the *Staphylococcus aureus* fibronectin receptor. *J. Biol. Chem.* **266**, 8343–8347 (1991).

19. McGavin, M. J. *et al.* Fibronectin receptors from *Streptococcus dysgalactiae* and *Staphylococcus aureus*. Involvement of conserved residues in ligand binding. *J. Biol. Chem.* **268**, 23946–23953 (1993).

20. Patti, J. M., Allen, B. L., McGavin, M. J. & Hook, M. MSCRAMM-mediated adherence of microorganisms to host tissues. *Annu. Rev. Microbiol.* **48**, 89–115 (1994).

21. Springer, T. A. The sensation and regulation of interactions with the extracellular environment: the cell biology of lymphocyte adhesion receptors. *Annu. Rev. Cell Biol.* **6**, 359–402 (1990).

22. Wesson, C. A. *et al.* *Staphylococcus aureus* Agr and Sar global regulators influence internalization and induction of apoptosis. *Infect. Immun.* **66**, 5238–5243 (1998).

23. Patti, J. M. *et al.* Molecular characterization and expression of a gene encoding a *Staphylococcus aureus* collagen adhesin. *J. Biol. Chem.* **267**, 4766–4772 (1992).

24. Smeltzer, M. S., Gillaspy, A. F., Pratt, F. L. J., Thames, M. D. & Iandolo, J. J. Prevalence and chromosomal map location of *Staphylococcus aureus* adhesin genes. *Gene* **196**, 249–259 (1997).

25. Snodgrass, J. L. et al. Functional analysis of the Staphylococcus aureus collagen adhesin B domain. Infect. Immun. 67, 3952–3959 (1999).

26. Switalski, L. M. et al. A collagen receptor on Staphylococcus aureus strains isolated from patients with septic arthritis mediates adhesion to cartilage. Mol. Microbiol. 7, 99–107 (1993).

27. Ryding, U., Flock, J. I., Flock, M., Söderquist, B. & Christensson, B. Expression of collagen-binding protein and types 5 and 8 capsular polysaccharide in clinical isolates of Staphylococcus aureus. J. Infect. Dis. 176, 1096–1099 (1997).

28. McDevitt, D., Francois, P., Vaudaux, P. & Foster, T. J. Molecular characterization of the clumping factor (fibrinogen receptor) of Staphylococcus aureus. Mol. Microbiol. 11, 237–248 (1994).

29. McDevitt, D., Francois, P., Vaudaux, P. & Foster, T. J. Identification of the ligand-binding domain of the surface-located fibrinogen receptor (clumping factor) of Staphylococcus aureus. Mol. Microbiol. 16, 895–907 (1995).

30. McDevitt, D. et al. Characterization of the interaction between the Staphylococcus aureus clumping factor (ClfA) and fibrinogen. Eur. J. Biochem. 247, 416–424 (1997).

31. Hartford, O., Francois, P., Vaudaux, P. & Foster, T. J. The dipeptide repeat region of the fibrinogen-binding protein (clumping factor) is required for functional expression of the fibrinogen-binding domain on the Staphylococcus aureus cell surface. Mol. Microbiol. 25, 1065–1076 (1997).

32. Ní Eidhin, D. et al. Clumping factor B (ClfB), a new surface-located fibrinogen-binding adhesin of Staphylococcus aureus. Mol. Microbiol. 30, 245–257 (1998).

33. Josefsson, E. et al. Three new members of the serine-aspartate repeat protein multigene family of Staphylococcus aureus. Microbiol. 144, 3387–3395 (1998).

34. Josefsson, E., O'Connell, D., Foster, T. J., Durussel, I. & Cox, J. A. The binding of calcium to the B-repeat segment of SrdD, a cell surface protein of Staphylococcus aureus. J. Biol. Chem. 273, 31145–31152 (1998).

35. Vaudaux, P. E. et al. Use of adhesion-defective mutants of Staphylococcus aureus to define the role of specific plasma proteins in promoting bacterial adhesion to canine arteriovenous shunts. Infect. Immun. 63, 585–590 (1995).

36. Nilsson, M. et al. A fibrinogen binding protein of Staphylococcus epidermidis. Infect. Immun. 66, 2666–2673 (1998).

37. Sjöquist, J., Meloun, B. & Hjelm, H. Protein A isolated from Staphylococcus aureus after digestion with lysostaphin. Eur. J. Biochem. 29, 572–578 (1972).

38. Lofdahl, S., Guss, B., Uhlén, M., Philipson, L. & Lindberg, M. Gene for staphylococcal protein A. Proc. Natl. Acad. Sci. USA 80, 697–701 (1983).

39. Uhlén, M. et al. Complete sequence of the staphylococcal gene encoding protein A. J. Biol. Chem. 259, 1695–1702 and 13628 (Corr.) (1984).

40. Uhlén, M., Guss, B., Nilsson, B., Gotz, F. & Lindberg, M. Expression of the gene encoding protein A in Staphylococcus aureus and coagulase-negative staphylococci. J. Bacteriol 159, 713–719 (1984).

41. Deisenhofer, J., Jones, T. A., Huber, R., Sjödahl, J. & Sjöquist, J. Crystallization, crystal structure analysis and atomic model of the complex formed by a human Fc fragment and fragment B of protein A from Staphylococcus aureus. Hoppe-Seyl. Zeitsch. Physiol. Chem. 359, 975–985 (1978).

42. Navarre, W. W. & Schneewind, O. Surface proteins of Gram-positive bacteria and the mechanisms of their targeting to the cell wall envelope. Microbiol. Mol. Biol. Rev. 63, 174–229 (1999).

43. Sjöquist, J., Movitz, J., Johansson, I.-B. & Hjelm, H. Localization of protein A in the bacteria. Eur. J. Biochem. 30, 190–194 (1972).

44. Schneewind, O., Model, P. & Fischetti, V. A. Sorting of protein A to the staphylococcal cell wall. *Cell* **70**, 267–281 (1992).
45. Schneewind, O., Mihaylova-Petkov, D. & Model, P. Cell wall sorting signals in surface protein of Gram-positive bacteria. *EMBO* **12**, 4803–4811 (1993).
46. Navarre, W. W. & Schneewind, O. Proteolytic cleavage and cell wall anchoring at the LPXTG motif of surface proteins in gram-positive bacteria. *Mol. Microbiol.* **14**, 115–121 (1994).
47. Schneewind, O., Fowler, A. & Faull, K. F. Structure of the cell wall anchor of surface proteins in *Staphylococcus aureus*. *Science* **268**, 103–106 (1995).
48. Mazmanian, S. K., Liu, G., Ton-That, H. & Schneewind, O. *Staphylococcus aureus* sortase, an enzyme that anchors surface proteins to the cell wall. *Science* **285**, 760–763 (1999).
49. Ton-That, H. & Schneewind, O. Anchor structure of staphylococcal surface proteins. IV. Inhibitors of the cell wall sorting reaction. *J. Biol. Chem.* **274**, 24316–24320 (1999).
50. Ton-That, H., Faull, K. F. & Schneewind, O. Anchor structure of staphylococcal surface proteins. I. A branched peptide that links the carboxyl terminus of proteins to the cell wall. *J. Biol. Chem.* **272**, 22285–22292 (1997).
51. Navarre, W. W., Ton-That, H., Faull, K. F. & Schneewind, O. Anchor structure of staphylococcal surface proteins. II. COOH-terminal structure of muramidase and amidase-solubilized surface protein. *J. Biol. Chem.* **273**, 29135–29142 (1998).
52. Jones, C. L. & Khan, S. A. Nucleotide sequence of the enterotoxin B gene from *Staphylococcus aureus*. *J. Bacteriol.* **166**, 29–33 (1986).
53. Tweten, R. K. & Iandolo, J. J. Transport and processing of staphylococcal enterotoxin B. *J. Bacteriol.* **153**, 297–303 (1983).
54. Wang, P.-Z. & Novick, R. P. Nucleotide sequence and expression of the β-lactamase gene from *Staphylococcus aureus* plasmid pI258 in *Escherichia coli*, *Bacillus subtilis*, and *Staphylococcus aureus*. *J. Bacteriol.* **169**, 1763–1766 (1987).
55. Navarre, W. W. & Schneewind, O. Cell wall sorting of lipoproteins in *Staphylococcus aureus*. *J. Bacteriol.* **178**, 441–446 (1996).
56. Schindler, C. A. & Schuhardt, V. T. Lysostaphin: a new bacteriolytic agent for the staphylococcus. *Proc. Natl. Acad. Sci. USA* **51**, 414–421 (1964).
57. Recsei, P. A., Gruss, A. D. & Novick, R. P. Cloning, sequence, and expression of the lysostaphin gene from *Staphylococcus simulans*. *Proc. Natl. Acad. Sci. USA* **84**, 1127–1131 (1987).
58. Heath, H. E., Heath, L. S., Nitterauer, J. D., Rose, K. E. & Sloan, G. L. Plasmid-encoded lysostaphin endopeptidase resistance of *Staphylococcus simulans* biovar *staphylolyticus*. *Biochem. Biophys. Res. Com.* **160**, 1106–1109 (1989).
59. Thumm, G. & Götz, F. Studies on prolysostaphin processing and characterization of the lysostaphin immunity factor (*lif*) of *Staphylococcus aureus* biovar *staphylolyticus*. *Mol. Microbiol.* **23**, 1251–1265 (1997).
60. Baba, T. & Schneewind, O. Target cell specificity of a bacteriocin molecule: a C-terminal signal directs lysostaphin to the cell wall of *Staphylococcus aureus*. *EMBO J.* **15**, 4789–4797 (1996).
61. Samuelson, P. *et al.* Cell surface display of recombinant proteins on Staphylococcus carnosus. *J. Bacteriol.* **177**, 1470–1476 (1995).
62. Pozzi, G., Contorni, M., Oggioni, M. R., Manganeli, R. & Fischetti, V. A. Expression of the M6 protein gene of *Streptococcus pyogenes* in *Streptococcus gordonii* after chromosomal integration and transcriptional fusion. *Infect. Immun.* **60**, 1902–1907 (1992).
63. Piard, J. C. *et al.* Cell wall anchoring of the *Streptococcus pyogenes* M6 protein in various lactic acid bacteria. *J. Bacteriol.* **179**, 3068–3072 (1997).

64. Strauss, A. & Gotz, F. *In vivo* immobilization of enzymatically active polypeptides on the cell surface of *Staphylococcus carnosus*. *Mol. Microbiol.* **21**, 491–500 (1996).

65. Gunneriusson, E., Samuelson, P., Uhlen, M., Nygren, P. A. & Stähl, S. Surface display of a functional single-chain Fv antibody on staphylococci. *J. Bacteriol.* **178**, 1341–1346 (1996).

66. Berger-Bachi, B. Expression of resistance to methicillin. *Trends Microbiol.* **2**, 389–309 (1994).

67. Hartman, B. J. & Tomasz, A. Low affinity penicillin binding protein associated with b-lactam resistance in *Staphylococcus aureus*. *J. Bacteriol.* **158**, 513–516 (1984).

68. Matsuhashi, M. *et al.* Molecular cloning of the gene for penicillin-binding protein supposed to cause high resistance to b-lactamase antibiotics in *Staphylococcus aureus*. *J. Bacteriol.* **167**, 975–980 (1986).

69. Berger-Bachi, B., Barberis-Maino, L., Strassle, A. & Kayser, F. H. FemA, a host-mediated factor essential for methicillin resistance in *Staphylococcus aureus*: molecular cloning and characterization. *Mol. Gen. Genet.* **219**, 263–269 (1989).

70. Berger-Bachi. Mapping and characterization of multiple chromosomal factors involved in methicillin resistance in *Staphylococcus aureus*. *Antimicrob. Agents Chemother.* **36**, 1367–1373 (1992).

71. DeLencastre, H. & Tomasz, A. Reassessment of the number of auxiliary genes essential for expression of high-level methicillin resistance in *Staphylococcus aureus*. *Antimicrob. Agents Chemother.* **38**, 2590–2598 (1994).

72. de Jonge, B. L. M. *et al.* Altered muropeptide composition in *Staphylococcus aureus* strains with an inactivated *femA* locus. *J. Bacteriol.* **175**, 2779–2782 (1993).

73. Henze, U., Sidow, T., Wecke, J., Labischinski, H. & Berger-Bachi, B. Influence of *femB* on methicillin resistance and peptidoglycan metabolism in *Staphylococcus aureus*. *J. Bacteriol.* **175**, 1612–1620 (1993).

74. Maidhof, H., Reinicke, B., Blumel, P., Berger-Bachi, B. & Labischinski, H. *femA*, which encodes a factor essential for expression of methicillin resistance, affects glycine content of peptidgylcan in methicillin-resistant and methicillin susceptible *Staphylococcus aureus* strains. *J. Bacteriol.* **173**, 3507–3513 (1991).

75. Stranden, A., Ehlert, K., Labischinski, H. & Berger-Bachi, B. Cell wall monoglycine cross-bridges and methicillin hypersusceptibility in a *femAB* null mutant of methicillin-resistant *Staphylococcus aureus*. *J. Bacteriol.* **1997**, 9–16 (1997).

76. Gustafson, J., Strassle, A., Hachler, H., Kayser, F. H. & Berger-Bachi, B. The *femC* locus of *Staphylococcus aureus* required for methicillin resistance includes the glutamine synthetase operon. *J. Bacteriol.* **176**, 1460–1467 (1994).

77. Jolly, L. *et al.* The *femR315* gene from *Staphylococcus aureus*, the interruption of which results in reduced methicillin resistance, encodes a phosphoglucosamine mutase. *J. Bacteriol.* **179**, 5321–5325 (1997).

78. Kopp, U., Roos, M., Wecke, J. & Labischinski, H. Staphylococcal peptidoglycan interpeptide bridge biosynthesis: a novel antistaphylococcal target? *Microb. Drug Resist.* **2**, 29–41 (1996).

79. Rohrer, S., Ehlert, K., Tschierske, M., Labischinski, H. & Berger-Bächi, B. The essential *Staphylococcus aureus* gene *fmhB* is involved in the first step of peptidoglycan pentaglycine interpeptide formation. *Proc. Natl. Acad. Sci. USA* **96**, 9351–56 (1999).

80. Matsuhashi, M., Dietrich, C. P. & Strominger, J. L. Incorporation of glycine into the cell wall glycopeptide in *Staphylococcus aureus*: Role of sRNA and lipid intermediates. *Proc. Natl. Acad. Sci. USA* **54**, 587–594 (1965).

81. Matsuhashi, M., Dietrich, C. P. & Strominger, J. L. Biosynthesis of the peptidoglycan of bacterial cell walls. III. *J. Biol. Chem* **242**, 3191–3206 (1967).

82. Petit, J.-F., Munoz, E. & Ghuysen, J. M. Peptide cross-links in bacterial cell wall peptidoglycans studied with specific endopeptidases from Streptomyces albus G. *Biochemistry* **5**, 2764–2776 (1966).

83. Ton-That, H., Labischniski, H., Berger-Bachi, B. & Schneewind, O. Anchor structure of staphyococcal surface proteins. III. The role of the FemA, FemB, and FemX factors in anchoring surface proteins to the bacterial cell wall. *J. Biol. Chem.* **273**, 29143–29149 (1998).

84. Mazmanian, S. K., Liu, G., Jensen, E. R., Lenoy, E. & Schneewind, O. *Staphylococcus aureus* mutants defective in the display of surface proteins and in the pathogenesis of animal infections. *Proc. Natl. Acad. Sci. USA* **97**, 5510–5515 (2000).

85. Ton-That, H., Liu, G., Mazmanian, S. K., Faull, K. F. & Schneewind, O. Purification and characterization of sortase, the transpeptidase that cleaves surface proteins of *Staphylococcus aureus* at the LPXTG motif. *Proc. Natl. Acad. Sci. USA* **96**, 12424–12429 (1999).

86. Lipmann, F. & Tuttle, L. C. The detection of activated carboxyl groups with hydroxylamine as interceptor. *J. Biol. Chem.* **161**, 415–416 (1945).

87. Ton-That, H., Mazmanian, H., Faull, K. & Schneewind, O. Anchoring of surface proteins to the cell wall of *Staphylococcus aureus*. I. Sortase catalyzed in vitro transpeptidation reaction using LPXTG peptide and NH2-Gly3 substrates. *J. Biol. Chem.* **275**, 9876–9881 (2000).

88. Ghuysen, J.-M. Use of bacteriolytic enzymes in determination of wall structure and their role in cell metabolism. *Bacteriol. Rev.* **32**, 425–464 (1968).

89. Tipper, D. J. & Strominger, J. L. Mechanism of action of penicillins: a proposal based on their structural similarity to acyl-D-alanyl-alanine. *Proc. Natl. Acad. Sci. USA* **54**, 1133–1141 (1965).

90. Ghuysen, J.-M. & Strominger, J. L. Structure of the cell wall of *Staphylococcus aureus*, strain Copenhagen. II. Separation and structure of the disaccharides. *Biochemistry* **2**, 1119–1125 (1963).

91. Ghuysen, J.-M., Tipper, D. J., Birge, C. H. & Strominger, J. L. Structure of the cell wall of *Staphylococcus aureus* strain Copenhagen. VI. The soluble glycopeptide and its sequential degradation by peptidases. *Biochemistry* **4**, 2245–2254 (1965).

92. Ghuysen, J.-M. Serine beta-lactamases and penicillin binding proteins. *Annu. Rev. Microbiol.* **45**, 37–67 (1991).

93. Strominger, J. L., Izaki, K., Matsuhashi, M. & Tipper, D. J. Peptidoglycan transpeptidase and D-alanine carboxypeptidase: penicillin-sensitive enzymatic reactions. *Fed. Proc.* **26**, 9–18 (1967).

94. Strominger, J. L. Penicillin-sensitive enzymatic reactions in bacterial cell wall synthesis. *Harvey Lectures* **64**, 179–213 (1968).

95. Rasmussen, J. R. & Strominger, J. L. Utilization of depsipeptide substrate for trapping acyl-enzyme intermediates of penicillin-sensitive D-alanine carboxypeptidases. *Proc. Natl. Acad. Sci. USA* **75**, 84–88 (1978).

96. Kozarich, J. W., Tokuzo, N., Willoughby, E. & Strominger, J. L. Hydroxylaminolysis of penicillin binding components is enzymatically catalyzed. *J. Biol. Chem.* **252**, 7525–7529 (1977).

97. Kozarich, J. W. & Strominger, J. L. A membrane enzyme from Staphylococcus aureus which catalyzes transpeptidase, carboxypeptidase, and penicillinase activities. *J. Biol. Chem.* **253**, 1272–1278 (1978).

98. Ferguson, M. A. J., Homans, S. W., Dwek, R. A. & Rademacher, T. W. Glycosylphosphatidylinositol moiety that anchors Trypanosoma brucei variant surface glycoprotein to the membrane. *Science* **239**, 753–759 (1988).

99. Borst, P. & Cross, G. A. Molecular basis for trypanosome antigenic variation. *Cell* **29**, 291–303 (1982).

100. Ferguson, M. A., Duszenko, M., Lamont, G. S., Overath, P. & Cross, G. A. Biosynthesis of *Trypanosoma brucei* variant surface glycoproteins. N-glycosylation and addition of a phosphatidylinositol membrane anchor. *J. Biol. Chem.* **261**, 356–362 (1986).

101. Fox, J. A., Duszenko, M., Ferguson, M. A., Low, M. G. & Cross, G. A. Purification and characterization of a novel glycan-phosphatidylinositol-specific phospholipase C from *Trypanosoma brucei*. *J. Biol. Chem.* **261**, 15767–15771 (1986).

102. Cross, G. A. Glycolipid anchoring of plasma membrane proteins. *Annu. Rev. Cell Biol.* **6**, 1–39 (1990).

103. Cross, G. A. Structure of the variant glycoproteins and surface coat of *Trypanosoma brucei*. *Phil. Trans. Royal Soc.* **307**, 3–12 (1984).

104. Hoeijmakers, J. H., Frasch, A. C., Bernards, A., Borst, P. & Cross, G. A. Novel expression-linked copies of the genes for variant surface antigens in trypanosomes. *Nature* **284**, 78–80 (1980).

105. Menon, A. K., Mayor, S., Ferguson, M. A., Duszenko, M. & Cross, G. A. Candidate glycophospholipid precursor for the glycosylphosphatidylinositol membrane anchor of *Trypanosoma brucei* variant surface glycoproteins. *J. Biol. Chem.* **263**, 1970–1977 (1988).

106. Kodukula, K., Gerber, L. D., Amthauer, R., Brink, L. & Udenfriend, S. Biosynthesis of glycosylphosphatidylinositoal (GPI)-anchored membrane proteinsin intact cells: specific amino acid requirements adjacent to the site of cleavage and GPI attachment. *J. Cell Biol.* **120**, 657–664 (1993).

107. Caras, I. W., Weddell, G. N. & Williams, S. R. Analysis of the signal for attachment of a glycophospholipid membrane anchor. *J. Cell Biol.* **108**, 1387–1396 (1989).

108. Udenfriend, S. & Kodukula, K. How glycosylphosphatidylinositol-anchored membrane proteins are made. *Annu. Rev. Biochem.* **64**, 563–591 (1995).

109. Benghezal, M., Lipke, P. N. & Conzelmann, A. Identification of six complementation classes involved in the biosynthesis of glycosylphosphatidylinositol anchors in *Saccharomyces cerevisiae*. *J. Ce. Biol.* **130**, 1333–1344 (1995).

110. Leidich, S. D. & Orlean, P. Gpi1, a *Saccharomyces cerevisiae* protein that participates in the first step in glycosylphosphatidylinotisol anchor synthesis. *J. Biol. Chem.* **271**, 27829–27837 (1996).

111. Benghezal, M., Benachour, A., Rusconi, S., Aebi, M. & Conzelmann, A. Yeast Gpi8 is essential for GPI anchor attachment onto proteins. *EMBO J.* **15**, 6575–6583 (1996).

112. Hamburger, D., Egerton, M. & Riezman, H. Yeast Gaa1p is required for attachment of a complete GPI anchpr onto proteins. *J. Cell Biol.* **129**, 629–639 (1995).

113. Ramalingam, S. *et al.* COOH-terminal processing of nascent polypeptides by the glycosylphosphatidylinositol transamidase in the presence of hydrazine is governed by the same parameters as glycosylphosphatidylinositol addition. *Proc. Natl. Acad. Sci. USA* **93**, 7528–7533 (1996).

114. Yu, J. *et al.* The affected gene underlying the class K glycosylphosphatidylinositol (GPI) surface protein defect codes for the GPI transamidase. *Proc. Natl. Acad. Sci. USA* **94**, 12580–12585 (1997).

115. Yeung, M. K. & Cisar, J. O. Sequence homology between the subunits of two immunologically and functionally distinct types of fimbriae of *Actinomyces spp. J. Bacteriol.* **172**, 2462–2468 (1990).

116. Yeung, M. K., Donkersloot, J. A., Cisar, J. O. & Ragsdale, P. A. Identification of a gene involved in assembly of *Actinomyces naeslundii* T14V type 2 fimbriae. *J. Bacteriol.* **66**, 1482–1491 (1998).

117. Dhar, G., Faull, K. F. & Schneewind, O. Anchor structure of cell wall surface proteins in *Listeria monocytogenes. Biochemistry* **in press** (2000).

118. Yeung, M. K., Donkersloot, J. A., Cisar, J. O. & Ragsdale, P. A. Identification of a gene involved in assembly of Actinomyces naeslundii T14V type 2 fimbriae. *Infection & Immunity* **66**, 1482–1491 (1998).

10

Pore-forming Cytolysins α- and γ-Hemolysins and Leukocidin from *Staphylococcus aureus*

YOSHIYUKI KAMIO, TOSHIO TOMITA, and JUN KANEKO

1. INTRODUCTION

Staphylococcus aureus produces a variety of extracellular proteins including five cytolytic toxins (i.e., α-, β-, γ, δ-hemolysins, and leukocidin), coagulase, enterotoxins A-E, toxin shock syndrome toxin-1, and others. These exoproteins may play important roles in establishing and maintaining infections of the bacterium.

α-Hemolysin (Hla) is a 33-kDa polypeptide secreted by most of clinically isolated *S. aureus*, and it has been shown to be a major virulence determinant in animal models of infection. This toxin has been proven to form pores in the cytoplasmic membranes of target cells.[1] Recently, the structure of Hla have been determined to 1.9Å resolution. γ-Hemolysin (Hlg), leukocidin (Luk) and Panton-Valentine leukocidin (**PVL**) have been isolated as the bi-component cytolysins from *S. aureus*.[2] These toxins have also been proven to be pore-forming toxins. Hlg consists of Hlg1 and Hlg2 components that cooperatively lyse erythrocytes from mammalian species. Luk and PVL, which are composed of LukS and LukF, and LukS-PV and LukF-PV, respectively, exhibit a narrow cell specificity for polymorphonuclear leukocytes (PMNLs) and monocytes/macrophages. Recently, it was demonstrated that Hlg shares a common component with Luk (i.e., Hlg1 of Hlg

---

Abbreviations: Hla, α-hemolysin; Hlg, γ-hemolysin; Luk, leukocidin; PVL, Panton-Valentine leukocidin; PMNLs, polymorphonuclear leukocytes binding to Hlg2 and LukS of the toxins.

YOSHIYUKI KAMIO, TOSHIO TOMITA, and JUN KANEKO • Department of Molecular and Cell Biology, Graduate School of Agricultural Science, Tohoku University, Sendai 981-8555, Japan.

Staphylococcus aureus *Infection and Disease*, edited by Allen L. Honeyman *et al.* Kluwer Academic/Plenum Publishers, New York, 2001.

is identical with LukF of Luk) and that the genes encoding PVL exist on the genome of a lysogenic bacteriophage φPVL. Most recently, the 3-dimensional structures of the water-soluble LukF and LukF-PV have been determined.

In the first part of this article, we will depict the roles of cell membranes in the pore formation by Hla as well as the molecular dissection of the toxin for understanding its pore-forming nature. Subsequently, we will refer to the current status of knowledge of molecular cloning of the genes coding, for PVL, Luk, and Hlg, molecular domains of the toxins which determine the cell specificities, 3-dimensional structure of LukF, mode of action of these bi-component toxins, and a clinical aspect of PVL. Finally, we will describe vitronection and its fragments as serum inhibitors of Hlg and Luk, and their specific.

2. MOLECULAR BASIS FOR THE MEMBRANE PORE FORMATION BY HLA

Chemical Nature of Hla

Hla is a hydrophilic 33-kDa polypeptide lacking cysteine. The *hla* gene was cloned from the *S. aureus* Wood 46 strain and sequenced. The deduced sequence of the 293 amino acids in the toxin does not have extensive stretches of hydrophobic amino acids. Circular dichroism spectroscopy indicates that Hla is predominatly β-sheet. In 1996, crystals of the Hla heptamer have been obtained using the nonionic detergent n-decyldimethyl- and n-decyldiethlphosphine oxide, and its structure has been determined to 1.9 Å resolution.[3,4] However, three-dimensional structure of water soluble monomer of Hla remains to be elucidated, mainly because of the difficulty in preparation of crystals of Hla monomer (i.e., Hla has a tendency to form amorphous and filamentous aggregates at higher concent-rations). The detail information on the structure of Hla heptamer as a transmembrane pore will be described in the later section.

Hla as a Prototype of Pore-forming Cytolysins

Early functional studies indicated that Hla induces the leakage of internal potassium ions from erythrocytes, followed by the ultimate colloid osmotic lysis of the cells. Important findings for understanding this hemolytic process were reported in late 1960s that Hla forms an annular structure with a diameter of approximately 10 nm on the surface of erythrocytes. Subsequent studies showed that the ring-shaped structures represented 12S oligomers, possibly hexamers, which were formed through aggregation of native 3S mono-meric toxin. The concept of Hla as a pore-forming cytolysin was proposed by Bhakdi and his colleagues in early 1980s on the basis of the findings that the annular structures of Hla formed on erythrocytes appeared to form transmembrane pores which allowed small molecules and ions to pass through. The membrane pore formed by Hla has been shown to be a nonselective ion channel with functional diameter of 1.1–2.5 nm. Image processing of electron micrographs and cross-linking of Hla oligomers on membranes suggested that the membrane pore is a hexamer. However, recent studies demonstrated a heptameric stoichiometry by the analysis of X-ray diffraction of single crystals of toxin oligomers. Heptamerization of the toxin on membranes was also shown by the gel-shift electrophoresis of the toxin molecules which were chemically-modified before and after oligomerization on the cell surface of rabbit erythrocytes.[3]

Molecular Domains of Hla Involved in Pore Formation

The central portion of Hla contains a glycine-rich region from residue 119 to residue 143. Based on the resistance to protease digestion, this region has been suggested to be occluded during the assembly of monomeric toxin into heptamer. Bayley and his colleagues developed an *in vitro* transcription and translation system for the production of truncation mutants of Hla encompassing the N-terminal or C-terminal half of the polypeptide, and they used this system for the functional complementation between the truncation mutants.[5] Their data suggested that the glycine-rich central region is not directly involved in oligomer formation, but it is more important for the final step in pore assembly. More recently, Palmer *et al.* deviced hemolytically active, site-selectively modifiable toxin by introduction of a cysteine residue (which is not contained in the wild-type toxin), followed by cross-linking of a fluorescent dye (6-acryloyl-2-dimethyl-amino-naphthalene, or acrylodan) to the cysteine.[6] By use of the mutant toxin carrying a cysteine at position 130, they showed that the fluorescent acrylodan linked to the cysteine was inserted into the lipid bilayer during pore formation, and that it possibly moved in close proximity to the internal membrane surface. Furthermore, they assigned the residues 126–140 for a trans-membrane sequence in the pore by the analysis of a series of single cysteine replacement mutants.[7, 8]

It has been shown that Hla fragments encompassing its N-terminal or C-terminal half exhibit binding activity towards rabbit erythrocytes, although they do not form oligo-mers.[14,18,19] Recent studies using a series of cysteine replacement mutants suggested that the C-terminal third part of Hla as well as the second half of the N-terminal third part of the toxin are responsible for toxin binding, and that the C-terminal third segment of the toxin is involved in the interaction between toxin protomers.[8] The crystal structure of heptamer pore revealed a mushroom-like shape with a diameter of 100 Å and a height of 100 Å in which the lower half of the stem, a 14 strand β-barrel, forms a transmembrane channel made up of residues from the seven central glycine-rich regions of the polypeptide chains (Figures 1A and 10). The interior of the β-barrel is hydrophilic, and the exterior has a hydrophobic belt with 28 Å in width. The N- and C-terminal thirds of the polypeptides form the cap of the mushroom, which is also rich in structure and residues outside the target cell. Interactions between the heptamer and the lipid head groups involve both the stem and the rim domains. When R200 residue was changed to a cysteine and chemically modified, the monomer of Hla binding to rabbit erythrocytes is abolished. X-ray analysis of the crystals of Hla heptamer also revealed that a cleft lined by W179 and R200 residues is a binding site for phospholipid head groups.

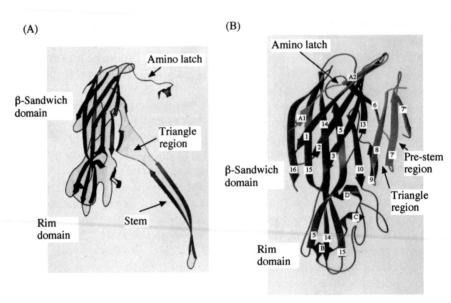

FIGURE 1. Ribbon representations of the single protomer of Hla taken from the Hla heptamer structure (A) and LukF water-soluble monomer (B). The pre-stem region of LukF makes hydrophobic contacts with the inner sheet of the β-sandwich domain. Hla protomer and LukF comparison will be depicted later. (A) and (B) were modified from the figures described by R. Olson *et al.* (reference 45). Reprints were permitted by the publisher.

Physical and Chemical Properties of Membranes that Affect the Pore-forming Process of Hla

It has been suggested that the susceptibility of mammalian erythrocytes to Hla is determined by the existence of putative receptor(s) (or high affinity binding sites). The putative receptor(s) for Hla are considered to be present on rabbit erythrocytes but absent on human erythrocytes. However, all attempts so far failed to isolate receptor molecule(s) from erythrocyte membranes, so that the molecular entity of the high affinity binding sites on rabbit erythrocytes is still enigmatic.

By use of multilamellar liposomes with defined physical and chemical properties, the roles of cell membranes in binding, assembly and pore formation of Hla were studied.[9-11] In order to avoid the exposure of hydrophobic surface on membranes, we employed multi-lamellar liposomes whose curvatures were in the size comparable with that of erythrocytes. The liposomes had mean diameters of 5–8 μm, and they responded thermotrophically well.

Assay for toxin binding to liposomes of various compositions showed that Hla binds much more (>100-fold) efficiently to the choline-type phospholipids (or phosphatidyl-choline and sphingomyelin) than to the other phospholipids and sphingoglycolipids.[9] The idea of the choline-type phospholipids as the binder molecules for Hla is consistent with the assymmetrical, preferential distribution of these lipids in the outer leaflet of the cell membrane of erythrocytes. Furthermore, these lipids may play a role for binding of Hla to lipid bilayers, even though the other molecule(s) would serve as receptor(s) for Hla.

Subsequently, we studied influence of membrane fluidity on the post-binding steps of the pore-forming process of Hla by using phosphatidylcholine liposomes of different acyl composition and cholesterol content.[10,11] We prepared liposome-bound toxin under conditions using solid and fluid membranes, and then assayed accessibility (or hemolytic activity) of the membrane-bound toxin to rabbit erthrocytes added, oligomerization of the membrane-bound toxin using SDS-polyacrylamide gel electrophoresis without preheating at 100°C, and susceptibility of liposome-bound toxin to trypsin digestion. The data showed the followings: [1] Hla binds to membranes as a hemolytically-active (reversibly-bound) state. [2] When phosphatidycholine membranes are fluidized either by phase transition or by inclusion of cholesterol over 20 mol%, hemolytic activity of the membrane-bound toxin is irreversibly decreased in a fashion of first-order kinetics with a half time of about 1 min, and thereafter assembly of the toxin gradually proceeds in the following 60 min. [3] Coexistence of unsaturated acyl chain-carrying phosphatidylcholine and cholesterol in membranes is a prerequisite for efficient oligomerization of Hla.[10] Interaction of Hla with these lipids in membranes remains to be elucidated at the molecular level. [4] Depending on the presence or absence of cholesterol, toxin oligomers may have different topology on/in membranes. Trypsin digestion liberated the N-terminal 8-amino-acid segment from membrane-bound oligomers only when the membranes included cholesterol. This finding implies that cholesterol may play a role in the final step for the formation of functional heptamer.

A working hypothesis for the membrane pore formation by Hla mainly on the basis of our data was summarized (Figure 2): [1] Hla binds to the exposed lipid bilayers composed of choline-type phospholipids as a hemolytically-active (or reversibly-bound) monomer. [2] When membrane is fluidized, the membrane-bound, hemolytically-active monomer is rapidly and irreversibly converted to nonhemolytic monomer. [3] The irreversively-bound monomer gradually assembles into stable but nonfunctional heptameron/in the fluidized membrane. [4] Unsaturated

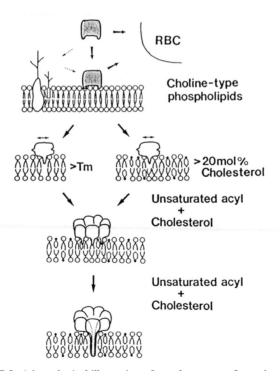

FIGURE 2. A hypothetical illustration of membrane pore formation by Hla.

acyl residue-carrying phospholipids and cholesterol cooperatively promotes the heptamerization of Hla and the following insertion of the transmembrane segment of the toxin into lipid bilayers, leading to the formation of functional pore. Recently, Gouaux *et al.* reported that from the analysis of the aligned sequence of Hla that the protomeric structures of Hla, PVL, and Luk components are quite similar.[12] Eventually, the X-ray analysis of the crystal structure of membrane-bound form of Hla and the water-soluble form of LukF and LukF-PV of PVL found to be quite similar in structure except only for the stem domain of each component. We will describe it later.

3. MOLECULAR CLONING OF THE GENES ENCODING STAPHYLOCOCCAL BI-COMPONENT CYTOLYSINS AND MOLECULAR DISSECTION OF THESE CYTOLYSINS FOR UNDERSTANDING THEIR CELL SPECIFICITIES

Description of a Family of Staphylococcal Bi-component Toxins

Four bi-component cytolysins have been isolated so far from the culture fluids of *Staphylocuccus aureus*. In this section, we will refer to the isolation and characterization of these toxins and their structure genes.

The first toxin is PVL that has been first purified by Woodin from the culture super-natants of *S. aureus* V8.[13] It contained two separate and synergistic protein components of 32 kDa and 38 kDa, which were refered to as S (for slow-eluted) and F (for fast-eluted), respectively, on the basis of their migration on carboxymethyl cellulose column. Later, Noda *et al.* purified leukocidin from the same bacterial strain using another purification procedure and crystallized the two components of the toxin.[14] PVL causes cytotoxic changes in PMNLs and monocytes from human and rabbit, and its cytotoxic activity towards target cells is highly specific. The genes *(lukF-PV* and *lukS-PV)* have been cloned (Figure 3A) and sequenced.[15]

The second is Luk which is secreted from *S. aureus* RIMD 310925. The genes coding for F and S components were first cloned and sequenced by our group in 1991 and 1992, and they were designated as *lukS* and *lukF*, respectively (Figure 3B).[16,17] We found that these genes are located in one cluster.[18] LukF and LukS should be destinguished from LukF-PV and LukS-PV, because LukF and LukS cooperatively lyse rabbit erythrocytes (but not human erythrocytes), whereas PVL (LukF-PV and LukS-PV) does not exhibit any hemolytic activity.

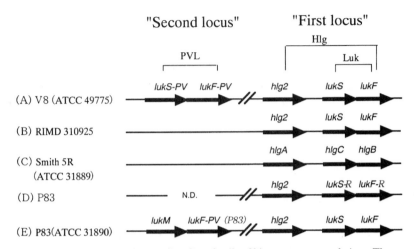

FIGURE 3. Staphylococcal genes coding for a family of bi-component cytolysines. The genes encoding staphylococcal leukocidin and γ-hemolysin are illustrated for five *S. aureus*. N.D., not determined.

The third cytolysin is Hlg that was first isolated from the culture supernatants of *S. aureus* Smith 5R as a bi-component hemolysin. Hlg consists of two distinct proteins of 32 kDa and 36 kDa. It is hemolytic to mammalian erythrocytes and cytolytic towards mammalian cultured cells. The Hlg genes (*hlg*), which were recently cloned and sequenced, are found to be in a gene cluster composed of *hlgA*, *hlgB*, and *hlgC* genes (Figure 3C).[19] Of the three *hlg* genes of *S. aureus* Smith 5R, *hlgB* and *hlgC* were found to have 97% homology with *lukF* and *lukS*, respectively, which have been previously cloned by our group from *S. aureus* RIMD 310925. HlgA (32 kDa) and HlgC (32 kDa) cause lysis of rabbit erythrocytes in combination with HlgB (36 kDa).[19]

The fourth bi-component toxin is leukocidin R (LukR) from *S. aureus* P83 strain, which was isolated from a bovine infected udder.[20] Two genes encoding LukR (*lukS-R* and *lukF-R*) were cloned and sequenced (Figure 3D). LukS-R and LukF-R are considered to correspond to HlgC and HlgB, respectively, because of the very high (97%) identity in their amino acid sequences. LukS-R and LukF-R can be distinguished from our Luk (LukS and LukF) and Hlg (HlgC and HlgB) of Smith 5R strain, because LukR can lyse human erythrocytes as well as PMNLs.[20] Recently, the gene coding for LukS-R, designated as *hlg2(P83)*, was cloned and sequenced (Figure 3E).[20] DNA sequencing data indicated that Hlg2(P83) corresponds to HlgA obtained from Smith 5R. However, Hlg2(P83) showed markedly low hemolytic activity in combination with LukF. This low activity of Hlg2(P83) is attributable to the replacement of arginine at position of 217 with lysine in HlgA.[21,22] Thus, Hlg2(P83) may be a single amino acid replacement mutant of HlgA. In 1995, a new protein component (LukM) was isolated and its gene (*lukM*) was cloned from the strain P83.[23] The *lukM* was found to be linked with *lukF-PV* in this strain.[24] We also found that LukM is a variant of LukS-PV.[25] In 1995, *S. aureus* V8 (ATCC 49775) was found to produce three more protein components besides LukS-PV and LukF-PV.[15] All three components were identified to be structural variants of the Hlg (see Figure 5). Purification of the five proteins and cloning of the corre-sponding genes provided evidence for the presence of two genetic loci in the strain (Figure 3). The "First locus" contains *hlg2*, *lukS*, and *lukF* genes (cloned from RIMD 310925 strain), which corre-sponds to *hlgA*, *hlgC*, and *hlgB* (cloned from Smith 5R). The "Second locus" contains *lukS-PV* and *lukF-PV* (cloned from ATCC 49775). In the following sections, we describe the current knowledge on the structural and biological properties of the bi-component toxins from *S. aureus*, mainly on the basis of our studies. Recently, we clarified that *lukM* and *lukF-PV* exist on the "Second locus" (Figure 3E) of the chromosome of the strain *S. aureus* ATCC 31890 as co-transcribed ORFs.[24]

Genes Coding PVL Exist on the Genome of a Temperate Bacteriophage (φPVL)[25,26]

It was known that only a few percents of *S. aureus* strains have the "Second locus" consisting of *LukS-PV* - *LukF-PV* cluster, and that these genes seems to be easily lost away from the cells. This fact led many investigators to study the origin of the "Second locus". However, no infor-mation about its origin was available. We found that the strains ATCC 49775 and 31890 have two common characteristics in the nucleotide sequences of the "Second locus" genes and their flanking regions, i.e., [1] there is a new open reading frame (ORF) upstream of the *lukS-PV* (or *lukM*) translation start codon. The amino acid sequence of the N-terminal 99 amino acid residues of this peptide showed more than 34% homology to the N-terminal region of a staphylococcal peptidoglycan hydrolase that is known to be from a prophage; and [2] one pair of 6-bp sequences, which resemble the core sequence of the φ11 phage attachment site, were located in the structural gene of *lukF-PV*. The data suggested, therefore, that the "Second locus" genes might be located on some extrachromosomal genetic element(s) specific to a few *S. aureus*. In 1997, we showed evidence that a phage-like particle (designated as φPVL) was isolated from the cleared lysate of mitomycin C-treated *S. aureus* ATCC 49775, and that the genome of φPVL contains *cos*, *attP* [*LukS -PV-LukF-PV*], *int*, and five direct repeat DNA sequences in close proximity. In 1998, the complete nucleotide sequence of the φPVL genome was analyzed, and the *att* sites (*attL*, *attR*, and *attB*) required for site-specific integration of φPVL into the host chromosome were also determined (Figure 4). The linear double-stranded φPVL genome comprised 41,401 bp with 3′ staggered cohesive ends (*cos*) of 9 bases, and it cotained 63 ORFs, among which regulatory proteins involved in DNA replication, structural proteins, a holin, a lysin, an integrase, and dUTPase, were tentatively identified by the comparison of the deduced amino acid sequences and by the analysis of the proteins isolated from φPVL particles. The [*lukS-PV-lukF-PV*], *attP*, and *int* (integrase gene) of φPVL were all located very close to one another within a 4.0 kb-segment on the genome in the order given, and this segment is located at the center from the left and the right *cos* sites. In addition, the *attP* region contained 5 direct repeat sequences which show high homology with the recombinase-binding sites of some other *S. aureus* bacteriophages. The φPVL genome was found to integrate into an ORF encoding an unknown protein com-prising 725 amino acid residues with two leucine zipper-like motifs.

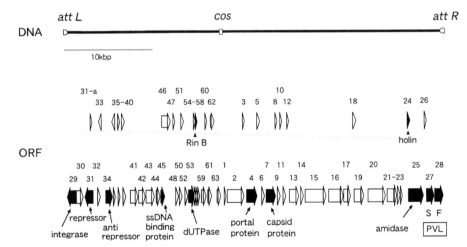

FIGURE 4. Schematic representation of the genome of φPVL with its identical ORFs and features. The numbered ORFs are depicted as arrows or arrowheads depending on their orientation. Putative functions of ORFs are indicated by closed arrows.

Luk and Hlg Share One Component

Luk and Hlg have previously been studied as distinct toxins with no structural or functional similarities. In 1993, however, we surprisingly found that LukF is identical with Hlg1 while purifying and characterizing Luk and Hlg from *S. aureus* RIMD 310925:[27] [1] Purified Hlg1 and LukF had a similarity in molecular size (34 kDa) as well as pI value (9.1). [2] The determined amino acid sequences for the N-terminal 59 amino acids and the C-terminal 2 amino acids of Hlg1 were identical to those of LukF. [3] In an Ouchterlony double diffusion test using anti-LukF and anti-Hlg1 antibodies, LukF and Hlg1 formed a fused line without spur, indicating that there is no apparent difference in antigenicity between them. [4] Combination of LukF with Hlg2 (instead of LukS) exhibited hemolytic activity, whereas Hlg1 and LukS (instead of Hlg2) cooperatively lysed human PMNLs. Thus, LukF and Hlg1 are interchangeable for expression of their cytolytic actvities.

To confirm the identity between LukF and Hlg1, we performed the following molecular genetical studies. *Hind*III fragments were obtained from the *Hind*III-digested chromosomal DNA of the strain RIMD310925, fractionated by agarose gel electrophoresis and used for hybridization with a *lukS*-containing probe (i.e., the 1.1 kbp *Eco*RI-*Xba*I frag-ment from plasmid pSA9-36).[18] The *lukS* probe recognized two *Hind*III fragments, the 12 kbp fragment containing *lukS* and *lukF* and another 3-kbp unknown fragment. DNA sequencing of these *Hind*III fragments indicated that the chromosomal region covering these fragments contains only three open reading frames for Hlg2, LukS, and LukF, which are aligned in this order.[18] Cloned LukS and cloned Hlg2 exhibited leukocytolytic and hemolytic activities, respectively, in the cooperation with the product of the third ORF (i.e., LukF or Hlg1). Thus, it is now evident that LukF is identical with Hlg1 of Hlg, so that the cell specificities of Luk and Hlg are determined by LukS and Hlg2, respectively.

Methods for Simultaneous Purification of Luk, PVL, and Hlg Components from *S. aureus*

The previously published procedures for purification of Luk are complicated and the final recoveries of both components are low. On the other hand, Hlg was partially purified by many groups and used for characterization of this toxin. However, the use of partially purified toxin preparations produced somewhat confusing data of the physiological properties of this toxin. The genetic studies by Foster and his colleagues have clearly shown that Hlg consists of two components,[19] and this was later confirmed by us.[33] The deduced amino acid sequences from the genes encoding LukS and Hlg2 indicated 72% amino acid homology between them.[16] This similarity of the primary structure in LukS and Hlg2 suggested us an application of the previous method (which was used for separation of Hlg2 from LukF) to the separation of LukS from LukF. By using an improved two-step method, we succeeded in the simultaneous purification of LukF, LukF-PV, LukS, LukS-PV, and Hlg2.[23] This procedure contains only two high performance column chromatographies using hydroxylapatite and cation exchange columns, and it yields more than 90% recovery of the toxin proteins from the stationary-growth-phased culture of *S. aureus.*

C-terminal Region of LukS is Essential for the Biological Activity of this Toxin Component[28]

LukS has been shown to bind specifically to monosialoganglioside GM1 (GM1) on the leukocyte membrane and activates phospholipase A2.[29] However, the nature of this binding was only poorly understood. While purifying LukF and LukS from a culture medium of *S. aureus*, we noticed that two protein peaks (LS1 and LS2) were eluted from the HPLC column at the position where LukS is usually eluted. We therefore purified these proteins to homogeneity and analyzed their chemical properties. On the basis of the N-terminal and C-terminal amino acid sequences of LS1 and LS2, it was concluded that LS1 is LukS itself whereas LS2 is a truncated form of LukS, which has lost the C-terminal 17-residue segment. LS2 was eluted after LukS from the cation exchange column, even though LS2 is more acidic than LukS because of the loss of 5 basic and 2 acidic residues from the C-terminus of LukS. This suggested the possibility that LukS and LS2 are in different conformations. Interestingly, LS2 showed no leukocytolytic activity in the presence of LukF, indicating that the C-terminal 17-residue segment of LukS is essential for Luk activity. LukS or LS2 was incubated with [$_3$H]-labelled GM1, and applied to a gel filtration. The radioactive ganglioside was co-eluted with LukS in the fraction corresponding to a molecular mass of about 30 kDa, and the molar ratio of LukS to GM1 in the fraction was determined to be about 1:1. In contrast, LS2 provides no evidence for its association to GM1. Therefore, we concluded that the C-terminal 17 amino acid residues of LukS play a pivotal role in the binding of the protein to GM1. To specify the amino acid residue(s) responsible for the binding of LukS to GM1, we constructed a mutant in which a glycine residue was substituted for W275 in LukS (see Figure 5), and assayed its binding to GM1 as well as its leukocytolytic activity.[30] The mutant showed neither the binding activity to GM1 nor cytolytic activity.

```
LukS      1:ANDTEDIGKGSDIEIIKRTEDKTSNKWGVTQNIQFDFVKDTKYNKDALILKMQGFISSRT
Hlg2      1:ENKIEDIGQGA--EIIKRTQDITSKRLAITQNIQFDFVKDKKYNKDALVVKMQGFISSRT
LukS-PV   1:DNNIENIGDGA--EVVKRTEDTSSDKWGVTQNIQFDFVKDKKYNKDALILKMQGFINSKT

         61:TYYNYKKTNHVKAMRWPFQYNIGLKTNDKYVSLINYLPKNKIESTNVSQTLGYNIGGNFQ
         59:TYSDLKKYPYIKRMIWPFQYNISLKTKDSNVDLINYLPKNKIDSADVSQKLGYNIGGNFQ
         59:TYYNYKNTDHIKAMRWPFQYNIGLKTNDPNVDLINYLPKNKIDSVNVSQTLGYNIGGNFN

        121:SAPSLGGNGSFNYSKSISYTQQNYVSEVEQQNSKSVLWGVKANSFATESGQKSAFDSDLF
        119:SAPSIGGSGSFNYSKTISYNQKNYVTEVESQNSKGVKWGVKANSFVTPNGQVSAYDQYLF
        119:SGPSTGGNGSFNYSKTISYNQQNYISEVEHQNSKSVQWGIKANSFITSLGKMSGHDPNLF

        181:VGYKPHSKDPRDYFVPDSELPPLVQSGFNPSFIATVSHEKGSSDTSEFEITYGRNMDVTH
        179:AQ-DPTGPAARDYFVPDNQLPPLIQSGFNPSFITTLSHERGKGDKSEFEITYGRNMDATY
        179:VGYKPYSQNPRDYFVPDNELPPLVHSGFNPSFIATVSHEKGSGDTSEFEITYGRNMDVTH

        241:AIKRSTHYGNSYLDGHRVHNAFVNRNYTVKYEVNWKTHEIKVKGQN            286
        238:A-----YVTRHRLAVDRKHDAFKNRNVTVKYEVNWKTHEVKIKSITPK           280
        239:ATRRTTHYGNSYLEGSRIHNAFVNRNYTVKYEVNWKTHEIKVKGHN            284
```

FIGURE 5. Comparison of the deduced amino acid sequence among LukS, Hlg2, and LukS-PV. In the residues in Hlg2 and LukS-PV, the identical residues with that of LukS are shaded. Dashed lines indicate deleted amino acids. The 5-residue segment KRLAI and R217 residue of Hlg2, the 2-residue segment DI of LukS, and the 5-residue segment IKRST of LukS and TRRTT of LukS-PV (Black boxes) are pivotal regions for the hemolytic activity of Hlg towards human erythrocytes, for the hemolytic activity of LukS towards rabbit erythrocytes, and the leukocytolytic activity of LukS and LukS-PV towards human and rabbit PMNLs, respectively. The residue W275 of LukS is a binding site of GM1.

Thus, it was concluded that the W275 residue of LukS is essential for its GM1 binding as well as its leukocytolytic activity.

Since LukS contains 4 tryptophan residues per molecule, conformational change of LukS upon binding to GM1 was examined by measuring intrinsic tryptophan fluorescence. When excited at 280 nm, LukS showed fluorescence with an emission maximum at 318 nm. The addition of GM1 to the LukS solution resulted in the reduction of fluorescence intensity and a blue shift of the emission maximum. At a 1 : 1 molar ratio of LukS to GM1, the reduction in fluorescence intensity was 33%, and the wave length for the maximum emission was 310 nm. Further addition of GM1 did not affect the fluorescence. Since it has been reported that occlusion of tryptophan residues from the protein surface is accompanied by a blue shift of tryptophan fluorescence, the above finding indicates that tryptophan residues in LukS become less exposed to the protein surface upon binding to GM1. The decreased fluorescence intensity might be due to the moving of the tryptophan residues in proximity to the quenching-inducible hydrophobic amino acids in the interior of the LukS molecule. The tryptophan fluorescence of LS2 also showed a emission maximum at 318 nm. However, this fluorescence was not affected by the addition of GM1 at any concentrations, providing further evidence that LS2 does not bind to GM1. These findings clearly indicate that a conformational change of LukS takes place on contact with GM1.

Hlg2 was also inactivated by the contact with GM1 at a molar ratio of 1:1, but not by any of the related glycolipids including monosialoganglioside G_{M2}, monosialoganglioside G_{M3}, disialoganglioside G_{D1a}, disialoganglioside G_{D1b}, disialoganglioside G_{D3}, cerebro-side sulfate, globoside, sialylparagloboside.[31] Gel filtration assay indicated that Hlg2 forms a Hlg2-GM1 complex.[31] Analysis of an intrinsic aromatic amino acid fluorescence of Hlg2 indicated that binding of GM1 to Hlg2 reduces the fluorescence intensity by 15% without changing the wavelength of maximum emission (or 325 nm). These findings suggest that GM1 is a possible receptor for the Hlg2 component on human red blood cells, and that Hlg2 protein takes a different conformation when bound to GM1.

Sequential Binding of the Two Components of Luk and Hlg to Their Target Cells

Woodin has first studied mode of action of leukocidin using purified two components of PVL, S and Figure.[13] He demonstrated that the two components of PVL synergistically lyse human PMNLs. Furthermore, he showed that preceding binding of the 32 kDa-component (corresponding to the S component) is a prerequisite for subsequent binding of 38 kDa-component (corresponding to the F component), leading to the lysis of leukocytes. Later, Noda et al. showed the sequential binding of the two components of another Luk, LukS and LukF, to rabbit PMNLs.[29] They showed that LukS binding induces LukF binding and subsequent activation of phospholipase A2 in rabbit PMNLs. Colin et al. also confirmed the Woodin's results.[32]

Since mode of action of Hlg was poorly understood, we first studied binding of its components to human erythrocytes.[33,34] Surprisingly, the precedence of the LukF (or Hlg1) binding was shown by the following evidence: LukF binding occurred irrespective of whether or not human erythrocytes have been preincubated with Hlg2, whereas no significant binding of Hlg2 took place without the preincubation of the erythrocytes with LukF. Thus, it was concluded that the LukF binding is a prerequisite for the subsequent binding of Hlg2 to erythrocytes, in contrast with the sequential binding of LukS and LukF to leukocytes.

Pore-forming Nature of Hlg and Luk[35,36]

When monitored the Hlg-induced hemolysis for single cells of human erythrocytes under a phase contrast microscope, it was observed that intact, disc-shaped erythrocytes became swollen and round-shaped cells with clear edge after the incubation with LukF and Hlg2 for 10 min, and the swollen cells lysed thereafter. Since swelling of cells is generally caused by the permeabilization of cell membranes, it was presumed that Hlg induced colloid osmotic lysis of human erythrocytes through pore formation. This assumption was supported by the following findings[35] [1] Hlg-induced hemolysis was prevented by the extracellular nonelectrolytes (such as polyethylene glycols) with the diameters of >2.5 nm, suggesting that the toxin forms a hydrophilic pore with a functional diameter of approximately 2.5 nm. [2] Electron microscopy of the negatively-stained, toxin-treated erythrocytes revealed that Hlg forms a ring-shaped structure, whose outer and inner diameters are approximately 7 and 3 nm, respectively. Therefore, the complex formation of Hlg on human erythrocytes was examined as follows: Cell-bound toxin was solubilized with SDS from erythrocyte membranes and it was then analyzed by SDS-polyacrylamide gel electrophoresis, followed by Western immunoblot using specific antisera raised against LukF and Hlg2. The data indicated that Hlg forms high-molecular-sized complex(es) of approximately 200 kDa, which contain LukF and Hlg2 at a molar ratio of 1:1 on the surface of human erythrocytes. Recently, the [LukF-Hlg2] complex was isolated. It was also demonstrated that the preceding binding of LukF is essential for the complex formation as well as for the Hlg2 binding. Furthermore, our recent data suggested that the membrane component(s), which are accessible by proteinase K, may be required for the complex formation of Hlg on human erythrocytes.[34] Taken together, Hlg may assemble into a annular complex on target membranes, forming a transmembrane pore with a functional diameters of approximately 2.5 nm.

Finck-Barbancon *et. al.* have reported that PVL causes influx of ethidium chloride, an impermeable ion to cell membrane, into human PMNLs.[37] Recently, Stalli *et al.* reported that PVL may stimulate intrinsic calcium channel(s) of human PMNLs, and the toxin may thereafter form membrane pore, leading to influx of extracellular ethidium ions.[38] Thus, PVL has been suggested to form membrane pores in the early stage its leukocytolytic action. However, molecular architecture of the membrane pore formed by PVL remained to be studied, and it should be also be elucidated whether or not the pore contains intrinsic membrane protein(s) of leukocytes. We studied membrane pore formation by Luk in the cell membrane of human PMNLs and rabbit erythrocytes and the following findings are evident. [1] Luk caused efflux of potassium ions from rabbit erythrocytes and swelling of the cells before hemolysis. However, ultimate lysis of the toxin-treated swollen erythro-cytes did not occur when polyethylene glycols with hydrodynamic diameters of ≥2.1 nm were present in the extracellular space. [2] Electron microscopy showed the presence of a ring-shaped structure with outer and inner diameters of 9 and 3 nm, respectively, on the Luk-treated human PMNLs and rabbit erythrocytes. [3] Ring-shaped structures of the same dimension were isolated from the target cells, and they contained LukS and LukF in a molar ratio of 1:1. [4] A single ring-shaped toxin complex had a molecular size of approximately 200 kDa. These results indicated that LukS and LukF assemble into a ring-shaped oligomer of approximately 200 kDa on the target cells, forming a membrane pore with a functional diameter approximately 2 nm.

Identification of the Essential Regions in LukS and Hlg2 for Their Specific Functions of the Toxins[39–42]

As stated above, we have demonstrated that LukF of Luk is identical with Hlg1 of Hlg, so that LukS and Hlg2 (Figure 5) should determine the specificities of these toxins towards their target cells. What region(s) of LukS and Hlg2 are pivotal for the cell specificities? To answer this question, we produced a series of chimeric proteins (LukS/Hlg2) and assayed these chimeric proteins for their specific cytolytic activity. We constructed 26 different plasmids which harbored chimeric genes (lukS/hlg2).[30] The chimeric genes of these plasmids were cloned down the lac promoter of pUC119 and expressed in E. coli. We intensively characterized six of the expressed chimeric proteins, which were designated as MHLS1, MHLS3, MHLS4, MHLS5, MHLS7, and MHLS8 (Figure 6): [1] The chimeric protein MHLS3, in which the N-terminal 164-residue segment of Hlg2 (which accounts for 60% of the entire residues of Hlg2) was replaced with the corresponding one of LukS, showed no hemolytic activity (Figure 6, lane 3). In contrast, the chimeric protein MHLS7, in which the first 60% of the N-terminal residues of LukS were replaced with the corre-sponding fragment of Hlg2, retained leukocytolytic activity (Figure 6, lane 6). [2] The chimeric protein MHLS4, in which the C-terminal 24 amino acid residues of LukS (V263NRNYTVKYEVNWKTHEIKVKGQN286) were replaced with those of Hlg2 (K255NRNVTVKYEVNWKTHEVRIK-SKSITPK280), lost leukocytolytic activity (Figure 6, lane 4). [3] Regardless of the substitution of the C-terminal 226 amino acid residues out of 286 residues of LukS for the corresponding residues of Hlg2, the chimeric protein MHLS5 showed full activity of Hlg (Figure 6, lane 5). On the

(A)   (B)

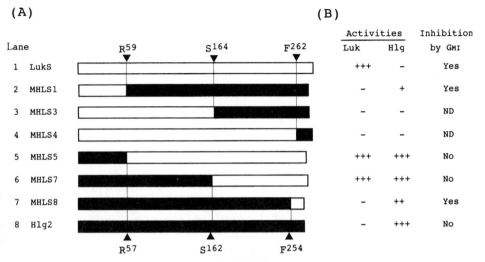

FIGURE 6. Schematic representation of LukS/Hlg2 chimeric proteins (A), and the results of the activities of leukocidin and γ-hemolysin, and the inhibition of the toxin activity by GM1 (B). Black and white boxes in (A) indicate the Hlg2- and LukS-segments, respectively. Triple, double, and single plus signs indicate 100%, 70%, and 10% or less activities compared with that of intact LukS and Hlg2, respectively. A minus indicates no detectable activity. N.D., not determined.

contrary, the substitution of the N-terminal 59 amino acid residues of LukS for those of Hlg2 lost almost all the hemolytic activity (Figure 6, lane 2). [4] The replacement of the C-terminal 26 amino acids of Hlg2 with the corresponding segment of LukS lowered the hemolytic activity to 70%, compared with that of intact Hlg2 (MHLS8; Figure 6, lane 7). The findings of [1], [2], and [3] clearly indicate that the essential regions for LukS- and Hlg2-specific functions are located within the C-terminal 24 residues of LukS and the N-terminal 59 residues of Hlg2, respectively. The data of [4] suggest that Hlg2 needs the amino acid sequence(s) between the S162 residue and the C-terminus for presentation of its full activity. Furthermore, it should be also noted that three chimeric proteins, or MHLS5, MHLS7, and MHLS8 were not inactivated by the addition of GM1 (Figure 6). The insusceptibility of these chimeric protein to the added GM1 remains to be explained.

In the 59-residue and 57-residue segments of the LukS and Hlg2, respectively, we found six regions which contain different amino acid residues between LukS and Hlg2 (Figure 5) i.e., (i) A1NDT4/E1NKI4 (Region A), (ii) K9GSDI13/Q9GA11 (—, deletion, Region B), (iii)

E21DK23/Q18DI20 (Region C), (iv) N25KWGV29/K23RLAI27 (Region D), (v)T41/K39 (Region E), and (iv) I49L50/V47V48 (Region F). To identify the segment(s) responsible for the γ-hemolysin activity, we constructed plasmids containing a series of mutant genes for each region, and inserted them into pUC119 to have a high level of lac-inducible expression in *E. coli*. As a result of these manipulations, four different plasmids that contained mutant genes were obtained and they were designated as pMLS-A, pMLS-D1, pMLS-AD1, and pMLS-D (Figure 7). The mutant protein expressed in *E. coli* harboring the appropriate plasmid was prepared from the sonicated extract of the cells, and purified to the degree of electrophoretic homogeneity.

The amino acid sequences from 1st to 35th of all mutant proteins coincided with that predicted from the nucleotide sequences found. When leukocytolytic and hemolytic activities of the purified mutant components were measured in the presence of LukF, the following findings became evident: [1] Mutant proteins MLS-A, MLS-D1, MLS-AD1, and MLS-D had full leukocytolytic activity as well as intact LukS (Figure 7, lanes 2–5). It is reasonable that they have the Luk activity, because they have the C-terminal 121-residue segment from Ser164 responsible for the leukocytolytic activity of intact LukS and the chimeric protein MHLS5 (Figure 7, lanes 1

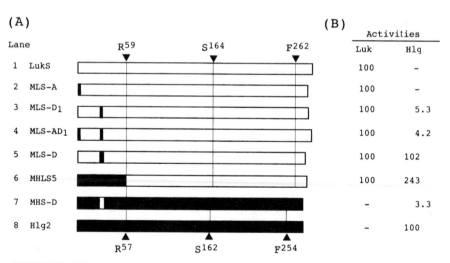

FIGURE 7. Schematic representation of LukS, Hlg2 and mutant proteins (A), and the resulting leukocidin and γ-hemolysin activities (B). Black and white boxes in (A) indicate the Hlg2- and LukS-segments, respectively. Percentage leukocytolysis and hemolysis indicate the activities compared with that of intact LukS (lane 1) and Hlg2 (lane 8). A minus indicates no detectable activity.

and 6). [2] Mutant protein MLS-A has no hemolytic activity (Figure 7, lane 2). [3] Mutants MLS-D1 and MLS-AD1, in which the entire 4-residue in Region A and 3-residue in Region D1 of the LukS were replaced by that of Hlg2, showed 5.3% and 4.2% hemolytic activity, respectively, compared with that of intact Hlg2 (Figure 7, lanes 3 and 4). [4] Mutant protein of LukS, MLS-D, in which 5-residue segment N25KWGV29 of LukS was replaced by the 5-residue segment K23RLAI27 of Hlg2, had full hemolytic activity (Figure 7, lane 5). The findings clearly indicate that the 5-residue segment K23RLAI27 in Region D of Hlg2 is necessary for the Hlg2 function. If γ-hemolysin-specific activity is decided by the 5-residue segment K23RLAI27 in Region D of Hlg2, γ-hemolysin activity should be lost or weakened by substituting the 5-residue segment N25KWGV29 of LukS for K23RLAI27 of Hlg2. Accordingly, we created the mutant protein MHS-D, in which the 5-residue segment K23RLAI27 of Hlg2 was replaced by N25KWGV29 of LukS (Figure 7, lane 7). The MHS-D lost almost all the hemolytic activity (Figure 7, lane 7). Thus, it was concluded that the 5-residue K23RLAI27 in Region D of Hlg2 is the minimum segment essential for the Hlg2-specific function of Hlg.

The binding order of the mutant protein MLS-D and LukF to the human erythrocytes was identified. The following findings are evident. [1] The initial binding of MLS-D as well as LukS is essential for the leukocytolytic activity. [2] In contrast, the binding of LukF is a prerequisite for the subsequent binding of MLS-D to human erythrocytes forming the [LukF-MLS-D] complex of about 200 kDa on the human erythrocytes for the hemolytic activity. [3] However, MHS-D could bind to LukF that had been initially bound to the erythrocytes. Thus, it is demonstrated that the 5-residue segment K23RLAI27 of Hlg2 has binding activity to LukF on the erythrocytes.

Luk can be distinguished from PVL with respect to its cytolytic spectrum, i.e., Luk lyses rabbit erythrocytes (but not human erythrocytes), whereas PVL reveals no hemolytic activity. We have recently showed that the D12 I13 of LukS is the determinant for its hemolytic activity towards rabbit erythrocytes: Deletion of D12 I13 residues from LukS abolished its hemolytic activity towards rabbit erythrocytes, whereas LukS-PV obtained hemolytic activity by the insertion of DI residues in between the 11th and the 12th positions (Figure 8).[42] Furthermore, we constructed the LukS-PV mutants having LukS-function towards rabbit erythrocytes to the same extent by the insertion of D, I, or AA residues between A11 and E12 of LukS-PV (Figure 8).

As shown above, an essential region for LukS-specific function is within C-terminal 122-residue segment (between S164 and the C-terminus) of LukS (see Figure 6, lane 6). After homology study of the deduced amino

198   YOSHIYUKI KAMIO *et al.*

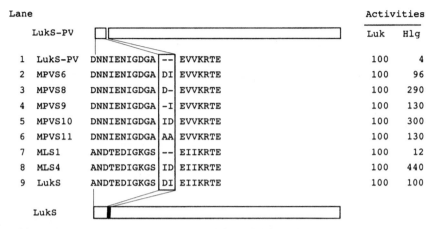

FIGURE 8. Schematic representation of LukS-PV, LukS, and mutant proteins, and the resulting hemolytic activity towards rabbit erythrocytes. Percentage hemolysis indicates the activities compared with that of intact LukS (lane 9). N.D. indicates no detectable activity.

acid sequence from the structure genes for LukS and Hlg2, we found a unique 5-residue sequence I242K243R244S245T246 within C-terminal 122-residue segment of LukS, of which 4-residue KRST is identical with a recognition site of protein phosphorylated by protein kinase A. This segment was deleted in Hlg2 (see Figure 5). To study whether or not the 5-residue segment (IKRST) is essential for the LukS-function, we created a series of mutant genes in the segment. Three different plasmids that contained mutant genes corresponding to the 5-residue segment were obtained and they were designated as pMLS-TS, pMLS-TA, and pMLS-TY. The mutant proteins expressed in *E. coli* harboring the appropriate plasmid were prepared from the sonicated extract of the cells and purified to the degree of electrophoretic homogeneity. After measuring leukocytolytic activity of the purified mutant components in the presence of LukF, the following findings became evident: [1] Mutant proteins MLS-TS, showed 10 times higher leukocytolytic activity than that of intact LukS (Figure 9, lanes 4 and 5). [2] Neither mutant protein MLS-TA nor MLA-TY has any Luk activity (Figure 9, lanes 6 and 7). The findings clearly indicate that the T246 residue of the 5-residue segment of LukS is pivotal for the LukS function. It is known that, for the recognition site-motifs of the protein phosphorylated by protein kinase A, serine residue is more suitable than threonine as a final amino acid residue in the 4-residue, R/K-R/K-X-S/T. If Luk-specific activity is decided by the 5-residue segment IKRST of LukS, the leukocytolytic activity might be endowed into Hlg2 by being inserted the 5-residue segment of LukS into between A238 and Y239 residues of Hlg2 (Figure 5). Accordingly, we created the mutant protein (MHS-Z)

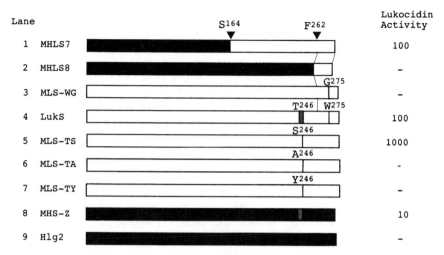

FIGURE 9. Schematic representation of LukS, Hlg2 and mutant proteins, and the resulting leukocidin activity. White and black boxes indicate the LukS- and Hlg2-segments, respectively. Shaded box in lane 4 represents 5-residue IKRST segment. Shaded box in MHS-Z (lane 8) represents the 5-residue I242K243R244S245T246 segment inserted into between A238 and Y239 residues of Hlg2 (see Figure 5). Percent leukocytolysis indicates the activity compared with that of intact LukS (lane 4). A minus indicates no detectable activity.

containing the 5-residue segment into between A238 and Y239 residues of Hlg2. The MHS-Z showed leukocytolytic activity with LukF, although not full activity (Figure 9, lane 8). Thus, it was concluded that the 5-residue IKRST is the minimum segment essential for the LukS-specific function of leukocidin.

Phosphorylation of LukS by Protein Kinase A Is Crucial for the LukS-specific Function of Luk on Human PMNLs[43]

The denatured LukS by heating at 100°C, but not intact LukS was strongly phosphorylated by $[\gamma_{-32}P]$ ATP in the presence of protein kinase A in cell-free system.[40] How-ever, neither both mutants MLS-TY and MLS-TA in which T246 was replaced by Y or A residue, respectively, nor Hlg2 itself in which the 5-residue segment of LukS was deleted, were phosphorylated by protein kinase A in cell-free system, even though they were de-natured by heating at 100°C. They had no leukocytolytic activity in the presence of LukF. The Hlg2 mutant MHS-Z in which the 5-residue segment was inserted at the position that the segment is deleted in Hlg2, was phosphorylated by protein kinase A and conferred leukocytolytic activity co-operatively with LukF. The results obtained indicate that the 5-residue segment IKRST is the pivotal segment of LukS responsible for the LukS function of Luk. The data also suggest that the phosphorylation of LukS occurs in human PMNLs and this reaction is crucial for the LukS-specific function of Luk. However, no direct evidence of the phosphorylation of LukS in human PMNLs was available. Recently, it was examined whether LukS is phosphorylated by exogenous $_{32}$P-H$_3$PO$_4$ on human PMNLs and whether the phosphorylation is prevented by H-89 which is a selective inhibitor of protein kinase A with an inhibition constant of 0.048 µM. It was shown that exposure of the cells to 0.05 µM and 0.5 µM H-89 caused 50% and 100% inhibition of $_{32}$P-H$_3$PO$_4$ incorporation into LukS, respectively, compared to that in the unexposed cells. The IC$_{50}$ value of H-89 in the incorporation of $_{32}$P-H$_3$PO$_4$ into LukS was 0.05 MM which was coincided with its inhibition constant of 0.048 µM. These results indicate that LukS is phosphorylated by protein kinase A on human PMNLs. This also suggested that H-89 should inhibit the leukocytolytic activity, if the phosphorylation of LukS by protein kinase A is crucial for the LukS-specific function of Luk. Accordingly, the effect of H-89 on the leukocytolytic activity of Luk was examined by observing the Luk-induced leukocytolysis of HMNLs microscopically after staining the cells with trypan blue. The cells which were exposed to 50 µM H-89 without Luk components showed no change of their morphology. The addition of H-89 at the concentration over a range of 50 to 0.5 µM to the reaction mixture containing LukS and LukF remained the cells to be swollen but not lysed for at least 20 min observed at 37°C. The cells exposed to 0.05 µM H-89, that lead to 50% inhibition of the phosphorylation of LukS, began to lysing with a loosened edge. However, the cell lysis remained incomplete for 10 min. Thus, it was concluded that the phosphorylation of LukS is crucial for the LukS-specific function of Luk. Although the mechanism of the lysis of human PMNLs by Luk remains to be elucidated, it is feasible that the modification of LukS to the phosphorylated one by protein kinase A on human PMNLs after its initial binding to human PMNLs followed by the subsequent binding of LukF is essential for inducing the cell lysis, because Luk in the presence of H-89 induced human PMNLs to be swollen but not be lysed. We observed the same phenomena in human PMNLs which were treated with both LukF and the mutant of LukS without phosphorylated site in itself. It could be proposed two possibilities of the involvement of the phosphorylation of LukS in its leukocytolytic activity. One is the fragile of the membrane of human PMNLs that was caused by the induction of some lytic enzyme, such as an autolytic enzyme or phospholipase which degrades the membrane. As mentioned above, the binding of LukS to rabbit PMNLs induced an activation of phospholipase A$_2$ in the leukocytes.[29] Taken together with our data, if any, the phosphorylated LukS-mediated signal transduction might be required for an activation of phospholipase A_2. The other is the possibility that the membrane pore consisting of LukF and phosphorylated LukS on human PMNLs might regulate the ion such as calcium current through the membrane. It is known that Luk induces an increase in the free intracellular Ca_{2+} under the physiological conditions ($[Ca_{2+}]$ = 1 to 1.5 μM) in human PMNLs. Gouaux *et al.* have analyzed the aligned sequences of Hla and Luk components in the context of the Hla heptamer structure determining by the crystallographical analysis and suggested that even though the level of sequence identity among Hla and Luk components (LukS and LukF) is distant, the three-dimensional structures of the protomers are conserved.[12] Based on their suggestion, we might propose that the phosphorylated residue T246 of LukS is at the bottom of rim domain which spans the hydrophobic domain of membrane bilayer of human PMNLs and that the T246 residue is phosphorylated by protein kinase A at the contact point of inner leaflet of the membrane and cytoplasm of human PMNLs. As mentioned above, LukF and LukS of Luk assemble into a ring-shaped 200 kDa complex in a molar ratio of 1:1, which form a membrane pore with a functional diameter of 2.1–2.4 nm. We examined complex formation of LukF with either LukS, MLS-TS, MLS-TA, MLS-TY, or MHS-Z on the human PMNLs. Our data showed that all of the mutants as well as LukS in combination with LukF assembled into approximately 200 kDa complex on the surface of human PMNLs. From these findings, we could distinguish the leukocytolytic function from the complex formation which forms the membrane pore on the surface of human PMNLs. We monitored the change of morphology of the cells of human PMNLs under a phase contrast microscope. Intact cells became swollen after the incubation at 37°C with LukF and Hlg2 for 10 min. However, any lysed cell was not observed by the incubation for more 20 min. The data indicated that LukF and Hlg2 cooperatively caused only swelling of the human PMNLs without lysis. Recently, Ferreras *et al.* reported that LukS + LukF and Hlg2 + LukF can form pores via oligomerization and are able to induce permeabilization of calcein on a artificial lipid membrane. However, the combination of LukS-PV + LukF-PV are not able to induce calcein permiability.[44]

Crystal Structure of LukF Delineates Conformational Changes Accompanying Formation of a Transmembrane Channel[45]

LukF Architecture

LukF has the shape of a prolate ellipsoid with dimensions of 72 Å × 34 Å × 25 (Figure 1B). In LukF the amino latch and the pre-stem adopt

dramatically different conformations when compared to the corresponding regions of an Hla protomer. Excluding these areas, the fold of LukF is
identical to the fold of an Hla protomer. The residues that comprise the
amino latch (E2–K16) adopt a β-strand conformation and extend the inner
β-sheet of the β-sandwich by one strand in LukF (Figure 1B). Measured in
terms of solvent accessible surface area, binding amino latch to the LukF
core buries 414_2. In striking contrast ot the Hla protomer, the glycine-rich
region of LukF forms a three-strand antiparalleled β-sheet that packs
against the inner β-sheet of the β-sandwich domain. The pre-stem β-sheet,
which includes the seven disordered residues spanning strand 7″ and
strand 8 (Figures 1C and 10), has an a(β)b(β)c(coil)d(β) fold. Hydrophobic residues predominate in the pre-stem interface with the β-sandwich
domain: there are 24 van der Walls interactions and the buried surface area
is 852_2, which is close to the 670_2 buried by the Hla amino latch when
bound at a similar site on an adjacent protomer in the heptamer structure.
Direct contact between the pre-stem and the amino latch is mediated by a
cluster of hydrophobic residues that includes V13, V17, Y117, and F119. In
Hla, the residues that occupy the latter two positions are predicted to lie
at the interfacial region of the lipid bilayer. The juxtaposition of Y117 and
F119 between the pre-stem and the amino latch makes direct "communication" between these two key regions possible.

LukF Surface Properties and Phospholipid Binding Site

The surface of the pre-stem β-sheet facing the LukF core is primarily
hydrophobic while the side directed toward the solvent is polar. Like Hla,
the LukF rim domain contains a lot of exposed aromatic residues. Located

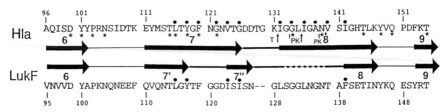

FIGURE 10. Alignment of the amino acid sequences within the triangle and stem (or
pre-stem) regions for Hla and LukF and demarcation of secondary structure elements. For
LukF, the dotted line defines the residues for which there is no electron density. Symbols are
defined as follows: dots in Hla, residues facing the lipid bilayer in Hla; asterisks, conserved
amino acids; arrows are trypsin (T) and proteinase K (PK) sites in the Hla water soluble
monomer; and dots in LukF are residues that are in the pre-stem/β-sandwich interface in
LukF.

in a cleft lined by W177 and R198 is a binding site for phospholipid head groups. In the Hla heptamer, there is a similar lipid binding site, i.e., W179 and R200 residues of Hla, and the latter residue is critical for binding of Hla to an erythrocyte membrane.

LukF Monomer and Hla Protomer Comparison

Superposition of the LukF and Hla protomer structures reinforces the conclusion that the cores are very similar despite a sequence identity of only 31.7% for the mature polypeptides. The comparison also emphasizes the divergence in conformation at the amino latch and glycine-rich "stem" regions, as illustrated in Figure 1A. Fitting of individual domains demonstrated that the r.m.s deviation between Cα positions for the β-sandwich and rim are 2.1Å and 2.4Å, respectively. To a first approximation, the β-sandwich and rim domains behave as rigid bodies that adopt different relative conformations in the monomer (LukF) and heptamer (Hla) due to small changes spread over a number of residues at the β sandwich/rim domain juncture. Recently, the 3-dimensional structure of the water-soluble LukF-PV monomer also analyzed and was found to be basically similar to that of LukF.[46]

Major conformational differences between LukF and the Hla protomer structures occur in the triangle region (see Figure 1, A and B). In contrast to the diffuse nature of the conformational differences relating the β-sandwich and rim domains, there are larger differences in main chain phi and psi angles for 4 residues in the triangle region which allow the LukF pre-stem to fold against the inner surface of the β -sandwich domain. In the Hla protomer, these main chain dihedral angles differ by >90° and are associated with a triangle conformation in which the polypeptide chain extends from the protomer core. The LukF pre-stem occupies approximately the same site that the amino latch of a neighboring protomer occupies in the oligomeric toxin, based on the analogy with the Hla heptamer.

The point of conformational divergence for the amino latch region is localized to residue K16 in LukF and N17 in the Hla protomer. Large differences in the phi and psi angles at these sites cause the polypeptide chain either to fold back on the β-sandwich core to interact with β-strand 1 (LukF), or to extend from the core to interact with a neighboring protomer (Hla heptamer). There are additional large differences in the conformation of residues within the amino latches of LukF and Hla. Recently, the 3-residue segment, L18Y19K20 of LukF was reported to be crucial for the biological activity of the toxin. In detail, see references 45 and 47.

Mechanism of Assembly

Combining salient features from the water-soluble monomer of LukF and the water-insoluble heptamer of Hla structures with data from studies of wild-type and mutant proteins provides molecular detail to and assembly mechanism for staphylococcal channel-foaming proteins (Figure 11). Although LukF does not form a homoheptamer, the similarity in structure and function between LukF and Hla and the similar size of the Hlg (LukF + Hlg2) oligomer and the Hla heptamer predict that LukF and Hla share elements of structure and mechanism. The Hla heptamer structure is a reasonable starting point from which to build a model of the pre-pore assembly intermediate and the LukF monomer structure may serve as a starting point for models of the Hla, LukS and Hlg2 water soluble and membrane-

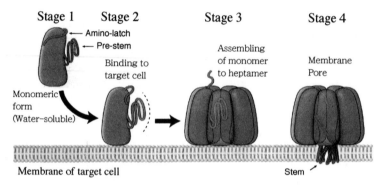

FIGURE 11. Mechanism of assembly for Hla using the structure of LukF as a model for the water soluble and membrane-bound monomers, as well as for the pre-pore subunits.[45] It is likely that the mechanism by which LukF assembles into oligomeric complexes will have features in common with the Hla assembly process. In the water soluble, monomeric state (1), the amino latch and pre-stem regions are folded against the protein core in β-strand and β-sandwich conformations, respectively. Upon membrane binding (2), the pre-stem becomes resistant to proteolysis, suggesting that protease access to the previously scissile pre-stem is prevented by either conformational rearrangement or by steric block from the membrane, as indicated by the dashed line. Contact with the membrane occurs, at least in part, through interactions between W177 and R198 (LukF) or W179 and R200 (Hla) and phospholipid headgroups. Assembly of the pre-pore (3) probably involves inclusion of the pre-stem regions within the lumen of the cap domain. The amino latch is still sensitive to proteolysis. Formation of the lytic pore (4) involves refolding of the pre-stem region and insertion into the membrane as well as rearrangement of the amino latch to the lumen of the cap domain. The amino latch is located at the same site on the inner surface of a neighboring β-sandwich domain as had been occupied by the pre-stem region. This fugure was modified one described by R. Olson *et al.* (reference 45). Reprint was permitted by publisher.

bound monomers. It is suggested that the membrane-bound monomer resembles the water soluble form of LukF except that interaction with the bilayer induces modest conformational changes in the rim and pre-stem regions. In addition, membrane binding renders the pre-stem resistant to proteolysis either through conformational changes, occlusion via the bilayer surface, or both. An important feature of the model shown in Figure 11 for the structure of the oligomeric pre-pore intermediate is that the glycine-rich pre-stem is located within the cap domain pore. This model stands in contrast to previous models[4] in which the glycine-rich pre-stem region is located on the periphery of the oligomer and in contact with the membrane surface.

This mechanism explains how the toxins exhibit solubility in aqueous solution and resist assembly until membrane binding triggers formation of the pre-pore. In the pre-pore state, the pre-stem has probably undergone partial rearrangement, the amino latch has moved from its β-strand position to enable productive protomer-protomer contact and the protomers assemble to a heptamer which is somewhat large in diameter compared to the final pore form. Insertion of the pre-stem into the membrane may occur by a cooperative "extrusion" of the polypeptide from the base of the cap at the same time as the amino latch folds into the lumen of the cap domain. By forming a pre-pore oligomer and associating with the membrane the pre-pore may thin the bilayer and thus facilitate stem insertion.

Since the LukF, LukS, and Hlg2 proteins form heteromers that may be hexames, there will certainly be differences in their assembly compared to Hla. However, given the structural and functional similarities among Hla, LukF, LukS and Hlg2, they will undoubtedly share many mechanistic features in common. Although the mechanism shown in Figure 11 is focused on Hla, we predict that LukF, LukS, and Hlg will assemble to form oligomers that have cap, rim, and stem domains like the Hla heptamer and that Hla and Luk will assemble via an oligomeric intermediate in which the pre-stem regions are clustered in the interior of the cap domain. Insights obtained from the studies of LukF and Hla may also be applicable to other non-staphylococcal channel forming toxins such as aerolysin and anthrax protective antigen. In more general terms, structural studies of Hla and LukF have shown how the exchange and sequential unmasking of specific protein in and protein-solvent interfaces plays a central role in the assembly of these oligomeric transmembrane toxins: the water soluble form is stabilized by interactions within a single subunit while the oligomeric form is stabilized by interactions between subunits and between the oligomer and the membrane.

4. PVL IN HUMAN INFECTIONS: A VIRULENCE DETERMINANT ASSOCIATED WITH NECROTIC LESIONS THAT HAVE POTENTIALLY SEVERE PROGNOSES

PVL is thought to be a virulence factor which responsible for the necrosis of infected tissues. The production of this toxin results from a lysogenic conversion occurring in less than 5% of *S. aureus* strains of clinical origin. When the presence of the PVL genes was determined by PCR amplification in a collection of 172 *S. aureus* strains obtained by the French National Reference Center for Staphylococcal Infections, the PVL genes were detected in 93% of strains associated with furuncles and in 85% of those associated with severe necrotic hemorrhagic pneumonias which were all community-acquired (Y. Piemont, personal communication). They were also detected in 55% of cellulitis strains, 50% of cutaneous abscess strains, 23% of osteomyelitis strains, and 13% of whitlow strains. The *pvl* genes were neither detected in strains responsible for other infections such as infective endocarditis, mediastinitis, hospital-acquired pneumonia, urinary tract infections and enterocolitis, nor in those associated with toxic-shock syndrome (Y. Piemont, personal communication). Hence, it appeared that PVL is mainly associated with skin or mucous membranes necrotic lesions and sometimes with osteomyelitis. These results underline the potential role of PVL as the causative agent of numerous staphylococcal clinical syndromes and suggest the development of new therapeutic tools for curing these infections which appear sometimes difficult to treat, despite the usual antibiotic susceptibility of the causative strains.

5. VITRONECTIN AND ITS FRAGMENTS PURIFIED AS SERUM INHIBITORS OF HLG AND LUK, AND THEIR SPECIFIC BINDING TO HLG2 AND LUKS OF THE TOXINS

Most recently, vitronectin which is a 75-kDa multifunctional glycoprotein and its fragments with 62, 57, and 38 kDa have been isolated from human serum as an inhibitor with an ability to fix Hlg and Luk.[48] The purified vitronectin and its fragments specifically bound to Hlg2 and LukS to prevent the toxin-induced lysis of human erythrocytes and human PMNLs, respectively. The vitronectin fragments and Hlg2 (or LukS) formed high-molecular weight complexes that co-sedimented in a sucrose gradient centrifugation and co-migrated on a native polyacrylamide gel electrophoresis. Intact vitronectin was 15-fold less active than the purified inhibitors, but its inhibitory activity was raised to a comparable level to that of the purified inhibitors when partially digested with human plasmin. Based on these results, vitronectin and its fragments are considered to be possible host components for fixation of Hlg and Luk in the loci of staphylococcal infections. The vitronectin-binding ability of Hlg and Luk is a novel function of the pore-forming cytolysins.

Since vitronectin is considered to regulate proteolytic enzyme cascades including the complement, coagulation and fibrinolysis systems, it would act as an ambivalent factor for hosts depending on the local and the systemic conditions of defense systems: [1] Provided Hlg and Luk are produced in the loci of staphylococcal infections, Hlg2 and LukS would be captured by vitronectin and its fragments in the extracellular matrix of fibroblasts and tissue macrophages, followed by integrin-mediated endocytosis and degradation by the cells. [2] Extracellular-matrix-associated vitronectins would be liberated by the action of plasmin in the sites of interstitial inflammation, and the liberated vitronectin fragments would fix and opsonize Hlg and Luk. [3] However, consumption of vitronectin by Hlg and Luk would cause an imbalance in the regulation of coagulation, fibrinolysis, and complement cascade, leading to tissue injuries by an excess level of terminal complex of complement and hyperproduction of plasmin. [4] Vitronectin is an acute phase protein, and it is synthesized predominantly in liver in response to interleukin 6, and delivered to peripheral tissues through blood circulation and transcytosis by the endothelial cells. Once extracellular-matrix-associated vitronectin is consumed by Hlg and Luk in the sites of staphylococcal infections, it would remain at lower levels there for a while. In the circumstances, staphylococcal cytolysins including Hlg and Luk might play a key role in skin and mucosal infections with severe prognosis. [5] Vitronectin has been shown to bind specifically to the cells of *S. aureus*, and it is considered to be a binding molecule for the bacterium. Production of Hlg and Luk by *S. aureus* would induce detachment and spreading of tissue-bound staphylococci by replacing the vitronectin-binding sites of the bacteria with Hlg2 and/or LukS as well as by the cytolytic activity of the toxins. Hlg2 and LukS would also neutralize the opsonic function of soluble vitronectin to prevent phagocytosis of *S. aureus* by professional phagocytes in the loci of inflammation. Thus, not only the cytolytic activity but also the vitronectin-binding activity of Hlg and Luk are the putative pathophysiological functions of the staphylococcal bicomponent toxins.

ACKNOWLEDGMENTS. Our works cited in this article were supported in part by the Grant-in Aid for Scientific Research from the Ministry of Education, Science, Sports and Culture of Japan (05304028, 06670280, 07660089, 08307004, 8660086, 09460042, 11694191, and 11460034 to Y. K.;

05670248, 06240212, 08670298, and 08219203 to T. T.; 09760064 and 11760050 to J. K.), The Naito Foundation, Yamada Science Foundation, Takeda Science Foundation, Intelligent Cosmos Academic Foundation, and Japanisch-Deutsches Kulturinstitute Foundation.

REFERENCES

1. S. Bhakdi and J. Tranum-Jensen, α-toxin of *Staphylococcus aureus*. *Microbiol. Rev.*, 55:733 (1991).

2. T. Tomita and Y. Kamio, Molecular biology of the pore-forming cytolysins from *Staphylococcus aureus*, α- and γ-hemolysin and leukocidin, *Biosci. Biotechnol. Biochem.*, 61:565 (1997).

3. J. E. Gouaux, O., Braha, M., Hobaugh, L., Song, S., Cheley, C. Shustak, and H. Bayley, Subunit stoichiometry of staphylococcal γ-hemolysin in crystals and on membranes: A heptamer trans-membrane pore, *Proc. Natl. Acad. Sci.*, 91:12828 (1994).

4. L. Song, M. R. Hobaugh, C. Shustak, S. Cheley, H. Bayley, and E. Gouaux, Structure of staphylococcal α-hemolysin, a heptameric transmembrane pore, *Science*, 274:1859 (1996).

5. B. Walker, M. Krishnasastry, and H. Bayley, Functional complementation of staphylococcal α-hemolysin fragments overlaps, nick, and gaps in the glycine-rich loop, *J. Biol. Chem.*, 268:5285 (1993).

6. M. Palmer, R. Jursch, U. Weller, A. Valeva, K. Hilgert, M. Kehoe, and S. Bhakdi, Production of functionally intact site-specifically modifiable protein by introduction of cysteine at positions 69, 130, and 186, *J. Biol. Chem.*, 268:11959 (1993).

7. A. Valeva, A. Weisser, B. Walker, M. Kehoe, H. Bayley, S. Bhakdi, and M. Palmer, Molecular architecture of a toxin pore: A 15-residue sequence lines the transmember ane channel of staphylococcal α-toxin, *EMBO J.*, 15:1857(1996).

8. B. Walker and H. Bayley, Key residues for membrane binding, oligomerization, and pore forming activity of staphylococcal α-hemolysin indetified by cysteine scanning mutagenesis and targeted chemical modification, *J. Biol. Chem.*, 270:23065 (1995).

9. M. Watanabe, T. Tomita, and T. Yasuda, Membrane-damaging action of staphylococcal α-toxin on phospholipid-cholesterol liposomes, *Biochim. Biophys. Acta*, 898:257 (1987).

10. T. Tomita, M. Watanabe and T. Yasuda, Influence of membrane fluidity on the assembly of *staphylococcus aureus* α-toxin, a channel-forming protein, in liposome membrane, *J. Biol. Chem.*, 267:13391 (1992).

11. T. Tomita, M. Watanabe, and T. Yasuda, Effect of fatty acyl domain of phospholipids on the membrane-channel formation of *Staphylococcus aureus* α-toxin in liposome membrane, *Biochim. Biophys. Acta*, 1104:325 (1992).

12. E. Gouaux, M. Hobaugh, and L. Song, α-Hemolysin, γhemolysin, and leukocidin from *Staphlococcus aureus*: Distant in sequence but similar in structure, *Protein Sci.*, 6:2631 (1997).

13. A. M. Woodin, Purification of the two components of leukocidin from *Staphylococcus aureus*, *Biochem. J.*, 75:158 (1960).

14. M. Noda, T. Hirayama, I. Kato, and F. Matsuda, Crystallization and properties of Staphylococcal leukocidin, *Biochem. Biophys. Acta*, 633:33 (1980).

15. G. Prevost, G. Cribier, P. Couppie, P. Petiau, G. Supersac, V. Finck-barbancon, H. Monteil, and Y. Peimont, Panton-Valentine leukocidin and γ-hemolysin from *Staphylococcus aureus* ATCC 49775 are encoded by distinct genetic loci and have different biological activities, *Intfect. Immun.*, 63:4121 (1995).

16. A. Rahman, K. Izaki, I. Kato, and Y. Kamio, Nucleotide sequence of leukocidin S-component gene (*lukS*) from methicillin resistant *Staphylococcus aureus*, *Biochem. Biophys. Res. Commun.*, 181:138 (1991).

17. A. Rahman, H. Nariya, K. Izaki, I. Kato, and Y. Kamio, Molecular cloning and nucleotide sequence of leukocidin F-component gene (*lukF*) from methicillin resistant *Staphylococcus aureus*, *Biochem. Biophys. Res. Commun.*, 184:640 (1992).

18. A. Rahman, K. Izaki, and Y. Kamio, γ-Hemolysin genes in the same family with lukF and lukS genes in methicillin resistant *Staphylococcus aureus*, *Biosci. Biotechnol. Biochem.*, 57:1234 (1993).

19. J. Cooney, S. Kiele, T. J. Foster, W. Otoole, The γ-hemolysin locus of *Staphylococcus aureus* comprises three genes, two of which are identical to the genes for the F and S components of leukocidin, *Infec. Immun.*, 61:768 (1993).

20. G. Supersac, G. Prevost, and Y. Piemont, Sequencing of leukocidin R from *Staphylococcus aureus* P83 suggests that staphylococcal leukocidins and γ-hemolysin are member of a single, two component family of toxins, *Infec. Immun.*, 61:580 (1993).

21. K. Sudo, W. Choorit, I. Asami, J. Kaneko, K. Muramoto, and Y. Kamio, Substititution of lysine for arginine in the N-terminal 217th amino acid residue of the H γ II of staphylococcal γ-hemolysin lowers the activity of the toxin, *Biosci. Biotechnol. Biochem.*, 59:1786 (1995).

22. K. Yokota, N. Sugawara, H. Nariya, J. Kaneko, T. Tomita, and Y. Kamio, Further study on the two pivotal parts of Hlg2 for the full hemolytic activity of staphylococcal γ-hemolysin, *Biosci. Biotechnol. Biochem.*, 62:1745 (1998).

23. W. Choorit, J. Kaneko, K. Muramoto, and Y. Kamio, Existence of a new protein component with the same function as LukF component of leukocidin or γ-hemolysin and its gene in *Staphylococcus aureus* P83, *FEBS Lett.*, 357:260 (1995).

24. J. Kaneko, K. Muramoto, and Y. Kamio, Gene of LukF-PV-like component of Panton-Valentine leukocidin in *Staphylococcus aureus* P83 is linked with *lukM*, *Biosci. Biotechnol. Biochem.*, 61:541 (1997).

25. J.Kaneko, T. Kimura. Y. Kawakami, T. Tomita, and Y. Kamio, Panton-Valentine leukocidin genes in a phage-like particle isolated from mitomycin C-treated *Staphylococcus aureus* V8 (ATCC 49775), *Biosci. Biotechnol. Biochem.*, 61:1960 (1997).

26. J. Kaneko, T. Kimura, S. Narita, T. Tomita, and Y. Kamio, Complete nucleotide sequence and molecular characterization of the temperate staphylococcal bacteriophage φPVL carring Panton-Valentine leukocidin genes, *Gene*, 215:57 (1998).

27. Y. Kamio, A. Rahman, H. Nariya, T. Ozawa, and K. Izaki, The two staphylococcal bicomponent toxins, leukocidin and γ-hemolysin, share one component in common, *FEBS Lett.*, 321:15 (1993).

28. H. Nariya, K. Izaki, and Y. Kamio, The C-terminal region of S component of staphylococcal leukocidin is essential for the biological activity of the toxin, *FEBS Lett.*, 329:219 (1993).

29. M. Noda, I. Kato, I. T. Hirayama, and F. Matsuda, Fixation and inactivation of staphylococcal leukocidin by phosphatidyl cholin and ganglioside G_{M1} in rabbit polymorphonuclear leukocytes, *Infec. Immun.*, 29:678 (1980).

30. H. Nariya and Y. Kamio, Identification of the essential regions for lukS- and H γ II-specific function of staphylococcal leukocidin and γ-hemolysin, *Biosci. Biotechnol. Biochem.*, 59:1603 (1995).

31. T. Ozawa, T. H. Nariya, J. Kaneko, K. Izaki, and Y. Kamio, Inactivation of γ-hemolysin activity by exogenous addition of monosialoganglioside G_{M1} in human erythrocyte, *Biosci. Biotechnol. Biochem.*, 58:602 (1994).

32. D. A. Colin, I. Mazurier, S. Sire, and V. Fink-Barbacon, Interaction of the two components of leukocidin from *Staphylococcus aureus* with human polymorphonuclear leukocyte membrane: sequential binding and subsequent activation, *Infect. Immu.*, 62:3184 (1994).

33. T. Ozawa, J. Kaneko, and Y. Kamio, Essential binding of LukF of staphylococcal γ-hemolysin followed by the binding of H γ II for the hemolysin of human erythrocytes, *Biosci. Biotechnol. Biochem.*, 59:1181 (1995).

34. J. Kaneko, T. Ozawa, T. Tomita, and Y. Kamio, Sequential binding of staphylococcal γ-hemolysin to human erythrocytes and complex fornmation of the hemolysin on the cell surface, *Biosci. Biotechnol. Biochem.*, 61:846 (1997).

35. N. Sugawara, T. Tomita, and Y. Kamio, Assembly of *Staphylococcus aureus* γ-hemolysin into a pore-forming ring-shaped complex on the surface of human erythrocytes, *FEBS Lett.*, 410:333 (1997).

36. N. Sugawara, T. Tomita, T. Sato, and Y. Kamio, Assembly of *Staphylococcus aureus* leukocidin into a pore-forming ring-shaped oligomer on human polymorphonuclear leukocytes and rabbit erythrocytes, *Biosci. Biotechnol. Biochem.*, 63:884 (1999).

37. V. Finck-Barbancon, G. Duportail, O. Meunier, and D. A. Colin, Pore formation by a two-component leukocidin from *Staphylococcus aureus* within the membrane of human polymorphonuclear leukocytes, *Biochim. Biophys. Acta*, 1182:275 (1993).

38. L. Stalli, H. Monteil, and D. A. Colin, The staphylococcal pore-forming leukotoxins open Ca_{2+} channel in the membrane of human polymorphonuclear neutrophiles, *J. Membr. Biol.*, 162:209 (1998).

39. H. Nariya and Y. Kamio, Identification of the minimum segment essential for the H γ II-specific function of staphylococcal γ-hemolysin, *Biosci. Biotechnol. Biochem.*, 61:1786 (1997).

40. H. Nariya, A. Nishiyama, and Y. Kamio, Identification of the minimum segment in which threonine[246] ,esidue is phosphorylated by protein kinase A for the LukS-specific function of staphylococcal leukocidin, *FEBS Lett.*, 415:96 (1997).

41. H. Nariya, A. Shimatani, T. Tomita, and Y. Kamio, Identification of the essential amino acid residues in LukS for the hemolytic activity of staphylococcal leukocidin towards rabbit erythrocytes, *Biosci. Biotechnol. Biochem.*, 61:2095 (1997).

42. A. Shimatani, J. Kaneko, T. Tomita, and Y. Kamio, Construction of a LukS-PV mutant of a staphylococcal Panton-Valentine leukocidin component having a high LukS-like function, *Biosci. Biotechnol. Biochem.*, 63:1828 (1999).

43. A. Nishiyama, H. Nariya, and Y. Kamio, Phosphorylation of LukS by protein kinase A is crucial for the LukS function of the staphylococcal leukocidin on human polymorphonuclear leukocytes, *Biosci. Biotechnol, Biochem.*, 62:1834 (1998).

44. M. Ferreras, F. Hoper, M.D. Serra, D. A. Colin, G. Prevost, and G. Menestrina, The interaction of *Staphylococcus aureus* bi-component γ-hemolysin and leucocidin with cells and lipid membranes, *Biochim. Biophy. Acta*, 1414:108 (1998).

45. R. Olson, H. Nariya, K. Yokota, Y. Kamio, and E. Gouaux, Crystal structure of staphylococcal LukF delineates conformational changes accompanying formation of a transmembrane channel, *Nature Structural Biology*, 6:134 (1999).

46. J. D. Pedelacq, L. Maveyraud, G. Prevost, L. Baba-Moussa, A. Gonzalez, E. Courcelle, W. Shepard, H.Monteil, J-P. Samama, and L. Mourey, The structure of a *Staphylococcus aureus* leucocidin component (LukF-PV) reveals the fold of the water-soluble species of a family of transmembrane pore-forming toxins, *Structure*, 7:277 (1999).

47. J. Kaneko, Ma A. L. Mascarenas, Md. N. Huda, T. Tomita, and Y. Kamio, An N-terminal region of LukF of staphylococcal leukocidin/gamma-hemolysin crucial for the biological activity of the toxin, Biosci. Biotechnol. Biochem., 62:1465 (1998).
48. H. Katsumi, T. Tomita, J. Kaneko, and Y. Kamio, Vitronectin and its fragments purified as serum inhibitors of *Staphylococcus aureus* γ-hemolysin and leukocidin, and their specific binding to the Hlg2 and the LukS components of the toxins, *FEBS Lett.*, In press (1999).

11

Osteomyelitis and Septic Arthritis

MARK S. SMELTZER and CARL L. NELSON

1. INTRODUCTION

The bacterial etiology of osteomyelitis was first recognized in the mid-19th century.[90] Since that time, repeated studies have confirmed that the primary cause is *Staphylococcus aureus*.[62] Although *S. epidermidis* has recently emerged as a prominent musculoskeletal pathogen, its emer-gence is due almost entirely to its remarkable capacity to colonize indwelling medical devices.[39] In fact, its ability to colonize biomaterials is so closely correlated with its capacity to cause disease that *S. epidermidis* has been appropriately referred to as a "pathogen of medical progress".[106] The contrast between the historical association of *S. aureus* with musculoskeletal infection and the recent emergence of *S. epidermidis* correctly implies that these two species are not equivalent pathogens either with respect to the infections they cause or the virulence factors they employ. It is convenient based on this disparate etiology to divide musculoskeletal infections into those involving bone (osteomyelitis), those confined to the joints (septic arthritis) and those involving indwelling medical devices. In the case of osteomyelitis, *S. aureus* is clearly the predominant pathogen.[62,83] With respect to infections involving indwelling medical devices, *S. epidermidis* takes on a more prominent role although *S. aureus* does not lag far behind.[20] The etiology of septic arthritis is more diverse, however, *S. aureus* remains among the most prominent causes, and *S. aureus* infections are

MARK S. SMELTZER • Department of Microbiology and Immunology and Department of Orthopaedic Surgery, University of Arkansas for Medical Sciences, Little Rock, AR 72205. CARL L. NELSON • Department of Orthopaedic Surgery, University of Arkansas for Medical Sciences, Little Rock, AR 72205.

Staphylococcus aureus *Infection and Disease*, edited by Allen L. Honeyman *et al.* Kluwer Academic/Plenum Publishers, New York, 2001.

generally more serious because they can cause extensive damage within a very short period of time.[63]

Although the focus of this text is on staphylococcal infection, we would be derelict in our duty if we focused so intently that we failed to note that a diverse group of other bacteria collectively cause a significant number of musculoskeletal infections. This group includes other Gram-positive cocci (e.g., *Streptococcus pyogenes*), a variety of Gram-negative bacteria (e.g., *Neisseria gonorrhoeae, Pseudomonas aeruginosa* and *Haemophilus influenzae*) and some anaerobic species (e.g. *Clostridium* spp.).[62,63,83] Like the correlation between *S. epidermidis* infection and indwelling medical devices, the tendency of non-staphylococcal species to cause musculoskeletal disease is generally restricted to relatively well defined clinical situations. For example, *N. gonorrhoeae* is a prominent cause of septic arthritis among young, sexually active adults suffering from disseminated gonococcal infection.[63] Other Gram-negative bacteria cause infection primarily in severely compromised and elderly patients.[62] The streptococci and anaerobic species are most often associated with injuries involving bites or some other form of trauma that includes contact with the mouth (e.g. fist injuries).[62] Not surprisingly, many of these species are also among the most prominent causes of peridontitis.[83] Finally, it is not uncommon to have a polymicrobial etiology, particularly in the case of post-traumatic osteomyelitis.[20] While these observations emphasize the complex nature of musculoskeletal infection, they do not preclude the conclusion that the staphylococci are the preeminent musculoskeletal pathogens.

2. THE CLINICAL SYNDROMES OF OSTEOMYELITIS AND SEPTIC ARTHRITIS

Osteomyelitis is a term generally applied to any infection involving bone. However, the use of a single term is somewhat misleading since such infections can have diverse clinical features. To reflect that fact, a number of classification schemes have been proposed. The simplest of these distinguishes between "acute" and "chronic" osteomyelitis, with acute infections being loosely defined as the first clinical episode and chronic infections being defined as those that were either left untreated or were not resolved by the initial therapy.[62] Although the distinction between acute and chronic osteomyelitis is certainly not definitive, it does provide some indication of clinical status in that patients with acute infection are more likely to present with systemic signs of disease and have a better chance of recovery without surgical intervention. In contrast, chronic infections are associated with a disrupted blood flow that compromises the ability to deliver antibiotics to the site of infection. The persistence of clinical signs for as little as 10 days has been associated with the formation of sufficient necrotic bone to compromise the blood flow and clinically categorize the infection as chronic.[62]

Lew and Waldvogel[62] proposed an alternative classification scheme that distinguishes between infections that arise via hematogenous seeding of the bone (hematogenous osteomyelitis) and infections that arise as an extension of an adjacent soft-tissue infection (osteomyelitis secondary to a contiguous focus of infection). Hematogenous osteomyelitis is most often seen in children and is typically localized to the metaphyseal region of dia-physeal bones, most notably the femur and tibia (Figure 1). Localization to these regions is thought to arise from the circulatory architecture of the metaphyseal vessels.[68] Specifically, the end-artery capillary loops turn acutely to join large sinusoidal intramedullary veins (Figure 2) This results in a reduced and turbulent blood flow that allows bacteria to accumulate and eventually escape through the fenestrated layer of endothelial cells lining the ends of the metaphyseal capillaries (Figure 3A). Also, phagocytes are absent or only weakly active in this region.[68] Although the circulatory architecture of the metaphysis contributes to disease, it also provides blood flow to the infected region. For that reason, such infections can often be resolved by antibiotic therapy as long as diagnosis and treatment are not delayed.

Hematogenous osteomyelitis in adults is rare and is most often local-ized to the spine.[62] Because the blood vessels that supply the spine are bifur-cated, the disease often involves two adjacent vertebrae and the intervening disk space (Figure 3B). The more common form of bone infection in adults is secondary osteomyelitis.[62] The prototype is an infection that arises via invasion of the bone from an adjacent soft tissue infection or an infected implant, however, those cases in which bacteria are introduced directly into the bone as a result of trauma (post-traumatic osteomyelitis) are usually included.[62,69] A variant that is common enough to have been given its own subcategory is "osteomyelitis secondary to vascular insufficiency".[62] The prototype example is a diabetic patient in which the blood flow to the lower extremities is compromised to the point that infected soft tissue wounds do not heal and bacteria eventually invade to the underlying bone. Such infections are typically localized in the feet (Figure 3C). Although secondary osteomyelitis is more likely to have a polymicrobial etiology, particularly in the case of post-traumatic osteomyelitis, S. aureus remains the most frequently isolated pathogen.[62,68,83]

The Waldvogel classification system remains both useful and widely used. However, Mader et al.[69] proposed a more descriptive system (the Cierny-Mader classification system) based on the extent of anatomic

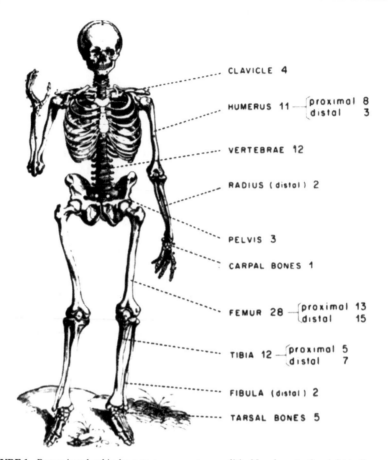

CLAVICLE 4

HUMERUS 11 — proximal 8
                        distal   3

VERTEBRAE 12

RADIUS (distal) 2

PELVIS 3

CARPAL BONES 1

FEMUR 28 — proximal 13
                      distal   15

TIBIA 12 — proximal 5
                    distal   7

FIBULA (distal) 2

TARSAL BONES 5

FIGURE 1. Bones involved in hematogenous osteomyelitis. Numbers to the right indicate the relative frequency of infection in a sampled population of 62 patients, some of which had multiple bone involvement. Infection of the long bones (humerus, femur and tibia) was most common in children while vertebral infections was most common in adults. *Reprinted with permission from Waldvogel, F.A., Medoff, G. and Swartz, M.N.: Osteomyelitis: A review of clinical features, therapeutic considerations and unusual aspects (first of three parts). New England Journal of Medicine 282:198–206, 1970.*

damage. This system includes the four categories of medullary (stage 1), superficial (stage II), localized (stage III) and diffuse (stage IV) osteomyelitis. Medullary osteomyelitis is confined to the endosteal space and most closely approximates the hematogenous disease seen in children.

   Superficial osteomyelitis arises from an adjacent soft tissue infection and is confined to the outer surface of the bone. This form is analogous to "osteomyelitis secondary to a contiguous focus of infection".[62] Localized

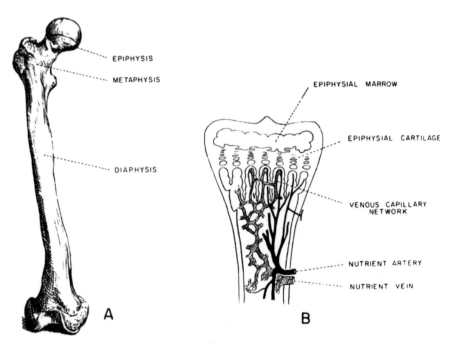

FIGURE 2. Circulatory architecture in long bones. (A) Femur, showing epiphysis, metaphysis and diaphysis. (B) Schematic representation of the vascular supply of long bone in the region of the epiphyseal growth plate. *Reprinted with permission from Waldvogel, F.A., Medoff, G. and Swartz, M.N.: Osteomyelitis: A review of clinical features, therapeutic considerations and unusual aspects (first of three parts). New England Journal of Medicine 282:198–206, 1970.*

osteomyelitis is characterized by full-thickness cortical sequestration and can arise as an extension of either the medullary or superficial forms of the disease. It is distinguished from diffuse osteomyelitis by the presence of sufficient healthy bone to allow surgical excision of the sequestrum without compromising structural stability. In contrast, diffuse osteomyelitis is a "through-and-through" infection that cannot be resolved without segmental resection.[68,69] It is important to emphasize, however, that the treatment of superficial or even medullary osteomyelitis may require some degree of surgical intervention.[62,69]

Alderson *et al.*[5] argued that hematogenous osteomyelitis and septic arthritis can be considered different manifestations of the same disease. While it is true that *S. aureus* can invade the joint from an adjacent bone lesion, septic arthritis arises more commonly by direct seeding of the synovium with blood-borne bacteria or by the direct introduction of bacteria due to penetrating trauma or intra-articular injections.[25,46] For that reason,

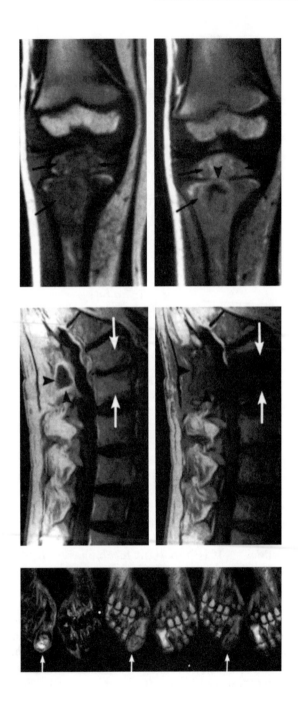

a consistent correlation between septic arthritis and osteomyelitis is limited primarily to infections in neonates and infants, which have transphyseal capillaries that cross the growth plate to directly connect the metaphysis and epiphysis, thereby providing bacteria with direct access to the joint.[68] Indeed, studies that have specifically examined the issue suggest that osteomyelitis and septic arthritis occur together in about 15% of the cases and that almost all of these involve neonates or children less than 2 years old.[46] In such cases, the symptoms are usually systemic rather than local, and it is sometimes possible to resolve the infection without surgery assuming prompt diagnosis and treatment.

In adults, the association between osteomyelitis and septic arthritis is largely limited to those cases in which the metaphysis is intracapsular. Examples include infections of the proximal femur, radius and humerus, which sometimes spread to the hip, elbow or shoulder joints respectively (Figure 1).[68] More commonly, septic arthritis in adults results from hematogenous seeding of the joint, usually in conjunction with trauma or some underlying disability (e.g., rheumatoid arthritis).[25] Nevertheless, it is reasonable to consider septic arthritis and osteomyelitis together because recent data suggests that the *S. aureus* virulence factors that contribute to the two infections are similar if not identical. These virulence factors are the primary focus of this chapter.

3. THE ECONOMIC IMPACT OF BONE AND JOINT INFECTION

Hedstrom and Lidgren[46] summarized recent epidemiological statistics of bone and joint infection, citing an incidence of "bacterial arthritis acute osteomyelitis" in Sweden of 1 in 10,000. They also noted that the incidence

◄──

FIGURE 3. Appearance on magnetic resonance imaging (MRI) of various types of osteomyelitis. The top panel shows acute osteomyelitis of the right tibia in a four-year-old boy. In a T_1-weighted image (left), a large area of signal hypointensity in bone marrow is seen (arrows). The intravenous injection of gadolinium enhances the signal (arrows) and reveals a small abscess (arrowhead). The middle panel shows vertebral osteomyelitis with a soft-tissue abscess one week after an L4–L5 diskectomy. In a T_1-weighted image (left) and after the intravenous injection of gadolinium (right), abnormalities of bone marrow in the vertebral bodies (arrows) and a posterior fluid collection (arrowheads) are evident. The bottom panel shows three views of acute osteomyelitis of the left big toe in a patient with diabetes mellitus. Abnormalities of bone marrow (arrows) are seen as an area of signal hypointensity in a T_1-weighted image (right), as an area of enhanced signal after the intravenous injection of gadolinium (center), and as an area of hyperintensity in an inversion-recovery sequence with fat suppression (left). *Reprinted with permission from Lew, D.P. and Waldvogel, F.A.: Current concepts: osteomyelitis. New England Journal of Medicine 336:999–1007, 1997.*

is higher (up to 1 in 1,000) in warmer, more humid climates. In the United States, the incidence of hematogenous ostemyelitis in children under 13 is approximately 1 in 5,000.[116] Early diagnosis followed by surgical decompression and antibiotic therapy has reduced the proportion of acute infections that develop into chronic disease from as high as 20% to approximately 2%.[46] The number of new cases of chronic osteomyelitis of either hematogenous or secondary origin has been estimated at between 1.5 and 3.0 per 10,000.[46] In a comprehensive survey of New York City hospital admissions in 1995, Rubin et al.[105] reported 2,000 cases of staphylococcal osteomyelitis and 700 cases of septic arthritis. That translates to an incidence ranging between 1 in 4,000 for osteomyelitis and 1 in 10,000 for septic arthritis. The average hospital stay ranged from 22.0 days with septic arthritis to 23.9 days with osteomyelitis at a total cost of approximately $93.9 million.[105]

In recent years, there has been a general decline in the number of hematogenous infections and a general increase in the number of post-traumatic and post-operative infections.[25,33,46] These trends are based on absolute numbers rather than changes in the infection rate. More directly, the increase in the number of post-operative infections reflects a relatively constant infection rate superimposed on an increase in the number of invasive orthopaedic procedures. Indeed, even with antibiotic prophylaxis, the incidence of prosthetic joint infections has remained relatively constant at between 1 and 2%.[46] It has been estimated that the number of surgical procedures performed worldwide for joint replacement or repair of hip fractures exceeds 2,000,000.[46] Based on this estimate and an infection rate between 1 and 2%, the number of infections would be expected to range between 20,000 and 40,000 per year. These infections often result in severe impairment and are rarely resolved without removal of the implant.

4. HOST FACTORS THAT CONTRIBUTE TO MUSCULOSKELETAL INFECTION

The staphylococci are opportunistic pathogens, which clearly implies that the status of the host plays an important role in the development of staphylococcal disease. The most obvious example is the implantation of biomaterials, which provide an inviting substrate for colonization by both S. epidermidis and S. aureus. The general physiological and immunological status of the host is also of paramount importance. For this reason, the Cierny-Mader classification system also defines three categories of patient, with the extremes being patients with normal physiological, metabolic and immunological functions (the A host) and severely compromised patients in which the treatment is deemed worse than the disease itself (the C host).[69] Thus, the best case scenario in the Cierny-Mader system would be the A host (no compromising debilities) suffering from medullary (class I) osteomyelitis. The worst case would be the C host (severe systemic compromise) suffering from diffuse (class IV) osteomyelitis. Between the extremes is the B host, which has varying degrees of local (the B_L host) or systemic compromise (the B_S host). Included among the factors contributing to systemic compromise are malnutrition, renal or hepatic failure, malignancy, age extremes, diabetes, and immunosuppression. Examples of local compromise include disrupted blood flow, extensive scarring, and tobacco abuse, which tends to restrict capillary blood flow.[69] In cases involving B hosts, attempts to resolve the infection should be preceded by efforts to overcome the compromise to an extent that approximates the A host as closely as possible. The same can be said of the C host although the primary clinical efforts in such cases are often directed at maintaining function rather than eradication of the infection.

5. BACTERIAL FACTORS THAT CONTRIBUTE TO INFECTION

General Considerations

The primary characteristic that distinguishes *S. aureus* from other staphylococcal species is its ability to produce a diverse array of virulence factors. Indeed, *S. aureus* is a remarkably well-armed pathogen capable of causing a diverse array of infections ranging from superficial infections of the skin (e.g., folliculitis) to serious and even-life threatening systemic disease (e.g., endocarditis). In contrast, *S. epidermidis* and the other coagulase-negative species produce a much more limited set of virulence factors and cause more indolent infections that are most often associated with implanted biomaterials.

Although musculoskeletal infections are generally not life threatening, they must be considered among the more serious forms of staphylococcal disease based on the potential for permanent disability and the extensive measures required to resolve the infection. Importantly, the need for such extensive intervention is largely independent of the resistance status of the infecting strain. That is due to the compromised blood flow associated with chronic infections and to formation of a biofilm, which contains bacterial microcolonies encased within a protective barrier generally referred to as the glycocalyx.[35,71] The glycocalyx further compromises the ability to deliver antibiotics to the biofilm-embedded bacteria[7] and is a primary reason why surgical debridement and/or removal of infected implants is usually required. Based on these considerations, it seems clear that meaningful advances in the control of musculoskeletal infection will require the development of prophylactic protocols capable of preventing the infection from becoming established in the first place. The development of such protocols will require a comprehensive understanding of the virulence factors that define the staphylococci as the preeminent musculoskeletal pathogens.

Staphylococcal virulence factors can be subdivided into two general categories.[25,101] The first are the surface-associated factors, which include both capsular and noncapsular polysaccharides as well as a group of surface-exposed proteins that act as adhesins by virtue of their ability to bind host proteins present in the extracellular matrix. The protein adhesins have been collectively referred to as "microbial surface components recognizing adhesive matrix molecules" or MSCRAMMs.[94] The second category of staphylococcal virulence factors contains extracellular proteins, which play a predominant role in tissue invasion and are responsible for most of the pathological consequences of S. aureus infection, largely by virtue of their impact on the host immune response.[101] This group, which includes both degradative enzymes (e.g., lipase, protease) and exotoxins (e.g., toxic shock syndrome toxin, the exfoliative toxins and the enterotoxins), is largely absent in S. epidermidis and the other coagulase-negative staphylococci.[101]

It is convenient to discuss staphylococcal virulence factors in the context of these two groups because it reflects the overall view of the molecular pathogenesis of staphylococcal infection. More directly, the surface-associated virulence factors appear to function during the early stages of infection when the most important consideration for the bacterium is avoiding host phagocytes and establishing a focus of infection. In contrast, production of the extracellular virulence factors is delayed until the density of bacteria at a localized site of infection results in limited nutrient availability and the need to invade additional tissues.[101] This two-stage scenario implies that the regulatory elements that control expression of staphylococcal virulence factors are of paramount importance. In S. aureus, the two most prominent regulatory loci are the accessory gene regulator (agr) and the staphylococcal accessory regulator (sar). These loci are discussed elsewhere in this text, however, it is important to emphasize that mutation of either or both has been shown to result in reduced virulence using animal models of both osteomyelitis and septic arthritis.[1,41,87] Because sar is required for optimal expression of agr, and because agr is required for exoprotein synthesis, it is generally assumed that the reduced virulence of sar and agr regulatory mutants is a function of their reduced capacity to produce extracellular virulence factors.[101] *S. epidermidis* encodes homologs of both *sar* and *agr*,[37,91] however, perhaps because the coagulase-negative staphylococci rarely produce exotoxins, their role in musculoskeletal infection has not been assessed.

Factors That Promote Colonization

The staphylococcal virulence factors that promote colonization are of particular importance for two reasons. First, they serve their primary functions during the earliest stages of infection. Given the difficulties associated with the effective treatment of established infections, it seems reasonable to target these early events in an effort to impair the bacterium's ability to gain its initial foothold. The second reason is that recent data suggests that at least some of the most relevant colonization factors are conserved among all staphylococcal species.[24,49,75] That suggests that it might be possible to develop a single prophylactic protocol capable of limiting the ability of all staphylococcal species to cause musculoskeletal infection.

Christensen *et al.*[18] subdivided the process of colonizing biomaterials into the four stages of exposure, attachment, aggregation and dispersion (Figure 4). There is no reason to think that the same stages are not applicable to the colonization of host tissues including bone and cartilage. The impact of exposure is obvious and may account for the predominance of *S. epidermidis* as the primary pathogen of device-related infections. More directly, because *S. epidermidis* is the most prominent staphylococcal species on human skin, its predominance over *S. aureus* as a device-related pathogen may reflect the fact that implanted biomaterials are exposed to *S. epidermidis* more often and in larger numbers.[18] However, exposure merely provides the opportunity for colonization, which implies that both *S. epidermidis* and *S. aureus* produce specific adhesins that promote the subsequent processes of attachment and aggregation. These adhesins may well be the primary factors that define the staphylococci as musculoskeletal pathogens.

The staphylococci appear to make two classes of adhesins. The first are surface-exposed proteins, most of which are covalently anchored to the cell wall peptidoglycan. Included in this group are the MSCRAMMs, which appear to be the primary adhesins responsible for the attachment of *S. aureus* to both host tissues and biomaterials.[94] Although they do not necessarily qualify as MSCRAMMs, *S. epidermidis* also produces protein adhesins (see below). The second category are exopolysaccharides, which make an indirect contribution during the early stages of infection by virtue of their ability to inhibit phagocytosis.[85] That is particularly true with respect to

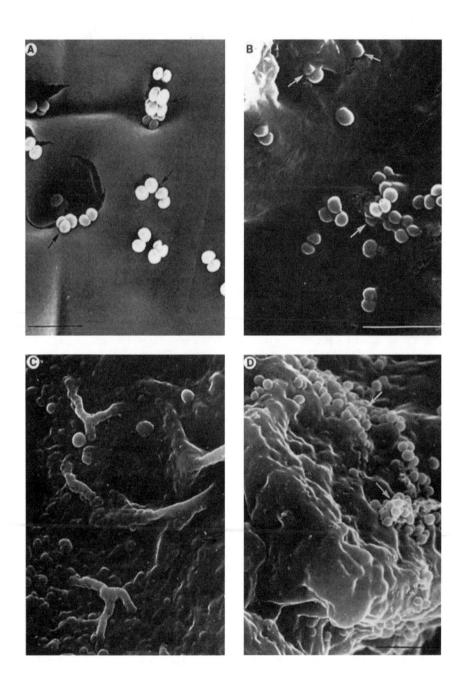

capsular polysaccharides, which clearly serve an important, antiphagocytic role.[119] However, the staphylococci also produce exopolysaccharides that function as adhesins.[108] Importantly, at least some exopolysaccharide adhesins are conserved and appear to serve the same functions in all staphylococcal species.[24,49,75]

Surface Protein Adhesins

The most extensively studied staphylococcal protein adhesins are the *S. aureus* MSCRAMMs. To date, *S. aureus* has been shown to exhibit specific, high-affinity binding of collagen,[118] fibronectin,[45] fibrinogen,[72,84] elastin,[92] laminin,[64] von Willebrand factor,[50] vitronectin,[58] thrombospondin[51] and bone sialoprotein.[109] Genes encoding MSCRAMMs that bind collagen (Cna), fibronectin (FnbpA and FnbpB), fibrinogen (ClfA and ClfB) and elastin (EbpS) have been cloned.[59,72,84,93,96] There is also evidence to suggest the existence of additional MSCRAMMs. Specifically, Josefsson *et al.*[60] described three genes (*sdrC, sdrD* and *sdrE*) that appear to encode MSCRAMMs based on a conserved region of serine-aspartate repeats (Sdr) like those found in ClfA and ClfB.[84] Although the putative ligand-binding domains of the Sdr MSCRAMMs exhibit little similarity,[60] the ligand-binding domains of ClfA and ClfB also exhibit relatively little similarity despite the fact that they both bind fibrinogen.[84] Based on that, it is unclear whether the differences in SdrC, SdrD and SdrE reflect a binding specificity for different host proteins or for different regions of the same protein.

The primary focus of studies aimed at assessing the role of MSCRAMMs in bone and joint infection has been directed at the

◄───

FIGURE 4. Stages involved in the colonization of biomaterials. The microphotographs demonstrate the colonization of *n*-butyl-cyanoacrylate by a strain of *S. epidermidis* recovered from a patient with endocarditis. (A) After 2 h of exposure. The cells have collected in surface pits and have formed small microcolonies. (B) After 4 h of exposure. The surface texture of the plastic has noticeably changed, and the cells have developed "foot processes." These changes are due to condensation of a newly formed thin covering sheet of polysaccharide-rich extracellular material ("glycocalyx"). (C) After 8 h of exposure. The surface of the plastic is totally obscured by a thick mat of bacteria, known as "slime," which consists of individual cells buried in the amorphous extracellular material. (D) After 24 h exposure. Nonadherent daughter cells, representing spontaneous phenotypic variants, have emerged from the slime and are now free to break away and drift to new colonization sites. *Reprinted with permission from Christensen G.D., Baldassarri, L., and Simpson, W.A.: Colonization of medical devices by coagulase-negative staphylococci. In: Bisno, A. L. and Waldvogel, F. A. Infections Associated with Indwelling Medical Devices, ASM Press, Washington, D.C., 1994:45–78.*

Cna collagen-binding protein. That focus is based on reports suggesting that the ability to bind collagen is a conserved characteristic of muscusloskeletal isolates.[54] That is an important observation since most *S. aureus* strains do not encode *cna* and do not bind collagen.[42] Although other reports have failed to find any correlation between collagen binding and musculoskeletal disease,[120] Cna is present on the surface of *S. aureus* cells growing in bone,[43] and infection with a *cna*-positive strain elicits an anti-Cna antibody response.[110] These results confirm that Cna is expressed *in vivo* during the course of *S. aureus* infection. Additionally, Nilsson *et al.*[86] demonstrated that active immunization with recombinant Cna and passive immunization with Cna-specific antibodies protects mice against intravenous challenge with *S. aureus*. Other studies have confirmed that *S. aureus* binds directly to collagen fibrils in cartilage[124] and that the Cna adhesin is both necessary and sufficient for this binding.[96] Most importantly, a *cna* mutant was shown to be less virulent than its isogenic parent strain in animal models of septic arthritis[95] and endocarditis.[53] Conversely, introduction of *cna* into a *cna*-negative strain enhanced virulence in the septic arthritis model.[95]

Although the focus has been on Cna and its role in musculoskeletal disease, *S. aureus* also produces MSCRAMMs that bind fibronectin and fibrinogen. That is important since both of these proteins occur in soluble form in plasma and are deposited on the surface of implanted biomaterials.[123] The ability to bind fibronectin is a highly conserved characteristic of *S. aureus*. It is a function of two MSCRAMM adhesins encoded by closely linked but independently expressed genes designated *fnbA* and *fnbB*.[38] Most strains appear to express both genes, and expression of either gene is sufficient to confer a level of fibronectin binding comparable to that observed in those strains that encode and express both genes.[45] The *fnbA* and *fnbB* genes are very similar and presumably arose by gene duplication. Fibronectin is a large glycoprotein found in soluble form in plasma and other body fluids and in a less soluble form in the extracellular matrix. It promotes clot formation and wound healing by binding to fibrin clots and promoting the adherence of platelets and fibroblasts to sites of inflammation. The binding of soluble fibronectin could provide the bacterium with a means to escape immune recognition or, based on the interaction between bound fibronectin and other host proteins found within the extracellular matrix, could serve as a bridge between the bacterium and host tissues.[102] Mutants of *S. aureus* unable to bind fibronectin have been shown to have a reduced capacity to colonize implanted coverslips.[45] Although it has not been directly examined using animal models of osteomyelitis or septic arthritis, Scheld *et al.*[112] reported a correlation between the ability to bind fibronectin and the propensity to cause endocarditis.

S. aureus also encodes at least two fibrinogen binding MSCRAMMs.[84] Because they promote the clumping of S. aureus in the presence of soluble fibrinogen, these MSCRAMMs are referred to as clumping factor A (ClfA) and clumping factor B (ClfB).[72,84] In contrast to FnbpA and FnbpB, the fibrinogen-binding MSCRAMMs do not bind the same regions of the fibrinogen molecule.[73,111] Soluble fibrinogen promotes the adherence of S. aureus to human endothelial cells by acting as a bridge between the bacterium and surface receptors present on the surface of the target cells.[17] S. aureus also induces platelet aggregation via a fibrinogen-dependent mechanism.[11] The observation that a recombinant form of the ClfA ligand-binding A domain inhibits platelet aggregation clearly implies that ClfA is more important than ClfB in that regard.[73] ClfA has also been shown to facilitate the adherence to immobilized fibrinogen deposited on the surface of implanted medical devices.[73] The fact that mutation of clfA results in a reduced capacity to adhere to platelet/fibrin clots and a reduced capacity to cause endocarditis[79] suggests that the contribution made by ClfB is relatively minor by comparison to ClfA. On the other hand, comparison of clfA and clfB mutants confirmed that ClfB promotes cell clumping and adherence to immobilized fibrinogen even in the absence of ClfA.[84] The production of two fibrinogen-binding proteins may reflect the fundamental nature of the need to bind fibrinogen. Indeed, Dickenson et al.[28] demonstrated that clfA, coa double mutants were not displaced from a fibrinogen-coated surface even under shear forces simulating blood flow. That clearly suggests that ClfB is sufficient to maintain contact with a fibrinogen-coated substrate. The production of two different fibrinogen-binding adhesins may also allow the bacterium to adhere to fibrin clots even in the presence of antibodies that block the activity of one adhesin.[84]

Although they do not necessarily qualify as MSCRAMMs, S. epidermidis also produces a number of surface protein adhesins. For example, Timmerman et al.[121] described a 220 kDa surface protein that promotes attachment of S. epidermidis to uncoated biomaterials. Other studies have identified a fibrinogen-binding protein[89] and an autolysin (AtlE) that not only promotes the primary attachment to polystyrene but also binds vitronectin.[48] The ability to bind serum proteins may promote the attachment to protein-coated implants and the subsequent aggregation of bacteria. Interestingly, Baldassarri et al.[9] demonstrated that the production of exopolysaccharide "slime" (see below) interferes with host protein receptors of S. epidermidis. That is consistent with reports suggesting that blood proteins do not promote the adherence of S. epidermidis to biomaterials.[81] However, it should be emphasized that this conclusion may apply only to strains that produce relatively large amounts of exopolysaccharides. Indeed, there are adherent strains of *S. epidermidis* that do not produce slime, and these strains exhibit greater surface hydrophobicity and the ability to adhere to biomaterials coated with host proteins including fibrinogen and fibronectin.[9] There are also reports suggesting that slime is not produced during the earliest stages of attachment.[97] Taken together, these results suggest that *S. epidermidis* surface proteins may be particularly important during the earliest stages of attachment before slime production becomes a factor. On the other hand, Hussain *et al.*[55] described a 140 kDa extracellular protein, the production of which was restricted to sessile bacteria and was closely associated with the ability to form a biofilm. Based on that, this protein was designated the "accumulation-associated protein".[55]

Staphylococcal Exopolysaccharides

It is clear that both *S. aureus* and *S. epidermidis* produce surface protein adhesins that promote their attachment to host tissues and biomaterials. It is also clear that at least some of these adhesins can promote the aggregation of bacterial cells by virtue of their ability to bind soluble proteins that are subsequently bound by other bacteria. Nevertheless, more recent data strongly suggests that the primary determinants required for the later stages of aggregation and biofilm formation are exopolysaccharides. In contrast to the MSCRAMMs, these have been most extensively studied in the coagulase-negative staphylococci, where they have been ambiguously referred to as capsule or "slime."[21] Early studies attempting to characterize "slime" were complicated by contamination with media components,[29] which lead to a great deal of confusion about its chemical composition. Although Hussain *et al.*[56] recently suggested that slime consists of techoic acid fragments rather than exopolysaccharides, other reports disagree with that conclusion,[10] and the term "slime" is still applied to the accumulated exopolysaccharides (Figure 5) associated with *S. epidermidis* biofilms.[6]

Christensen *et al.*[21] was among the first to report a correlation between the production of slime and the ability of *S. epidermidis* to adhere to plastic. It was noted that some strains did not produce slime and that slime production was dependent on growth conditions, most notably the inclusion of carbohydrates in the growth medium. It was also noted that slime production was more common among bacteremia isolates than among commensal isolates from the skin.[6] Based on that, it was suggested that slime may be an important factor that distinguishes between "virulent" and "avirulent" strains of *S. epidermidis*. Subsequent studies confirmed the existence of a "slime-associated antigen" (SAA) that was both heat and protease

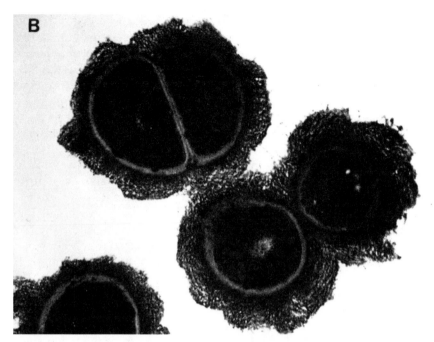

FIGURE 5. Staphylococcal exopolysaccharides. Transmission electron micrograph of *S. epidermidis* strain RP12 showing a highly organized thick layer of extracellular material covering the bacterial cell. The extracellular material stains with Alcian blue, indicating that the material is a polysaccharide. *Reprinted with permission from Christensen G.D., Baldassarri, L., and Simpson, W.A.: Colonization of medical devices by coagulase-negative staphylococci. In: Bisno, A. L. and Waldvogel, F. A. Infections Associated with Indwelling Medical Devices, ASM Press, Washington, D.C., 1994:45–78.*

stable.[19] However, Baldassarri *et al.*[10] found that SAA was produced by only 59% of slime-positive strains, which strongly suggests that additional "slime-associated" antigens exist. Tojo *et al.*[122] subsequently purified a polysaccharide adhesin (designated CPA or, more commonly, PS/A) that was distinct from SAA[19] and was also produced by some, but not all, adherent strains of *S. epidermidis*. Like SAA, slime-positive strains that do not produce PS/A have been identified,[82] and PS/A mutants are still able to colonize indwelling catheters and cause endocarditis.[113]

More definitive characterization of the exopolysaccharide adhesins was greatly enhanced by the development of efficient protocols for the genetic manipulation of the staphylococci. For instance, Muller *et al.*[80] described a set of transposon-insertion mutants that did not produce slime or PS/A and were deficient with respect to both the initial attachment phase and accumulation into biofilms. The close association of the two phenotypes, together with the fact that all of the transposon insertions mapped to the same 11.6 kb region of the chromosome, clearly suggests that PS/A production is closely associated with slime production.[80] However, because mutants unable to attach would presumably also be deficient with respect to the subsequent steps that lead to biofilm formation, these results are inconclusive with respect to the relative contribution of PS/A and slime to the separate steps of attachment and aggregation.

Heilmann *et al.*[47] provided convincing genetic evidence that the attachment and aggregation of *S. epidermidis* occur via a two-step process mediated by distinct adhesins. Specifically, they identified two classes of mutants, one of which (class A) lacked five surface proteins, was less hydrophobic, and was deficient in the primary attachment to polysytrene despite the fact that they could still form multi-layered cell clusters.[47,48] It was subsequently demonstrated class mutants were deficient in the production of five proteins, all of which were derived from the 120 kDa AtlE progenitor.[48] The 60 and 52 kDa proteins derived from AtlE were identified as an amidase and a glucosaminidase respectively.[48] The other two proteins were smaller (45 and 38 kDa) and were thought to be degradation products of the 60 and 52 kDa proteins. Complementation studies revealed that the 60 kDa amidase was sufficient to restore the ability to attach to polystyrene.[47] As noted above, these results strongly suggest that AtlE is a primary mediator of the initial events leading to the colonization of biomaterials.

The second class of mutants (class B) could attach to polystyrene but could not form multi-layered clusters.[47] They did not exhibit any change in surface proteins or hydrophobicity. Mack *et al.*[67] also identified *S. epidermidis* mutants that exhibited a wild-type phenotype with respect to the initial adherence events but were defective in the accumulative phase of biofilm formation. Based on the phenotype of these mutants, it was suggested that the adhesin, which was identified as a β-1,6-linked glucosaminoglycan, be referred to as the polysaccharide intercellular adhesin or PIA.[65] Subsequent studies confirmed that class B mutants were PIA-deficient and that PIA production was restored by introduction of a plasmid carrying the *ica* (intercellular adhesin) operon.[49] The *ica* locus contains four genes (*icaA, icaB, icaC* and *icaD*). IcaA and IcaD are membrane proteins that are responsible for the N-acetylglucosaminyl transferase activity that appears to be the primary determinant of PIA biosynthesis.[40] IcaB includes a signal sequence and appears to be transported out of the cell although its function remains unknown.[49] IcaC also appears to be an integral membrane protein and is required, along with

IcaA and IcaD, for long chain PIA biosynthesis.[40,49] A comparison of 179 strains of *S. epidermidis* confirmed that 86.8% of the biofilm-producing strains produced PIA while 88.6% of the biofilm-negative strains did not.[66] Interestingly, the *ica* operon is also present in *S. aureus* and also contributes to biofilm formation in that species.[24,49]

More recent studies have suggested that SAA and PIA may be the same thing.[10] Also, McKenney *et al.*[74] recently demonstrated that PS/A is encoded by the *ica* locus and suggested that the only difference between PIA and PS/A is the nature of the substituent groups attached to the β-1,6-linked polyglucosamine backbone. Moreover, Rupp *et al.*[107] identified an *S. epidermidis* hemagglutinin that also appears to be closely related if not identical to PIA.[108] These results certainly do not preclude the hypothesis that the adherence of *S. epidermidis* to biomaterials is a two-stage process involving multiple adhesins. However, the convergence of several investigators on PIA clearly implies that the *ica* locus and the production of PIA plays a predominant role with respect to biofilm formation and the pathogenesis of *S. epidermidis* foreign-body infections.[108] Interestingly, McKenney *et al.*[75] recently demonstrated that immunization with PIA, which they referred to as PNSG (poly-*N*-succinyl β-1-6 glucosamine), protected mice against hematogenous challenge with *S. aureus*. They also demonstrated that PIA was produced by *S. aureus* but only when the bacterium was growing *in vivo*. Since the challenge was done by intravenous infection, it is unclear whether the effect was a function of the enhanced phagocytosis of *S. aureus* in the bloodstream or an impaired capacity to colonize host tissues and form a biofilm. The latter possibility has particular relevance since biofilm formation is a hallmark feature of staphylococcal musculoskeletal infection.[23,35] Indeed, formation of a biofilm is a primary factor complicating the ability to resolve musculoskeletal infections without surgical debridement.[34,35,62] Moreover, conservation of *ica* and PIA production in both *S. aureus* and *S. epidermidis* suggests that it might be possible to develop therapeutic protocols that would encompass all of the primary staphylococcal musculoskeletal pathogens.[75]

Finally, several studies have confirmed that PIA production is subject to phase variation.[126] This variation occurs at both the physiological and the genetic level. For instance, the presence of exogenous sugars (e.g., glucose) is required for biofilm formation *in vitro*.[6] Also, Ziebuhr *et al.*[128] demonstrated genetic phase variation that is dependent on the insertion and excision of a transposable element (IS256) into the *ica* locus. Although these studies were done in *S. epidermidis*, it is clear that the *ica* locus is more highly conserved in *S. aureus* than the ability to produce a biofilm, at least with respect to *in vitro* growth conditions.[24] The same can be said of *S. aureus* capsular polysaccharides,[61] however, it is important to emphasize that PIA and capsular polysaccharides are not the same thing. Moreover, while the absence of a capsule does reduce the capacity of *S. aureus* to cause septic arthritis, this effect appears to be a function of the antiphagocytic properties of the capsule rather than a direct contribution to the colonization of cartilage.[85] Indeed, there is no direct evidence to suggest that *S. aureus* capsular polysaccharides function as adhesins that promote the colonization of host tissues or biomaterials.[49,113] That is consistent with the observation that we have been unable to demonstrate a virulence difference between heavily-encapsulated serotype 1 and 2 strains and their corresponding capsule mutants using a rabbit model of acute, post-traumatic osteomyelitis (data not shown). Moreover, when we used the same model to compare the virulence of a heavily-encapsulated strain (Smith diffuse) with a microencapsulated, serotype 8 strain (UAMS-1) obtained directly from the bone of a patient suffering from osteomyelitis, we found that UAMS-1 was significantly more virulent.[114] Importantly, the opposite was true (i.e., Smith diffuse was more virulent than UAMS-1) when the comparison was done using a murine peritonitis model.[114] Although not definitive, these results suggest that capsule production is not an important factor contributing to the pathogenesis of osteomyelitis. These results also emphasize the existence of specific, strain-dependent characteristics that are directly relevant to the pathogenesis of musculoskeletal infection.

Interestingly, subsequent studies revealed that heavily-encapsulated strains *of S. aureus* do not bind collagen even if they produce the Cna MSCRAMM.[42] Comparisons with isogenic capsule mutants indicate that the inability to bind collagen is due to masking of Cna on the cell surface. As noted above, a similar masking effect has been described in *S. epidermidis*.[9] To the extent that the Cna adhesin is thought to make an important contribution to the colonization of bone and cartilage,[54,118,124] this suggests that capsule mutants might actually have enhanced virulence, at least with respect to non-hematogenous forms of infection. However, it is important to emphasize that heavily-encapsulated, serotype 1 and 2 strains are not representative of the micro-encapsulated serotype 5 and 8 strains that cause the overwhelming majority of *S. aureus* infections.[8] Indeed, our comparisons between serotype 8 strains and their corresponding capsule mutants have not revealed any significant difference in the ability to bind collagen[42] or the ability to cause osteomyelitis (data not shown).

Factors That Damage The Host

While the protein and exopolysaccharide adhesins play a pivotal role in the initiating events leading to infection, they are not responsible for the pathological effects observed as the infection progresses. Nair *et al.*[83] pointed out that bacteria cause bone destruction by one of three mechanisms. The first is the production of degradative products that destroy the noncellular components of bone. Although *S. aureus* produces a number of degradative enzymes, the role of these proteins in bone loss has not been investigated. The second is the production of bacterial products that promote cellular processes that stimulate the degradation of bone. The third is inhibition of bone synthesis. There is mounting evidence to suggest that the last two are responsible for most of the bone loss associated with *S. aureus* musculoskeletal infection.

Nair *et al.*[76] reported the existence of a "surface-associated material" (SAM) that could be extracted from *S. aureus* by gentle stirring in saline and was capable of promoting bone resorption as evidenced by the release of calcium in a murine calvarial bone resorption assay. This material was found to contain at least 15 proteins ranging in size from 14 to 90 kDa.[76] Fractionation revealed that the most active component contained a 35 kDa protein that appeared to be a heterodimer of 16–18 kDa proteins. Subsequent studies revealed that the *S. aureus* SAM induces bone resorption by stimulating osteoclast proliferation and fusion of osteoclast precursors to form multinucleated cells.[76] This activity was inhibited in the presence of antibodies against TNF-α and IL-6. *S. epidermidis* was also recently shown to produce SAM although the proteins involved appear to be larger (50–66 kDa) and the *S. epidermidis* SAM appears to promote bone resorption by a slightly different mechanism.[77]

These studies raise the possibility that much of the bone pathology associated with staphylococcal infection results from the induction of cytokines that alter the process of bone remodeling. That is consistent with the fact that *S. aureus* is a much more virulent pathogen than *S. epidermidis* and the fact that, unlike *S. epidermidis*, *S. aureus* produces a diverse array of exotoxins, many of which are known to be potent inducers of cytokine production. Specific exotoxins shown to contribute to the pathogenesis of musculoskeletal infection include toxic shock syndrome toxin-1 (TSST-1),[2,3] the enterotoxins,[15] and the α and γ hemolytic toxins.[88] The effect of the α and γ hemolytic toxins, both of which are pore-forming toxins, appears to be synergistic since mutants unable to produce only one of these toxins were not significantly attenuated with respect to their ability to cause septic arthritis.[88]

Most of the aforementioned toxins, as well as the superantigens TSST-1 and the enterotoxins, induce production of IL-1β, IL-6 and TNFα, which has the direct effect of inducing osteoclast activation and the indirect effect of triggering synovial macrophages to produce additional proinflammatory mediators.[15,88] Superantigen induction of cytokine production is due to the stimulation of large numbers of CD4[+] T lymphocytes, which also has the effect of inducing polyclonal B cell activation.[2,4] Indeed, antibodies against CD4 and the Vβ region of the T cell receptor inhibit the development of arthritis.[3] Peptidoglycan and/or polysaccharides also appear to contribute to B cell activation, particularly during the early stages of infection.[4] As confirmed using animal models of both septic arthritis[13] and osteomyelitis,[125] the combined effect results in massive infiltration of phagocytes and T cells. Based on these considerations, Bremell *et al.*[13] proposed a three-step process to explain the pathogenesis of *S. aureus* septic arthritis. The first step is the introduction of bacteria either directly or by seeding from the bloodstream. In the latter case, the MSCRAMMs adhesins (e.g., Cna) presumably guide homing of the bacterium to the synovium. The second step involves a nonspecific inflammatory response in which bacteria are phagocytosed by macrophages and polymorphonuclear neutrophils (PMNs). Whether or not the infection progresses beyond this point depends largely on the phagocytic capacity of the host and the specific properties of the infecting strain. If, for instance, the strain produces TSST-1 or one of the other superantigens, a massive infiltration of T cells ensues resulting in T cell proliferation and induction of cytokine synthesis. As noted above, IL-1β, IL-6 and TNFα appear to be particularly important in that regard. The results obtained with a mouse osteomyelitis model are entirely consistent with this overall hypothesis.[125]

Internalization and Small Colony Variants

One of the hallmark features of staphylococcal osteomyelitis is its tendency to recur even after long periods of apparent quiescence. Although it has not been proven, there is a general presumption that subsequent infections represent an actual recurrence of the primary infection rather than a second, etiologically unrelated infection. That raises the question of how the bacteria managed to persist in the host for an extended period in the absence of any clinical evidence of disease. Recent data suggests two intriguing possibilities. First, although *S. aureus* is generally considered a prototypical extracellular pathogen, *in vitro* studies have recently confirmed that it can invade and persist within host cells.[30] Importantly, osteoblasts are included among the host cell targets.[31,57,103] Internalization appears to be dependent on a receptor-mediated pathway[57] that requires host cell tyrosine kinase activity.[30] Studies with mutants unable to produce either fibronectin-binding protein also demonstrated that the ability to bind fibronectin was required for efficient internalization.[30] The fact that these mutants retained the capacity to adhere to epithelial cells suggests that internalization is probably a multi-step process that may also involve other *S. aureus* adhesins. Also, the observation that excess fibronectin blocked internalization suggests that the interaction between *S. aureus* and the host cell surface probably occurs via a direct interaction with an as yet unidentified host cell receptor rather than an indirect bridging mechanism mediated by fibronectin.[30]

The second possibility that could account for the long-term persistence of *S. aureus* is the formation of small-colony variants (SCVs). Interestingly, Proctor[98] noted that many of the characteristics of SCVs are also observed among bacteria growing on the surface of implanted biomaterials. Included among these characteristics are a reduced growth rate, the failure to produce hemolytic toxins, decreased oxidative metabolism and a reduced susceptibility to antibiotics.[98] Transient deficiencies in electron transport appear to be responsible for the reduced capacity to produce hemolytic toxins and the increased resistance to antibiotics, particularly with respect to the aminoglycosides.[98,99] Indeed, von Eiff *et al.*[99] reported that the use of gentamicin-impregnated beads in the treatment of patients suffering from osteomyelitis may actually select for SCVs. Although the SCV phenotype is reversible, it has been associated with growth *in vivo* and with growth in the presence of antibiotics.[98] Most importantly, SCVs have been isolated from patients suffering from recurrent infections including osteomyelitis.[100] Finally, it has been suggested that the issues of internalization by host cells and SCVs may be directly related in that the SCV phenotype may promote survival of bacteria within the intracellular environment.[98]

Animal Models of Musculoskeletal Infection

The ability to assess the contribution of individual virulence factors to the pathogenesis of staphylococcal musculoskeletal infection depends on the availability of appropriate animal models. That has proven a formidable task both because *S. aureus* produces a remarkable array of virulence factors, many of which are functionally redundant, and because the conditions that contribute to musculoskeletal infection are extremely difficult to mimic in model systems. That is particularly true with respect to osteomyelitis, where most animal models have relied on the direct introduction of bacteria into bone, usually after traumatizing the bone and usually in the presence of schlerosing agents and/or foreign bodies. For example, Rissing *et al.*[104] developed a rat model in which *S. aureus* and sodium morrhuate were introduced directly into the bone marrow either by direct injection or via a hole drilled in the tibial metaphysis. Spagnolo *et al.*[117] avoided the use of schlerosing agents and foreign-body implants by sealing bacteria into the bone with fibrin glue. Because *S. aureus* produces

fibrinogen-binding proteins, the fibrin glue would presumably provide
an alternative substrate for colonization that would effectively mimic the
presence of a foreign-body implant. The model we use does not employ
schlerosing agents or implants but does rely on the introduction of bacteria directly into a devascularized bone segment.[114] Despite the severity of
these models, it is important to recognize that *S. aureus* osteomyelitis is
often a consequence of trauma that results in the formation of necrotic
bone. Additionally, resolution of the infection often requires reconstruc-
tive surgery that requires the use of orthopaedic implants. Based on these
observations, such models should not be dismissed as wholly inappropriate. Indeed, our model was successfully used to demonstrate that *agr*
mutants are less virulent than their wild-type counterparts.[41] Such models
have also proven remarkably useful with respect to the evaluation of alternative therapeutic protocols.[34,44]

Models that mimic the hematogenous seeding of bone have proven
inordinately difficult to develop even after subjecting animals to extreme
procedures like those discussed above. An exception are avian models that
take advantage of the fact that the circulatory architecture in the avian wing
is similar to that observed in growing human bones.[32] However, there are
important differences between avian and mammalian systems that suggest
that these models may not be representative of human infection.[27] That
is perhaps best evidenced by the fact that models of hematogenous
osteomyelitis that employ mammalian species are inconsistent in the
absence of prior trauma. For instance, Hienz *et al.*[52] described a hematogenous model in rats that required drilling a hole in the tibia or mandible
and introducing sodium morrhuate into the defect prior to introducing
bacteria via the femoral vein. Although Matsushita *et al.*[70] described a
mouse model of hematogenous infection that did not require pretreatment
of the mice, the model was highly strain dependent both in terms of "lodge-
ment" of bacteria in the bone marrow and the ability to cause clinical evidence of osteomyelitis. More recently, Chadha *et al.*[16] described a mouse
model in which hematogenous infection was established following the
introduction of an "incomplete cartilaginous fracture of the right proximal
tibial growth plate". This model appeared to be more reproducible than
other models and has the distinct advantage of allowing the use of the
diverse immunological tools available for murine systems.[125] It could
also be argued that such fractures are representative of the precipitating
traumas that often lead to osteomyelitis.

By comparison, models of staphylococcal septic arthritis are relatively
straightforward. For example, Bremell *et al.*[14] described a murine model
that achieved a high infection rate (80–90%) by simply introducing
S. aureus into the tail vein. This model was used to characterize the

histological progression of septic arthritis and the nature of the host immune response.[12,13] It was also used to demonstrate that the capacity of *S. aureus* to cause septic arthritis is reduced by mutation of the *sar* or *agr* regulatory loci[1,87] and by mutation of *cna*.[95]

Adherence of staphylococci to biomaterials has been assessed *in vitro* using plastic (e.g., polystyrene microtiter plates), glass and various polymers (e.g., polyethylene or polyvinyl chloride tubing).[47] These surfaces are not necessarily equivalent. For instance, Heilmann *et al.*[47] isolated *S. epidermidis* mutants that were deficient with respect to attachment to polystyrene but were still able to form a biofilm on glass. They also isolated mutants with the opposite phenotype (i.e. able to attach to polystyrene but unable to form a biofilm on glass). The impact of serum proteins on attachment has been assessed by precoating surfaces either with whole blood or purified proteins (e.g. fibrinogen, fibronectin).[45,84] The ability of *S. aureus* to bind collagen has been studied using collagen-coated glass coverslips exposed to shear forces that approximate those observed in the blood.[78,115] The ability to bind cartilage has been studied directly using disks of bovine nasal cartilage.[118]

Several *in vivo* models have also been described including some that specifically assess the impact of implants on musculoskeletal infection.[26,36,108] For example, Fischer *et al.*[36] utilized a guinea pig model in which titanium plates were attached to the iliac bones to demonstrate that *S. aureus* strains unable to bind fibronectin have a reduced capacity for colonization. Darouiche *et al.*[26] used a rabbit model in which a stainless steel screw was inserted into a hole drilled through the intracondylar notch and into the medullary canal of the femur. Using this model, these authors were unable to demonstrate a significant difference between a wild-type strain of *S. aureus* and isogenic mutants unable to bind fibrinogen, fibronectin or collagen. The ability of *S. epidermidis* to bind orthopaedic implants has not been specifically addressed, however, Rupp *et al.*[108] recently demonstrated that mutants unable to produce the polysaccharide intercellular adhesin (PIA) have a reduced capacity to adhere to subcutaneously-implanted catheters and are less likely to cause abscess formation.

6. TREATMENT OF STAPHYLOCOCCAL MUSCULOSKELETAL INFECTION

The treatment of staphylococcal musculoskeletal infections is remarkably intrusive. Indeed, the difficulties associated with the resolution of musculoskeletal infections are so pronounced that Mader and Calhoun[68] have suggested that it is more appropriate to refer to the successful treatment of osteomyelitis as having "arrested" rather than "cured" the infection. Moreover, Cierny[22] found that the treatment protocol required to "arrest" the infection was worse than the infection itself in 10–15% of adult osteomyelitis patients. The best option in an additional 10% of patients was amputation.

The treatment and prognosis of adult osteomyelitis is directly related to the physiological, anatomical and psychosocial factors that dictate whether the surgical treatment is simple, complex, curative, palliative or ablative. The site of the infection and the amount of tissue necrosis dictate the appropriate type of therapy. As discussed above, the amount of tissue necrosis is defined by the Cierny-Mader classification system. From this staging system, the two key factors in treatment are proper identification of the infecting bacterium and its antibiotic-susceptibility profile and determination of the method to be employed for delivery of the antibiotic. However, at least in the case of chronic osteomyelitis, it is clear that adequate debridement of necrotic bone is a fundamental requirement that must be completed for antibiotic therapy to be effective.

Surgical debridement is a complicated process that can take several forms depending on the extent of bone destruction. In the case of acute osteomyelitis, surgical intervention may be limited to decompression to release intramedullary or subperiosteal pressure.[62] In chronic osteomyelitis, it is generally necessary to remove all necrotic bone and soft tissue irrespective of the size of the resulting defect. In such cases, it may be necessary to employ bone grafts to fill the dead space and revascularization procedures (e.g., muscle flaps) to enhance the ability to ward off recurrent infection.[62] In the case of osteomyelitis secondary to vascular insufficiency, the primary factor determining whether amputation can be avoided is whether revascularization is successful enough to raise the oxygen tension in the infected tissue to a level that will allow the wound to heal.[62] Based on these considerations, the overall treatment protocol can be summarized by the sequential steps of 1) identification of the infecting bacterium and determination of its antibiotic susceptibility profile, 2) implementation of steps aimed at optimizing the condition of the host, 3) debridement and stabilization of the defect, 4) systemic and/or local delivery of antibiotics and 5) reconstruction of the defect.

The issue of localized delivery of antibiotics within a bone defect remains somewhat controversial. It is clear that the use of antibiotic-laden bone cement can result in localized concentrations of antibiotics that exceed those that can be achieved by the use of intravenous drugs. However, it is unlikely that localized antibiotic delivery systems will eliminate the need for systemic antibiotic therapy. Indeed, using a rabbit osteomyelitis model, Evans and Nelson[34] demonstrated that the highest success rate was dependent on the implantation of antibiotic-impregnated beads and the concomitant use of systemic antibiotics. Parenteral antibiotics are usually administered for at least four and more commonly six weeks.[62] In the case of hematogenous osteomyelitis in children, parenteral antibiotics followed by several weeks of oral therapy is usually sufficient provided that diagnosis and treatment is not delayed and patient compliance is high.[62] However, it remains imperative that the infection be closely monitored and that surgical decompression be employed in a timely fashion if the symptoms of the infection do not abate.[62]

In those cases involving infected orthopaedic implants, it is almost imperative that the implant be removed. A primary question is whether to employ "two-stage exchange arthroplasty" or "one-stage exchange arthroplasty", the difference being that the former employs a period of parenteral antimicrobial therapy between removal and implantation of a new prosthesis while the latter incorporates removal and reconstruction into a single procedure.[62] In the case of a one-stage procedure, antibiotic-laden bone cement is always used, however, one-stage arthroplasty does have a higher rate of recurrence than the two-stage procedure.[62]

REFERENCES

1. Abdelnour, A., Arvidson, S., Bremell, T., et al.: The accessory gene regulator (agr) controls Staphylococcus aureus virulence in a murine arthritis model. Infection and Immunity 61:3879–3885, 1993.
2. Adelnour A. and Bremell, T.: Toxic shock syndrome toxin 1 contributes to the arthritogenecity of Staphylococcus aureus. Journal of Infectious Diseases 170:94–99 (1994).
3. Abdelnour, A., Bremell, T., Holmdahl, R., et al.: Clonal expansion of T lymphocytes causes arthritis and mortality in mice infected with toxic shock syndrome toxin 1-producing staphylococci. European Journal of Immunology 24:1161–1166, 1994.
4. Abdelnour A. and Tarkowski, A.: Polyclonal B-cell activation by an arthritogenic Staphylococcus aureus strain: contribution of T-cell and monokines. Cellular Immunology 147:279–293, 1993.
5. Alderson, M., Speers, D., Emslie, K., et al.: Acute haematogenous osteomyelitis and septic arthritis—a single disease: an hypothesis based upon the presence of transphyseal blood vessels. Journal of Bone and Joint Surgery 68-B:268–274, 1986.
6. Ammendolia, M. G., Di Rosa, R., Montanaro, L., et al.: Slime production and expression of the slime-associated antigen by staphylococcal clinical isolates. Journal of Clinical Microbiology 37:3235–3238, 1999.
7. Amorena, B., Gracia, E., Monzon, M., et al.: Antibiotic susceptibility assay for Staphylococcus aureus in biofilms developed in vitro. Journal of Antimicrobial Chemotherapy 44:43–55, 1999.
8. Arbeit, R. D., Karakawa, W. W., Vann, W. F., et al.: Predominance of two newly described capsular polysaccharide types among clinical isolates of Staphylococcus aureus. Diagnostic Microbiology and Infectious Diseases 2:85–91, 1984.

9. Baldassarri, L., Donelli, G., Gelosia, A., *et al.*: Expression of slime interferes with *in vitro* detection of host protein receptors of *Staphylococcus epidermidis. Infection and Immunity* 65:1522–1526, 1997.

10. Baldassarri, L., Donelli, G., Gelosia, A., *et al.*: Purification and characterization of the Staphylococcal slime-associated antigen and its occurrence among *Staphylococcus epidermidis* clinical isolates. *Infection and Immunity* 64:3410–3415, 1996.

11. Bayer, A. S., Sullam, P. M., Ramos, M., *et al.*: *Staphylococcus aureus* induces platelet aggregation via a fibrinogen-dependent mechanism which is independent of principal platelet glycoprotein independent of principal platelet glycoprotein IIb/IIIa fibrinogen-binding domains. *Infection and Immunity* 63:3634–3641, 1995.

12. Bremell, T., Abdelnour, A., and Tarkowski, A.: Histopathological and serological progression of experimental *Staphylococcus aureus* arthritis. *Infection and Immunity* 60:2976–2985, 1992.

13. Bremell, T., Lange, S., Holmdahl, R., *et al.*: Immunopathological features of rat *Staphylococcus aureus* arthritis. *Infection and Immunity* 62:2334–2344, 1994.

14. Bremell, T., Lange, S., Yacoub, A., *et al.*: Experimental *Staphylococcus aureus* arthritis in mice. *Infection and Immunity* 59:2615–2623, 1991.

15. Bremell, T. and Tarkowski, A.: Preferential induction of septic arthritis and mortality by superantigen-producing staphylococci. *Infection and Immunity* 63:4185–4187, 1995.

16. Chadha, H. S., Fitzgerald, R. H., Jr., Wiater, P., *et al.*: Experimental acute hematogenous osteomyelitis in mice. I. Histopathological and immunological findings. *Journal of Orthopaedic Research* 17:376–381, 1999.

17. Cheung, A. L., Krishnan, M., Jaffe, E. A., *et al.*: Fibrinogen acts as a bridging molecule in the adherence of *Staphylococcus aureus* to cultured human endothelial cells. *The Journal of Clinical Investigation* 87:2236–2245, 1991.

18. Christensen, G. D., Baldassarri, L., and Simpson, W. A.: Colonization of medical devices by coagulase-negative staphylococci. *In:* Bisno, A. L. and Waldvogel, F. A. *Infections Associated with Indwelling Medical Devices*, ASM Press, Washington, D.C., 1994: 45–78.

19. Christensen, G. D., Barker, L. P., Mawhinney, T. P., *et al.*: Identification of an antigenic marker of slime production for *Staphylococcus epidermidis. Infection and Immunity* 58:2906–2911, 1990.

20. Christensen, G. D. and Simpson, W. A.: Gram-positive bacteria: Pathogenesis of staphylococcal musculoskeletal infections. *In:* Esterhai, J. L., Jr., Gristina, A. G., and Poss, R. (Eds.), *Musculoskeletal Infection*, American Academy of Orthopaedic Surgeons, Park Ridge, Il, 1990:57–78.

21. Christensen, G. D., Simpson, W. A., Bisno, A. L., *et al.*: Adherence of slime-producing strains of *Staphylococcus epidermidis* to smooth surfaces. *Infection and Immunity* 37:318–326, 1982.

22. Cierny, G. III.: Classification and treatment of adult osteomyelitis. *In:* Evarts, C. M. (Ed.), *Surgery of the Musuloskeletal System*, Churchill Livingston, New York, 1990:4337–4379.

23. Costerton, J. W., Stewart, P. S., and Greenberg, E. P.: Bacterial biofilms: a common cause of persistent infections. *Science* 284:1318–1322, 1999.

24. Cramton, S. E., Gerke, C., Schnell, N. F., *et al.*: The intercellular adhesion (*ica*) locus is present in *Staphylococcus aureus* and is required for biofilm formation. *Infection and Immunity* 67:5427–5433, 1999.

25. Cunningham, R., Cockayne, A., and Humphreys, H.: Clinical and molecular aspects of the pathogenesis of *Staphylococcus aureus* bone and joint infections. *Journal of Medical Microbiology* 44:157–164, 1996.

26. Darouiche, R. O., Landon, G. C., Patti, J. M., et al.: Role of Staphylococcus aureus surface adhesins in orthopaedic device infections: are results model-dependent? Journal of Medical Microbiology 46:75–79, 1997.

27. Daum, R. S., Davis, W. H., Farris, K. B., et al.: A model of Staphylococcus aureus bacteremia, septic arthritis, and osteomyelitis in chickens. Journal of Orthopaedic Research 8:804–813, 1990.

28. Dickinson, R. B., Nagel, J. A., McDevitt, D., et al.: Quantitative comparison of clumping factor-and coagulase-mediated Staphylococcus aureus adhesion surface-bound fibrinogen under flow. Infection and Immunity 63:3143–3150, 1995.

29. Drewry, D. T., Galbraith, L., Wilkinson, B. J., et al.: Staphylococcal slime: a cautionary tale. Journal of Clinical Microbiology 28:1292–1296, 1990.

30. Dziewanowska, K., Patti, J. M., Deobald, C. F., et al.: Fibronectin binding protein and host cell tyrosine kinase are required for internalization of Staphylococcus aureus by epithelial cells. Infection and Immunity 67:4673–4678, 1999.

31. Ellington, J. K., Reilly, S. S., Warner, K. R., et al.: Mechanims of Staphylococcus aureus invasion of cultured osteoblasts. Microbial Pathogenesis 26:317–323, 1999.

32. Emslie, K. R. and Nade, S.: Acute hematogenous staphylococcal osteomyelitis: a description of the natural history in an avian model. American Journal of Pathology 110:333–345, 1983.

33. Espersen, F., Frimodt-Moller, N., Rosdahl, V. T., et al.: Changing pattern of bone and joint infections due to Staphylococcus aureus: study of cases of bacteremia in Denmark, 1959–1988. Reviews of Infectious Diseases 13:347–358, 1991.

34. Evans, R. P. and Nelson, C. L.: Gentamicin-impregnated polymethylmethacrylate beads compared with systemic antibiotic therapy in the treatment of chronic osteomyelitis. Clinical Orthopaedics and Related Research 295:37–42, 1993.

35. Evans, R. P., Nelson, C. L., Bowen, W. R., et al.: Visualization of bacterial glycocalyx with a scanning electron microscope. Clinical Orthopaedics and Related Research 347:243–249, 1998.

36. Fischer, B., Vaudaux, P., Magnin, M., et al.: Novel animal model for studying the molecular mechanisms of bacterial adhesion to bone-implanted metallic devices: role of fibronectin in Staphylococcus aureus adhesion. Journal of Orthopaedic Research 14:914–920, 1996.

37. Fluckiger, U., Wolz, C., and Cheung, A. L.: Characterization of a sar homolog of Staphylococcus epidermidis. Infection and Immunity 66:2871–2878, 1998.

38. Foster, T. J. and Hook, M.: Surface protein adhesins of Staphylococcus aureus. Trends in Microbiology 6:484–488, 1998.

39. Foster, T. J. and McDevitt, D.: Molecular basis of adherence of staphylococci to biomaterials. In: Bisno, A. L. and Waldvogel, F. A. (Eds.), Infections Associated with Indwelling Medical Devices, ASM Press, Washington, D.C., 1994:31–44.

40. Gerke, C., Kraft, A., Süßmuth, R., et al.: Characterization of the N-acetylglucosaminyl-transferase activity involved in the biosynthesis of the Staphylococcus epidermidis polysaccharide intercellular adhesin. Journal of Biological Chemistry 273:18586–18593, 1998.

41. Gillaspy, A. F., Hickmon, S. G., Skinner, R. A., et al.: Role of the accessory gene regulator (agr) in pathogenesis of staphylococcal osteomyelitis. Infection and Immunity 63:3373–3380, 1995.

42. Gillaspy, A. F., Lee, C. Y., Sau, S., et al.: Factors affecting the collagen binding capacity of Staphylococcus aureus. Infection and Immunity 66:3170–3178, 1998.

43. Gillaspy, A. F., Patti, J. M., and Smeltzer, M. S.: Transcriptional regulation of the Staphylococcus aureus collagen adhesin gene, cna. Infection and Immunity 65:1536–1540, 1997.

242			MARK S. SMELTZER and CARL L. NELSON

44. Gracia, E., Lacleriga, A., Monzon, M., *et al.*: Application of a rat osteomyelitis model to compare *in vivo* and *in vitro* the antibiotic efficacy against bacteria with high capacity to form biofilms. *Journal of Surgical Research* 79:146–153, 1998.
45. Greene, C., McDevitt, D., Francois, P., *et al.*: Adhesion properties of mutants of *Staphylococcus aureus* defective in fibronectin-binding proteins and studies on the expression of *fnb* genes. *Molecular Microbiology* 17:1143–1152, 1995.
46. Hedström, S. Å. and Lidgren, L.: Septic arthritis and osteomyelitis. *In*: Klippel, J. H. and Dieppe, P. A. (Eds.), *Rheumatology*, Mosby, London, 1998:6.2.1–6.2.10.
47. Heilmann, C., Gerke, C., Perdreau-Remington, F., *et al.*: Characterization of Tn*917* insertion mutants of *Staphylococcus epidermidis* affected in biofilm formation. *Infection and Immunity* 64:277–282, 1999.
48. Heilmann, C., Hussain, M., Peters, G., *et al.*: Evidence for autolysin-mediated primary attachment of *Staphylococcus epidermidis* to a polystyrene surface. *Molecular Microbiology* 24:1013–1024, 1997.
49. Heilmann, C., Schweitzer, O., Gerke, C., *et al.*: Molecular basis of intercellular adhesion in the biofilm-forming *Staphylococcus epidermidis*. *Molecular Microbiology* 20:1083–1091, 1996.
50. Herrmann, M., Hartleib, J., Kehrel, B., *et al.*: Interaction of von Willebrand factor with *Staphylococcus aureus*. *Journal of Infectious Diseases* 176:984–991, 1997.
51. Herrmann, M., Suchard, S. J., Boxer, L. A., *et al.*: Thrombospondin binds to *Staphylococcus aureus* and promotes staphyloccal adherence to surfaces. *Infection and Immunity* 59:279–288, 1991.
52. Hienz, S. A., Sakamoto, H., Flock, J. I., *et al.*: Development and characterization of a new model of hematogenous osteomyelitis in the rat. *Journal of Infectious Diseases* 171:1230–1236, 1995.
53. Hienz, S. A., Schennings, T., Heimdahl, A., *et al.*: Collagen binding of *Staphylococcus aureus* is a virulence factor in experimental endocarditis. *Journal of Infectious Diseases* 174:83–88, 1996.
54. Holderbaum, D., Spech, T., Ehrhart, L. A., *et al.*: Collagen binding in clinical isolates of *Staphylococcus aureus*. *Journal of Clinical Microbiology* 25:2258–2261, 1987.
55. Hussain, M., Herrmann, M., vonEiff, C., *et al.*: A 140-kd extracellular protein is essential for the accumulation of *Staphylococcus epidermidis* strains on surfaces. *Infection and Immunity* 65:519–524, 1997.
56. Hussain, M., Wilcox, M. H., and White, P. J.: The slime of coagulase-negative staphylococci: biochemistry and relation to adherence. *FEMS Microbiol Rev* 104:191–208, 1993.
57. Jevon, M., Guo, C., Ma, B., *et al.*: Mechanism of internalization of *Staphylococcus aureus* by cultured human osteoblasts. *Infection and Immunity* 67:2677–2681, 1999.
58. Jonsson, K., McDevitt, D., McGavin, M. H., *et al.*: *Staphylococcus aureus* expresses a major histocompatibility complex class II analog. *Journal of Biological Chemistry* 270:21457–21460, 1995.
59. Jonsson, K., Signas, C., Muller, H. P., *et al.*: Two different genes encode fibronectin binding proteins in *Staphylococcus aureus*: the complete nucleotide sequence and characterization of the second gene. *The European Journal of Biochemistry* 202:1041–1048, 1991.
60. Josefsson, E., McCrea, K. W., Eidhin, D. N., *et al.*: Three new members of the serine-aspartate repeat protein multigene family of *Staphylococcus aureus*. *Microbiology* 144:3387–3395, 1998.
61. Lee, J. C., Takeda, S., Livolsi, P. J., *et al.*: Effects of *in vitro* and *in vivo* growth conditions on expression of type 8 capsular polysaccharide by *Staphylococcus aureus*. *Infection and Immunity* 61:1853–1858, 1993.

62. Lew, D. P. and Waldvogel, F. A.: Current concepts: osteomyelitis. *New England Journal of Medicine* 336:999–1007, 1997.
63. Liu, N. Y. and Giansiracusa, D. F.: Septic arthritis. *In:* Gorbach, S. L., Bartlett, J. G., and Blacklow, N. R. (Eds.), *Infectious Diseases*, W. B. Saunders Co., Philadelphia, 1998:1344–1355.
64. Lopes, J. D., Dos Reis, M., and Brentani, R. R.: Presence of laminin receptors in *Staphylococcus aureus. Science* 229:275–277, 1985.
65. Mack, D., Fischer, W., Krokotsch, A., *et al.*: The intercellular adhesin involved in biofilm accumulation of *Staphylococcus epidermidis* is a linear β-1,6-linked glucosaminoglycan: purification and structural analysis. *Journal of Bacteriology* 178:175–183, 1996.
66. Mack, D., Haeder, M., Siemssen, N., *et al.*: Association of biofilm production of coagulase negative staphylococci with expression of a specific polysaccharide intercellular adhesin. *Journal of Infectious Diseases* 174:881–884, 1996.
67. Mack, D., Nedelmann, M., Krokotsch, A., *et al.*: Charaterization of transposon mutants of biofilm-producing *Staphylococcus epidermidis* impaired in the accumulative phase of biofilm production: genetic identification of a hexoasmine-containing polysaccharide intercellular adhesin. *Infection and Immunity* 62:3244–3253, 1994.
68. Mader, J. T. and Calhoun, J.: Osteomyelitis. *In:* Mandell, G. L., Bennett, J. E., and Dolin, R. (Eds.), *Principles and Practice of Infectious Diseases,* Churchill Livingstone, New York, 1995:1039–1051.
69. Mader, J. T., Shirtliff, M., and Calhoun, J. H.: Staging and staging application in osteomyelitis. *Clinical Infectious Diseases* 25:1303–1309, 1997.
70. Matsushita, K., Hamabe, M., Matsuoka, M., *et al.*: Experimental hematogenous osteomyelitis by *Staphylococcus aureus. Clinical Orthopaedics and Related Research* 334:291–297, 1997.
71. Mayberry-Carson, K. J., Tober-Meyer, B., Smith, J. K., *et al.*: Bacterial adherence and glycocalyx formation in osteomyelitis experimentally induced with *Staphylococcus aureus. Infection and Immunity* 43:825–833, 1984.
72. McDevitt, D., Francois, P., Vaudaux, P., *et al.*: Molecular characterization of the clumping factor (fibrinogen receptor) of *Staphylococcus aureus. Molecular Microbiology* 11:237–248, 1994.
73. McDevitt, D., Nanavaty, T., House-Pompeo, K., *et al.*: Characterization of the interaction between the *Staphylococcus aureus* clumping factor (ClfA) and fibrinogen. *European Journal of Biochemistry* 247:416–424, 1997.
74. McKenney, D., Hübner, J., Muller, E., *et al.*: The *ica* locus of *Staphylococcus epidermidis* encodes production of the capsular polysaccharide/adhesin. *Infection and Immunity* 66:4711–4720, 1998.
75. McKenney, D., Pouliot, K. L., Wang, Y., *et al.*: Broadly protective vaccine for *Staphylococcus aureus* based on an *in vivo*-expressed antigen. *Science* 284:1523–1527, 1999.
76. Meghji, S., Crean, S. J., Hill, P. A., *et al.*: Surface-associated protein from *Staphylococcus aureus* stimulates osteoclastogenesis: possible role in *S. aureus*-induced bone pathology. *British Journal of Rheumatology* 37:1–7, 1998.
77. Meghji, S., Crean, S. J., Nair, S., *et al.*: *Staphylococcus epidermidis* produces a cell-associated proteinaceous fraction which causes bone resorption by a prostanoid-independent mechanism: relevance to the treatment of infected orthopaedic implants. *British Journal of Rheumatology* 36:957–963, 1997.
78. Mohamed, N., Teeters, M. A., Patti, J. M., *et al.*: Inhibition of *Staphylococcus aureus* adherence to collagen under dynamic conditions. *Infection and Immunity* 67:589–594, 1999.

79. Moreillon, P., Entenza, J. M., Francioli, P., *et al.*: Role of *Staphylococcus aureus* coagulase and clumping factor in pathogenesis of experimental endocarditis. *Infection and Immunity* 63:4738–4743, 1995.

80. Muller, E., Hubner, J., Gutierrez, N., *et al.*: Isolation and characterization of transposon mutants of *Staphylococcus epidermidis* deficient in capsular polysaccharide/adhesin and slime. *Infection and Immunity* 61:551–558, 1993.

81. Muller, E., Takeda, S., Goldmann, D. A., *et al.*: Blood proteins do not promote adherence of coagulase-negative staphylococci to biomaterials. *Infection and Immunity* 59:3323–3326, 1991.

82. Muller, E., Takeda, S., Shiro, H., *et al.*: Occurence of capsular polysaccharide/adhesin among clinical isolates of coagulase-negative staphylococci. *Journal of Infectious Diseases* 168:1211–1218, 1993.

83. Nair, S. P., Meghji, S., Wilson, M., *et al.*: Bacterially induced bone destruction: mechanisms and misconceptions. *Infection and Immunity* 64:2371–2380, 1996.

84. Ni Eldhin, D., Perkins, S., Francois, P., *et al.*: Clumping factor B (ClfB), a new surface-located fibrinogen-binding adhesin of *Staphylococcus aureus*. *Molecular Microbiology* 30:245–257, 1998.

85. Nilsson, I-M., Lee, J. C., Bremell, T., *et al.*: The role of staphylococcal polysaccharide microcapsule expression in septicemica and septic arthritis. *Infection and Immunity* 65:4216–4221, 1997.

86. Nilsson, I-M., Patti, J. M., Bremell, T., *et al.*: Vaccination with a recombinant fragment of collagen adhesin provides protection against *Staphylococcus aureus*-mediated septic death. *The Journal of Clinical Investigation* 101:2640–2649, 1998.

87. Nilsson, I., Bremell, T., Ryden, C., *et al.*: Role of the staphylococcal accessory gene regulator (*sar*) in septic arthritis. *Infection and Immunity* 64:4438–4443, 1996.

88. Nilsson, I., Hartford, O., Foster, T., *et al.*: Alpha-toxin and gamma-toxin jointly promote *Staphylococcus aureus* virulence in murine septic arthritis. *Infection and Immunity* 67:1045–1049, 1999.

89. Nilsson, M., Frykberg, L., Flock, J.-I., *et al.*: A fibrinogen-binding protein of *Staphylococcus epidermidis*. *Infection and Immunity* 66:2666–2673, 1998.

90. Norden, C., Gillespie, W. J., and Nade, S.: Hematogenous osteomyelitis. *In*: Norden, C., Gillespie, W. J., and Nade, S. (Eds.), *Infections in Bones and Joints*, Blackwell Scientific Publications, Boston, 1994:137–165.

91. Otto, M., Süßmuth, R., Vuong, C., *et al.*: Inhibition of virulence factor expression in *Staphylococcus aureus* by the *Staphylococcus epidermidis* *agr* pheromone and derivatives. *FEBS Letters* 450:257–262, 1999.

92. Park, P. W., Roberts, D. D., Grosso, L. E., *et al.*: Binding of elastin to *Staphylococcus aureus*. *Journal of Biological Chemistry* 266:23399–23406, 1991.

93. Park, P. W., Rosenbloom, J., Abrams, W. R., *et al.*: Molecular cloning and expression of the gene for elastin-binding protein (*ebpS*) in *Staphylococcus aureus*. *Journal of Biological Chemistry* 271:15803–15809, 1996.

94. Patti, J. M., Allen, B. L., McGavin, M. J., *et al.*: MSCRAMM-mediated adherence of microorganisms to host tissue. *Annual Reviews of Microbiology* 48:585–617, 1994.

95. Patti, J. M., Bremell, T., Krajewska-Pietrasik, D., *et al.*: The *Staphylococcus aureus* collagen adhesin is a virulence determinant in experimental septic arthritis. *Infection and Immunity* 62:152–161, 1994.

96. Patti, J. M., Jonsson, H., Guss, B., *et al.*: Molecular characterization and expression of a gene encoding a *Staphylococcus aureus* collagen adhesin. *Journal of Biological Chemistry* 267:4766–4772, 1992.

97. Peters, G., Locci, R., and Pulverer, G.: Adherence and growth of coagulase-negative staphylococci on surfaces of intravenous catheters. *Journal of Infectious Diseases* 146:479–482, 1982.

98. Proctor, R. A.: Microbial pathogenic factors: small colony variants. In: Bisno, A. L. and Waldvogel, F. A. (Eds.), *Infections Associated with Indwelling Medical Devices*, ASM Press, Washington, D.C., 1994:79–90.

99. Proctor, R. A., Rolauffs, B., Lindner, N., et al.: Recovery of small colony variants of *Staphylococcus aureus* following gentamicin bead placement for osteomyelitis. *Clinical Infectious Diseases* 25:1250–1251, 1997.

100. Proctor, R. A., van Langevelde, P., Kristjansson, M., et al.: Persistent and relapsing infections associated with small-colony variants of *Staphylococcus aureus*. *Clinical Infectious Diseases* 20:95–102, 1995.

101. Projan, S. J. and Novick, R. P.: The Molecular Basis of Pathogenicity. In: Crossley, K. B. and Archer, G. L. (Eds.), *The Staphylococci in Human Disease*, Churchill Livingstone, New York, 1997:55–81.

102. Raja, R. H., Raucci, G., and Hook, M.: Peptide analogs to a fibronectin receptor inhibit attachment of *Staphylococcus aureus* to fibronectin-containing substrates. *Infection and Immunity* 58:2593–2598, 1990.

103. Reilly, S. S., Ramp, W. K., Zane, S. F., et al.: Internalization of *Staphylococcus aureus* by embryonic chicken osteoblasts *in vivo*. *Journal of Bone and Mineral Research* 12:S231, 1997.

104. Rissing, J. P., Buxton, T. B., Weinstein, R. S., et al.: Model of experimental chronic osteomyelitis in rats. *Infection and Immunity* 47:581–586, 1985.

105. Rubin, R. J., Harrington, C. A., Poon, A., et al.: The economic impact of *Staphylococcus aureus* infection in New York City hospitals. *Emerging Infectious Diseases* 5:9–17, 1999.

106. Rupp, M. E. and Archer, G. L.: Coagulase-negative Staphylococci: pathogens associated with medical progress. *Clinical Infectious Diseases* 19:231–245, 1994.

107. Rupp, M. E., Sloot, N., Meyer, H. G. W., et al.: Characterization of the hemagglutinin of *Staphylococcus epidermidis*. *Journal of Infectious Diseases* 172:1509–1518, 1995.

108. Rupp, M. E., Ulphani, J. S., Fey, P. D., et al.: Characterization of the importance of polysaccharide intercellular adhesin/hemagglutinin of *Staphylococcus epidermidis* in the pathogenesis of biomaterial-based infection in a mouse foreign body infection model. *Infection and Immunity* 67:2627–2632, 1999.

109. Ryden, C., Yacoub, A. I., Maxe, I., et al.: Specific binding of bone sialoprotein to *Staphylococcus aureus* isolated from patients with osteomyelitis. *Journal of Biological Chemistry* 184:331–336, 1989.

110. Ryding, U., Christensson, B., Soderquist, B., et al.: Antibody response to *Staphylococcus aureus* collagen binding protein in patients with *S. aureus* septicaemia and collagen binding properties of corresponding strains. *Journal of Medical Microbiology* 43:328–334, 1995.

111. Savage, B., Bottini, E., and Ruggeri, Z. M.: Interaction of integrin $\alpha_{IIb}\beta_3$ with multiple fibrinogen domains during platelet adhesion. *Journal of Biological Chemistry* 270: 28812–28817, 1995.

112. Scheld, W. M., Strunk, R. W., Balian, G., et al.: Microbial adhesion to fibronectin *in vitro* correlates with production of endocarditis in rabbits. *Proceedings of the Society for Experimental Biology and Medicine* 180:474–482, 1985.

113. Shiro, H., Meluleni, G., Groll, A., et al.: The pathogenic role of *Staphylococcus epidermidis* capsular polysaccharide/adhesin in a low-inoculum rabbit model of prosthetic valve endocarditis. *Circulation* 92:2715–2722, 1995.

114. Smeltzer, M. S., Thomas, J. R., Hickmon, S. G., *et al.*: Characterization of a rabbit model of staphylococcal osteomyelitis. *Journal of Orthopaedic Research* 15:414–421, 1997.

115. Snodgrass, J. L., Mohamed, N., Ross, J. M., *et al.*: Functional analysis of the *Staphylococcus aureus* collagen adhesin B domain. *Infection and Immunity* 67:3952–3959, 1999.

116. Sonnen, G. M. and Henry, N. K.: Pediatric bone and joint infections. Diagnosis and antimicrobial management. *Pediatric Clinics of North America* 43:933–947, 1996.

117. Spagnolo, N., Greco, F., Rossi, A., *et al.*: Chronic staphylococcal osteomyelitis: a new experimental rat model. *Infection and Immunity* 61:5225–5230, 1993.

118. Switalski, L. M., Patti, J. M., Butcher, W. G., *et al.*: A collagen receptor on *Staphylococcus aureus* strains isolated from patients with septic arthritis mediates adhesin to cartilage. *Molecular Microbiology* 7:99–107, 1993.

119. Thakker, M., Park, J-S., Carey, V., *et al.*: *Staphylococcus aureus* serotype 5 capsular polysaccharide is antiphagocytic and enhances bacterial virulence in a murine bacteremia model. *Infection and Immunity* 66:5183–5189, 1998.

120. Thomas, M. G., Peacock, S., Daenke, S., *et al.*: Adhesion of *Staphylococcus aureus* to collagen is not a major virulence determinant for septic arthritis, osteomyelitis, or endocarditis. *Journal of Infectious Diseases* 179:291–293, 1999.

121. Timmerman, C. P., Fleer, A., Besnier, J. M., *et al.*: Characterization of a proteinaceous adhesin of *Staphylococcus epidermidis* which mediates attachment to polystyrene. *Infection and Immunity* 59:4187–4192, 1991.

122. Tojo, M., Yamashita, N., Goldmann, D. A., *et al.*: Isolation and characterization of a capsular polysaccharide adhesin from *Staphylococcus epidermidis*. *Journal of Infectious Diseases* 157:713–722, 1988.

123. Vaudaux, P. E., Pittet, D., Haeberli, A., *et al.*: Host factors selectively increase staphylococcal adherence on inserted catheters: a role for fibronectin and fibrinogen or fibrin. *Journal of Infectious Diseases* 160:865–875, 1989.

124. Voytek, A., Gristina, A. G., Barth, E., *et al.*: Staphylococcal adhesion to collagen in intra-articular sepsis. *Biomaterials* 9:107–110, 1988.

125. Yoon, K. S., Fitzgerald, R. H., Jr., Sud. S., *et al.*: Experimental acute hematogenous osteomyelitis in mice. II. Influence of *Staphylococcus aureus* infection on T-cell immunity. *Journal of Orthopaedic Research* 17:382–391, 1999.

126. Ziebuhr, W., Heilmann, C., Gotz, F., *et al.*: Detection of the intercellular adhesion gene cluster (*ica*) and phase variation in *Staphylococcus epidermidis* blood culture strains and mucosal isolates. *Infection and Immunity* 65:890–896, 1997.

127. Ziebuhr, W., Krimmer, V., Rachid, S., *et al.*: A novel mechanism of phase variation of virulence in *Staphylococcus epidermidis*: evidence for control of the polysaccharide intercellular adhesin synthesis by alternating insertion and excision of the insertion sequence element IS*256*. *Molecular Microbiology* 32:345–356, 1999.

Internalization of *Staphylococcus aureus* by Nonprofessional Phagocytes

KENNETH W. BAYLES and GREGORY A. BOHACH

1. INTRODUCTION

One general means of grouping pathogenic microorganisms is based on their location relevant to host cells during infection. Some organisms such as the rickettsia, chlamydia, and viruses are considered to be obligate intracellular pathogens since they are unable to replicate outside of host cells. Other pathogens may be grown on axenic media in the laboratory and do not require an intracellular environment. Within this second group are two subgroups, extracellular pathogens and the facultative intracellular pathogens. Many facultative intracellular organisms are known for their ability to survive, and even replicate, in an intracellular environment. These include organisms within a variety of genera such as *Mycobacterium*, *Salmonella*, *Shigella*, and *Listeria*, in addition to certain fungi and protozoa. Some of these species are typically engulfed by actively phagocytic cells such as neutrophils or macrophages. These pathogens have evolved unique mechanisms for evading the host cell killing mechanisms. Other organisms are internalized by nonprofessional phagocytes such as epithelial or endothelial cells. By necessity, these organisms have developed mechanisms by which they induce cytoskeletal rearrangements leading to uptake of the organism. Extracellular pathogens are becoming less well defined for several reasons and the distinction between facultative intracellular organisms and extracellular pathogens is becoming unclear. The main reason is that many pathogens long considered to be extracellular

KENNETH W. BAYLES and GREGORY A. BOHACH • Department of Microbiology, Molecular Biology and Biochemistry, University of Idaho, Moscow, ID 83844-3052.

Staphylococcus aureus *Infection and Disease*, edited by Allen L. Honeyman *et al.* Kluwer Academic/Plenum Publishers, New York, 2001.

pathogens have been shown, in recent years, to have properties similar to facultative intracellular pathogens. Thus as we now see, the designation of organisms as to their cellular location is a useful but imperfect classification system.

Staphylococcus aureus is one such organism that is not internalized efficiently by nonprofessional phagocytes and has been traditionally considered to be an extracellular pathogen.[1,2] However, as new information is obtained, it is becoming clearer that S. aureus and many other organisms traditionally considered to be extracellular have an intracellular niche that may be important for pathogenesis. Our understanding of the mechanisms and consequences of internalized staphylococci is currently somewhat limited. However, techniques developed for the study of other organisms are generally applicable to S. aureus and crucial events employed by internalization of this organism often overlap those of other well-characterized pathogens. The purpose of this review is to summarize our current knowledge concerning the mechanisms by which S. aureus is internalized by nonprofessional phagocytes and the potential effects of this interaction in pathogenesis.

2. EARLY KEY STUDIES DEMONSTRATING THE INTERNALIZATION OF S. AUREUS BY VARIOUS TYPES OF NONPROFESSIONAL PHAGOCYTES

The study of intracellular S. aureus in nonprofessional phagocytic cells is a relatively new field of investigation. Prior to 1990, only a few published reports on this topic existed in the literature. Although there have been numerous descriptions of intracellular staphylococci from clinical specimens, the organisms were typically shown to be localized in phagocytic cells or their location was not designated. The initial demonstration of internalization of S. aureus by nonprofessional phagocytes was made using endothelial cells. Since then, other investigators have employed a number of model systems including various sources of epithelial cells, osteoblasts, and fibroblasts. Each cell line has its own unique advantage as far as serving as a model for a particular infectious disease or clinical situation.

Endothelial Cells

The first clear demonstration of active internalization by endothelial cells was a report in 1985 by Ogawa et al.[3] These investigators, while assessing the adherence of S. aureus to cells, demonstrated internalized organisms in primary cultures of endothelial cell monolayers derived from human heart valves or umbilical cords. They reported a close association between staphylococcal cells and the endothelial cell membranes, invagination of the membranes and subsequent internalization of the cells, which became localized within vacuoles. Since then, several investigators have studied internalization of *S. aureus* by endothelial cells from a variety of sources, such as human umbilical vein endothelial cells (HUVEC). The major impetus for these studies has been an attempt to understand the role of internalization in development of infections within the cardiovascular system, i.e., staphylococcal endocarditis. Hamill *et al.*[4] and Lowy *et al.*[5] extended the initial work of Ogawa *et al.*[3] by investigating the internalization of *S. aureus* by human, bovine and rabbit endothelial cells. Combined, these studies showed that staphylococcal internalization is a multistep process. Adherence is followed by formation of appendages on the endothelial cells, which elongate and eventually enclose the organism in a vacuole. The authors noted that internalization of *S. aureus* displayed ultrastructural characteristics similar to uptake of obligate intracellular pathogens such as rickettsial species. It was noted that, not only were the bacteria not killed by the endothelial cell, they seemed to be multiplying in an intracellular environment.

Epithelial Cells

The interaction of *S. aureus* with epithelial cells could have important implications for colonization of certain sites within the host. However, until recently, reports of internalization of *S. aureus* by epithelial cells have been quite limited. Schmidt *et al.*[6] investigated the internalization of several staphylococcal species from urinary tract infections for the ability to enter HEp-2 cells. Murai *et al.*[7] later showed that primary glomerular epithelial cells ingest *S. aureus* in vitro. Almeida *et al.*,[8] studying infectious bovine mastitis, demonstrated that *S. aureus* is actively internalized by bovine mammary epithelial cells using both primary cell cultures and the bovine mammary epithelial cell line, MAC-T.[9] Bayles *et al.*[10] subsequently characterized the internalization process and showed that many of the cell surface and intracellular events are similar to those displayed by well-established facultative intracellular pathogens.[11]

Other Cell Types

Significant contributions to our understanding of the importance of intracellular staphylococci have come from investigations using other cell types. For example, a great deal of information has resulted from the investigation of *S. aureus* internalization by osteoblasts as a model system for studying osteomyelitis. As early as 1995, Hudson and colleagues[12] showed that *S. aureus* associated with cultured chick osteoblasts and were then internalized. Several investigators have also demonstrated internalization of *S. aureus* by fibroblasts. The first reported study was published by Usui *et al*.[13] in 1992 who employed fibroblasts from primary murine skin cultures or NIH 3T3 cells. Sinha *et al*.[14] also studied internalization of *S. aureus* in fibroblast cell cultures and has provided important insights into the mechanisms of staphylococcal internalization (see below) using this system.

Ingestion of Other Staphylococcal Species

Species of *Staphylococcus* other than *S. aureus* may be internalized by nonprofessional phagocytes. The rate of internalization is generally low compared to *S. aureus* although there are differences among the various types of cells used. For example, in addition to *S. aureus*, mouse glomerular epithelial cells are reportedly able to ingest the coagulase negative staphylococci, *S. epidermidis*, and *S. saprophyticus*.[7] In contrast, other cell types from the kidney internalize only *S. aureus*. Schmidt *et al*.[6] also compared the invasion of HEp-2 cells by *S. aureus*, *S. epidermidis* and *S. saprophyticus*. These investigators demonstrated that adherence and internalization were strongly correlated. *S. saprophyticus* was the most invasive and the three species differed significantly in regard to their ability to induce cytotoxicity.

3. CELLULAR EFFECTS OF INTRACELLULAR *S. AUREUS*

General Features

Many features associated with internalization of *S. aureus* by nonprofessional phagocytes are similar regardless of the host cell type involved. Several investigators[3-5] described ultrastructural characteristics of human or rabbit endothelial cells infected with *S. aureus*. The internalization process is a multi-step sequence of events beginning with intimate contact between the host and bacterial cell surfaces and typically ending with lysis of the host cell membrane. There is general agreement that in most situations, *S. aureus* is metabolically active inside host cell nonprofessional phagocytes. The organism was noted to replicate intracellularly and eventually cause host cell disruption and death. The staphylococcal cells remain intact in endothelial cells despite lysosomal fusion.[5] Other evidence of metabolic activity includes the demonstration that *S. aureus* escapes from the endosome and induces physiological alterations such as apoptosis, necrosis, and inflammatory cytokines in epithelial cells.[10,55] Similar experiments confirmed that the results obtained with epithelial cells are also applicable to endothelial cells,[15] fibroblasts[16] and osteoblasts.[17]

Some of the ultrastructural features associated with the staphylococcal internalization cycle of bovine mammary epithelial cells are demonstrated in Figure 1. Transmission electron microscopy reveals that bacteria in close contact with the cell surface become associated with pseudopod-like structures (Figure 1, panels A and C). The surface appendages eventually engulf the bacteria, leading to the formation of membrane-bound endosomes. The morphology of the host cell membrane during uptake of *S. aureus* resembles that induced by other organisms including *Yersinia*

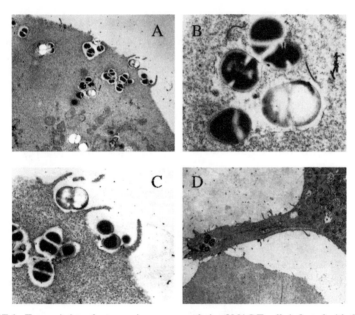

FIGURE 1. Transmission electron microscopy analysis of MAC-T cells infected with *S. aureus* strain Novel. All panels represent a 3-hr co-culture of MAC-T cells with *S. aureus*. (A) Invasion of a MAC-T cell by *S. aureus* illustrating contact with the MAC-T cell surface, formation of pseudopod-like structures, engulfment of bacteria, endosome formation and degradation of the endosomal membrane in the interior of the cell (5,000×). (B) Enlargement (30,000×) of panel A showing endosomal membrane fragments. (C) Enlargement (15,000×) of pseudopod-like structures and engulfment of bacteria. (D) Cytoplasmic membrane contortion (4,000×) associated with many of the infected MAC-T cells. Reproduced from reference 10 with permission.

species[1] and Group A streptococci.[18] Because of these similarities, Sinha et al.[14] and Murai et al.[16] suggested that *S. aureus* becomes internalized by cells via the "zipper-type" mechanism.[19] Additional characterization of the molecules involved and signal transduction pathways will be required to confirm this possibility. Careful observation of high magnification electron micrographs reveals the presence of fibrilar-like material that appears to link the bacterial and host cell surfaces (Figure 1). These presumably represent receptor-ligand complexes (see below) and were also evident in electron micrographs of *S. aureus* interactions with human valvular endothelial cells.[3]

An endosomal membrane is clearly evident around bacteria that had recently entered the cell (Figure 1, panels A and C). However, vacuoles farther from the cytoplasmic membrane of the host cell, presumably those internalized for longer periods of time, typically begin to degrade. Some bacteria are adjacent to vacuolar fragments, while others are entirely free in the cytoplasm (Figure 1, panels A and B), an observation that has also been confirmed by other investigators.[15,16,20] Many of the infected cells displayed cytoplasmic membrane contortions (Figure 1, panel D) similar to protrusions produced by intracellular *Shigella* and *Listeria* undergoing actin tailing. However, studies using phalloidin-based staining performed in our laboratories have not revealed actin tailing associated with intracellular *S. aureus* and the reasons for formation of these structures is currently unknown. Since *S. aureus* resides within the MAC-T cytoplasm, we have hypothesized that release from the vacuole is mediated by one (or more) of at least four different staphylococcal hemolysins known to damage membranes (α-, β-, γ- and δ-toxins; see Bohach et al.[21]).

Kinetics of Uptake and Survival

Several investigators have quantified the internalization of *S. aureus* by a variety of cells. In one representative study, we examined the ability of a highly transmissible *S. aureus* bovine mastitis isolate, designated strain Novel,[22] to enter MAC-T cells. The invasion assay employed was based on the principle that bacteria inside host cells are protected from the antimicrobial effects of gentamicin added to the medium.[23] While this is a versatile method, gentamicin can be substituted with lysostaphin for the analysis of intracellular *S. aureus*.[4,7,15] *S. aureus* enters either epithelial or endothelial cells in a dose-dependent fashion (Figure 2, see Almeida et al.,[8] Bayles et al.[10] and Menzies et al.[15]). With MAC-T cells and the Novel strain of *S. aureus*, a linear increase in the number of intracellular bacteria was observed up to a multiplicity of infection (MOI) of 53. Above this dose, substantial increases in bacterial survival are not observed,

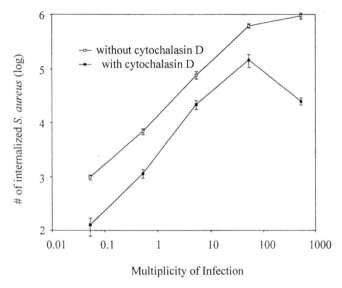

FIGURE 2. Internalization of *S. aureus* strain Novel by MAC-T cells. A dose response invasion assay was performed by exposing MAC-T cell monolayers to various concentrations of *S. aureus* so that the MOI was altered within the range indicated. Culture media were supplemented with either gentamicin alone or gentamicin plus cytochalasin D. Reproduced from reference 10 with permission.

indicating that saturation of the internalization mechanism or death of the host cell had occurred. Similar to results of other investigators working with different systems,[4,8] treatment with 0.5 µg/ml cytochalasin D reduced the survival of *S. aureus* approximately 10-fold indicating that cytoskeletal rearrangements were involved in the internalization process (Figure 2, see Bayles *et al.*[10]).

Time course experiments have shown that internalization is quite rapid. Using available techniques, it is possible to monitor the increase in the number of internalized bacteria from 30 minutes to 3 hours.[7,13,15,24] Studies have also been performed by a number of investigators to assess the long-term survival of intracellular staphylococci. These experiments are hampered because of the membrane lytic action of *S. aureus* cytotoxins exposing viable bacteria to either gentamicin or lysostaphin. Therefore, because of the differential ability of *S. aureus* strains to express membrane active toxins, results may vary considerably from one laboratory to another. However, despite the limitations of this technique, *S. aureus* has been shown to increase in numbers within cells for at least 10 hours.[24] Using MAC-T cells, microscopic analysis can show that some individual

epithelial cells contained large numbers of viable and dividing staphylococci for at least three days following infection with *S. aureus* (our unpublished results). *S. aureus* also persists in other types of nonprofessional
phagocytes. Within osteoblasts, the number of viable intracellular organisms remains constant for at least 7.5 hours.[12] Endothelial cells[25] and
keratinocytes[26] have also been shown to harbor intracellular *S. aureus* for
extended periods.

Small Colony Variants

One potential consequence of intracellular growth is the induction of
S. aureus small colony variants (SCVs), which are thought to be responsible for the persistent and recurrent infections commonly caused by *S.
aureus*.[27] SCVs represent nonpigmented and nonhemolytic subpopulations
of *S. aureus* that grow slowly on standard growth medium.[27] Many of the
clinical and laboratory-generated *S. aureus* SCVs are defective in components of the electron transport chain resulting in the slow growth
phenotype. Vesga *et al.*[28] have reported that SCV formation is induced by
prolonged exposure to the intracellular milieu. Stable SCVs were isolated
72 hr after infection of bovine aortic endothelial cells at a frequency of
10^{-3}. This represents a 1,000-fold greater rate of SCV formation compared
to the spontaneous rate (1.11×10^{-7}) suggesting that the intracellular environment induces the formation of SCVs. Whether the induction of SCV
formation is a consequence of selective pressure for slow growing variants
that do not produce α-toxin or whether there exists a defined SCV-
inducing signal has not been determined. Regardless of the mechanism by
which SCVs arise, greater than 200-fold more SCVs persisted intracellularly
after 24 or 48 hr relative to wild type cells.[25] The relationship between
intracellular metabolism and SCV formation is an intriguing area of
staphylococcal research that is likely relevant to persistent infections.
However, much remains to be done to understand the role that SCVs play
during infection and the molecular mechanisms by which they arise.

4. STAPHYLOCOCCAL FACTORS REQUIRED FOR INTERNALIZATION

The main *S. aureus* adhesion factor responsible for the signal transduction initiating pseudopod formation and endocytosis is one or both of
its fibronectin (Fn)-binding proteins (FnBPs). Although the role of FnBP
in internalization has clearly been shown, a requirement for accessory molecules has not been ruled out. To assess the role of FnBPs in the entry of

eukaryotic cells by *S. aureus*, a well-characterized laboratory *S. aureus* strain (8325-4) was used. This strain, which expresses both FnBPs A and B,[29] was compared to its double isogenic mutant strain (DU5883), which does not express either FnBP due to an allelic replacement of both structural genes.[29] As shown in Figure 3, the parental 8325-4 strain is efficiently internalized, while the mutant (DU5883) demonstrates a dramatic reduction in number of bacteria internalized.[30] These results, which are consistent with the results generated by several other groups,[14,31,32] indicate that FnBP is required for efficient internalization of *S. aureus* 8325-4 cells. Interestingly, mutations in several other surface protein genes (i.e., protein A and fibrinogen binding protein) did not significantly alter internalization.[30] Although, the absence of FnBPs in the strain DU5883 dramatically reduced internalization, adhesion was reduced to a much lesser extent (Figure 3). Compared to the parental strain, DU5883 exhibited a 98% reduction in internalization and only a 37% reduction in adherence to MAC-T cells. Similar effects of the FnBP mutations on adherence and invasion were also observed by Lammers *et al.*[32] Combined, these results suggest that other MSCRAMMs (Microbial Surface Components Recognizing Adhesive Matrix Molecules) can override the loss of Fn binding and allow adherence

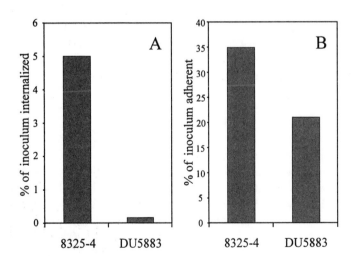

FIGURE 3. Role of FnBPs in adherence vs. internalization. Compared to 8325-4, adherence of DU5883 to MAC-T cells (B) was reduced by 37%. In contrast, internalization of DU5883 (A) was reduced by >90% compared to 8325-4. This suggests that other MSCRAMMs can compensate for adherence but not internalization and that adherence alone does not promote internalization. The data presented are representative of one experiment performed three times. Reproduced from reference 30 with permission.

to host cells, but that adherence via other MSCRAMMs does not lead to efficient internalization.[30]

The receptors most commonly utilized by several bacterial pathogens for binding and internalization are integrins, which are large $\alpha\beta$ heterodimeric membrane proteins found on the surface of a wide range of mammalian cells. Integrins are involved in promoting adhesion to extracellular matrix proteins, such as Fn, collagen and laminin.[33] Evidence that Fn was involved in the binding of *S. aureus* to host cells was generated by demonstrating that anti-Fn antibodies inhibited internalization by greater than 95% and that soluble Fn (at all concentrations tested) blocked internalization into MAC-T cells.[30,34] Preincubation of either the bacteria or MAC-T cells with medium containing soluble Fn inhibited both adherence and internalization of *S. aureus* 8325-4 by MAC-T cells.[30] In contrast, internalization into host cells, such as HEp-2 cells, that do not normally produce Fn, revealed a different picture. Unlike MAC-T cells, which produce low levels of Fn, internalization into HEp-2 cells is stimulated by the addition of low levels of soluble Fn and inhibited by higher concentrations, presumably above the levels that saturate the integrin molecules.[34] Thus, low levels of Fn appear to be necessary for internalization but high levels (presumably above that normally produced by MAC-T cells) is inhibitory. A role for integrins in this process was demonstrated in studies by Dziewanowska *et al.*[34] and Sinha *et al.*[14] using antibodies directed against $\alpha_5\beta_1$ integrin. Incubation of the host cells with the anti-integrin antibodies significantly reduced internalization of *S. aureus.* Based on the results presented above, a model for the interaction of *S. aureus* FnBP with the host cell has been proposed.[14,30,35,36] In this model, fibronectin functions as a bridging molecule by simultaneously binding to *S. aureus* FnBP and the host cell receptor, integrin.

Recent studies support the bridge model but go on to suggest the presence of a coreceptor that is involved in the *S. aureus*-host cell interaction.[34] Using ligand blotting of cell membrane proteins to a functional fragment of FnBP, an approximately 55-kDa protein that binds to FnBP was identified from both human and bovine epithelial cells. This 55-kDa protein was subsequently shown to be displayed on the surface of the host cells and was identified as heat shock protein (Hsp) 60. A similar coreceptor model has also been proposed for *Neisseria gonorrhoea* internalization by van Putten *et al.*[37] in which a Fn bridge linking OpaA and $\beta 1$ integrin, is stabilized by a host cell glycosaminoglycan co-receptor. In both of these systems, a co-ligand may be necessary for binding since Fn alone is likely to be insufficient to induce bacterial uptake.[38]

Once the appropriate molecular interactions have been made, host cell signaling via a protein tyrosine kinase (PTK)-dependent mechanism[30]

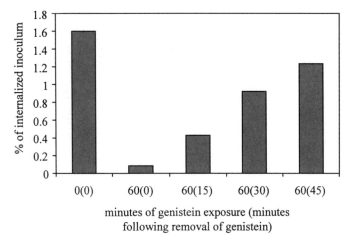

FIGURE 4. Effects of genistein on internalization of *S. aureus*. MAC-T cells were incubated with genistein for 60 minutes, washed and allowed to recover for the period of time shown (in parenthesis) prior to adding bacteria. The data presented are from a representative experiment performed three times. Reproduced from reference 30 with permission.

initiates cytoskeletal rearrangements that result in engulfment of the bacteria and uptake into the cell. Several groups have demonstrated the importance of microfilaments during internalization by showing that cytochalasin D, a microfilament depolymerizing agent, dramatically inhibits uptake of *S. aureus*.[8,10,15,35,39] Two groups have also provided evidence that microtubules and clathrin coated pits are involved in *S. aureus* internalization by osteoblast cells.[35,39] In many cases the pathways leading to cytoskeletal rearrangement are initiated by PTK activation induced by bacterial binding to host cell receptors. As shown in Figure 4, internalization of *S. aureus* requires PTK activity since uptake is reversibly blocked by a 60 min exposure to genistein, a specific inhibitor of PTKs. This inhibitory effect of genistein is not a result of toxicity since removal of the genistein results in partial recovery of the ability of the host cells to internalize the bacteria.

5. INFECTION BY *S. AUREUS* INDUCES APOPTOSIS IN NONPROFESSIONAL PHAGOCYTES

As shown in Figure 5, *S. aureus* induces a dramatic change in the morphology of infected epithelial cells. Some infected cells detach from the plates within two hours after adding staphylococci to the monolayers.[10]

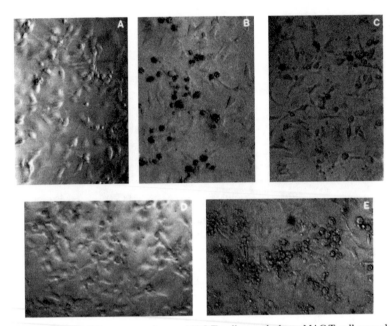

FIGURE 5. Effects of *S. aureus* strains on MAC-T cell morphology. MAC-T cell monolayers were either uninfected (A) or were infected with *S. aureus* strain RN6390 (parental control strain) (B), RN6911 (an *agr⁻* mutant) (C), ALC135 (an *agr⁻*, *sar⁻* mutant) (D), or ALC136 (a *sar⁻* mutant) (E) for 2 hr prior to the addition of gentamicin. Photomicrographs were taken at 22 hr following the addition of gentamicin. Reproduced from reference 24 with permission.

Detachment from the substrate is accompanied by rounding of the cells and a mottled appearance of the cell membrane (Figure 5, panel B). By 20 hr post-infection, the majority of cells (typically, at least 80% of the population) exhibit the rounded morphology.[10] This correlates with the percentage of infection, which was also estimated to be approximately 80%. The uninfected control cells adhere normally and maintain normal cellular morphology (Figure 5, panel A).

The morphology of epithelial cells infected with *S. aureus* resembles cells undergoing apoptosis.[40,41] One hallmark of apoptotic cells is the fragmentation of the DNA by specific endonucleases.[41–43] This phenomenon can be visualized as a characteristic ladder pattern in which each fragment increases in size by approximately 180 bp. As shown in Figure 6, DNA laddering occurs in *S. aureus*-infected MAC-T cells (Figure 6, lane 3), but not in uninfected MAC-T control cells (Figure 6, lane 2). In confirmation that internalized *S. aureus* cells induced the bovine epithelial host cells

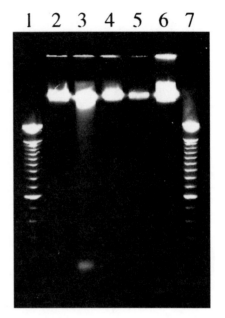

FIGURE 6. Effects of *agr* and *sar* on the induction of apoptosis. DNA was extracted from MAC-T cells infected with RN6390 (parental control strain; lane 3), RN6911 (an *agr* mutant; lane 4), ALC135 (an *agr*, *sar* mutant; lane 5), or ALC136 (a *sar* mutant; lane 6). MAC-T cells were exposed to bacteria for 2 h prior to the addition of gentamicin and then incubated for an additional 22 hr prior to the DNA extraction. Electrophoretic separation of the DNA was performed using a 1.8% agarose gel. The DNA in lane 2 was extracted from the uninfected control MAC-T cells treated with gentamicin for 22 h. Lanes 1 and 7 contain a 100-bp DNA ladder. Reproduced from reference 24 with permission.

to become apoptotic, some *S. aureus*-infected MAC-T cells were observed to exhibit an intense green positive fluorescence using the TUNEL method,[10] which is based on the specific staining of the 3′ hydroxyl ends of the fragmented DNA within apoptotic cells.[44–47] Since the initial observation that internalized *S. aureus* induces apoptosis,[10] several other subsequent studies have demonstrated similar findings with other cell lines, including endothelial cells,[15] fibroblasts,[16] osteoblasts[48] and keratinocytes.[26]

Assessment of Caspase Activity and Cytokine Induction

To determine whether caspases could be involved in apoptosis induced by intracellular *S. aureus*, we first examined caspase 3, a central effector caspase, which can be proteolytically cleaved and activated by several initiator caspases. Internalized *S. aureus* caused a 6.6-fold increase in caspase 3 activity by MAC-T cells compared to the uninfected control after 6 h of infection (Figure 7). This indicated that indeed *S. aureus* induces apoptosis via a caspase dependent mechanism similar to that recently reported for activation of caspase 3 in apoptosis induced by *Legionella pneumophila*.[49]

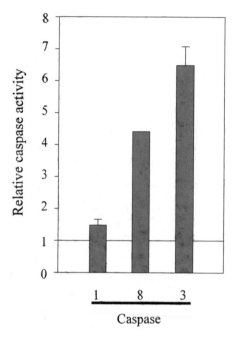

FIGURE 7. Caspase 1, 8 and 3 activities in MAC-T cells infected with *S. aureus*. Increase in caspase activity (n-fold) was calculated by dividing the relative fluorescence value obtained from analysis of infected cells by that of the uninfected control. The value obtained from uninfected cells is represented by 1. Values from four (caspases 1 and 3) and two (caspase 8) separate experiments were used to calculate the mean relative activity (±S.E.M.). Reproduced from reference 55 with permission.

Caspase 1 and caspase 8 each utilizes a different pathway to activate caspase 3.[50] Although caspase 1 has been shown to be the target for the induction of apoptosis by *Shigella*[51] and *Salmonella*,[52] we found only minimal stimulation of caspase 1 activity in MAC-T cells after 6 h of infection (Figure 7) and no significant caspase 1 activity at 3 h after infection (unpublished results). In contrast, caspase 8 activity in MAC-T cells increased 4.4-fold after 6 h of infection (Figure 7). Thus, unlike *Shigella* and *Salmonella*, data from this study indicate that the induction of apoptosis by *S. aureus* in our system does not involve activation of caspase 1. Instead, these data suggest that *S. aureus* induces apoptosis through a mechanism involving caspases 8 and 3, similar to the pathway induced in macrophages by Sendai virus.[53]

Caspase 8 is thought to be the most apical of the caspases that initiate apoptosis. The pathway initiated by caspase 8 is also known as "death receptor-mediated" since binding of TNF or Fas ligand to their cell surface receptors can result in the proteolytic activation of associated caspase 8.[54] Thus, the induction of cytokines by intracellular *S. aureus* could play an important role in the induction of apoptosis.

To examine cytokine expression in MAC-T cells infected with *S. aureus*, a quantitative RT-PCR technique was used. In this study, internalization of *S. aureus* consistently increased the transcript levels of the pro-inflammatory cytokines TNF-α and IL-1β[55] compared to the uninfected controls. Viable staphylococci were required to induce cytokine expression since equivalent numbers of UV-killed RN6390 cells were unable to elevate any cytokine transcript accumulation above basal levels. Although it is currently unknown whether activation of caspases 8 and 3 occurs through signaling by TNF-α (as illustrated in Figure 8), the observation that TNF-α transcripts accumulate in cells infected with *S. aureus* makes this an

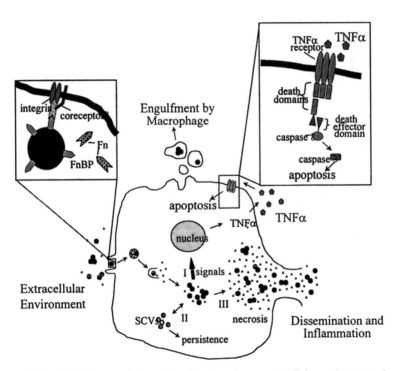

FIGURE 8. Model of Agr regulation during invasion. In an extracellular environment, levels of *agrD*-encoded octapeptide (triangles) are low and *S. aureus* (solid circles) expresses cell surface-associated adhesins. These adhesins are proposed to interact with host plasma membrane-associated integrin and Hsp-60 molecules via a Fn bridge. Once internalized, a rapid accumulation of octapeptide within the endosome causes a shift to expression of exoproteins. Some exoproteins could affect escape from the endosome, resulting in the dilution of the octapeptide and a shift away from expression of exoproteins. Once *S. aureus* resides in the cytoplasm, we envision three possible outcomes: I) induction of apoptosis, II) formation of small colony variants (hatched circles), or III) host cell necrosis. The model for induction of apoptosis could involve a TNFα-mediated pathway through caspases 8 and 3 as described by Cohen.[66]

intriguing possibility. After infection with *S. aureus*, transcripts for the pro-inflammatory cytokine IL-6 were slightly elevated (1.26-fold increase), whereas levels of transcripts encoding the anti-inflammatory cytokines, IL-8 and TGF-β, were similar to the uninfected controls.[55] In osteoblast cells, IL-6 and IL-12 expression was enhanced upon *S. aureus* internalization.[17] Furthermore, in contrast to our results, Yao *et al.*[56] demonstrated a clear stimulation of IL-8 and protein levels by internalized *S. aureus*, a difference that may be cell specific.

The results of our studies with MAC-T cells suggest that infection with *S. aureus* causes a significant increase in the expression of the pro-inflammatory cytokines, TNF-α and IL-1β, (and possibly IL-6) while the expression of the anti-inflammatory cytokines, IL-8 and TGF-β appears to be unaffected. Effects of other pathogens on cytokine expression in response to internalization have been well documented and, in some cases, characterized. *Shigella flexneri* causes release of IL-1β through an inter-action with caspase 1 to initiate an inflammatory response.[51] In contrast, *Yersinia* spp. inhibits production of TNF-α to suppress inflammation.[57] Interestingly, strains of *S. aureus* are variable in their ability to induce inflammation. For example, *S. aureus* is typically considered to be pyogenic and many infections with *S. aureus* increase the level of pro-inflammatory cytokines in different cell types.[58,59] However, the lack of an inflammatory response frequently associated with certain types of *S. aureus* infections, such as subclinical bovine mastitis[60] and human toxic shock syndrome,[61] suggests that mechanisms to suppress the inflammatory response might also exist.

Effects of Regulatory Mutations on Invasion and Apoptosis

It is well established that, when bacteria are exposed to changing environmental conditions, an adaptive response is elicited that enables them to adjust to their new surroundings. This adaptive response can include responses to a variety of changing conditions such as nutrient availability, oxygen tension, or the presence of toxic substances. Clearly, the host cell endosomal compartment and cytoplasm provide unique environments to which *S. aureus* must adapt to allow it to survive (and possible multiply). A recent study by Vriesema *et al.*[62] is consistent with the notion that a variety of genes are specifically induced upon entry into a host cell. These genes could be divided into four different categories and include those involved in transport, catabolism, biosynthesis and DNA repair. How *S. aureus* is able to adapt to an initial encounter with a eukaryotic cell and then to an intra-cellular lifestyle is unknown, although recent studies have shed some light on this as well.

Based upon our results, internalization of *S. aureus* by MAC-T cells is associated with at least three features. First, internalization involves PTK activity and actin reorganization via mechanism(s) requiring expression of FnBPs. Second, the bacteria escape from the endosome and gain access to the cytoplasm. Third, internalized staphylococci induce host cell apoptosis. Like most aspects of pathogenesis, we found several or all of these features to be coordinately regulated.

Several published studies describe staphylococcal loci that regulate multiple phenotypic traits.[63,64] One such locus, designated *agr* for accessory gene regulator, affects the expression of several virulence factors. In an *agr* mutant, the expression of extracellular (secreted) virulence factors, including α-, β-, γ- and δ-hemolysins, leukocidin, toxic shock syndrome toxin-1, enterotoxins B and C, lipase, hyaluronate lyase, V8 protease, capsular polysaccharide and fatty acid-metabolizing enzyme are reduced.[65] The same mutation, however, causes the overexpression of specific cell wall-associated proteins, including protein A, FnBPs, clumping factor, and vitronectin-binding protein.[65] A second locus, called *sar* for staphylococcus accessory regulator, has also been shown to affect virulence factor production, largely by regulating the expression of *agr*.

In simple preliminary experiments, the effects of different *S. aureus* virulence factor regulatory systems (Agr and Sar) on infection of MAC-T cells was assessed. Consistent with elevated surface protein expression, each mutant strain tested was internalized by MAC-T cells with numbers consistently greater than the wild-type strain.[24] Photographs of the MAC-T cells infected by each of the different strains used above were taken after 22 hr to evaluate the effects of intracellular staphylococci on MAC-T cells. Substantial differences were observed in MAC-T cell morphology depending on the strain used for infection (Figure 5). Uninfected MAC-T cells appeared normal. Internalization of the parental strain RN6390 resulted in the generation of morphological changes similar to those observed with the MAC-T cells infected with strain Novel (see above). However, internalization of the *agr* mutant strain RN6911 or the *agr, sar* double mutant strain ALC135 produced no visible changes in morphology. MAC-T cells which had internalized the *sar* mutant strain ALC136 exhibited dramatically altered cellular morphology but were distinctly different compared to cells infected with the parental strain (RN6390). The *sar* mutant-infected cells appeared slightly larger and did not have the mottled cell surface that was a characteristic of the MAC-T cells infected with RN6390. Consistent with the induced morphological changes observed, only the parental strain induced apoptosis as suggested by the DNA laddering in the RN6390-infected MAC-T cells (Figure 6, lane 3). Thus, the ability to induce apoptosis is dependent on *agr*- and *sar*-regulated factors. The identity of these factors remains unknown.

Suspected Mechanisms

A model for the function of Agr-mediated quorum sensing in staphylococcal disease has recently been proposed.[65] In this model, extracellular concentration of the AgrD octapeptide controls expression of the *agr* operon and thereby mediates differential expression of cell wall-associated factors and exoproteins. Low levels of octapeptide (Agr down-regulated) lead to the expression of cell wall-associated factors (negatively regulated by Agr) while high octapeptide levels (Agr up-regulated) trigger a shift to the expression of exoproteins (positively regulated by Agr). According to this model, *S. aureus* cells that have recently entered a host would be expected to express cell wall-associated proteins since the initial octapeptide concentration would be low. The bacteria would be in a state to resist host defense mechanisms (presumably due to the production of surface factors such as protein A) while being primed to bind tissue surfaces (due to the production of fibronectin- and/or collagen-binding MSCRAMMs). Once a focus of infection had been established, they would multiply and form a characteristic barrier (abscess) that would provide additional protection against host defenses. As the number and concentration of bacteria increased within the abscess, the *agrD*-encoded octapeptide would reach a "threshold" concentration that would promote a shift to the expression of tissue-damaging exoproteins and escape from the abscess barrier. This then would lead to a corresponding shift to a more progressive and invasive infection.

Based on our current information, we propose a modification of this model to accommodate staphylococci in an intracellular niche. According to our model (Figure 8), upon entry into the host or previously sterile body site, extracellular *S. aureus* cells are likely to express cell surface-associated adherence factors including FnBPs which promote both adherence to and uptake by host cells. At this stage of infection, the AgrD octapeptide is low since it would be diluted in the surrounding fluids and the bacteria would be in a physical state that is optimal for binding to cell surfaces and subsequent internalization. Upon internalization by the host cell, the bacteria are immediately surrounded by an endosomal membrane.[3–5,10,12,15] Since this could simulate a state of extremely high cell density, an almost immediate accumulation of octapeptide within the confined space of the endosome could trigger expression of Agr and its up-regulated exoproteins.

Some of these exoproteins (particularly the hemolysins) could play a role in escape from the endosome. We have shown that, shortly after internalization, *S. aureus* escapes from the endosome via a process that results in lysis of the endosomal membrane (Figure 1).[10] Outside of the endosome, the octapeptide is immediately diluted again, resulting in an Agr-mediated shift away from the expression of exoproteins, and toward a physiological state that is more adapted to promote survival and growth within the cytoplasm.

Once the bacteria have gained access to the cytoplasm, we envision three possible outcomes that could have dramatically different effects on pathogenesis (Figure 8). These outcomes are based on the different effects that were observed with the MAC-T cells when infected by the *S. aureus* strains used in our studies and the results of Proctor *et al.*[27] One pathway (pathway I) could lead to the production of an Agr-regulated factor that triggers the development of apoptosis. The resulting apoptotic bodies would then be engulfed by resident macrophages. Engulfment of membrane-bound bacteria could provide a protective environment (analogous to the Trojan horse) within the macrophage resulting in its inability to produce an appropriate bactericidal response. This is supported by the observation that macrophages isolated from infected bovine udders often contain viable *S. aureus* cells.[67] It is also becoming well-established that induction of apoptosis by bacteria can have significant effects on cytokine regulation and hence the status of the host immune response.[51,68] Alternatively, metabolically inactive small colony variants could be formed (pathway II), causing little damage to the host cell and leading to a more chronic and persistent disease.[27] Finally, if the bacteria accumulated to a high enough concentration in the cytoplasm, AgrD octapeptide levels could reach a concentration sufficient to shift expression to exoproteins. Activation of cytolytic proteins (hemolysins) would result in lysis of the host cell (pathway III), spread to adjacent cells, generating an abscess or possibly a more progressive and invasive disease. The occurrence of this final phase would be dependent on the ability of *S. aureus* to replicate, allowing the accumulation of enough octapeptide to shift gene expression back to the exoproteins. According to our model, any inhibition of growth in the cytoplasm would reduce the accumulation of octapeptide and subsequently delay lysis of the host cell. Thus, the commitment to advance toward a more progressive infection, in contrast to a more persistent and chronic infection (two conditions that would not be mutually exclusive), would be made within the cytoplasm and could be based on the immunological state of the host.

Effects on Pathogenesis

Although experimental results that conclusively show a role for intra-cellular *S. aureus* in pathogenesis or persistence are limited, there has been much speculation as to the role that intracellular *S. aureus* plays during an infection. Schmidt *et al.*[6] proposed that intracellular staphylococci might be responsible for the failure of certain antimicrobial treatments in human infections. Similarly, Craven *et al.*[69] suggested that difficulty in treating staphylococcal bovine mastitis may be due to intracellular organisms. It has also been proposed that an intracellular environment could provide pro-tection against a host immune response. Compounding the problem for the host is the possibility that staphylococcal superantigens may induce a type of immune response that does not efficiently deal with intracellular pathogens.[72] Other possible roles for intracellular *S. aureus* also exist. Studies by Drake and Pang[73] indicate that internalized *S. aureus* results in increased levels of procoagulant activity in cultured human cardiac valve endothelial (HCVE) cells. A model describing a potential mechanism of vegetation formation in infective endocarditis implicates the procoagulant activity of infected endothelial cells in the initiation of vegetation formation.

The role of apoptosis during staphylococcal infection is quite specu-lative and therefore it is prudent to attempt to learn from other related systems. Although the number of bacterial pathogens that have been shown to induce apoptosis is growing rapidly,[74] its role in disease is known for only a few organisms. For example, the ability of *S. flexneri* to induce apoptosis is thought to be important for pathogenesis by inducing an acute inflam-matory response that promotes massive secondary invasion of the bacte-ria.[75] In *Salmonella* infections, there is a correlation between the ability to induce apoptosis and the progression of disease.[76]

Is the ability to induce apoptosis a virulence mechanism or simply a defense response of the host cell? The presence of pro- and anti-apoptosis mechanisms in several pathogens suggests that organisms manipulate the host cell apoptotic pathway, both positively and negatively, to the benefit of the bacteria.[77-79] In all of these systems, it is speculated that the molec-ular control of apoptosis allows the bacteria to take advantage of the intra-cellular environment while, at the same time, providing a mechanism to exit the host cell. Whether *S. aureus* uses pro- and anti-apoptosis mecha-nisms as a switch between acute and chronic disease is an intriguing possibility, but one that has not yet been confirmed.

ACKNOWLEDGMENTS. This work was supported by U.S.D.A. (NRICGP) (GAB) and PHS grants AI28401 (GAB) and AI38901 (KWB), the United

Dairymen of Idaho (GAB) and the Idaho Agricultural Experiment Station.

REFERENCES

1. Isberg, R. R. Discrimination between intracellular uptake and surface adhesion of bacterial pathogens. *Science* **252**, 934–938 (1991).
2. Rankin, S., Isberg, R. R. & Leong, J. M. The integrin-binding domain of invasin is sufficient to allow bacterial entry into mammalian cells. *Infect. Immun.* **60**, 3909–3912 (1992).
3. Ogawa, S. K., Yurberg, E. R., Hatcher, V. B., Levitt, M. A. & Lowy, F. D. Bacterial adherence to human endothelial cells *in vitro*. *Infect. Immun.* **50**, 218–224 (1985).
4. Hamill, R. J., Vann, J. M. & Proctor, R. A. Phagocytosis of *Staphylococcus aureus* by cultured bovine aortic endothelial cells: model for postadherence events in endovascular infections. *Infect. Immun.* **54**, 833–836 (1986).
5. Lowy, F. D., Fant, J., Higgins, L. L., Ogawa, S. K. & Hatcher, V. B. *Staphylococcus aureus*—human endothelial cell interactions. *J. Ultrastruct. Mol. Struct. Res.* **98**, 137–146 (1988).
6. Schmidt, H., Bukholm, G. & Holberg-Petersen, M. Adhesiveness and invasiveness of staphylococcal species in a cell culture model. *APMIS* **97**, 655–660 (1989).
7. Murai, M., Usui, A., Seki, K., Sakurada, J. & Masuda, S. Intracellular localization of *Staphylococcus aureus* within primary cultured mouse kidney cells. *Microbiol. Immunol.* **36**, 431–443 (1992).
8. Almeida, R. A., Matthews, K. R., Cifrian, E., Guidry, A. J. & Oliver, S. P. *Staphylococcus aureus* invasion of bovine mammary epithelial cells. *J. Dairy Sci.* **79**, 1021–1026 (1996).
9. Hyunh, H. T., Robitaille, G. & Turner, J. D. Establishment of bovine mammary epithelial cells (MAC-T): an *in vivo* model for bovine lactation. *Exp. Cell Res.* **197**, 191–199 (1991).
10. Bayles, K. W. *et al.* Intracellular *Staphylococcus aureus* escapes the endosome and induces apoptosis. *Infect. Immun.* **66**, 336–342 (1998).
11. Falkow, S., Isberg, R. R. & Portnoy, D. A. The interaction of bacteria with mammalian cells. *Annu. Rev. Cell Biol.* **8**, 333–363 (1992).
12. Hudson, M. C., Ramp, W. K., Nicholson, N. C., Williams, A. S. & Nousiainen, M. T. Internalization of *Staphylococcus aureus* by cultured osteoblasts. *Microb. Path.* **19**, 409–419 (1995).
13. Usui, A., Murai, M., Seki, K., Sakurada, J. & Masuda, S. Conspicuous ingestion of *Staphylococcus aureus* organisms by murine fibroblast *in vitro*. *Microbiol. Immunol.* **36**, 545–550 (1992).
14. Sinha, B. *et al.* Fibronectin-binding protein acts as a *Staphylococcus aureus* invasin via fibronectin bridging to integrin a5b1. *Cell. Microbiol.* **1**, 101–117 (1999).
15. Menzies, B. E. & Kourteva, I. Internalization of *Staphylococcus aureus* by endothelial cells induces apoptosis. *Infect. Immun.* **66**, 5994–5998 (1998).
16. Murai, M. *et al.* Apoptosis observed in BALB/3T3 cells having ingested *Staphylococcus aureus*. *Microbiol. Immunol.* **43**, 653–661 (1999).
17. Bost, K. L. *et al.* *Staphylococcus aureus* infection of mouse or human osteoblasts induces high levels of interleukin-6 and interleukin-12 production. *J. Infect. Dis.* **180**, 1912–1920 (1999).
18. Dombek, P. E. *et al.* High-frequency intracellular invasion of epithelial cells by serotype M1 group A streptococci: M1 protein-mediated invasion and cytoskeletal rearrangements. *Mol. Microbiol.* **31**, 859–870 (1999).

19. Griffin, F. M., Jr., Griffin, J. A., Leider, J. E. & Silverstein, S. C. Studies on the mechanism of phagocytosis. I. Requirements for circumferential attachment of particle-bound ligands to specific receptors on the macrophage plasma membrane. *J. Exp. Med.* **142**, 1263–1282 (1975).

20. Reilly, S. S., Hudson, M. C., Kellam, J. F. & Ramp, W. K. *In vivo* internalization of *Staphylococcus aureus* by embryonic chick osteoblasts. *Bone* **26**, 63–70 (2000).

21. Bohach, G., Dinges, M. M., Mitchell, D. T., Ohlendorf, D. H. & Schlievert, P. M. Exotoxins. in *The Staphylococci in human disease* (eds. Crossley, K. B. & Archer, G. L.) 83–111 (Churchill Livingstone, New York, 1997).

22. Smith, T. H., Fox, L. K. & Middleton, J. R. Outbreak of mastitis caused by one strain of *Staphylococcus aureus* in a closed dairy herd. *J. Am. Vet. Med. Assoc.* **212**, 553–556 (1998).

23. Isberg, R. R., Voorhis, D. L. & Falkow, S. Identification of invasin: a protein that allows enteric bacteria to penetrate cultured mammalian cells. *Cell* **50**, 769–778 (1978).

24. Wesson, C. A. *et al.* The *Staphylococcus aureus* Agr and Sar global regulators influence internalization and induction of apoptosis. *Infect. Immun.* **66**, 5238–5243 (1998).

25. von Eiff, C. *et al.* A site-directed *Staphylococcus aureus hemB* mutant is a small-colony variant which persists intracellularly. *J. Bacteriol.* **179**, 4706–4712 (1997).

26. Nuzzo, I., Sanges, M. R., Folgore, A. & Carratelli, C. R. Apoptosis of human keratinocytes after bacterial invasion. *FEMS Immunol. Med. Microbiol.* **27**, 235–240 (2000).

27. Proctor, R. A., Balwit, J. M. & Vesga, O. Variant subpopulations of *Staphylococcus aureus* as cause of persistent and recurrent infections. *Infect. Agents Dis.* **3**, 302–312 (1994).

28. Vesga, O. *et al. Staphylococcus aureus* small colony variants are induced by the endothelial cell intracellular milieu. *J. Infect. Dis.* **173**, 739–742 (1996).

29. Greene, C. *et al.* Adhesion properties of mutants of *Staphylococcus aureus* defective in fibronectin-binding proteins and studies on the expression of *fnb* genes. *Mol. Microbiol.* **17**, 1143–1152 (1995).

30. Dziewanowska, K. *et al.* Fibronectin binding protein and host cell tyrosine kinase are required for internalization of *Staphylococcus aureus* by epithelial cells. *Infect. Immun.* **67**, 4673–4678 (1999).

31. Peacock, S. J., Foster, T. J., Cameron, B. J. & Berendt, A. R. Bacterial fibronectin-binding proteins and endothelial cell surface fibronectin mediate adherence of *Staphylococcus aureus* to resting human endothelial cells. *Microbiology* **145**, 3477–3486 (1999).

32. Lammers, A., Nuijten, P. J. & Smith, H. E. The fibronectin binding proteins of *Staphylococcus aureus* are required for adhesion to and invasion of bovine mammary gland cells. *FEMS Microbiol. Lett.* **180**, 103–109 (1999).

33. Isberg, R. R. & Tran Van Nhieu, G. Binding and internalization of microorganisms by integrin receptors. *Trends Microbiol.* **2**, 10–14 (1994).

34. Dziewanowska, K. *et al.* Staphylococcal fibronectin binding protein interacts with heat shock protein 60 and integrins: role in internalization by epithelial cells. *Infect. Immun.* In press (2000).

35. Ellington, J. K. *et al.* Mechanisms of *Staphylococcus aureus* invasion of cultured osteoblasts. *Microb Pathog* **26**, 317–323 (1999).

36. Joh, D., Wann, E. R., Kreikemeyer, B., Speziale, P. & Hook, M. Role of fibronectin-binding MSCRAMMs in bacterial adherence and entry into mammalian cells. *Matrix Biol.* **18**, 211–223 (1999).

37. van Putten, J. P., Duensing, T. D. & Cole, R. L. Entry of OpaA+ gonococci into HEp-2 cells requires concerted action of glycosaminoglycans, fibronectin and integrin receptors. *Mol. Microbiol.* **29**, 369–379 (1998).

38. Tran Van Nhieu, G. & Isberg, R. R. Bacterial internalization mediated by beta 1 chain integrins is determined by ligand affinity and receptor density. *Embo J.* **12**, 1887–1895 (1993).

39. Jevon, M. *et al.* Mechanisms of internalization of *Staphylococcus aureus* by cultured human osteoblasts. *Infect. Immun.* **67**, 2677–2681 (1999).

40. Kerr, J. F. R., Wylie, A. H. & Currie, A. R. Apoptosis: a basic biological phenomenon with wide-ranging implications in tissue kinetics. *Br. J. Cancer* **26**, 239–257 (1972).

41. Majno, G. & Joris, I. Apoptosis, oncosis and necrosis. *Am. J. Pathology* **146**, 3–15 (1995).

42. Peitsch, M. C., Mannherz, H. G. & Tschopp, J. The apoptosis endonucleases: cleaning up after cell death? *Trends in Cell Biol.* **4**, 37–41 (1994).

43. Wyllie, A. H. Glucocorticoid-induced thymocyte apoptosis is associated with endogenous endonuclease activation. *Nature (London)* **284**, 555–556 (1980).

44. Facchinetti, A. *et al.* An improved method for the detection of DNA fragmentation. *J. Immunol. Methods* **136**, 1251–1256 (1991).

45. Gavrieli, Y., Sherman, Y. & Ben-Sasson, S. A. Identification of programmed cell death *in situ* via specific labeling of nuclear DNA fragmentation. *J. Cell. Biol.* **119**, 493–501 (1992).

46. Piqueras, B., Autran, B., Debre, P. & Gorochov, G. Detection of apoptosis at the single-cell level by direct incorporation of fluorescein-dUTP in DNA strand breaks. *BioTechniques* **20**, 634–640 (1996).

47. Wijsman, J. H. *et al.* A new method to detect apoptosis in paraffin sections: *In situ* end-labeling of fragmented DNA. *J. Histochem. Cytochem.* **41**, 7–12 (1993).

48. Tucker, K. A., Reilly, S. S., Leslie, C. S. & Hudson, M. C. Intracellular *Staphylococcus aureus* induces apoptosis in mouse osteoblasts. *FEMS Microbiol. Lett.* **186**, 151–156 (2000).

49. Gao, L. Y. & Abu Kwaik, Y. Activation of caspase 3 during *Legionella pneumophila*-induced apoptosis. *Infect. Immun.* **67**, 4886–4894 (1999).

50. Thornberry, N. A. & Lazebnik, Y. Caspases: enemies within. *Science* **281**, 1312–1316 (1998).

51. Chen, Y., Smith, M. R., Thirumalai, K. & Zychlinsky, A. A bacterial invasin induces macrophage apoptosis by binding directly to ICE. *EMBO J.* **15**, 3853–3860 (1996).

52. Hersh, D. *et al.* The Salmonella invasin SipB induces macrophage apoptosis by binding to caspase-1. *Proc. Natl. Acad. Sci. USA* **96**, 2396–2401 (1999).

53. Bitzer, M. *et al.* Sendai virus infection induces apoptosis through activation of caspase-8 (FLICE) and caspase-3 (CPP32). *J. Virol.* **73**, 702–708 (1999).

54. Kidd, V. J. Proteolytic activities that mediate apoptosis. *Annu. Rev. Physiol.* **60**, 533–573 (1998).

55. Wesson, C. A. *et al.* Apoptosis induced by *Staphylococcus aureus* in epithelial cells utilizes a mechanism involving caspases 8 and 3. *Infect. Immun.* **68**, 2998–3001 (2000).

56. Yao, L., Lowy, F. D. & Berman, J. W. Interleukin-8 gene expression in *Staphylococcus aureus*-infected endothelial cells. *Infect. Immun.* **64**, 3407–3409 (1996).

57. Palmer, L. E., Hobbie, S., Galan, J. E. & Bliska, J. B. YopJ of *Yersinia pseudotuberculosis* is required for the inhibition of macrophage TNF-a production and downregulation of the MAP kinases p38 and JNK. *Mol. Microbiol.* **27**, 953–965 (1998).

58. Yao, L. *et al.* Internalization of *Staphylococcus aureus* by endothelial cells induces cytokine gene expression. *Infect. Immun.* **63**, 1835–1839 (1995).

59. Persson-Waller, K. Accumulation of leucocytes and cytokines in the lactating ovine udder during mastitis due to *Staphylococcus aureus* and *Escherichia coli*. *Res. Vet. Sci.* **62**, 63–66 (1997).

60. Pyorala, S. Staphylococcal and streptococcal mastitis. in *The Bovine Udder and Mastitis* (ed. Sandholm, M., Honkanen-Buzalski, T., Kaartineu, L. & Pyoral, S.) 143–148 (University of Helsinki, Helsinki, 1995).

61. Fast, D. J., Schlievert, P. M. & Nelson, R. D. Nonpurulent response to toxic shock syndrome toxin 1-producing *Staphylococcus aureus*. Relationship to toxin-stimulated production of tumor necrosis factor. *J. Immunol.* **140**, 949–953 (1988).

62. Vriesema, A. J. *et al.* Altered gene expression in *Staphylococcus aureus* upon interaction with human endothelial cells. *Infect. Immun.* **68**, 1765–1772 (2000).

63. Recsei, P. *et al.* Regulation of exoprotein gene expression in *Staphylococcus aureus* by *agr. Mol. Gen. Genet.* **202**, 58–61 (1985).

64. Cheung, A. L., Koomey, J. M., Butler, C. A., Projan, S. J. & Fischetti, V. A. Regulation of exoprotein expression in *Staphylococcus aureus* by a locus (*sar*) distinct from *agr. Proc. Natl. Acad. Sci. USA* **89**, 6462–6466 (1992).

65. Projan, S. J. & Novick, R. P. The molecular basis of pathogenicity. in *The staphylococci in human disease* (eds. Crossley, K. B. & Archer, G. L.) 55–81 (Churchill Livingstone, New York, NY, 1997).

66. Cohen, G. M. Caspases: the executioners of apoptosis. *Biochem. J.* **326**, 1–16 (1997).

67. Craven, N. & Anderson, J. C. The location of *Staphylococcus aureus* in experimental chronic mastitis in the mouse and the effect on the action of sodium cloxacillin. *British Journal of Experimental Pathology* **60**, 453–459 (1979).

68. Schesser, K. *et al.* The *yopJ* locus is required for Yersinia-mediated inhibition of NF-kappaB activation and cytokine expression: YopJ contains a eukaryotic SH2-like domain that is essential for its repressive activity. *Mol. Microbiol.* **28**, 1067–1079 (1998).

69. Craven, N. & Anderson, J. C. Phagocytosis of *Staphylococcus aureus* by bovine mammary gland macrophages and intracellular protection from antibiotic action *in vitro* and *in vivo*. *J. Dairy Res.* **51**, 513–523 (1984).

70. Lew, D. P. & Waldvogel, F. A. Osteomyelitis. *N. Engl. J. Med.* **336**, 999–1007 (1997).

71. Lowy, F. D. *Staphylococcus aureus* infections. *N. Engl. J. Med.* **339**, 520–532 (1998).

72. Ferens, W. A. & Bohach, G. A. Persistence of *Staphylococcus aureus* on mucosal membranes: superantigens and internalization by host cells. *J. Lab. Clin. Med.* **135**, 225–230 (2000).

73. Drake, T. A. & Pang, M. *Staphylococcus aureus* induces tissue factor expression in cultured human cardiac valve endothelium. *J. Infect. Dis.* **157**, 749–756 (1988).

74. Gao, L. Y. & Kwaik, Y. A. The modulation of host cell apoptosis by intracellular bacterial pathogens. *Trends Microbiol.* **8**, 306–313 (2000).

75. Zychlinsky, A. & Sansonetti, P. J. Apoptosis as a proinflammatory event: what can we learn from bacteria-induced cell death? *Trends Microbiol.* **5**, 201–204 (1997).

76. Richter-Dahlfors, A., Buchan, A. M. J. & Finlay, B. B. Murine salmonellosis studied by confocal microscopy: *Salmonella typhimurium* resides intracellularly inside macrophages and exerts a cytotoxic effect on phagocytes *in vivo*. *J. Exp. Med.* **186**, 569–580 (1997).

77. Aliprantis, A. O. *et al.* Cell activation and apoptosis by bacterial lipoproteins through toll-like receptor-2. *Science* **285**, 736–739 (1999).

78. Clifton, D. R. *et al.* NF-kappa B-dependent inhibition of apoptosis is essential for host cellsurvival during *Rickettsia rickettsii* infection. *Proc. Natl. Acad. Sci. USA* **95**, 4646–4651 (1998).

79. Fan, T. *et al.* Inhibition of apoptosis in chlamydia-infected cells: blockade of mitochondrial cytochrome c release and caspase activation. *J. Exp. Med.* **187**, 487–496 (1998).

13

Staphylococcus aureus Mastitis

LARRY K. FOX, KENNETH W. BAYLES, and GREGORY A. BOHACH

1. INTRODUCTION

Contagious mastitis is spread from cow to cow generally by fomites. Historically, *Streptocococcus agalactiae* has been the major etiological agent. Concerted management efforts to eradicate this otherwise obligate udder pathogen, such as milking time hygiene, dry cow therapy, and blitz treatment of infected udders, has led to a marked reduction in the prevalence of *S. agalactiae*; many herds have been free of *S. agalactiae* mastitis for several years. Today, the major contagious mastitis pathogen is *Staphylococcus aureus*, where estimates of prevalence exceed 5% of cows.[1,2] Recently, dairy managers have become more aware of *S. aureus* mastitis infections and have made additional efforts to remove this pathogen from their herds. Such efforts have been hampered by the inability of dairy managers to detect all infections consistently due to their inability to detect multiple and perhaps some unknown reservoirs, and by the resistance this pathogen has shown to many antibiotic therapy regimens. These issues, together with the pathogenesis of *S. aureus* bovine mastitis, the defense mechanisms of the host, virulence factors, identification of reservoirs of infection, and control through prevention, treatment, and vaccination, will be addressed.

LARRY K. FOX • Department of Veterinary Clinical Medicine and Surgery, Washington State University, Pullman, WA 99164. KENNETH W. BAYLES and GREGORY A. BOHACH • Department of Microbiology, Molecular Biology and Biochemistry, University of Idaho, Moscow, ID 83844-3052.

Staphylococcus aureus *Infection and Disease*, edited by Allen L. Honeyman *et al.* Kluwer Academic/Plenum Publishers, New York, 2001.

2. PATHOGENESIS

Mastitis is a general term for inflammation of the mammary gland. Inflammation, in the classical sense, is seen as redness, heat, swelling, and pain. Thus, the clinical signs of mastitis are a hard, red tinged, warmer than normal, udder, which may elicit a painful reaction when touched. The presentation of mastitis can take many forms, namely the acute form, which is accompanied by systemic signs of fever and mild depression, and the more severe peracute form, which is characterized by the presence of fever, depression, shivering, loss of appetite, and loss of weight. There is also a gangrenous form where the affected quarter becomes markedly swollen and the teat becomes cold and cyanotic. A line of demarcation forms separating the living from the dead tissue.[3] Although mastitis can exhibit many forms, greater than 95% of the cases of mastitis are subclinical, where macroscopic changes to the udder are not seen. In cases of subclinical mastitis, there are changes in milk composition and milk production.[4] Milk production, a sign of loss of function, decreases with mastitis. The inflammatory changes associated with mastitis are correlated with intramammary infection. Often *S. aureus* mastitis is associated with a mild form of inflammation as noted by a Virginia Tech study where it was reported that approximately 40% of all cows with *S. aureus* mastitis infections had milk somatic cell counts of less than 400,000 cells/ml.[5] It has been noted that less than 100 colony forming units (cfu) of *S. aureus*/ml of milk can be isolated from infected quarters.[6,7] The lack of somatic cell response, associated inflammatory mediators, and the low population of *S. aureus* within the gland are suggestive of mild cases of this disease. In chronic, either clinical or subclinical disease, there is loss of parenchymal and ductular tissue. Gudding et al.[8] reported that *S. aureus* attaches to epithelium and appears to induce eroded and ulcerative tissue. Nickerson and Heald[9] noted that neutrophil extravasion is associated with the damaged epithelium. Presumably the neutrophil influx is a primary or secondary cause of the loss of milk production associated with increased milk somatic cell counts. *S. aureus* intramammary infections can be persistent[10] and the organism can be quite contagious. A recent report indicates that *S. aureus* prevalence of this disease could rise from <5% to greater than 30% in a year's period, causing a marked elevation of milk somatic cell counts, even in a herd practicing excellent mastitis control procedures.[11]

3. IDENTIFICATION AND DIAGNOSIS

S. aureus bovine isolates are gram positive, catalase positive cocci. Isolation of the pathogen and identification of the virulence factors have been the traditional methods used to diagnose *S. aureus* mastitis infections. Like strains from other hosts, *S. aureus* bovine isolates are defined, classically, as those staphylococci that caused plasma to coagulate. With respect to mastitis, two other coagulase positive staphylococcal species are now recognized.[12] Although the coagulase test will not definitively identify *S. aureus*,[13] more than 95% of all coagulase positive staphylococcal mastitis isolates were classified as *S. aureus*.[14] The remaining isolates are, with rare exception, *Staphylococcus hyicus* and *Staphylococcus intermedius*. Hemolysis patterns, termed alpha and beta, have also been used to speciate the staphylococci, although this is a less reliable method than coagulase. Hemolytic patterns can be influenced by different blood agar lots. Additionally, not all *S. aureus* produce detectable hemolysins while some coagulase negative isolates do produce hemolysins. A simple means to identify *S. aureus* mastitis isolates from other coagulase positive isolates is through growth on "P" agar, supplemented with 7 ug acriflavine per ml of agar.[15] Tests for heat-stable nuclease and thermonuclease can also be used to identify *S. aureus*.[13]

Recently the Staph-antibody or *S. aureus* antibody Test Kit has been marketed as a diagnostic tool for *S. aureus* mastitis.[16] The basis of this test is the identification of local synthesis of immunoglobulin G produced against *S. aureus* antigens.[17] Our research group has determined that the test cannot be used to identify the *S. aureus* positive quarter since the antibody levels are elevated in all four quarters, although the highest antibody levels are found in the infected quarter. Additionally, the test can not reliably identify *S. aureus* infected quarters in cows producing less than 13.6 kg in less than 30 days of milk. Moreover the results of the test sometimes fall within a "grey-zone," where the antibody level is deemed to be in a range that can not distinguish between an infected and non-infected gland. The sensitivity and specificity of this test has been reported to have a wide range. One report indicates the sensitivity may be as low as 59%, and another suggests the specificity is as low as 61%.[16] However, specificity as high as 100% and sensitivity as high as 92% have also been reported.[6,18]

4. PREVALENCE

Cows

As indicated above, *S. agalactiae* was the most prevalent major contagious mastitis pathogen. With the advent of milking time hygiene, teat dip and dry cow therapy, this pathogen has been eradicated from many if not most US dairies. Thus, *S. aureus* has emerged as the most prevalent major contagious mastitis pathogen. A survey of Pacific Northwest US dairies during the 1980s indicated that 84% were infected with S. aureus.[19] A survey done in Britain at approximately the same time period suggested that 93% of herds were affected.[20] These two surveys relied on the aseptic collection of composite milk from cows at milking to estimate herd prevalence. They both estimated that 20% of the cows were infected. More current estimates in the US suggest lower herd and cow prevalence. A California study suggests that approximately 8% of the cows are infected in 100% of the herds.[21] A Pennsylvania State University study[22] examined the prevalence of S. aureus in herds that used excellent or poor milking time hygiene techniques. The excellent control herds had 0.6% of the mammary quarters infected, while the poor control herds had a quarter prevalence of 6.6%, 11 times greater. A similar survey indicated a 3.0% and 14.6% prevalence of S. aureus mastitis in excellent and poorer mastitis control herds, respectively.[23] Since the primary reservoir of S. aureus is the cow with mastitis, microbiologic culture of bulk tank farm milk can be used to estimate the prevalence of S. aureus in a herd. The appearance of S. aureus in the farm bulk tank milk generally indicates that there are cows with S. aureus mastitis in the herd. Results from a survey where bulk tank samples of milk from Vermont dairies suggested that approximately 50% of herds have S. aureus mastitis cows.[24] These bulk tank surveys clearly are lower estimates of S. aureus prevalence than surveys where individual cows were sampled suggesting that bulk tank milk culture is a less sensitive measure of estimating S. aureus prevalence. Yet all the data clearly reveals that S. aureus mastitis is widely prevalent in the US, in herds with both excellent and poor mastitis control procedures. Thus, years of milking time hygiene and dry cow therapy usage has not led to the eradication of this disease. However, these control procedures are clearly effective in reducing the prevalence, as evidenced by the lower estimates of S. aureus prevalence in the most recent surveys.[1,2]

Heifers

One explanation as to why milking time hygiene and dry cow therapy have rarely led to the eradication of this disease in dairy herds is the continuous reservoir of freshening heifers. Heifers appear to introduce new strains of this disease to their herds.[25] Herds with a higher prevalence of S. aureus mastitis in the lactating cows tended to have higher prevalence among the heifers at freshening.[26] However, this relationship was not excessively strong. Heifers with S. aureus colonizing the teat skin area prepartum, and as early as preweaning, were 3.34 times more likely to have S. aureus mastitis infections than heifers without such colonization. Some heifers were persistently colonized by *S. aureus* at several body sites, primarily mucosal external orifices. This research suggested that these persistently colonized heifers might represent a primary reservoir of *S. aureus* for other farm heifers, especially when that colonization includes the teat skin area.

A study conducted in Washington, Vermont, California, and Louisiana was designed to determine the prevalence of mastitis in heifers at calving as affected by location and season.[27] The prevalence of *S. aureus* mastitis in heifers was consistently highest in Louisiana, with as high as 9% of all freshening heifers having this disease. It appeared that climate might have an influence on *S. aureus* mastitis in heifers at freshening. All states reported less than 2% prevalence in the winter, and states other than Louisiana consistently reported prevalence of less than 3%. These other states have milder and colder climates than Louisiana, which can often be exceptionally hot and humid (subtropical) in the late spring through early fall period. The Louisiana research group has suggested that biting flies may lead to the transmission of *S. aureus* to teat skin, and that colonization of injured skin occurs.[28] Colonization of *S. aureus* on teat skin is enhanced by injury,[29] and evidence has demonstrated that colonization of the teat skin will predispose the heifer to *S. aureus* mastitis at freshening.[15] Some data from the Louisiana research group does suggest that fly control may reduce the incidence of *S. aureus* mastitis in heifers (Owens, unpublished data, 1999).

5. INTERACTIONS OF *S. AUREUS* WITH THE BOVINE IMMUNE SYSTEM

Since *S. aureus* actively colonizes the external portions of the mammary gland, dairy cattle are at frequent risk of infection particularly in situations which compromise the ability of their normal immune system to block new infections. Once established, typical staphylococcal infections may ascend to the duct system and eventually reach the alveoli, although they generally remain localized in the mammary gland by the bovine immune system. Combined the innate and specific immune responses constitute a normally formidable barrier to the entry and replication of *S. aureus* and other potential mastitis pathogens. However, the continued problem that staphylococcal mastitis poses to the dairy industry is evidence that the bovine immune system provides protection that is only partial and short lived. These problems have hampered the development of an effective vaccine for staphylococcal mastitis.

Innate Physical and Chemical Barriers

Physical barriers constitute a significant portion of the innate immune defenses against *S. aureus* in the mammary gland (Figure 1). The intact external surface of the healthy udder provides an effective barrier to entry into the interior of the mammary gland. This is as a result of concerted effects of physical barriers and certain chemical substances they contain. Like epithelial surfaces of other animals, the bovine mammary gland is covered by normally impenetrable fibrous layers on the external skin surface. Entry of external staphylococci into the udder through the streak

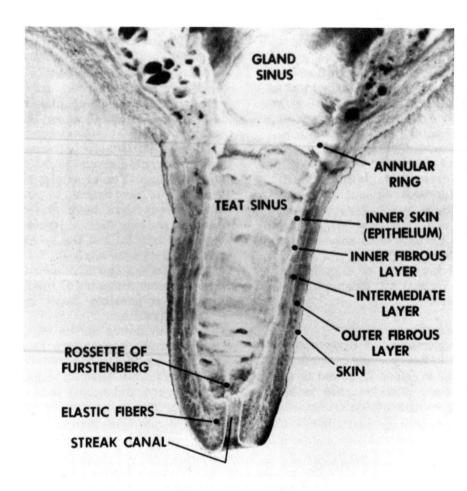

FIGURE 1. The anatomy of the bovine teat. Reprinted from Schalm *et al.*[3] with permission.

canal is blocked by the action of sphincter muscles and elastic fibers, which close the end of the teat apex after milking. In addition, keratin in the streak canal provides an additional physical barrier and harbors several antibacterial compounds.

Trauma to the teat end and streak canal facilitate development of mastitis for several reasons. Trauma is known to increase the colonization rate of *S. aureus* on the outer surface of the teat. This makes it more likely that a number of *S. aureus*, sufficient to initiate an infection, gain access to the area of the streak canal when it is opened during and immediately following milking. Even minor trauma, such as that associated with milking, can facilitate entry of *S. aureus* into the teat sinus. Once *S. aureus* enters the mammary gland, the normal flow of the milk could remove *S. aureus* from the udder unless the organism can establish counteractive mechanisms.

A variety of antibacterial chemical substances interfere with the ability of *S. aureus* to establish an infection once it gains access to the interior of the udder. Iron binding host proteins particularly lactoferrin interfere with *S. aureus* replication by limiting available iron. Lactoferrin which is normally found in moderate quantities in milk and another less abundant iron binding compound, transferrin, both increase in concentrations during the initial inflammatory response to *S. aureus* in the mammary gland. Lysozyme, the cell wall active compound is present in low but significant quantities in milk. Bovine milk has relatively high levels of lactoperoxidase, an enzyme which, in the presence of thiocyanate and hydrogen peroxidase, is cidal toward *S. aureus*. Milk also contains low levels of lysozyme and complement although their effects on *S. aureus* in the mammary gland are not well documented.

Phagocytic Cells

Upon entry into the mammary gland, staphylococci encounter a variety of cell populations that contribute to elimination of the organism. Bovine macrophages constitute a resident cell population of the normal mammary gland and, as a result, are the major cellular based anti-staphylococcal component at the earliest stages of infection. Macrophages have multiple functions and participate in both innate and specific immune functions. Although macrophages generally can ingest and kill staphylococci, opsonized bacteria are more efficiently killed. Macrophages also contribute to the specific immune response by processing antigens. Ingested staphylococci or their products such as exotoxins are expressed in association with MHC Class II on the cell surface for presentation to T cells.

Bacterial colonization of the mammary epithelium results initially in an inflammatory reaction characterized early on by the recruitment of neutrophils through the usual mechanisms involving host-derived or bacterial-derived chemotactic factors. These cells constitute the largest subpopulation of leukocytes in typical cases of mastitis caused by pyogenic organisms such as staphylococci. Typically, neutrophils are effective at killing most strains of opsonized S. aureus although the ability of certain more virulent strains to express various exotoxins including membrane active toxins (see below) impedes their effectiveness.

Lymphocytes and Immunoglobulins

There are significant differences between the peripheral blood and the mammary gland immune systems of dairy animals.[30] This is reflected perhaps most dramatically in the subpopulations of lymphocytes, which are important components of the specific immune response. Several staphylococcal exotoxins, particularly superantigens, dramatically affect the function and composition of bovine lymphocytes as discussed below. Bovine T lymphocytes subpopulations seem to share considerable functional similarities with T lymphocytes of other animals, including rodents and primates. For example, bovine peripheral blood and mammary gland secretions contain T cells expressing either the α/β or the γ/δ T cell receptor. The α/β T cells are divided functionally into CD4$^+$ and CD8$^+$ T cells and the ratio of these two cell types differ depending on the location. In the peripheral blood, similar to primates, the CD4:CD8 T cell ratio typically ranges from 1.0 and 2.0. In contrast, mammary gland secretions have substantially fewer CD4$^+$ cells relative to CD8$^+$ cells. The functional significance of these differences is unclear at the present time particularly since the CD8 marker is present on both suppressor and cytotoxic T cells. One unique characteristic of bovine species is the relatively large percentage of γ/δ T cells. The total of number γ/δ T cells varies with age. Young animals contain up to 80% γ/δ T cells, whereas levels in adult animals are substantially lower, albeit higher than in primates and rodents. The function of the γ/δ T cells in the bovine immune system is not well understood at the present time, although evidence exists to support the notion that they mediate their effects largely through cytotoxicity. Natural killer lymphocytes also display cytotoxic activity through antibody-dependant cell mediated cytotoxicity. They possess Fc receptors that recognize immunoglobulin-coated host cells bound to microbial antigens on the surface of infected cells and also possess direct antimicrobial killing ability for some organisms, including S. aureus.

Anti-staphylococcal antibody titers are elevated during staphylococcal mastitis. These antibodies facilitate, but are not sufficient for, resolution or prevention of mastitis. This is consistent with the failure of vaccines to prevent staphylococcal infections although they often result in reduced severity and duration of staphylococcal mastitis. Generally, induction of antibodies in milk correlates with peripheral levels although titers are usually lower in milk.[3] IgG1 is the most prevalent immunoglobulin in the mammary gland. Bovine IgG1, IgG2, and IgM have the ability to opsonize *S. aureus*. IgA is present in concentrations lower than IgG1 and acts largely as a neutralizing antibody and is non-opsonic. For T dependant antigens such as most *S. aureus* exoproteins and toxins, antibodies are expressed by B lymphocytes following antigen recognition, processing and MHC Class II presentation to T helper cells. T independent antigens such as some microbial surface molecules are T independent antigens and stimulate B cells without the involvement of T cells.

Effect of Lactation Stage on Mastitis

The incidence of *S. aureus* mastitis is affected by the bovine lactation cycle and increases as a result of immunosuppression in periparturient animals. Lactation stage-dependent changes in lymphocyte subpopulations and their responsiveness occur both systemically and in the mammary gland. During this period of time, differences in mononuclear cell subpopulations are greatest if healthy cows are compared to mastitic animals. Pregnant and periparturient cows have somewhat lower proportions of CD2+ and CD8+ cells in peripheral blood compared to non-pregnant, non-lactating cows, and also demonstrate lactation-dependent fluctuations in subpopulations of γ/δ T cells.[31] Expression of certain markers such as CD2, CD4, CD8, and WC1 decreases to a minimum level approximately three weeks prior to parturition and gradually increases afterwards.[31] The response of blood lymphocytes to mitogens is depressed at parturition.[32,33] Lymphocyte cultures from cows during mid and late lactation express primarily IFN-γ, whereas cultures from periparturient cows express mainly IL-4, and show a diminished cytotoxic potential.[33] Parturition is also associated with a pronounced depression of blood neutrophil function.[34–36] Compared to late lactation, periparturient cows exhibit reduced phagocytosis, migration, and bactericidal potential of neutrophils.[34] The composition of mammary lymphocyte populations is also lactation stage-dependent. Parturition is associated with an abrupt and major decrease of the CD4:CD8 ratio in mammary gland secretions.[37,38] The CD4:CD8 ratio remains depressed throughout most of lactation, although it gradually increases. The major increase takes place after drying off.[38]

6. SUBVERSION OF THE BOVINE MAMMARY GLAND DEFENSES

Once the physical and chemical barriers that the bovine udder presents have been breached, S. aureus can modulate the normal composition of immune cells in the mammary gland. For example, Park et al.[39] demonstrated that mammary gland secretions from cows with S. aureus mastitis, contain an activated CD8+ subpopulation that suppresses the function of bovine CD4+ cells. The ability of S. aureus to interfere with the bovine defenses results from the action of multiple virulence factors including surface molecules, hemolysins, enzymes, and a group of superantigen (SAg) exotoxins.[40]

Establishing an Infection

The first step in pathogenesis for any bacterial pathogen is to colonize its host. The ability of S. aureus to resist being washed out with the milk and succeed in establishing an initial infection has been attributed to numerous factors. Adaptation to nutrients and other environmental conditions in the udder are clearly necessary for replication of the organism. Lammers et al.[41] identified certain S. aureus genes induced specifically in milk that likely are involved in adapting to this new environment. Binding to milk fat globules has also been proposed as a mechanism by which S. aureus increase their buoyancy and ascend into the gland sinus.[42] However, probably one of the most critical steps in the initiation of an infection is binding to host tissues. S. aureus produces numerous surface proteins, or MSCRAMMs (microbial surface components recognizing adhesive matrix molecules) that are involved in the adhesion to various substrates. Although studies of the surface molecules required for adherence within the mammary gland are limited, mice immunized with fusion proteins encompassing the fibronectin-binding domain of a staphylococcal fibronectin-binding protein exhibit some protection against challenge with S. aureus using a mastitis model.[43] These data suggest that fibronectin present on the epithelial lining of the mammary gland are specifically recognized and bound by S. aureus and thus may be involved in colonization. In vitro experiments using fibronectin-binding protein deficient mutants are consistent with this hypothesis. In two separate studies, S. aureus strains that did not produce one or both of the fibronectin-binding proteins did not adhere to cultured bovine mammary epithelial cells as well as the parental strain.[44,45] Whether the fibronectin-binding protein mutants also exhibit reduced ability to colonize and produce disease in the mammary gland has not been examined.

Another key component required for colonization of host tissue (including the mammary gland) is the ability to resist the cellular immune response of the host. This may be particularly important for the development of *S. aureus* mastitis since cell-mediated immunity is a primary defense of the mammary gland against bacterial pathogens (see above). At least one surface-associated factor, protein A, may be involved in resisting phagocytosis. Based on its ability to bind the Fc portion of opsonizing antibodies, it is thought that protein A prevents a normal interaction of antibodies with the bacteria, thus, preventing opsonization. In fact, protein A does appear to contribute to the pathogenesis of mastitis. *S. aureus* strains that produced protein A exhibit increased virulence in a mouse mastitis model, resulting in an approximately 10-fold increase in bacterial recovery 30 hr postinfection.[46]

Another surface-associated factor that is presumed to be important in resistance to cell-mediated host defenses is capsular polysaccharides. At least eleven different capsule types have been isolated from different *S. aureus* strains. Most of these are referred to as "microcapsules" since they are produced at low levels *in vitro*. In a recent study, 59% of bovine mastitis isolates were found to produce either type 5 or 8 capsules,[47] a trend that is similar in human isolates. Thus, it is possible that these capsule types provide a selective advantage to the bacteria. Indeed, several studies indicate that the capsule produced by *S. aureus* has antiphagocytic properties *in vitro*.[48] However, there is currently no experimental evidence to suggest that staphylococcal capsule is protective in an infected udder.

Suppression of the Bovine Immune Response by *S. aureus* Superantigens

Several staphylococcal SAgs associated with a percentage of bovine mastitis isolates, particularly staphylococcal enterotoxin C (SEC) and toxic shock syndrome toxin-1 (TSST-1) belong to the SAg family and are prototypic microbial SAgs responsible for a variety of human and animal diseases.[49,50] There is some degree of host-specificity of staphylococcal SAgs. For example, SEC-bovine, the molecular variant produced by bovine mastitis isolates, has a slightly different amino acid sequence compared to SEC produced by staphylococci isolated from humans, sheep, or canines.[51] SAgs are potent activators of T cells and induce cell activation through a mechanism unique from conventional antigens. SAg binding to T cells is dependent mainly on the Vβ region of the T cell receptor. This site is located outside of the site involved in antigen recognition. Therefore, SAg activation is less specific than activation by conventional antigens, and a high proportion of T cells become activated. The result of this interaction is an abnormal signal transduction resulting in massive cytokine release, T cell proliferation, and a potential for anergy, or apoptosis of activated lymphocytes.

Until recently, very few studies were conducted to investigate the effects of these toxins on the bovine immune system. It is now known that bovine T cells proliferate upon exposure to SEC in a manner similar to that shown previously for primate and murine lymphocytes.[52] Specifically, they respond in a Vβ dependent fashion. Stimulation of bovine PBMC with SAgs in vitro causes a delayed proliferative response in which maximum stimulation occurs following 6 days. Rather than dividing, CD4+ cell numbers decline during the initial 96 hours of incubation as a result of selective apoptosis of this subpopulation.[53] This period is followed by a three day period of vigorous proliferation, although CD8+ cells increase more dramatically than CD4+ cells. As a result, after seven days of culture, the CD4:CD8 ratio declines to 0.3 in PBMC cultures from an initial normal value of 1.5. The activated CD8+ cells are enlarged and upregulate several activation markers including MHC II and Il-2α. Interestingly, another activation marker, designated ACT3, is expressed on the majority of bovine CD8+ T cells following stimulation by SEC.[54] The function of CD8+ T cells expressing ACT3 remains to be determined and is likely to be involved in immunosuppression. In other systems, CD8 cells resulting from SAg stimulation, inhibit proliferation of CD4+ cells,[55] induce FAS-ligand-mediated cell death of CD4+ cells,[56] or have depressed cytotoxic capacity.[57]

Exposure of bovine PBMCs to SEC causes upregulation of IL-4 and downregulation of IL-12. This pattern is suggestive of a Type 2 response induction and may be unique to the bovine system since in other animals SAgs typically induce primarily type 1 cytokines.[58] The potential consequences of this effect for mastitis are unclear although it suggests that dairy animals infected with a SAg producing strain may be less able to resolve intracellular infections.

Role of Other Staphylococcal Virulence Factors

Other *S. aureus* exoproteins may also be required for maintaining and/or escalating the infection. Although many of these exoproteins have been implicated in the pathogenesis of mastitis, only a few have actually been examined in any detail. A study by Bramley *et al.*,[59] again using a mouse mastitis model, revealed that strains producing α- and β-toxin led to significantly higher recovery of *S. aureus* from the infected mammary gland. Furthermore, the production of α-toxin was highly correlated with the ability to induce lethality within 48 hr, killing 60% of the inoculated mice. Strains that did not produce α-toxin produced acute mastitis but did not induce lethality.[59]

Because of the diversity of extracellular factors that *S. aureus* produces, it is difficult to establish the roles of each in the development of *S. aureus* mastitis. As described above, studies using purified toxin and site-directed mutagenesis strategies have been the primary methods utilized to demonstrate roles of specific staphylococcal factors in mastitis. Although these methods have proved useful, they are inefficient and do not assess the complexity of factors that are involved in pathogenesis. More recently, sophisticated molecular strategies have been applied to examine the factors involved in various staphylococcal diseases, including *in vivo* expression technology[60] and signature-tagged mutagenesis.[61,62] The results of these studies have begun to reveal the broad spectrum of factors that are required for staphylococcal pathogenesis.

Evasion of the Immune Response by Intracellular *S. aureus* in Bovine Epithelial Cells

Although antibodies seem to play a role in limiting the duration and severity of *S. aureus* infections in the mammary gland, they are not fully protective against colonization or new mastitis infections.[63] Some of the staphylococcal virulence factors such as protein A and the hemolysins probably contribute to the ineffectiveness of antibody mediated killing of staphylococci. However, work with isogenic mutants has failed to confirm this explanation for the ineffective function of antibodies.[64] The intracellular location of some staphylococci could provide an alternative explanation.

Although *S. aureus* is not internalized as efficiently as some other organisms such as *Salmonella* species and *Listeria monocytogenes*, its entry into bovine phagocytes and nonprofessional phagocytes cells is clearly documented in vitro and in vivo.[65] Much of the in vitro work in this area has been conducted with the MAC-T cell line derived from bovine mammary epithelium.[66] Uptake by these bovine cells requires intimate contact between staphylococcal fibronectin binding protein and its receptors on host cells (β1 integrins and heat shock protein 60),[67] host cell signal transduction and cytoskeletal rearrangements. Following internalization within a membrane-bound endosome, *S. aureus* cells eventually escape, multiply in the cytoplasm and induce inflammatory mediators and apoptosis.[68]

An intracellular environment could provide a mechanism where by *S. aureus* could evade the bovine immune response. Intracellular staphylococci would be more likely to evade macrophages. In addition, the bovine cytokine profiles induced by SAg exposure might further enhance the advantage of intracellular staphylococci.[69]

Regulation of Staphylococcal Virulence Factors

Like most staphylococcal diseases, the ability of S. aureus to infect the bovine udder is likely to be dependent on the staphylococcal virulence factor regulators, Agr and Sar.[70] The Agr locus encodes a transcription regulatory system that differentially regulates exoprotein and cell wall-associated genes under its control. The locus is comprised of a four-gene operon and a divergently transcribed regulatory RNA molecule, termed RNAIII. Two genes within the agr operon (agrA and agrC) encode a response regulator and a sensor histidine kinase, respectively, which are members of the two-component regulatory system family of proteins,[71] involved in sensing and responding to extracellular signals. The other two genes, agrD and agrB, encode an octapeptide signaling molecule and a protein that is believed to be involved in the processing and/or transport of the octapeptide, respectively. Studies indicate that high levels of octapeptide are recognized by the AgrC histidine kinase, leading to the activation of the AgrA response regulator. Activated AgrA then promotes the transcription of RNAIII, which, in turn, affects the expression of Agr-regulated genes.

The differential effect of Agr on extracellular and cell wall-associated protein production is best illustrated by analysis of gene expression in vitro. In general, Agr activates exoprotein production, while cell wall-associated protein production is repressed by this regulatory protein. During the exponential phase of growth, cell wall-associated proteins are produced while exoprotein production is repressed. As the cells enter stationary phase, a transition occurs in which cell wall protein expression diminishes and exoprotein production commences. The molecular mechanism of this growth phase regulation can be attributed to the accumulation of AgrD octapeptide in the culture medium. Once a "threshold" level of octapeptide has accumulated, the AgrC sensor protein is activated, triggering the stimulation of the Agr regulatory cascade. By measuring the octapeptide concentration within the surrounding medium, the Agr regulatory system senses, indirectly, bacterial cell density.

The role of the Agr regulatory system during pathogenesis has been hypothesized to enable the bacteria to differentially express various genes during the course of infection. For example, genes whose products are involved in establishing an infection (e.g., adherence and resistance to host immune responses) are expressed initially, while those genes whose

products are involved in maintaining the infection (e.g., toxins and proteases) are turned on later. Thus, an encounter of *S. aureus* with the bovine
udder would initially involve bacteria (which are relatively few in number)
that are in a state that maximizes adherence to the epithelial lining
(perhaps involving fibronectin-binding protein) and resistance to
opsinophagocytosis (protein A). Once the infection is established and the
bacterial cell density has reached a certain level, a shift in gene expression
occurs that results in the production of exoproteins involved in the tissue
destruction and inflammation that is associated with this disease. It should
be noted that the mammary alveoli and microabscesses associated with
staphylococcal mastitis could provide barriers for the rapid accumulation
of octapeptide, thus leading to bacterial exoprotein production in localized regions of the mammary gland. This would presumably promote the
progression of the disease at localized sites within the mammary gland and,
if unchecked, potentially lead to the acute or gangrenous forms of the
disease.

7. CONTROL

The milking time hygiene techniques of: 1) single service towels to
wash and dry udders, 2) pre- and post-milking teat disinfection, 3) use of
latex type gloves by milkers during milking, and 4) milking unit disinfection (backflush) were shown to be very effective in reducing the incidence
of *S. aureus* mastitis in dairy cattle. The fundamental studies surrounding
these control programs were well researched by the National Institute for
Research and Dairying (NIRD) in England.[72] Given the contagious nature
of *S. aureus*, and its ability to colonize the teat skin prior to causing infection, it should be clear why these techniques have been so successful. These
techniques prevent the spread of *S. aureus* from teat to teat at milking time
by isolating or removing the fomites that spread the disease. With these
procedures, single service towels are used to wash and dry udders, thus
reducing between cow contamination. Milkers wear disposable latex gloves,
providing for a smooth surface that can be cleaned between cow milkings
and disposed of thereafter. The between milking backflush system is
designed to disinfect the unit between cow milkings. Lastly, any residual
S. aureus remaining on the skin surface either before or after milking can
be removed with pre- and post-milking disinfectants. Along with dry cow
therapy, the milking time hygiene has a time-honored position as the most
effective mastitis control strategy. Some mastitis researchers have advocated
that these control practices should control all *S. aureus* mastitis. It has also
been advocated that segregation of *S. aureus* infected cows, and milking

these infected cows last, will remove the possibility of developing a *S. aureus* mastitis problem. Yet these milking time hygiene procedures coupled with segregation are not always as successful as suggested.[11,14] We have found that segregation will not be very effective until milking time hygiene mastitis control strategies are most rigorously practiced.

Culling *S. aureus* mastitis cows may be a more extreme measure of segregation. Whereas culling eliminates the problem cow, it does not eliminate the problem in management that leads to the cow's exposure to the disease. Clearly cows can develop *S. aureus* mastitis despite the application of excellent milking time hygiene and other mastitis control practices. However, these cows that occasionally develop *S. aureus* mastitis should be the exception, not the rule. The mastitis control practices should be robust and complete enough to withstand the occasional failure where a cow develops *S. aureus* mastitis. When these practices are not complete, and an outbreak of *S. aureus* mastitis does occur, then the mastitis control practices need to be evaluated before a program of culling is instituted. Most often weak links in the control program can be uncovered, and although strategic culling of *S. aureus* mastitis cows may reduce the prevalence most quickly, culling alone will do little to reduce the long term incidence of *S. aureus* mastitis. Development and implementation of a better mastitis control program is the best method to eliminate the *S. aureus* mastitis outbreak. Very contagious forms of *S. aureus* exist and may spread despite excellent milking time hygiene techniques.[11] Some *S. aureus* strains spread from cow to cow, while others are not transmitted.

There have been many attempts to develop a successful vaccine against *S. aureus* mastitis.[73] Problems typically encountered are the identification of the critical virulence factors that will stimulate an effective and protective immune response. The virulence factors associated with *S. aureus* mastitis that are both necessary and sufficient to cause disease have not been adequately determined. For example, the coagulase enzyme is a defining feature for *S. aureus* and those mastitis pathogens that are found to be coagulase negative are generally considered to be less pathogenic than *S. aureus*. This might suggest that coagulase is a necessary virulence factor. However, strains of *S. aureus* that are coagulase negative have been found to cause mastitis. In one study, the coagulase negative variant was found to be the most prevalent cause of this disease.[13] This might suggest that coagulase is not necessary for disease. Other virulence factors: protein A, adhesions, pseudocapsule, and β- and γ-toxins have been used as primary antigens in several *S. aureus* vaccines.[73] Yet despite some recently reported success with these vaccines, only two *S. aureus* vaccines are currently commercially available (Boehringer Ingelheim Vetmedica, Health, Inc., St. Joseph, MO), and both were developed more than 30 years ago. This would suggest that research in the field of *S. aureus* mastitis vaccine development holds promise, but is far from contributing to the abatement of this disease.

8. TREATMENT

Mastitis is generally a disease that in large part can be prevented or reduced in incidence. This is especially true for the contagious mastitis pathogens. Thus, treatment reflects the lack of ability to control or prevent the disease. Antibiotic therapies can be applied during subclinical or clinical cases of mastitis, during lactation or during the dry-period. The anecdotal success rate of antibiotic intramammary therapy for *S. aureus* mastitis has been rather poor. However many published reports suggest a reasonable success rate. In a total of 58 studies that examined the success of treatment of *S. aureus* mastitis, cure rates with dry cow therapy average 63% with a range of 14% to 100% (Fox, unpublished data). Success of clinical treatments of *S. aureus* mastitis suggests a 54% cure rate with a range of 26% to 92%. These studies included 16 trials of subclinical treatments of *S. aureus* mastitis, suggesting a 48% cure rate with a range of 17% to 95%. Thus it would appear that treatment during the dry-period is most successful, while treatment of subclinical cases is least successful. An explanation for these hierarchical results is that dry-cow therapies usually contain greater concentrations of antibiotics in longer acting preparations, than found in lactating cow therapies. Such formulations are logical given that there is less concern for meat withdrawal during the dry period and no concern for milk withholding times associated with antibiotic residues.

Yet many would argue that therapy of *S. aureus* mastitis in the field is rarely as successful as reported for research trials. Possible explanations for the disparity in success rates between that which is reported in the refereed literature and that reported by veterinarians and dairy managers may be due to several factors. Discussion by Erskine et al.[74] suggests that *S. aureus* infections may relapse after treatment. This would suggest that the antibiotic never fully eliminated the pathogen. Rather, the antibiotic was able to reduce the *S. aureus* to levels that were below the threshold of detection. This is quite plausible given that *S. aureus* characteristically causes intramammary infection with far fewer colony-forming units than other mastitis pathogens. It has been reported that even in the absence of treatment, *S. aureus* will be periodically shed in the milk at low levels, sometimes at levels which are below the standard methods of detection.[7] Thus, one may propose that antibiotic therapy induces a latent infection resulting in an apparent, but false positive, cure. Additionally, sometimes research models include experimental infections. An experimental infection that has not had time to cause pathological damage to the udder might be easier to eliminate than a natural chronic infection.

Why are *S. aureus* so refractory to treatment? Again there are several explanations, all of which may act together to make successful therapy one that is difficult to achieve. There is evidence to suggest that the pathologic damage caused by *S. aureus* will cause ductal occlusions and thus inhibit the diffusion of antibiotic to the various foci of infection (Nickerson, unpublished data). Histological findings indicate that micro-abscesses develop in response to *S. aureus* infection. The microabscesses might act as privileged sites for the bacteria to grow and protect them-selves from diffused antibiotic. For these reasons, some have studied the use of systemic treatment coupled with intramammary therapy.[75] Logically such an approach should increase treatment success. However, although research has found that most systemic/intramammary treatment regimens improve the cure rates against *S. aureus* mastitis, improved success may not always be achieved and often may not be great enough to off-set the added cost of drug and management. Another explanation of *S. aureus* resistance to therapy is the development of a genetic resistance to some antibiotics. Additionally, it has been demonstrated that *S. aureus* when exposed to penicillin can form progeny that lack cell walls, L-forms,[76] and thus become resistant to the beta-lactam (penicillin) type of antibiotic. Lastly, as discussed, it has been observed that internalized *S. aureus*, can resist killing and thus be unaffected by the surrounding antibiotic. Presumably these internalized *S. aureus* can then reinfect the gland when the host cell dies and lyses.

Treatment of Heifer *S. aureus* Mastitis

Treatment of preterm heifers with intramammary antibiotics has been suggested.[77,78] Most trials indicate that there is a significant cure rate of *S. aureus* mastitis infections when either dry-cow or lactation antibiotic therapy regimens are used in heifers. The dry-cow preparation has a better cure rate than does lactation therapy. Residue avoidance is the predomi-nant problem with intramammary treatment preterm in heifers. Perhaps if a herd has a definitive problem with *S. aureus* mastitis in heifers, then preterm therapy could become part of the control program. There are clearly problems (such as increased residues in milk at first calving) with suggesting the use of intramammary antibiotic therapy for all heifers preterm.

9. CONCLUSIONS

S. aureus is currently the most prevalent cause of contagious mastitis. Perhaps more than 90% of all herds and 5% of all cows in the US have this disease. Currently, the best method to control S. aureus mastitis is through prevention. The preventive techniques help block the transmission of S. aureus from one cow via a fomite to another cow. These techniques focus at milking time and include: single service towels to wash and dry udders during cow preparation, use of disinfectant in the premilking wash solution, use of gloves by milkers, use of milking unit backflush to disinfect units between cow milkings, and postmilking teat disinfection to remove any residual S. aureus that remain on the gland after milking. Dry cow antibiotic therapy is marginally effective in eliminating S. aureus mastitis infections. But dry cow therapy has the advantage of avoiding problems associated with antibiotic residues, i.e., milk withholding. Segregation of infected cattle has often been proposed as a control strategy. Segregation and selective culling of infected cattle can be effective control procedures for S. aureus mastitis when all the other control practices are first in place.

The current techniques utilized to prevent the transmission of S. aureus from cow to cow are time-consuming, labor intensive, and expensive. Combined, these factors exact a pronounced toll on the dairy industry. Clearly, a better strategy is needed to effectively reduce the prevalence of S. aureus mastitis in dairy herds. Although the vaccines developed to prevent mastitis have met with limited success, a better understanding of the physical and immunological defense mechanisms present within the bovine udder to combat bacterial infection, along with a broader knowledge of the staphylococcal factors that are important in the pathogenesis of this disease, should lead to improved methods for reducing these persistent infections.

ACKNOWLEDGMENTS. This work was supported by U.S.D.A. (NRICGP) (GAB) and PHS grants AI28401 (GAB) and AI38901 (KWB), the United Diarymen of Idaho (GAB), the Washington State Dairy Products Commission (LKF) and the Idaho Agricultural Experiment Station.

REFERENCES

1. Wilson, D. J., Gonzalez, R. N. & Das, H. H. Bovine mastitis pathogens in New York and Pennsylvania: prevalence and effects on somatic cell count and milk production. J. Dairy Sci. **80**, 2592–2598 (1997).

2. Hogan, J. S. & Smith, K. L. Occurrence of clinical and subclinical environmental streptococcal mastitis. In *Symposium on udder health management for environmental streptococci*, pg 36 (Ontario, Canada, 1997).

3. Schalm, O. W., Carroll, E. J. & Jain, N. C. *Bovine mastitis* (Lee & Febiger, Philadelphia, 1971).

4. Fox, L. K., Shook, G. E. & Schultz, L. H. Factors related to milk loss in quarters with low somatic cell counts. *J. Dairy Sci.* **68**, 2100–2107 (1985).

5. Jones, G. M., Pearson, R. E., Clabaugh, G. A. & Heald, C. W. Relationships between somatic cell counts and milk production. *J. Dairy Sci.* **67**, 1823–1831 (1984).

6. El-Rashidy, A. A., Fox, L. K. & Gay, J. M. Diagnosis of *Staphylococcus aureus* intramammary infection by detection of specific antibody titer in milk. *J. Dairy Sci.* **75**, 1430–1435 (1992).

7. Sears, P. M., Smith, B. S., English, P. B., Herer, P. S. & Gonzalez, R. N. Shedding pattern of *Staphylococcus aureus* from bovine intramammary infections. *J. Dairy Sci.* **73**, 2785–2789 (1990).

8. Gudding, R., McDonald, J. S. & Cheville, N. F. Pathogenesis of *Staphylococcus aureus* mastitis: bacteriologic, histologic, and ultrastructural pathologic findings. *Am. J. Vet. Res.* **45**, 2525–2531 (1984).

9. Nickerson, S. C. & Heald, C. W. Histopathologic response of the bovine mammary gland to experimentally induced *Staphylococcus aureus* infection. *Am. J. Vet. Res.* **42**, 1351–1355 (1981).

10. Anderson, J. C. Progressive pathology of staphylococcal mastitis with a note on control, immunization, and therapy. *Veterinary Journal* **110**, 372–376 (1982).

11. Smith, T. H., Fox, L. K. & Middleton, J. R. Outbreak of mastitis caused by one strain of *Staphylococcus aureus* in a closed dairy herd. *J. Am. Vet. Med. Assoc.* **212**, 553–556 (1998).

12. Hogan, J. S. *et al. Laboratory handbook on bovine mastitis*, (National Mastitis Council, Inc., Madison, WI, 1999).

13. Fox, L. K., Besser, T. E. & Jackson, S. M. Evaluation of a coagulase-negative variant of *Staphylococcus aureus* as a cause of intramammary infections in a herd of dairy cattle. *J. Am. Vet. Med. Assoc.* **209**, 1143–1146 (1996).

14. Fox, L. K. & Hancock, D. D. Effect of segregation on prevention of intramammary infections by *Staphylococcus aureus*. *J. Dairy Sci.* **72**, 540–544 (1989).

15. Roberson, J. R., Fox, L. K., Hancock, D. D. & Besser, T. E. Evaluation of methods for differentiation of coagulase-positive staphylococci. *J. Clin. Microbiol.* **30**, 3217–3219 (1992).

16. Fox, L. K. & Adams, D. S. Use of enzyme linked immunosorbent assay to detect antibody against *S. aureus* in milk: where are we today? In *National Mastitis Council Annual Meeting*, pg 58 (Arlington, VA, 1999).

17. Adams, D. S., McDonald, J. S., Hancock, D. & McGuire, T. C. *Staphylococcus aureus* antigens reactive with milk immunoglobulin G of naturally infected dairy cows. *J. Clin. Microbiol.* **26**, 1175–1180 (1988).

18. Matsushita, T. *et al.* Performance studies of an enzyme-linked immunosorbent assay for detecting *Staphylococcus aureus* antibody in bovine milk. *J. Vet. Diagn. Invest.* **2**, 163–166 (1990).

19. Fluharty, D. M. & Wright, D. Mobile lab hit the road to help Northwest dairyman. *Hoard's Dairyman* **127**, 1101 (1982).

20. Wilson, C. D. & Richards, M. S. A survey of mastitis in the British dairy herd. *Vet. Rec.* **106**, 431–435 (1980).

21. Gonzalez, R. N., Jasper, D. E., Farver, T. B., Bushnell, R. B. & Franti, C. E. Prevalence of udder infections and mastitis in 50 California dairy herds. *J. Am. Vet. Med. Assoc.* **193**, 323–328 (1988).

22. Erskine, R. J., Eberhart, R. J., Hutchinson, L. J. & Spencer, S. B. Herd management and prevalence of mastitis in dairy herds with high and low somatic cell counts. *J. Am. Vet. Med. Assoc.* **190**, 1411–1416 (1987).

23. Hutton, C. T., Fox, L. K. & Hancock, D. D. Mastitis control practices: differences between herds with high and low milk somatic cell counts. *J. Dairy Sci.* **73**, 1135–1143 (1990).

24. Goldberg, J. J., Pankey, J., Drechsler, P. A., Murdough, D. B. & Howard, P. A. An update survey of bulk tank milk quality in Vermont. *J. Food Prot.* **54**, 549 (1991).

25. Roberson, J. R. Epidemiology of Staphylococcus aureus intramammary infections in prepartum dairy heifers. In *3rd International mastitis seminar*, pg 13 (Tel Aviv, Israel, 1995).

26. Roberson, J. R., Fox, L. K., Hancock, D. D., Gay, C. C. & Besser, T. E. Coagulase-positive Staphylococcus intramammary infections in primiparous dairy cows. *J. Dairy Sci.* **77**, 958–969 (1994).

27. Fox, L. K. *et al.* Survey of intramammary infections in dairy heifers at breeding age and first parturition. *J. Dairy Sci.* **78**, 1619–1628 (1995).

28. Owens, W. E., Oliver, S. P., Gillespie, B. E., Ray, C. H. & Nickerson, S. C. Role of horn flies (*Haematobia irritans*) in Staphylococcus aureus-induced mastitis in dairy heifers. *Am. J. Vet. Res.* **59**, 1122–1124 (1998).

29. Fox, L. K., Nagy, J. A., Hillers, J. K., Cronrath, J. D. & Ratkowsky, D. A. Effects of postmilking teat treatment on the colonization of Staphylococcus aureus on chapped teat skin. *Am. J. Vet. Res.* **52**, 799–802 (1991).

30. Sordillo, L. M., Shafer-Weaver, K. & DeRosa, D. Immunobiology of the mammary gland. *J. Dairy Sci.* **80**, 1851–1865 (1997).

31. Van Kampen, C. & Mallard, B. A. Effects of peripartum stress and health on circulating bovine lymphocyte subsets. *Vet. Immunol. Immunopathol.* **59**, 79–91 (1997).

32. Soper, F. F., Muscoplat, C. C. & Johnson, D. W. In vitro stimulation of bovine peripheral blood lymphocytes: analysis of variation of lymphocyte blastogenic response in normal dairy cattle. *Am. J. Vet. Res.* **39**, 1039–1042 (1978).

33. Shafer-Weaver, K. A. & Sordillo, L. M. Bovine CD8+ suppressor lymphocytes alter immune responsiveness during the postpartum period. *Vet. Immunol. Immunopathol.* **56**, 53–64 (1997).

34. Kehrli, M. E., Jr., Nonnecke, B. J. & Roth, J. A. Alterations in bovine neutrophil function during the periparturient period. *Am. J. Vet. Res.* **50**, 207–214 (1989).

35. Cai, T. Q. *et al.* Association between neutrophil functions and periparturient disorders in cows. *Am. J. Vet. Res.* **55**, 934–943 (1994).

36. Guidry, A. J., Paape, M. J. & Pearson, R. E. Effects of parturition and lactation on blood and milk cell concentrations, corticosteroids, and neutrophil phagocytosis in the cow. *Am. J. Vet. Res.* **37**, 1195–1200 (1976).

37. Yang, T. J., Ayoub, I. A. & Rewinski, M. J. Lactation stage-dependent changes of lymphocyte subpopulations in mammary secretions: inversion of CD4+/CD8+ T cell ratios at parturition. *Am. J. Reprod. Immunol.* **37**, 378–383 (1997).

38. Asai, K. *et al.* Variation in CD4+ T and CD8+ T lymphocyte subpopulations in bovine mammary gland secretions during lactating and non-lactating periods. *Vet. Immunol. Immunopathol.* **65**, 51–61 (1998).

39. Park, Y. H., Fox, L. K., Hamilton, M. J. & Davis, W. C. Suppression of proliferative response of BoCD4+ T lymphocytes by activated BoCD8+ T lymphocytes in the mammary

gland of cows with *Staphylococcus aureus* mastitis. *Vet. Immunol. Immunopathol.* **36**, 137–151 (1993).

40. Sutra, L. & Poutrel, B. Virulence factors involved in the pathogenesis of bovine intramammary infections due to *Staphylococcus aureus*. *J. Med. Microbiol.* **40**, 79–89 (1994).

41. Lammers, A., Kruijt, E., van de Kuijt, C., Nuijten, P. J. & Smith, H. E. Identification of *Staphylococcus aureus* genes expressed during growth in milk: a useful model for selection of genes important in bovine mastitis? *Microbiology* **146**, 981–987 (2000).

42. Ali-Vehmis, T. & Sandholm, M. Balance between bacteria and host: the bacteria's point of view. in *The bovine udder and mastitis* (eds. Sandholm, M., Honkanen-Buzalski, T., Kaartinen, L. & Pyorala) 49–58 (Gummerus Kijapaino Oy, Jyvaskyla, 1995).

43. Mamo, W. *et al.* Vaccination against *Staphylococcus aureus* mastitis: immunological response of mice vaccinated with fibronectin-binding protein (FnBP-A) to challenge with S. aureus. *Vaccine* **12**, 988–992 (1994).

44. Dziewanowska, K. *et al.* Fibronectin binding protein and host cell tyrosine kinase are required for internalization of *Staphylococcus aureus* by epithelial cells. *Infect. Immun.* **67**, 4673–4678 (1999).

45. Lammers, A., Nuijten, P. J. & Smith, H. E. The fibronectin binding proteins of *Staphylococcus aureus* are required for adhesion to and invasion of bovine mammary gland cells. *FEMS Microbiol. Lett.* **180**, 103–109 (1999).

46. Foster, T. J. *et al.* Genetic studies of virulence factors of *Staphylococcus aureus*. Properties of coagulase and γ-toxin and the role of a toxin, β toxin, and protein A in the pathogenesis of S. aureus infections. in *Molecular biology of staphylococci*. (ed. Novick, R. P.) 403–417 (VCH, New York, 1990).

47. Guidry, A., Fattom, A., Patel, A. & O'Brien, C. Prevalence of capsular serotypes among *Staphylococcus aureus* isolates from cows with mastitis in the United States. *Vet. Microbiol.* **59**, 53–58 (1997).

48. Thakker, M., Park, J. S., Carey, V. & Lee, J. C. *Staphylococcus aureus* serotype 5 capsular polysaccharide is antiphagocytic and enhances bacterial virulence in a murine bacteremia model. *Infect. Immun.* **66**, 5183–5189 (1998).

49. Kenny, K., Reiser, R. F., Bastida-Corcuera, F. D. & Norcross, N. L. Production of enterotoxins and toxic shock syndrome toxin by bovine mammary isolates of *Staphylococcus aureus*. *J. Clin. Microb.* **31**, 706–707 (1993).

50. Schlievert, P. M. Role of superantigens in human disease. *J. Infect. Dis.* **167**, 997–1002 (1993).

51. Marr, J. C. *et al.* Characterization of novel type C staphylococcal enterotoxins: biological and evolutionary implications. *Infect. Immun.* **61**, 4254–4262 (1993).

52. Deringer, J. R., Ely, R. J., Monday, S. R., Stauffacher, C. V. & Bohach, G. A. Vβ-dependent stimulation of bovine and human T cells by host-specific staphylococcal enterotoxins. *Infect. Immun.* **65**, 4048–4054 (1997).

53. Ferens, W. A. *et al.* Induction of type 2 cytokines by a staphylococcal enterotoxin superantigen. *J. Nat. Toxins* **7**, 193–213 (1998).

54. Ferens, W. A. *et al.* Activation of bovine lymphocyte subpopulations by staphylococcal enterotoxin C. *Infect. Immun.* **66**, 573–580 (1998).

55. Noble, A., Pestano, G. A. & Cantor, H. Suppression of immune responses by CD8 cells. I. Superantigen-activated CD8 cells induce unidirectional Fas-mediated apoptosis of antigen-activated CD4 cells. *J. Immunol.* **160**, 559–565 (1998).

56. Damle, N. K., Leytze, G., Klussman, K. & Ledbetter, J. A. Activation with superantigens induces programmed death in antigen-primed CD4+ class II+ major histocompatibility complex T lymphocytes via a CD11a/CD18-dependent mechanism. *Eur. J. Immunol.* **23**, 1513–1522 (1993).

57. Sundstedt, A. *et al.* Superantigen-induced anergy in cytotoxic CD8+ T cells. *J. Immunol.* **154**, 6306–6313 (1995).

58. Litton, M. J., Sander, B., Murphy, E., O'Garra, A. & Abrams, J. S. Early expression of cytokines in lymph nodes after treatment in vivo with Staphylococcus enterotoxin B. *J. Immunol. Methods* **175**, 47–58 (1994).

59. Bramley, A. J., Patel, A. H., O'Reilly, M., Foster, R. & Foster, T. J. Roles of alpha-toxin and beta-toxin in virulence of *Staphylococcus aureus* for the mouse mammary gland. *Infect. Immun.* **57**, 2489–2494 (1989).

60. Lowe, A. M., Beattie, D. T. & Deresiewicz, R. L. Identification of novel staphylococcal virulence genes by in vivo expression technology. *Mol. Microbiol.* **27**, 967–976 (1998).

61. Coulter, S. N. *et al.* *Staphylococcus aureus* genetic loci impacting growth and survival in multiple infection environments. *Mol. Microbiol.* **30**, 393–404 (1998).

62. Mei, J. M., Nourbakhsh, F., Ford, C. W. & Holden, D. W. Identification of *Staphylococcus aureus* virulence genes in a murine model of bacteraemia using signature-tagged mutagenesis. *Mol. Microbiol.* **26**, 399–407 (1997).

63. Foster, T. J. Potential for vaccination against infections caused by *Staphylococcus aureus*. *Vaccine* **9**, 221–227 (1991).

64. Patel, A. H., Nowlan, E. D., Weavers, E. D. & Foster, T. J. Virulence of protein A-deficient and alpha-toxin-deficient mutants of *Staphylococcus aureus* isolated by allele replacement. *Infect. Immun.* **55**, 3103–3110 (1987).

65. Craven, N. & Anderson, J. C. Phagocytosis of *Staphylococcus aureus* by bovine mammary gland macrophages and intracellular protection from antibiotic action *in vitro* and *in vivo*. *J. Dairy Res.* **51**, 513–523 (1984).

66. Bayles, K. W. *et al.* Intracellular *Staphylococcus aureus* escapes the endosome and induces apoptosis. *Infect. Immun.* **66**, 336–342 (1998).

67. Dziewanowska, K., Edwards, V. M., Deringer, J. R. & Bohach, G. A. Comparison of the beta-toxin from *Staphylococcus aureus* and *Staphylococcus intermedius*. *Arch. Biochem. Biophys.* **335**, 102–108 (1996).

68. Wesson, C. A. *et al.* Apoptosis induced by *Staphylococcus aureus* in epithelial cells utilizes a mechanism involving caspases 8 and 3. *Infect. Immun.* **68**, 2998–3001 (2000).

69. Ferens, W. A. & Bohach, G. A. Persistence of *Staphylococcus aureus* on mucosal membranes: superantigens and internalization by host cells. *J. Lab. Clin. Med.* **135**, 225–230 (2000).

70. Novick, R. P. Pathogenicity factors and their regulation. in *Gram-positive pathogens* (eds. Fischetti, V. A., Novick, R. P., Ferretti, J. J., Portnoy, D. A. & Rood, J. I.) 392–407 (ASM, Washington, D.C., 2000).

71. Kornblum, J., Kreiswirth, B. N., Projan, S. J., Ross, H. & Novick, R. P. Agr: a polycistronic locus regulating exoprotein synthesis in *Staphylococcus aureus*. in *Molecular biology of the staphylococci* (ed. Novick, R. P.) 373–402 (VCH Publishers, Inc., New York, 1990).

72. Neave, F. K., Dodd, F. H., Kingwill, R. G. & Westgarth, D. R. Control of mastitis in the dairy herd by hygiene and management. *J. Dairy Sci.* **52**, 696–707 (1969).

73. Nickerson, S. C. Role of vaccination and treatment programs. In *National Mastitis Council Annual Meeting*, pg 76 (Arlington, VA, 1999).

74. Erskine, R. J., Bartlett, P. C., Crawshaw, P. C. & Gombas, D. M. Efficacy of intramuscular oxytetracycline as a dry cow treatment for *Staphylococcus aureus* mastitis. *J. Dairy Sci.* **77**, 3347–3353 (1994).

75. Owens, W. E., Watts, J. L., Boddie, R. L. & Nickerson, S. C. Antibiotic treatment of mastitis: comparison of intramammary and intramammary plus intramuscular therapies. *J. Dairy Sci.* **71**, 3143–3147 (1988).

76. Sears, P. M., Fettinger, M. & Marsh-Salin, J. Isolation of L-form variants after antibiotic treatment in *Staphylococcus aureus* bovine mastitis. *J. Am. Vet. Med. Assoc.* **191**, 681–684 (1987).
77. Trinidad, P., Nickerson, S. C., Alley, T. K. & Adkinson, R. W. Efficacy of intramammary treatment in unbred and primigravid dairy heifers. *J. Am. Vet. Med. Assoc.* **197**, 465–470 (1990).
78. Oliver, S. P., Lewis, M. J., Gillespie, B. E. & Dowlen, H. H. Influence of prepartum antibiotic therapy on intramammary infections in primigravid heifers during early lactation. *J. Dairy Sci.* **75**, 406–414 (1992).

14

Global Regulation of Virulence Determinants in *Staphylococcus aureus*

AMBROSE L. CHEUNG

1. INTRODUCTION

Staphylococcus aureus is an important pathogen both in the community and hospital settings.[1] The spectrum of diseases caused by this organism is extremely wide, ranging from superficial infections to deep-seated and systemic infections such as pneumonia, endocarditis, osteomyelitis and sepsis.[2] Despite the use of antibiotics to treat these infections, the morbidity and mortality remain high, in part due to this microorganism's consistent ability to develop resistance to multiple antibiotics.[3] The recent report of reduced susceptibility to vancomycin, first in Japan and subsequently in the United States[4] has raised significant concern because it may signify the spreading of resistant *S. aureus* strains that may be impossible to treat with preexisting antibiotics.

The pathogenicity of *S. aureus* is multifactorial. With the exception of toxin-mediated diseases, it has been difficult to implicate a single factor that would explain the myriad of staphylococcal syndromes. Not surprisingly, many animal studies with a single knockout of specific virulence determinants have failed to define individual factor responsible

AMBROSE L. CHEUNG • Department of Microbiology, Dartmouth Medical School, Hanover, NH 03755.

Staphylococcus aureus *Infection and Disease*, edited by Allen L. Honeyman *et al.*
Kluwer Academic/Plenum Publishers, New York, 2001.

for many disease states.[5] As with many Gram positive pathogens, *S. aureus* relies on a large set of extracellular and cell-wall associated proteins for its pathogenicity. Many of these extracellular virulence determinants are usually synthesized and secreted during the postexponential phase (e.g., α-hemolysin and toxin shock toxin) in laboratory cultures.[5] In contrast, cell-wall associated proteins (e.g., protein A, clumping factor A) are produced primarily during the exponential phase and are repressed postexponentially.[5,6] The coordinate synthesis of cell-wall proteins in the exponential phase and extracellular proteins during the postexponential phase suggests that many of these virulence determinants are under global regulatory control.[5] One of these loci is the *agr* regulon which up-regulates the synthesis of many extracellular toxins and enzymes while down-regulating cell-wall proteins postexponentially.[6] Besides the *agr* regulon, other global regulatory loci such as *sar* and *sae* may also participate to activate the synthesis of cell-wall proteins during the exponential phase.[7,8] However, the bacterial signals, in particular those generated in response to the host environment, are as yet unknown. Additionally, host constituents such as tissue factors and phagocytic cells may also modulate the expression of regulatory and target genes involved in bacterial pathogenesis. To elucidate some of these host-induced genes, several approaches have been devised to identify bacterial gene sequences that are differentially expressed within the host environment during infections. These methods include: a) **differential display** by identifying differentially expressed mRNA transcripts;[9] b) *in vivo* expression technology (**IVET**) for selecting promoter fragments linked to an indicator gene expressed in hosts;[10,11] 3) signature-tagged mutagenesis (**STM**) with a negative selection strategy to identify attenuated strains created by transposon mutagenesis;[12,13] and 4) differential fluorescent induction (**DFI**) in which promoter fragments are fused to the green fluorescent protein (GFP) of the jellyfish *Aequorea victoria* to be used as a selective marker in a fluorescence activated sorter (FACS), thus enabling selection of genes that are differentially expressed in the host environment.[14,15] Understanding the roles of these bacterial genes may lead to new insights into the pathogenic process and most certainly will facilitate the identification of additional regulatory factors.

In this chapter, available information on the regulation of pathogenicity in *S. aureus* is described. It should be understood that most of these data are generated from *in vitro* studies. It is highly likely that, as the roles of these pathogenicity genes are assessed *in vivo*, our perception of their relevance in infections may be transformed.

2. GLOBAL REGULATION OF VIRULENCE DETERMINANTS DURING THE GROWTH CYCLE BASED ON *IN VITRO* STUDIES

The coordinate regulation of extracellular and cell-wall virulence determinants during the growth cycle indicates that these factors are controlled by global regulatory elements. During the exponential phase, cell wall proteins, many of which carry adhesive functions, are synthesized. These cell wall proteins, also called MSCRAMMS (microbial surface components recognizing adhesive matrix molecules), include protein A, fibrinogen binding proteins, fibronectin binding proteins, collagen binding protein etc. (Table I). Based on phenotypic analyses, the synthesis of these surface adhesins is likely activated by global regulatory loci such as *sar* and *sae*.[7,8] Upon transition from the exponential to the postexponential phase, regulatory signals are generated from *agr*, *sar*, *sigB*, *sarR* and possibly other regulatory elements (Figure 1, see details below). Additional signals, such as those identified by *in vivo* selection strategies, probably modulate the contribution of these known regulatory elements. The *agr* locus plays an important role in up-regulating the synthesis of extracellular enzymes and toxins during the postexponential phase. Likewise, SarA, the major *sar* regulatory molecule, is capable of up-modulating the *agr* locus as well as binding directly to the promoter of the alpha-hemolysin gene (*hla*) to augment hemolysin production.[16] Furthermore, postexponentiallyinduced transcription factors, such as SigB, may also modulate the expression of SarA and possibly other stress-induced genes. More recently, a newly characterized protein, designated SarR, was found to bind to the *sar* promoter region to down-regulate SarA protein expression. As evaluated in liquid culture studies, the confluence of these regulatory signals likely contributes to an outburst in the synthesis of toxins and enzymes. With increased crowding of extracellular bacteria during the postexponential phase, the secretion of these toxins and enzymes presumably will facilitate host cell lysis, thereby allowing the bacteria to spread to new sites.

The *agr* Locus

The *agr* locus is the site of a transposon insertion in a pleiotropic exoprotein-defective mutant.[17,18] Cloning of the chromosomal sequence adjacent to this insertion has led to the identification of the *agr* global regulatory locus.[6,17] The *agr* locus up-regulates the synthesis of exoproteins while repressing cell wall protein synthesis postexponentially. The opposite regulation of two sets of genes by a single regulatory element is a salient feature of the *agr* system. The *agr* locus is composed of two divergent

TABLE I
Virulence factors of *S. aureus*

Factor	Putative Functions
Cell-wall constituents	
Clumping factor A (*clfA*)	Adhesin to fibrinogen
Clumping factor B (*clfB*)	Adhesin to fibrinogen
Coagulase (*coa*)	Binding to fibrinogen
FibA protein (*fibA*)	Binding to fibrinogen
Fibronectin binding protein A (*fnbA*)	Attachment to fibronectin
Fibronectin binding protein B (*fnbB*)	Attachment to fibronectin
Collagen binding protein (*cna*)	Adhesin to collagen
Elastin binding protein (*ebpS*)	Binding to elastin
MHC analogous protein (*map* or *eap*)	Binding to extracellular matrix proteins including fibronectin, fibrinogen, vitronectin, bone sialoprotein and thrombospondin
Polysaccharide intracellular adhesin (*pia*)	Intercellular adhesion and biofilm formation
Protein A (*spa*)	Possible evasion of host defenses
Capsular polysaccharides (types 1, 5 and 8) (*cap*)	Anti-phagocytic molecule
Extracellular toxins and enzymes	
Enterotoxins A-E, H (*sea-e, h*)	Evasion of host defenses with superantigen functions, causative agent for food-associated diarrhea
Toxin shock syndome toxin-1 (*tst*)	Evasion of host defenses with superantigen properties, causative agent for TSS
Exfoliative toxin A,B (*eta, etb*)	Evasion of host defenses, causative agents for staphylococcal scalded skin syndrome
Lipase (*geh*)	Evasion of host defense
V8 protease (*sasP* or *ssp*)	Tissue invasion and modification of surface proteins
Panton-Valentin leukocidin (*lukF, lukS*)	Evasion of host defenses, lysis of host phagocytes
Staphylokinase (*sak*)	Evasion of host defenses
α-hemolysin (*hla*)	Tissue invasion, form pores in host cell membrane
β-hemolysin (*hlb*)	Tissue invasion, sphingomyelinase
δ-hemolysin (*hld*)	Potentiation of β-hemolysin
γ-hemolysin (*hlgA, B, C*)	Potentiation of host cell lysis
Phospholipase C (*plc*)	Lysis of host cells
Elastase (*sepA*)	Tissue invasion
Hyaluronidase (*hysA*)	Tissue invasion

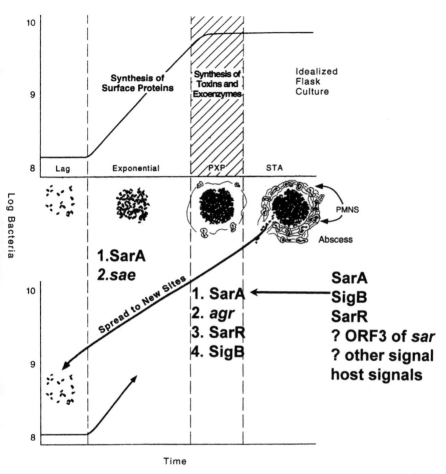

FIGURE 1. The expression of virulence determinants as controlled by global regulatory loci during the growth cycle based on mostly *in vitro* data.

transcripts (RNAII and RNAIII) driven by two distinct promoters (P2 and P3 promoters, respectively) (Figure 2). The P2 transcript encodes four genes, *agrB, D, C,* and *A,* all required for the normal activation of the RNAII and RNAIII transcripts in the *agr* system.[19–21] The P3 transcript encodes the 26 amino acid δ-hemolysin peptide which has no defined role in regulation.[19,20] A second regulatory molecule, SarA, also participates in the activation of the *agr* P2 and P3 promoters (Figure 2).[22] In contrast to many regulatory systems where the effector molecules are proteins, the *agr* regulatory molecule is the RNAIII transcript which acts mainly at the level of transcription.[19,20]

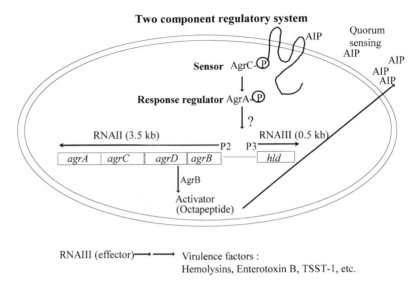

RNAIII (effector)⟶ ⟶ Virulence factors :
                            Hemolysins, Enterotoxin B, TSST-1, etc.

FIGURE 2. A model of the *agr* regulatory system.

Sequence analysis revealed that AgrC and AgrA are the membrane
sensor and the response activator of a two-component regulatory system
which is autoinduced by a post-translationally modified auto-inducing
peptide.[23,24] The peptide is processed from within the 46-residue *agrD* gene
product.[24] Accordingly, AgrB, a 26 kDa transmembrane protein, may be
involved in the secretion and processing of the octapeptide which undergoes cyclization (via a thiolactone bond) between the cysteine reside and
the C-terminal carboxyl group, thus resulting in the formation of a cyclic
peptide.[25,26] Structure-function studies have shown that the linear structure
is inactive[25] thus implying that the ring structure is essential for proper
function.

The autoinducing peptide (AIP), upon reaching a critical concentration as a result of bacterial accumulation in liquid culture, would activate
the 46 kDa transmembrane sensor protein, AgrC, by phosphorylating a specific histidine residue.[27] It is presumed that a second phosphorylation step
of the aspartic residue of AgrA, a 34 kDa cytoplasmic protein, would ensue,
thus activating the response regulator, AgrA, via transphosphorylation.
Although the primary function of AgrA is to activate the two *agr* promoters, purified recombinant AgrA has failed to demonstrate binding to the
intergenic region between the P2 and P3 promoter.[28] This lack of binding
may be explained by a need for AgrA phosphorylation in order for binding

to occur. Alternatively, AgrA may fail to re-nature during purification in the presence of a denaturing agent (i.e., urea).[28] Whether SarA, in conjunction with AgrA, is required for the activation of the dual *agr* promoters is not completely clear. More recently, Balaban *et al.*, reported the isolation of a 38 kDa protein that is not encoded by *agr*. However, the claim on the role of this protein, rather than a peptide, as an autoinducer is being disputed.[26] Irrespective of the mode of activation, the end result is that RNAIII, the *agr* regulatory molecule, is synthesized as a consequence of these signaling events.

Induction of the P2 operon is clearly required for the activation of the P3 promoter (i.e., production of the RNAIII transcript). Once RNAIII is synthesized, it is involved in the transcriptional up-regulation of exoprotein genes (e.g., hemolysins) and down-regulation of cell-wall protein genes (protein A and fibronectin binding protein genes). Whether the effect is direct on target gene promoters or via an intermediary such as AgrA or other unknown gene products has not been determined. Besides its transcriptional effect, studies by Morfeldt and colleagues[29] indicated that the effect of RNAIII on *hla* expression may be translational. It was proposed that the nascent *hla* transcript may have secondary structure in the 5' end which interferes with the initiation of translation. Pairing of RNAIII with *hla* mRNA will nullify this secondary structure, thus allowing the normal progression of translational signals.[29]

The *agr* locus is conserved among staphylococci. However, RNAIII homologs encoded by other staphylococcal species vary considerably in sequences.[30–32] Unlike *S. aureus*, the RNAIII species from *S. lugdenesis* do not encode δ-hemolysin.[31] Homologous *agrA*, *C*, *D*, and *B* sequences (encoded by RNAII) have been observed in *S. epidermidis*[30] and *S. lugdunensis*.[31] In particular, the C-terminal half of AgrC and N-terminal 1/3 of AgrB are conserved. In contrast, the C-terminal part of AgrB and all of AgrD are variable.[24,26] A survey of AgrDs among *S. aureus* strains from which the modified peptides are processed revealed that AIP can differ in sequence. Remarkably, AIP from some *S. aureus* strains can inhibit the *agr* response of others. Additionally, Otto and colleagues demonstrated that the *agr* peptide (or pheromone) from *S. epidermidis* can also suppress the expression of *agr*-mediated virulence factors in *S. aureus*. On the basis of these findings, Novick *et al.*[24] have divided the AIPs of *S. aureus* into 4 major groups (Group I, II, III and IV) such that an AIP can activate other strains in the same group whereas it would inhibit strains in divergent groups.[24] In that regard, Mayville *et al.* recently found that a synthetic Group II thiolactone peptide greatly attenuated a murine experimental skin abscess infection by a group I strain.[25] As the concentration of bacteria required to induce "reactive" concentrations of AIP is quite high (~10^8 CFU), the role of AIP in acute *S. aureus* bacteremic infections is not clear since the number of bacteria responsible for these infections is generally low (10^2–10^3 CFU/ml of blood).

Besides *S. aureus*, peptide-inducing quorum sensing systems have been found in the autoinduction of bacteriocin and lantibiotic synthesis in Lactobacilli[33] and in competence induction in *Streptococcus pneumonia*[34] and *Bacillus subtilis*.[35] As both Gram positive and Gram negative bacteria harbor quorum sensing systems, a comparison of the two systems is of interest. Wherein Gram positive bacteria signal receptors are activated by peptides, the autoinducers of Gram negative bacteria are mostly N-acyl homoserine lactones. The Gram negative class of autoinducers acts primarily intracellularly while the Gram positive counterparts interacts with signal transducer on the surface of the bacteria. These differences suggest that the evolutionary origin of the quorum sensing system between Gram positive and Gram negative species is quite diverse.

The *sar* Locus

The *sar* locus was originally identified by a Tn*917*LTV1 insertion that decreased the synthesis of hemolysins and fibrinogen binding proteins.[8] The *sar* locus is composed of three overlapping transcripts, designated sarA, sarC and sarB, originated from promoters P1, P3 and P2, respectively (Figure 3). The promoter boxes (−10 and −35) of P1 and P2 have sequence similarity to the σA and σ70 dependent promoters of *B. subtilis* and *E. coli*, respectively. In contrast, the *sar* P3 promoter possesses a striking homology to the σB-dependent promoter of *B. subtilis*.[36] Activation of these promoters have been shown to be involved in the general stress response of Gram positive bacteria.[37] Embedded within the interpromoter regions of P2-P3 and P3-P1 are two smaller ORFs, lying upstream of the major 372-bp *sarA* ORF. Due to their overlapping nature, each of the *sar* transcripts encodes SarA, a 14.7 kDa protein with a deduced pI of 8.52.[38] Complementation analysis indicated that SarA is the major regulatory molecule of the *sar* locus[22,39] hence responsible for the up-regulation in hemolysins (α and β toxins),[22,40] toxic shock toxin (TSST1),[41] enterotoxin B,[41] fibrinogen binding proteins (e.g., coagulase) and fibronectin binding proteins[42] and down-regulation of protein A,[43] collagen binding protein,[44] V8 protease[41] and lipase[8] (Table II). More recently, the *sar* locus has been shown to repress autolytic activity.[45] SarA has a limited but regional sequence similarity with VirF[38] a positive transcriptional regulator of virulence genes located in a large plasmid in *Shigella flexneri*.[46] Interestingly, the region of sequence similarity corresponds to the DNA binding domain of VirF.[38,46] Notably, a small molecular size, a high percentage of charged amino acids

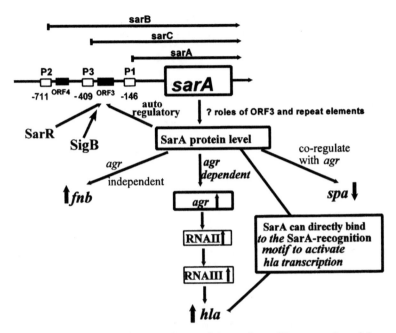

FIGURE 3. The putative regulatory pathways of the *sar* locus. The expression of the major regulatory molecule, SarA, is controlled by SarA (Heinrichs *et al.* 1996) and upstream promoter elements (e.g., ORFs) (Cheung *et al.* 1997a). The SarA protein levels likely determine the degree of activation (*hla, fnbB*) or repression (*spa*) of target genes. The SarA level is partially determined by the auto-regulatory activity of SarA and by a regulatory protein (SarR) which somehow suppresses sarA and increases sarC transcription. Additionally, the P3 promoter is SigB-dependent. The *sar* regulatory system can be divided into three major pathways based on its interaction with *agr*: 1) α-hemolysin activation pathway (*hla* via *agr*); 2) protein A repression pathway (co-regulate with *agr* to suppress *spa* transcription); and 3) fibronectin binding protein activation pathway (*fnbA* expression independent of *agr*). Our premise is that the SarA protein binds to a conserved SarA-recognition motif to initiate target gene transcription. This mode of gene activation/repression may explain how the *sar* locus can regulate target genes (e.g., *hla*) via both *agr*-dependent and *agr*-independent pathways.

(33%) and a net basic charge are molecular properties of SarA that are frequently found in DNA binding proteins in prokaryotes.[47]

Several lines of experimental evidence suggest that the *sar* locus regulates *agr*, thus putting *agr* downstream in the *sar* regulatory cascade (Figure 3). First, RNAII and RNAIII, two *agr*-encoded transcripts, are diminished in *sar* mutants but restored upon complementation with intact *sar* fragments.[48] Second, hemolysin production, which is diminished in *sar*

TABLE II
Virulence determinants regulated by *sar* and *agr*

	sar	*agr*
α-hemolysin	increased	increased
β-hemolysin	increased	increased
δ-hemolysin	increased	increased
TSST-1	increased	increased
Lipase	decreased	increased
V8 protease	decreased	increased
Enterotoxin B	increased	increased
Fibronectin binding protein A	increased	decreased
Clumping factor A	unknown	no effect
Coagulase	increased	decreased
Collagen binding protein	decreased	minimal decrease
Capsular polysaccharide (type 5)	increased	increased

These phenotypes are compiled from several souces (Kornblum *et al.* 1990; Cheung *et al.* 1992, 1994a; Chan and Foster, 1998a; Wolz *et al.* 2000; Blevin *et al.* 1999, and unpublished data).

mutants, can be restored to wild type levels by supplying a plasmid carrying RNAIII under an inducible promoter.[48] Third, gel shift and DNase I footprinting studies revealed binding of SarA to *agr* promoter fragments.[49] The SarA binding site on the *agr* promoter has been mapped to a 29-bp sequence, locating between the P2 (−73 to −101 upstream of the P2 transcription start) and P3 promoters of *agr* (−83 to −111 upstream of the P3 transcription start).[6] Rechtin *et al.* showed that SarA likely exists as a dimer.[50] However, this group mapped SarA to a wider binding site on the *agr* promoter than the 29-bp sequence.[50] Because greater amounts of SarA (requiring 6–50 nM of SarA corresponding to 88–735 μg of purified protein vs 1–5 μg in our studies) were employed in their footprinting reactions, it is conceivable that technical differences may have accounted for the divergent results. Nonetheless, deletion studies (below) indicated that the 29-bp binding site is required for the transcription of RNAII of the *agr* locus in *S. aureus*.

Besides regulating *hla* expression via the control of *agr*, phenotypic and transcriptional analyses of target genes such as *spa* (protein A gene)[43] and *fnbA* (fibronectin binding protein A gene)[42] indicate that the *sar* locus likely modulates the transcription of these genes via *agr* independent mechanisms. Based upon the interaction with *agr*, the *sar* locus likely regulates its target genes via at least three pathways (Figure 3). In addition to the *agr*-dependent *hla* pathway, the transcriptional suppression of *spa* (the protein A pathway) is dependent on co-regulation by *sar* and *agr*.

Remarkably, the up-regulation of *spa* in a *sar* mutant can be repressed by a plasmid supplying RNAIII (the *agr* regulatory molecule) in trans and vice versa.[43] These data are consistent with an RNAIII-dependent as well as a *sar*-dependent but RNAIII-independent mechanism. For the third pathway (*fnbA*), the *sar* locus upregulates the transcription of these genes via an *agr*-independent mechanism.[42]

The mechanism by which SarA, the major *sar* effector molecule, regulates its assortment of target genes has recently been elucidated. In aligning the sequence upstream of the −35 promoters of several target genes, a consensus sequence, homologous to the 29-bp SarA binding site (or recognition motif) on the *agr* promoter as mapped by the DNase I footprinting assay, emerges (Figure 4). The importance of the consensus sequence in activating the transcription of *hla* and *agr* in *S. aureus* has been confirmed by deletion studies in which a *hla* and an RNAII-containing fragments devoid of the SarA recognition motif failed to transcribe the respective genes as compared with the intact controls,[16] thus hinting at the essential role of the SarA binding site "*in vivo*". Remarkably, the transcription of *spa*, a gene normally repressed by the *sar* locus, also becomes de-repressed (as measured by a XylE reporter fusion assay) in a wild type strain containing a shuttle plasmid in which the SarA

SarA recognition motif:

agr   ATTTGTATTTAATATTTTAACATAAA 20/26
[nt mapped by footprinting analysis underlined (Chien et al.,1999)]

hla   ATTTTTATTTAATAGTTAATTAATTG   23/26

spa   AATTATAAATATAGTTTTTAGTATTG   17/26

fnbA   ACTTGAATACAATTTATAGGTATATT 16/26

sec   ATTTTCTTTTAATATTTTTTTAATTG 23/26

Consensus ATTTgTATtTAATATTTataTAAtTg
                        t t
                        g

FIGURE 4. Alignment of a putative common SarA recognition sequence from promoters of *sar* target genes. *hla*, α-hemolysin gene; *spa*, protein A gene; *fnbA*, fibronectin binding protein A gene; *fnbB*, fibronectin binding protein B gene; *sec*, enterotoxin C gene. The consensus sequence was derived as follows: 4/6, capital letter; 3/6, small letter; an even distribution of nucleotides at a specific position will be presented as combinations of small letters.

recognition motif has been deleted from the *spa* promoter region.[16] DNase I footprinting assays, however, disclosed that the SarA binding sites on the *hla* and *spa* promoters are wider than the consensus sequence, thus raising the possibility that the SarA recognition motif is an activation site within a larger binding domain.[16] On the basis of these findings, we formulated a unifying hypothesis for virulence gene activation in *S. aureus* whereby SarA is the regulatory protein that binds to the consensus SarA recognition motif to activate (e.g., *hla*) or repress (*spa*) the with a decrease in the extent of *agr* activation (RNAII and RNAIII). As definitive evidence for the translation of ORF3 is lacking, the likelihood that the sequence encoding transcription of *sar* target genes, thus accounting for both *agr*-dependent and *agr*-independent modes of regulation. Based on the proposed pathway, it can be observed that *hla* transcription can be up-regulated via dual pathways, first via an up-regulation of *agr*, second via direct binding of SarA to the *hla* promoter (Figure 3).

The expression of SarA, the *sar* effector molecule, is controlled by an 800-bp triple promoter region with extensive secondary structure (direct and inverted repeats) and potential coding regions (ORF3 and ORF4) among promoter elements (Figure 3). Nonsense mutations in ORF3 lead to a reduction in SarA protein level[49] which, in turn, correlates ORF3, rather than the translation product itself, modulates the expression of SarA cannot be ruled out. Besides these putative ORFs, the complexity of the *sar* promoters hints at the possibility that regulatory proteins may bind to the promoter region to modulate SarA expression, thus leading to varying levels of target gene activation or suppression.

The first evidence that additional transcription factor binds to the *sar* promoter region comes from the recognition that the P3 promoter (GGGTAT at the −10 promoter box), contrary to the *sar* P1 and P2 promoters, is maximally expressed during the postexponential phase,[36] a feature commonly found in δB-dependent promoters.[37] This observation was subsequently confirmed by the absence of the P3 transcript in a *sigB* mutant of *S. aureus*.[51] *In vitro* transcription assays also validated the SigB dependency of the *sar* P3 promoter.[52,53] Interestingly, the *sigB* mutant expressed higher levels of α-hemolysin, fibrinogen-binding[51] and fibronectin binding proteins than the parent (unpublished data), phenotypes consistent with enhanced SarA expression as confirmed by immunoblot and ELISA analyses.[51] Transcriptional fusion with a *gfp* reporter gene disclosed that the *sar* P1 promoter is more active in the *sigB* mutant than the parental strain while the P3 promoter is less active, as one would predict from its δB dependency. Based on these data, a model linking SigB to the expression of SarA can be proposed (Figure 5). Upon the induction of *sigB* in response to environmental stresses and/or ATP deprivation (e.g., anaerobic growth), free SigB protein will be available to activate the *sar* P3 promoter.[37] Activation of P3 is associated with down-regulation of the *sar* P1 promoter (unpublished observation). As P1 is the strongest promoter within the *sar* regulatory system,[54] the net effect is a decrease in SarA protein expression in response to SigB activation, thus accounting for the reduction in the expression of α-hemolysin, fibrinogen and fibronectin binding proteins in the parental strain as compared with the *sigB* mutant (Figure 5).

The *sar* locus is also auto-regulatory. This was evaluated in a pair of isogenic *sar* strains using transcriptional fusion of various *sar* promoters linked to the *xylE* reporter gene.[54] Based on XylE activity, the *sar* P1 promoter is most active, with ~40 fold more activity than the P2 and P3 promoters (Table III). Interestingly, P1 promoter activity can be down-modulated when it acts in concert with the *sar* P3 promoter (P3-P1 vs P1 in Table IIIa). Analysis of transcriptional fusions in a *sar* mutant (Table IIIa) disclosed that promoter activities for all three *sar* promoters are lower in the *sar* mutant than the parental control. Complementation of the *sar* mutant with single copies of *sar* fragments encoding sarA, sarC and sarB transcription units disclosed that each of these fragments augments *sar* P1 promoter activity (the strongest *sar* promoter) as assayed by XylE reporter fusions, with sarC and sarB transcription units disclosed that each of these fragments augments *sar* P1 promoter activity (the strongest *sar* promoter) as assayed by XylE reporter fusions, with the sarB

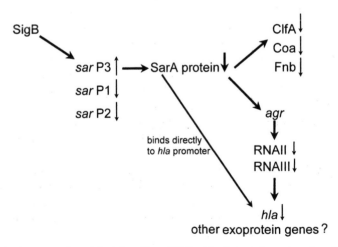

FIGURE 5. A proposed model of the effect of SigB activation on the expression of virulence determinants in *S. aureus*.

TABLE III
Expression of *sar* promoter-XylE fusions in a pair of
isogenic *sar* strains

A. Construct	XylE activity (mU/mg of protein)	
	RN6390	ALC488 (*sar* mutant)
P1	137.2	18.4
P3	3.0	0.4
P2	4.0	1.2
P3-P1	74.6	35.4
B. Strains	XylE activity of *sar* P1 promoter	
RN6390	314	
ALC488	27.6	
A88 (sarB)	408	
ALC488 (sarA)	272	
ALC488 (sarC)	178	

(A) Activity from each construct is defined as mU per mg of cellular
protein. The samples were taken at early stationary phase. (B)Expres-
sion of *xylE* fusions (mU/mg of cellular proteins) from the *sar* P1 promoter in *sar* mutant strain ALC488 complemented with single copies
of various *sar* fragments in the chromosome using the integration
vector pCL84 (Manna *et al.* 1998).

transcriptional unit being the most effective (Table IIIb). Recognizing
that each of these *sar* fragments encodes SarA, it is highly likely that SarA
acts a positive regulator of *sar* P1 promoter activity (Figure 3). Additionally, the effectiveness of a sarB-encoding fragment in restoring P1 promoter
activity also implies that the promoter sequence upstream of the *sarA*
ORF serves to modulate SarA expression (Table IIIb), possibly by
virtue of differential promoter activation or alterations in the secondary
structure of the promoter in response to DNA binding proteins.[22] In particular, there are regions of inverted and direct repeats that may conceiv-
ably alter SarA expression (e.g., by interfering with RNAP or ribosomal
RNA binding). Additionally, there are putative coding region (e.g., ORF3)
that may alter SarA protein expression.[49] Finally, there is a likelihood that
the promoter region may serve as a binding site for additional regulatory
proteins.

A novel protein that binds to the *sar* promoter was recently isolated
from cell lysates of *S. aureus* with a DNA-specific column containing a
49-bp sequence of the *sar* P2 promoter.[54] This P2 sequence shares
homology with a 34-bp sequence upstream of the *sar* P1 promoter.[54] The
putative gene, designated *sarR*, encodes a 115 a.a. protein (13.6 kDa) that
shares homology with SarA (51% similarity and 28% identity) (unpublished data).

The *sarR* gene is present in *S. aureus* strains and in *S. saprophyticus* as disclosed by hybridization studies under high stringency conditions. Purified SarR was found to bind *sar* P1, P3 and P2 promoters by gel shift and DNaseI footprinting assays. Allelic replacement of *sarR* with an *ermC* gene diminished P3 transcription and enhanced P1 transcription in the mutant (Figure 6a). As P1 is the strongest promoter within the *sar* locus, a mutation in *sarR* will be expected to yield an increase in SarA expression. This has been confirmed with an immunoblot probed with anti-SarR monoclonal antibodies (Figure 6B). More importantly, the *sarR* mutant, in correlation with an elevated SarA level, expressed higher levels of *agr* activation than the parental strain (Figure 6c). Taken together, these studies strongly support the notion that SarR is a repressor protein that binds to the *sar* promoter region to up-regulate P3 and down-regulate P1 transcription, with the net effect being a decrease in SarA protein expression (Figure 3).

To sum up these *in vitro* studies, it is evident that the *sar* locus is an integral part of the regulatory circuitry that coordinates the expression of virulence factors in *S. aureus* (Figure 7). The central player of the *sar* regulatory system is the SarA protein (Figure 3). In identifying a conserved SarA recognition motif among *sar* target genes such as *agr, hla, spa* and *fnbA*, we have put forward a unifying hypothesis whereby the "effector molecule," SarA, binds to conserved sequence motif upstream of the −35 promoter boxes of target genes to activate (*hla* and *agr*) or suppress (*spa*) gene transcription.[16] Besides the recognition motif, the other prominent feature of the *sar* regulatory system is that the SarA protein level correlates with the extent of target gene transcription.[49] As would have been expected of a complex regulatory system, both activator and repressor proteins provide "check and balance" to this system. In particular, the SarA protein, possibly in conjunction with regulatory elements upstream of the *sarA* coding region (e.g., ORF3, direct and repeated elements), provides positive input for SarA expression. Counteracting against these positive influences are regulatory proteins such as SarR and SigB. Expression of these two proteins serves to down-modulate transcription from the *sar* P1 promoter, which is the strongest promoter within the *sar* regulatory system. The net effect of SarR and SigB expression, both maximally expressed during the postexponential phase, is a decrease in SarA protein expression, probably in late exponential phase. In addition to its effect on SarA expression, there is preliminary evidence that SarR may bind to the target gene promoters (unpublished observation), thus possibly affecting target gene transcription directly. Despite a lower SarA level during late postexponential phase (due to SarR and SigB), transcriptional analysis clearly demonstrated the maximal expression

A: *sar* probe

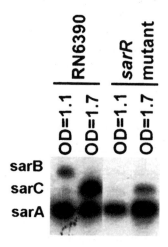

sarB
sarC
sarA

RN6390 | OD=1.1 OD=1.7
sarR mutant | OD=1.1 OD=1.7

B: anti-SarA antibody

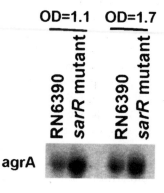

RN6390
sarR mutant

C: *agrA* probe

OD=1.1   OD=1.7

RN6390 *sarR* mutant   RN6390 *sarR* mutant

agrA

FIGURE 6. The effect of a *sarR* mutation on *sar* transcripts (A), SarA expression (B) and *agrA* (RNAII) transcription. Figure 6A displays a Northern blot (10 μg of total RNA each) probed with a *sarA* probe (nt 620–1349) (Bayer *et al.* 1996). Figure 6B shows an immunoblot of the cell extract (25 μg each) of RN6390 and the *sarR* mutant (harvested at early stationary phase) probed with anti-SarA monoclonal antibody 1D1 at 1:2000 dilution. A Northern blot of the RNAII (*agrA* probe) transcript in RN6390 and the *sarR* mutant was shown (C). The *agrA* probe corresponds to nt 3830–4342 according to published sequence (Kornblum *et al.* 1990).

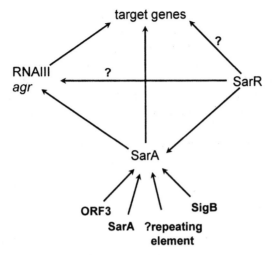

FIGURE 7. The global regulation of virulence determinants in *S. aureus.*

of RNAIII during this growth period. Thus, an additional signal is likely required for late postexponential up-regulation of RNAIII and ensuing *hla* expression.

The *sae* Locus

The *sae* locus was initially identified by a transposon Tn*551* insertion in strain ISP479.[7,55] Phenotypic analysis suggests that the *sae* gene product is probably required for the expression of many exoprotein genes. Remarkably, cell bound coagulase is down-regulated by a *sae* mutation while the expression of another cell-wall protein, protein A, is unaffected. More importantly, the transcription of *sar* and *agr* is not altered as a result of a *sae* mutation, thus implying that *sae* may act downstream of these two regulatory loci.[7] Alternatively, the *sae* locus may influence target gene transcription via an *agr/sar* independent mechanism.

Environmental Factors Affecting Global Regulation

Environmental factors play a role in *agr* and *sar* expression. For instance, 1 M NaCl has been shown to disrupt RNAIII transcription.[56,57] Chan and colleagues have described an *agr* independent mode of *spa, hla* and *tst* repression in the presence of 1 M NaCl.[56] Likewise, glucose appears to down-modulate *agr*-related genes, thus demonstrating catabolite repression of the *agr* locus.[58] Glycerol monolaurate, a surfactant, has also been found to inhibit postexponential phase activation of virulence factors (e.g., exoproteins) without affecting *agr* expression in *S. aureus*.[5] In the absence of any additional nutrient or exogenous constituents in minimal growth medium, the pH of the culture normally decreases as the cells enter the postexponential phase; if, however, the pH of the culture is kept at 5.5, RNAIII expression will decrease further than cultures maintained at pH 6.5.[58]

The effect of antibiotics on exoprotein gene expression is more variable. Subinhibitory concentrations of antibiotics were reported by Gemmel and Shibl to have a general inhibitory effect on exoprotein gene expression.[59] Contrary to this observation, recent studies by Ohlsen and colleagues disclosed that beta-lactams and fluoroquininones at subinhibitory concentrations result in an increase in *hla* expression while macrolides and aminoglycosides have mild inhibitory effects.[60] Whether this effect is mediated by global regulatory loci such as *sar, agr, sigB* or other unknown regulatory element is not clear. Bisognano *et al.* described increased expression of fibronectin binding proteins by fluoroquininone-resistant *S. aureus* exposed to subinhibitory concentrations of ciprofloxacin.[61] Presumably, changes in DNA supercoiling or possibly alterations in stress-induced transcription factors (e.g., SigB) may have modified surface protein expression. Whether global regulatory loci play an intermediary role in *fnb* expression in response to subinhibitory levels of fluoroquininones is not well defined. Importantly, many of these environmental and antibiotic studies utilized strain 8325-4[41,56,61,62] in which a defect in one of the anti-Sigma factor genes (*rsbU*) in the *sigB* operon has been found.[63,64] Additionally, most of these environmental studies were conducted in batch cultures. As numerous environmental variables may be altered as bacterial cultures transition from exponential to postexponential phase (e.g., pH, glucose limitation and altered oxygen tension), the interpretation of these data attributable a single environmental variable should be made with caution. Finally, these *in vitro* studies did not take into account the host forces at play *in vivo* (e.g., host proteins, phagocytic cells and local microenvironment within specific tissues). Thus, there is a strong rationale to examine some of these variables in an *in vivo* setting.

3. VIRULENCE GENE EXPRESSION IN HOST ENVIRONMENTS

To correlate *in vitro* findings with those *in vivo*, our laboratory has constructed a shuttle plasmid containing a promoterless green fluorescent protein reporter gene (*gfp$_{uv}$*).[65] Contrary to other reporter systems,

GFPuv, being relatively stable, can be easily detected as green fluorescence by long wavelength UV light excitation. As this detection method does not require cell lysis, the insertion of a gene promoter upstream of the *gfp*$_{uv}$ reporter gene renders this system useful for both *in vivo* and *in vitro* analyses.

Using this strategy, various *sar* promoter fragments was inserted upstream of the *gfp*$_{uv}$ reporter gene in a shuttle plasmid followed by electroporation into *S. aureus* strain RN6390.[65] Activation of these colonies with a hand held long wavelength UV light disclosed that only the *sar* P1 and the combined P2-P3-P1 promoters display green fluorescence while the *sar* P2 and the δB-dependent P3 promoters yield very little fluorescence.

We next introduced these bacteria in a rabbit endocarditis model to assess *in vivo* gene activation.[65] Experimentally, a polyethylene catheter was introduced across the aortic valve into the left ventricle via the right carotid artery. The challenging bacterial inoculum was then injected into the catheter. In most animals, successful induction of the disease was confirmed within 48 h of bacterial challenge as indicated by persistently positive blood culture and culture-positive bacterial vegetations at autopsy. Using this model, *S. aureus* bacteria containing the *sar* P1, P2 or P3 GFPuv fusions were injected intravenously into catheterized rabbits. Twenty four hours after iv infections, cardiac vegetations were removed and examined. The results revealed that the *sar* P1 promoter is active *in vitro* and *in vivo* (Table IV). In contrast, the P3 promoter is inactive in both instances. Surprisingly, the P2 promoter is silent *in vitro* but becomes highly active *in vivo*. These comparative data emphasize the differential activation of *sar* promoters between *in vivo* and *in vitro* settings. This finding also serves to stress that host signals are likely involved in activating global regulatory loci in *S. aureus*. As global regulatory elements activate or repress a subset of virulence genes, the response of the bacteria to selective host

TABLE IV
Activation of *sar* promoters *in vivo*

	in vitro (agar plate)	*in vivo* (rabbit endocarditis)
sar P1 promoter	active	active
sar P3 promoter	silent	silent
sar P2 promoter	silent	active

S. aureus strains (RN6390) containing shuttle plasmids with assorted *sar* promoter fragments were assessed with a long wavelenth UV light (*in vitro*). The cardiac tissues from infected rabbits were examined with UV fluorescence (Cheung *et al.* 1998).

microenvironments perhaps should be viewed in the context of a gene subset rather than as a specific virulence determinant.

Besides different patterns of promoter activation, the same promoter activated in one tissue may not be activated in another. As an example, the *sar* P2 promoter was activated in heart valve tissues but remained silent in the kidney in the rabbit endocarditis model despite the prevalence of bacteria in both tissues.[65] As opposed to the heart valve which adjoins the bloodstream, the kidney, as an area of high pH and osmolarity, likely presents a microenvironment not conducive to *sar* P2 activation.

The activation of a particular promoter also depends on the location within a single target tissue. In particular, the *sar* P2 promoter was found to be active only on the surface on the vegetation where the cells are metabolically active but not in the depth of the vegetation where the bacterial cells are metabolically quiescent. Presumably, activation of the P2 promoter, combined with the P1 promoter, would yield a higher level of hemolysin production,[54] exactly what metabolically active cells would need to propagate in infected tissues.

The Role of *agr*, *sar* and *sigB* in Virulence

As many of the virulence factors (e.g., hemolysins and fibronectin binding proteins) are regulated by *sar* and *agr*,[66] the contributory roles of *sar* and *agr* to virulence have been evaluated in several animal model systems including the rabbit endocarditis model,[48,66] the endophthalmitis models,[67-69] the mouse arthritis model,[70,71] the rabbit osteomyelitis model[72] and the mouse subcutaneous infection model.[25,62] The results of these published studies will not be described in full detail here. However, it suffices to say that all of these animal studies serve to demonstrate that *sar* and *agr* mutants are less able to cause infections than the parental control. Nevertheless, it is of interest that in the rabbit endocarditis model, which represents an acute/subacute endovascular infection model, the *sar* mutant displayed reduced infection rates (0 and 10% at 10^3 and 10^4 CFU as inocula) as compared with the parental strain (90 and 70%, respectively).[66] Remarkably, the double *sar/agr* mutant exhibited further reduction in infection rates (0, 0, 25 and 50% at 10^3-10^6 CFU as inocula) than single mutants alone (Table V).[66] Besides reduction in infectivity rates, the number of bacteria in the endocardial vegetations in the single and double mutants were significantly lower than the control, with the double mutant displaying a higher reduction.[66] Early adherence studies (30 min after infection) also disclosed reduced adherence to the heart valve by the double mutant.[66] These animal studies support the notion that *sar* and *agr* are important regulatory loci that control the expression of virulence

TABLE V
Infectivities of *agr*, *sar* and *agr/sar* mutants in the rabbit endocarditis model

	Parent	*agr* mutant	*sar* mutant	double mutant
10^3 CFU	9/10	4/10*	0/10†	0/10§
10^4 CFU	7/10	4/11	1/9†	0/10§
10^5 CFU	11/11	8/10	10/11	2/7§
10^6 CFU	9/9	8/11	9/12	4/8§

Bacteria were injected directly into the marginal ear veins of rabbits which had been catheterized 48 h earlier. All rabbits were sacrificed at 48 h after bacterial challenge. Values are given as number with endocarditis/total number of rabbits. *Statistically significant when compared with parental strain (P value ≤ 0.03; Fisher exact test). †The infection rates are significantly higher than the parental strain (P values ≤ 0.0001 and 0.015 at 10^3 and 10^4 inocula, respectively). §Induction rates are lower than that of the parental strain (P values of 0.00006, 0.0015. 0.002 and 0.03 at 10^3 – 10^6, respectively) (Cheung *et al.* 1994a).

determinants in *S. aureus* including those involved in initial adherence (e.g., *fnb* controlled by *sar*)[66] and intravegetation multiplication (e.g., *hla* by *sar* and *agr*) in the fibrin-platelet matrix on the valvular endothelium. With so many virulence determinants altered in these mutants, these studies clearly emphasize the multifactorial nature of pathogenicity in *S. aureus*. Due to the similarity in pathology between the rabbit endocarditis model and human subacute endocarditis,[73] it is likely that these regulatory loci play a major role in human infections as well.

Contrary to *sar* and *agr*, *sigB* has not been found to play any major roles in acute animal infection models involving a pair of isogenic *sigB* strains.[51,62,74] In examining the proposed SigB activation pathway (Figure 5), it can be argued that activation of SigB in acute infections, with its downmodulating effect on *hla*, *fnb* and *coa* expression (via reduced SarA), will be detrimental to the "well being" of the bacterium. Indeed, attempts to detect activation of the δB-dependent *sar* P3 promoter in heart, kidney and spleen tissues in the rabbit endocarditis model has failed (unpublished observations). Despite this finding, the role of SigB in persistent chronic infections (e.g., chronic abscess, osteomyelitis) has not been ruled out since one would expect the indolence of these infections to occur without a major outburst of hemolysins and enzymes, factors that are critical to microbial propagation in acute infections. Finally, small colony variants of *S. aureus* have been observed in patients with chronic but persistent *S. aureus* infections (e.g., cystic fibrosis lung, chronic but low-grade bacteremia and osteomyelitis).[75] Some of the these small colony variants have been linked to menadione, hemin and thymidine auxotrophies.[75] Whether small colony phenotype is modulated by regulatory loci such as *sigB*, *sar* and *agr* has not been determined.

The Role of *sar* and *agr* in Apoptosis

Chronic *S. aureus* infections are frequent in selected patient populations, especially those with diabetes[76] and cystic fibrosis.[77,78] It has been proposed that internalization of *S. aureus* by host cells may mediate persistent infections since the intracellular milieu, with its protected microenvironment, may shield the bacteria against antibiotics and antimicrobial agents.[79,80] More specifically, recent studies have shown that *S. aureus* can be internalized by bovine mammary epithelial cells[80] and human endothelial cells[79] and subsequently induces apoptosis. In contrast to necrosis, apoptosis is an innate cell suicide mechanism that proceeds without significant inflammatory responses.[81] Pathogen-induced apoptosis may serve to evade host defenses that may otherwise limit the extent of bacterial infections.

As with animal infection models, it is highly likely that a subset of genes are turned on once the *S. aureus* bacteria are inside mammalian cells. Studies by Wesson *et al.* revealed that *agr* and *sar* mutants were internalized by cultured bovine mammary epithelial cells at levels greater than the parental strain but, unlike the parent control, failed to induce apoptosis. Thus, *sar* and *agr* regulated proteins are critical to the induction of apoptosis in bovine mammary epithelial cells. Because of tissue and host cell specificity, it is not clear whether similar *S. aureus*-induced apoptotic pathways regulated by *sar* and *agr* would apply to other cell lines such as human endothelial cells and epithelial cells, especially those lining the respiratory epithelium.

With the use of GFP as a reporter in *S. aureus*, our laboratory recently demonstrated that *S. aureus* can be internalized by a pulmonary epithelial cell line derived from a cystic fibrosis patient (CFT-1).[82] Importantly, *S. aureus* is not a passive bystander in the internalization process but rather replicates actively inside pulmonary epithelial cells and induces apoptosis. Thus, bacterial replication precedes apoptosis of the infected cells. These studies suggest that *S. aureus*, by virtue of its internalization and replication inside pulmonary epithelial cells, may contribute to the pathogenesis of persistent *S. aureus* infections in susceptible patients (e.g., CF or elderly patients).

4. CONCLUSIONS AND FUTURE DIRECTIONS

Clearly, the *sar* and *agr* loci are an integral part of a regulatory circuitry that coordinately controls the expression of virulence determinants in *S. aureus*. The multifactorial nature of *S. aureus* pathogenicity implies that it may be useful to target a pleiotropic regulator rather than a specific determinant for the development of novel antimicrobial agents. Based on interactions with *agr*, the *sar* regulatory system can be divided into three distinct pathways for target gene activation: 1) the *hla* pathway (via *agr*); 2) the *spa* pathway (co-repression with *agr*); and 3) the *fnb* pathway (*agr*-independent). In identifying a conserved SarA recognition motif among *sar* target genes such as *agr*, *hla*, *spa* and *fnbA*, we propose a unifying hypothesis whereby SarA, the major *sar* regulatory molecule, binds to the conserved sequence upstream of the −35 promoter box of target genes to activate (e.g., *hla*) or repress (e.g., *spa*) gene transcription. As the SarA level is critical to the extent of target gene activation, the prediction is that there are multiple levels of inputs, with SarA and regulatory elements within the promoter system (e.g., ORF) serving as activators, and SigB and SarR acting as repressors for SarA expression (Figure 7). Superimposed upon these regulatory elements are host signals which likely perturb SarA expression, either via these *in vitro*-associated regulators or via novel control pathway that can only be detected with *in vivo* selection system. The end result is that SarA, upon reaching a threshold, will modulate target gene expression by binding to the respective promoter. Because of the intermediary role of *agr*, some of these target genes will have dual activation pathways (e.g., *hla*).

The expression of virulence determinants *in vivo* is clearly influenced by host signals. As the host milieu, with an interplay of tissue factors and host defense forces, is complex, an exciting part of future staphylococcal research clearly lies in novel approaches that identify virulence genes primarily expressed *in vivo*. One promising approach has been signature tagged mutagenesis (STM) in which transposon-tagged mutants of *S. aureus* that do not survive in a murine peritoneal challenge are identified.[12,13] Presumably, disruption of the *in vivo*-required gene has led to non-survivors in the murine peritoneal challenge, which can then be traced with specific oligonucleotide tags. Despite the identification of essential survival genes (e.g., genes for amino acid synthesis) with STM, early reports indicated that this approach has identified promising candidate genes with unknown functions (David Holden, personal communication). Another exciting approach has been differential fluorescence induction (DFI).[13] Contrasting to STM, this approach has the advantage of multiple *in vitro* and *in vivo* selections automated by cell sorting in flow cytometry.[14,15] In brief, a promoter library, consisting of random promoter fragments inserted upstream of a *gfp* reporter gene in a shuttle plasmid, was constructed in a *S. aureus* strain. Colonies with little fluorescence can be selected from *in vitro* grown bacteria. This will be followed by selection of highly fluorescent colonies in an infected animal model system (e.g., rabbit endocarditis). This procedure can then be repeated to enrich for colonies that are only fluorescent *in vivo* but not *in vitro*. These promoter fragments, presumably representing genes activated only *in vivo*, can then be identified.

It is reasonable to assume that *S. aureus*, upon encountering the host milieu, would initiate an appropriate network of virulence genes in response to host signals. The coordinate expression of these genes is likely to be precise since the sequence by which specific genes are expressed is critical to microbial survival. In this context, it is highly appropriate to envision bacterial response as a subset of genes activated by the host microenvironment. Clearly, *sar* and *agr* are not the only regulatory elements that controls the expression of virulence determinants *in vivo*.[25,66-72] Our challenge will be to identify those set of virulence genes selectively expressed *in vivo*. Presumably, these genes would be easily missed with *in vitro* screening methods. Understanding how these genes work will place us at the threshold of deciphering the precise interplay of microbial and host factors. With the impending threat of vancomycin resistance in *S. aureus*, these novel virulence genes may provide the basis for designing new antimicrobial agents and preventive vaccines.

REFERENCES

1. Lowy, F. D. Staphylococcus aureus infections [see comments]. *New England Journal of Medicine* **339**, 520–532 (1998).
2. Boyce, J. M. Epidemiology and prevention of nosocomial infections. in *The staphylococci in human diseases* (eds. Crossley, K. B. & Archer, G. L.) (Churchill Livingstone, New York, 1997).
3. Neu, H. C. The crisis in antibiotic resistance [see comments]. *Science* **257**, 1064–1073 (1992).
4. Hiramatsu, K. Vancomycin resistance in staphylococci. *Drug Resistance Updates* **1**, 135 (1998).
5. Projan, S. J. & Novick, R. P. The molecular basis of pathogenicity. in *The Staphylococci in Human Diseases* (eds. Crossley, K. B. & Archer, G. L.) (Churchill Livingstone, New York, 1997).
6. Kornblum, J., Kreiswirth, B., Projan, S. J., Ross, H. & Novick, R. P. *agr*: A polycistronic locus regulating exoprotein synthesis in *Staphylococcus aureus*. in *Molecular Biology of the Staphylococci* (ed. Novick, R. P.) (VCH Publishers, New York, 1990).
7. Giraudo, A. T., Cheung, A. L. & Nagel, R. The sae locus of Staphylococcus aureus controls exoprotein synthesis at the transcriptional level. *Archives of Microbiology* **168**, 53–58 (1997).
8. Cheung, A. L., Koomey, J. M., Butler, C. A., Projan, S. J. & Fischetti, V. A. Regulation of exoprotein expression in Staphylococcus aureus by a locus (sar) distinct from agr. *Proceedings of the National Academy of Sciences of the United States of America* **89**, 6462–6466 (1992).
9. Zhang, J. P. & Normark, S. Induction of gene expression in Escherichia coli after pilus-mediated adherence [see comments]. *Science* **273**, 1234–1236 (1996).

10. Mahan, M. J., Slauch, J. M. & Mekalanos, J. J. Selection of bacterial virulence genes that are specifically induced in host tissues [see comments]. *Science* **259**, 686–688 (1993).

11. Lowe, A. M., Beattie, D. T. & Deresiewicz, R. L. Identification of novel staphylococcal virulence genes by in vivo expression technology. *Molecular Microbiology* **27**, 967–976 (1998).

12. Mei, J. M., Nourbakhsh, F., Ford, C. W. & Holden, D. W. Identification of Staphylococcus aureus virulence genes in a murine model of bacteraemia using signature-tagged mutagenesis. *Molecular Microbiology* **26**, 399–407 (1997).

13. Schwan, W. R. *et al.* Identification and characterization of the PutP proline permease that contributes to in vivo survival of Staphylococcus aureus in animal models. *Infection & Immunity* **66**, 567–572 (1998).

14. Valdivia, R. H., Hromockyj, A. E., Monack, D., Ramakrishnan, L. & Falkow, S. Applications for green fluorescent protein (GFP) in the study of host-pathogen interactions. *Gene* **173**, 47–52 (1996).

15. Valdivia, R. H. & Falkow, S. Fluorescence-based isolation of bacterial genes expressed within host cells. *Science* **277**, 2007–2011 (1997).

16. Chien, Y., Manna, A. C., Projan, S. J. & Cheung, A. L. SarA, a global regulator of virulence determinants in Staphylococcus aureus, binds to a conserved motif essential for sar-dependent gene regulation. *Journal of Biological Chemistry* **274**, 37169–37176 (1999).

17. Morfeldt, E., Janzon, L., Arvidson, S. & Lofdahl, S. Cloning of a chromosomal locus (exp) which regulates the expression of several exoprotein genes in Staphylococcus aureus. *Molecular & General Genetics* **211**, 435–440 (1988).

18. Recsei, P. *et al.* Regulation of exoprotein gene expression in Staphylococcus aureus by agr. *Molecular & General Genetics* **202**, 58–61 (1986).

19. Janzon, L. & Arvidson, S. The role of the delta-lysin gene (hld) in the regulation of virulence genes by the accessory gene regulator (agr) in Staphylococcus aureus. *EMBO Journal* **9**, 1391–1399 (1990).

20. Novick, R. P. *et al.* Synthesis of staphylococcal virulence factors is controlled by a regulatory RNA molecule. *EMBO Journal* **12**, 3967–3975 (1993).

21. Novick, R. P. *et al.* The agr P2 operon: an autocatalytic sensory transduction system in Staphylococcus aureus. *Molecular & General Genetics* **248**, 446–458 (1995).

22. Cheung, A. L., Bayer, M. G. & Heinrichs, J. H. sar Genetic determinants necessary for transcription of RNAII and RNAIII in the agr locus of Staphylococcus aureus. *Journal of Bacteriology* **179**, 3963–3971 (1997).

23. Ji, G., Beavis, R. C. & Novick, R. P. Cell density control of staphylococcal virulence mediated by an octapeptide pheromone. *Proceedings of the National Academy of Sciences of the United States of America* **92**, 12055–12059 (1995).

24. Ji, G., Beavis, R. & Novick, R. P. Bacterial interference caused by autoinducing peptide variants. *Science* **276**, 2027–2030 (1997).

25. Mayville, P. *et al.* Structure-activity analysis of synthetic autoinducing thiolactone peptides from Staphylococcus aureus responsible for virulence. *Proceedings of the National Academy of Sciences of the United States of America* **96**, 1218–1223 (1999).

26. Novick, R. P. & Muir, T. W. Virulence gene regulation by peptides in staphylococci and other Gram-positive bacteria. *Current Opinion in Microbiology* **2**, 40–45 (1999).

27. Lina, G. *et al.* Transmembrane topology and histidine protein kinase activity of AgrC, the agr signal receptor in Staphylococcus aureus. *Molecular Microbiology* **28**, 655–662 (1998).

28. Morfeldt, E., Panova-Sapundjieva, I., Gustafsson, B. & Arvidson, S. Detection of the response regulator AgrA in the cytosolic fraction of Staphylococcus aureus by monoclonal antibodies. *FEMS Microbiology Letters* **143**, 195–201 (1996).

29. Morfeldt, E., Taylor, D., von Gabain, A. & Arvidson, S. Activation of alpha-toxin translation in Staphylococcus aureus by the trans-encoded antisense RNA, RNAIII. *EMBO Journal* 14, 4569–4577 (1995).
30. Van Wamel, W. J., van Rossum, G., Verhoef, J., Vandenbroucke-Grauls, C. M. & Fluit, A. C. Cloning and characterization of an accessory gene regulator (agr)-like locus from Staphylococcus epidermidis. *FEMS Microbiology Letters* 163, 1–9 (1998).
31. Vandenesch, F., Projan, S. J., Kreiswirth, B., Etienne, J. & Novick, R. P. Agr-related sequences in Staphylococcus lugdunensis. *FEMS Microbiology Letters* 111, 115–122 (1993).
32. Tegmark, K., Morfeldt, E. & Arvidson, S. Regulation of agr-dependent virulence genes in Staphylococcus aureus by RNAIII from coagulase-negative staphylococci. *Journal of Bacteriology* 180, 3181–3186 (1998).
33. Klein, C., Kaletta, C. & Entian, K. D. Biosynthesis of the lantibiotic subtilin is regulated by a histidine kinase/response regulator system. *Applied & Environmental Microbiology* 59, 296–303 (1993).
34. Havarstein, L. S., Coomaraswamy, G. & Morrison, D. A. An unmodified heptadecapeptide pheromone induces competence for genetic transformation in Streptococcus pneumoniae. *Proceedings of the National Academy of Sciences of the United States of America* 92, 11140–11144 (1995).
35. Solomon, J. M., Lazazzera, B. A. & Grossman, A. D. Purification and characterization of an extracellular peptide factor that affects two different developmental pathways in Bacillus subtilis. *Genes & Development* 10, 2014–2024 (1996).
36. Bayer, M. G., Heinrichs, J. H. & Cheung, A. L. The molecular architecture of the sar locus in Staphylococcus aureus. *Journal of Bacteriology* 178, 4563–4570 (1996).
37. Haldenwang, W. G. The sigma factors of Bacillus subtilis. *Microbiological Reviews* 59, 1–30 (1995).
38. Cheung, A. L. & Projan, S. J. Cloning and sequencing of sarA of Staphylococcus aureus, a gene required for the expression of agr. *Journal of Bacteriology* 176, 4168–4172 (1994).
39. Heinrichs, J. H., Bayer, M. G. & Cheung, A. L. Characterization of the sar locus and its interaction with agr in Staphylococcus aureus. *Journal of Bacteriology* 178, 418–423 (1996).
40. Cheung, A. L. & Ying, P. Regulation of alpha- and beta-hemolysins by the sar locus of Staphylococcus aureus. *Journal of Bacteriology* 176, 580–585 (1994).
41. Chan, P. F. & Foster, S. J. Role of SarA in virulence determinant production and environmental signal transduction in Staphylococcus aureus. *Journal of Bacteriology* 180, 6232–6241 (1998).
42. Wolz, C. *et al.* Regulation of fibronectin binding protein by the *agr* and *sar* regulatory loci of *Staphylococcus aureus.* *Molecular Microbiology* In Press (2000).
43. Cheung, A. L., Eberhardt, K. & Heinrichs, J. H. Regulation of protein A synthesis by the sar and agr loci of Staphylococcus aureus. *Infection & Immunity* 65, 2243–2249 (1997).
44. Blevins, J. S., Gillaspy, A. F., Rechtin, T. M., Hurlburt, B. K. & Smeltzer, M. S. The Staphylococcal accessory regulator (sar) represses transcription of the Staphylococcus aureus collagen adhesin gene (cna) in an agr-independent manner. *Molecular Microbiology* 33, 317–326 (1999).
45. Fujimoto, D. F. & Bayles, K. W. Opposing roles of the Staphylococcus aureus virulence regulators, Agr and Sar, in Triton X-100- and penicillin-induced autolysis. *Journal of Bacteriology* 180, 3724–3726 (1998).
46. Hale, T. L. Genetic basis of virulence in Shigella species. *Microbiological Reviews* 55, 206–224 (1991).

47. Smith, I. Regulatory proteins that control late-growth development. in *Bacillus subtilis and other Gram Positive Bacteria* (eds. Sonenshein, A. L., Hoch, J. A. & Losick, R.) (ASM Press, Washington, D.C., 1993).

48. Cheung, A. L., Yeaman, M. R., Sullam, P. M., Witt, M. D. & Bayer, A. S. Role of the sar locus of Staphylococcus aureus in induction of endocarditis in rabbits. *Infection & Immunity* **62**, 1719–1725 (1994).

49. Chien, Y., Manna, A. C. & Cheung, A. L. SarA level is a determinant of agr activation in Staphylococcus aureus. *Molecular Microbiology* **30**, 991–1001 (1998).

50. Rechtin, T. M. *et al.* Characterization of the SarA virulence gene regulator of Staphylococcus aureus. *Molecular Microbiology* **33**, 307–316 (1999).

51. Cheung, A. L., Chien, Y. T. & Bayer, A. S. Hyperproduction of alpha-hemolysin in a sigB mutant is associated with elevated SarA expression in Staphylococcus aureus. *Infection & Immunity* **67**, 1331–1337 (1999).

52. Deora, R., Tseng, T. & Misra, T. K. Alternative transcription factor sigmaSB of Staphylococcus aureus: characterization and role in transcription of the global regulatory locus sar. *Journal of Bacteriology* **179**, 6355–6359 (1997).

53. Miyazaki, E., Chen, J. M., Ko, C. & Bishai, W. R. The Staphylococcus aureus rsbW (orf159) gene encodes an anti-sigma factor of SigB. *Journal of Bacteriology* **181**, 2846–2851 (1999).

54. Manna, A. C., Bayer, M. G. & Cheung, A. L. Transcriptional analysis of different promoters in the sar locus in Staphylococcus aureus. *Journal of Bacteriology* **180**, 3828–3836 (1998).

55. Giraudo, A. T., Raspanti, C. G., Calzolari, A. & Nagel, R. Characterization of a Tn551-mutant of Staphylococcus aureus defective in the production of several exoproteins. *Canadian Journal of Microbiology* **40**, 677–681 (1994).

56. Chan, P. F. & Foster, S. J. The role of environmental factors in the regulation of virulence-determinant expression in Staphylococcus aureus 8325–4. *Microbiology* **144**, 2469–2479 (1998).

57. Regassa, L. B. & Betley, M. J. High sodium chloride concentrations inhibit staphylococcal enterotoxin C gene (sec) expression at the level of sec mRNA. *Infection & Immunity* **61**, 1581–1585 (1993).

58. Regassa, L. B., Novick, R. P. & Betley, M. J. Glucose and nonmaintained pH decrease expression of the accessory gene regulator (agr) in Staphylococcus aureus. *Infection & Immunity* **60**, 3381–3388 (1992).

59. Gemmel, C. G. & Shibl, A. M. A. The control of toxin and enzyme biosynthesis instaphylococci by antibiotics. in *Staphylococci and Staphylococcal Diseases* (ed. Jeljaszewicz, J.) (Gustav Fisher Verlag, Stuggart, 1976).

60. Ohlsen, K. *et al.* Effects of subinhibitory concentrations of antibiotics on alpha-toxin (hla) gene expression of methicillin-sensitive and methicillin-resistant Staphylococcus aureus isolates. *Antimicrobial Agents & Chemotherapy* **42**, 2817–2823 (1998).

61. Bisognano, C., Vaudaux, P. E., Lew, D. P., Ng, E. Y. & Hooper, D. C. Increased expression of fibronectin-binding proteins by fluoroquinolone-resistant Staphylococcus aureus exposed to subinhibitory levels of ciprofloxacin. *Antimicrobial Agents & Chemotherapy* **41**, 906–913 (1997).

62. Chan, P. F., Foster, S. J., Ingham, E. & Clements, M. O. The Staphylococcus aureus alternative sigma factor sigmaB controls the environmental stress response but not starvation survival or pathogenicity in a mouse abscess model. *Journal of Bacteriology* **180**, 6082–6089 (1998).

63. Kullik, I. & Giachino, P. The alternative sigma factor sigmaB in Staphylococcus aureus: regulation of the sigB operon in response to growth phase and heat shock. *Archives of Microbiology* **167**, 151–159 (1997).

64. Kullik, I., Giachino, P. & Fuchs, T. Deletion of the alternative sigma factor sigmaB in Staphylococcus aureus reveals its function as a global regulator of virulence genes. *Journal of Bacteriology* **180**, 4814–4820 (1998).

65. Cheung, A. L., Nast, C. C. & Bayer, A. S. Selective activation of sar promoters with the use of green fluorescent protein transcriptional fusions as the detection system in the rabbit endocarditis model. *Infection & Immunity* **66**, 5988–5993 (1998).

66. Cheung, A. L. *et al.* Diminished virulence of a sar-/agr-mutant of Staphylococcus aureus in the rabbit model of endocarditis. *Journal of Clinical Investigation* **94**, 1815–1822 (1994).

67. Giese, M. J., Berliner, J. A., Riesner, A., Wagar, E. A. & Mondino, B. J. A comparison of the early inflammatory effects of an agr-/sar-versus a wild type strain of Staphylococcus aureus in a rat model of endophthalmitis. *Current Eye Research* **18**, 177–185 (1999).

68. Booth, M. C., Atkuri, R. V., Nanda, S. K., Iandolo, J. J. & Gilmore, M. S. Accessory gene regulator controls Staphylococcus aureus virulence in endophthalmitis. *Investigative Ophthalmology & Visual Science* **36**, 1828–1836 (1995).

69. Booth, M. C. *et al.* Staphylococcal accessory regulator (sar) in conjunction with agr contributes to Staphylococcus aureus virulence in endophthalmitis. *Infection & Immunity* **65**, 1550–1556 (1997).

70. Abdelnour, A., Arvidson, S., Bremell, T., Ryden, C. & Tarkowski, A. The accessory gene regulator (agr) controls Staphylococcus aureus virulence in a murine arthritis model. *Infection & Immunity* **61**, 3879–3885 (1993).

71. Nilsson, I. M., Bremell, T., Ryden, C., Cheung, A. L. & Tarkowski, A. Role of the staphylococcal accessory gene regulator (sar) in septic arthritis. *Infection & Immunity* **64**, 4438–4443 (1996).

72. Gillaspy, A. F. *et al.* Role of the accessory gene regulator (agr) in pathogenesis of staphylococcal osteomyelitis. *Infection & Immunity* **63**, 3373–3380 (1995).

73. Durack, D. T. & Beeson, P. B. Pathogenesis of infective endocarditis. in *Infective Endocarditis* (ed. Rahimtoola, S. H.) (Grune and Stratton, Inc., New York, 1980).

74. Nicholas, R. O. *et al.* Isolation and characterization of a sigB deletion mutant of Staphylococcus aureus. *Infection & Immunity* **67**, 3667–3669 (1999).

75. Proctor, R. A. & Peters, G. Small colony variants in staphylococcal infections: diagnostic and therapeutic implications. *Clinical Infectious Diseases* **27**, 419–422 (1998).

76. Calhoun, J. H. *et al.* Treatment of diabetic foot infections: Wagner classification, therapy, and outcome. *Foot & Ankle* **9**, 101–106 (1988).

77. Albus, A. *et al.* Staphylococcus aureus capsular types and antibody response to lung infection in patients with cystic fibrosis. *Journal of Clinical Microbiology* **26**, 2505–2509 (1988).

78. May, J. R., Herrick, N. C. & Thompson, D. Bacterial infection in cystic fibrosis. *Archives of Disease in Childhood* **47**, 908–913 (1972).

79. Menzies, B. E. & Kourteva, I. Internalization of Staphylococcus aureus by endothelial cells induces apoptosis. *Infection & Immunity* **66**, 5994–5998 (1998).

80. Wesson, C. A. *et al.* Staphylococcus aureus Agr and Sar global regulators influence internalization and induction of apoptosis. *Infection & Immunity* **66**, 5238–5243 (1998).

81. Weinrauch, Y. & Zychlinsky, A. The induction of apoptosis by bacterial pathogens. *Annual Review of Microbiology* **53**, 155–187 (1999).

82. Yankaskas, J. R. *et al.* Papilloma virus immortalized tracheal epithelial cells retain a well-differentiated phenotype. *American Journal of Physiology* **264**, C1219–1230 (1993).

Index

Keep Your
Brain
Fit

KEEP YOUR BRAIN FIT

Puzzle text and content © 2000 British Mensa Limited
Introduction text, book design and artwork © 2007 Carlton Books Limited

Published by
Thunders Mouth Press
An Imprint of Avalon Publishing Group Incorporated
245 West 17th Street • 11th Floor
New York, NY 10011-5300

Library of Congress Cataloging-in-Publication data is available

ISBN-10: 1-56858-351-6
ISBN-13: 978-1-56858-351-8

10 9 8 7 6 5 4 3 2 1

Printed in Dubai
Distributed by Publishers Group West

Keep Your
Brain
Fit

THUNDER'S
MOUTH
PRESS

PUZZLE SYMBOLS

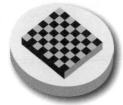

Logical
thinking

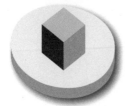

Spatial
awareness

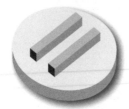

Pattern
recognition

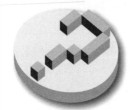

Deduction

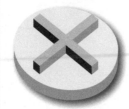

Numerical
awareness

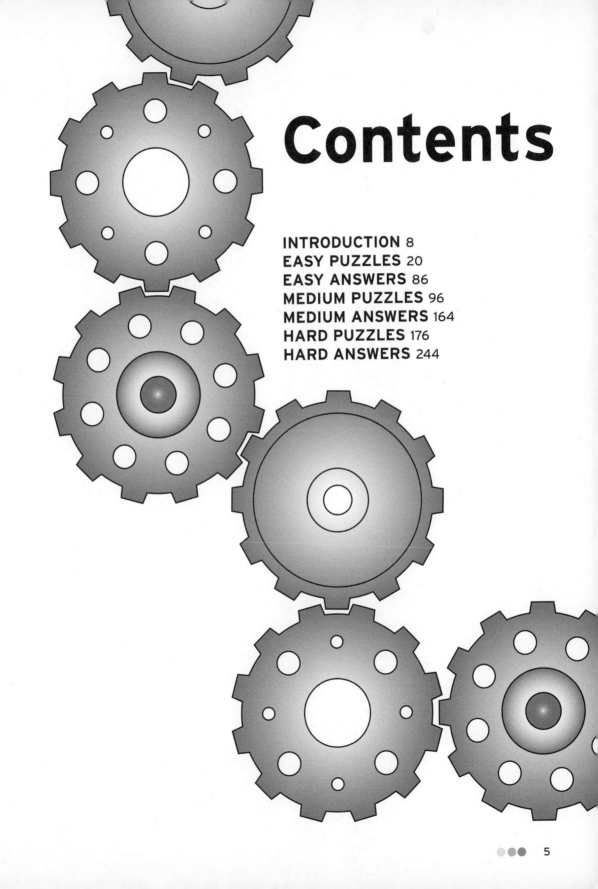

Contents

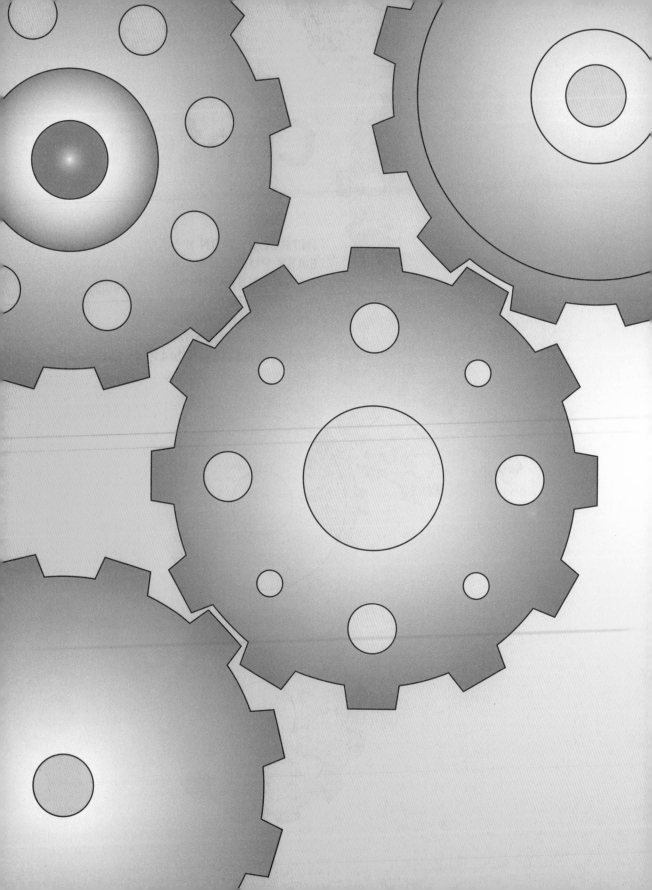

Introduction:
The Puzzle Reflex
by Tim Dedopulos

Puzzles are as old as humankind. It's inevitable – it's the way we think. Our brains make sense of the world around us by looking at the pieces that combine to make up our environment. Each piece is then compared to everything else we have encountered. We compare it by shape, size, colour, textures, a thousand different qualities, and place it into the mental categories it seems to belong to. Then also consider other nearby objects, and examine what we know about them, to give context. We keep on following this web of connections until we have enough understanding of the object of our attention to allow us to proceed in the current situation. We may never have seen a larch before, but we can still identify it as a tree. Most of the time, just basic recognition is good enough, but every time we perceive an object, it is cross-referenced, analysed, pinned down – puzzled out.

This capacity for logical analysis – for reason – is one of the greatest tools in our mental arsenal, on a par with creativity and lateral induction. Without it, science would be non-existent, and mathematics no more than a shorthand for counting items. In fact, although we might have made it out of the caves, we wouldn't have got far.

Furthermore, we automatically compare ourselves to each other – we place ourselves in mental boxes along with everything else. We like to know where we stand. It gives us an instinctive urge to compete, both against our previous bests and against each other. Experience, flexibility and strength are acquired through pushing personal boundaries, and that's as true of the mind as it is of the body. Deduction is something that we derive satisfaction and worth from, part of the complex blend of factors that goes into making up our self-image. We get a very pleasurable sense of achievement from succeeding at something, particularly if we suspected it might be too hard for us.

The brain gives meaning and structure to the world through analysis, pattern recognition, and logical deduction – and our urge to measure and test ourselves is an unavoidable reflex that results from that. So what could be more natural than spending time puzzling?

EARLY PUZZLES

The urge to solve puzzles appears to be a universal human constant. They can be found in every culture, and in every time that we have good archaeological evidence for. The earliest material uncovered so far that is indisputably a puzzle has been dated to a little after 2000BC – and the first true writing we know of only dates back to 2600BC. The puzzle text is recorded on a writing tablet, preserved from ancient Babylonia. It is a mathematical puzzle based around working out the sides of a triangle.

Other puzzles from around the same time have also been discovered. The Rhind Papyrus from ancient Egypt describes a puzzle that is almost certainly a precursor of the traditional English riddle "As I Was Going to St. Ives." In the Rhind Papyrus, a puzzle is constructed around the clearly unreal situation of seven houses, each containing seven cats – and every cat kills seven mice that themselves had each consumed seven ears of millet.

In a similar foreshadowing, a set of very early puzzle jugs – Phoenician work from around 1700BC, found in Cyprus – echo designs that were to become popular in medieval Europe. These particular jugs, belonging to a broad category known as Askoi, had to be filled from the bottom. This form of trick vessel would later become known as a Cadogan Teapot. These devices have no lid, and have to be filled through a hole in the base. Because the hole funnels to a point inside the vessel, it can be filled to about half-way without spilling when it is turned back upright.

Earlier finds do exist, but so much context is lost down through the years that it can be difficult to be certain that the creators were thinking of puzzles specifically, or just of mathematical demonstrations. A set of ancient Babylonian tablets showing geometric progressions – mathematical sequences – is thought to be from 2300BC. One of the very first mathematical finds though, thought to possibly be from as far back as 2700 BC, is a set of stone balls carved into the shapes of the Platonic solids. These are regular convex polyhedrons – three-dimensional solid shapes made up solely of identical regular polygons. The most familiar is the basic cube, made up of six squares, but there are just four others – the tetrahedron, made up of four equilateral triangles; the octahedron, made up of eight equilateral triangles; the dodecahedron, made from twelve pentagons, and the icosahedron, made of twenty equilateral triangles.

There's no way now of knowing whether the carvings were teaching aids, puzzle or game tools, demonstrations of a theory, artistic constructions or even religious icons. The fact they exist at all however shows that someone had previously spent time working out a significant abstract mathematical puzzle – discovering which regular convex polyhedrons could exist.

AMENEMHET'S LABYRINTH

One of the greatest physical puzzles ever engineered comes from the same time period. The Egyptian Pharaoh Amenemhet III constructed a funerary pyramid with a huge temple complex around it in the form of an incredible labyrinth. Designed to guard the Pharaoh's mummy and treasures from disturbance or robbery, the labyrinth was so lavish and cunning that it is said to have been both the inspiration and template for the famous labyrinth that Daedalus built at Knossos for King Minos of Crete – the one that supposedly contained the Minotaur.

PUZZLE HISTORY

Coming forward in time, the evidence for the variety and complexity of puzzles gets ever stronger – an inevitable fact of archaeological and historical research. Greek legend claims that numbered dice were invented at the siege of Troy around 1200BC. We know that there was a craze for lateral thinking puzzles and logical dilemmas in the Greek culture from the 5th to 3rd centuries BC. A lot of very important mathematical work also took place in Greece from the middle of the first millennium BC, moving across to Rome during the first centuries AD. At the same time, the Chinese were playing with numerical puzzles and oddities, most famously the magic square, which they called *Lo Shu* (River Map), and also doing more strong mathematical work.

Puzzles and puzzle-like games that survive through to modern times get more common as we get closer to modern times, naturally. The game of Go arose in China some time around 500 BC, spreading to Japan a thousand years later – it is still an important sport there. At the same time, Chess was first appearing, either in India (*Chaturanga*), China (*Xiang-qi*), or both. Puzzle rings that you have to find out how to separate also appeared in China, possibly in the 3rd century AD, as did Snakes & Ladders, around 700AD.

The first known reference to a game played with cards is in 969AD, in records reporting the activities of the Chinese Emperor Mu-tsung. These are not thought to be the playing cards now familiar in the west, however – it seems likely that those arose in Persia during the 11th or 12th century AD. The physical puzzle Solitaire is first reported in 1697AD. As the eighteenth century gave way to the nineteenth, the forces of the industrial revolution really started to transform the way that ideas propagated, and the puzzle world exploded. Some of the more notable highlights include the invention of the jigsaw puzzle by John Spilsbury in 1767; Tic-Tac-Toe's first formal discussion in 1820, by Charles Babbage; poker first appearing around 1830 in the USA; Lucas inventing the Tower of Hanoi puzzle in 1883; the first crossword appearing in New York World on December 21, 1913, created by Arthur Wynne; Erno Rubik's invention of his Cube in 1974; and the invention of Sudoku in 1979 for Dell Magazines by Howard Garns, an American, who first called it "Number Place".

PLASTICITY

It turns out that it's a good thing puzzles are such an important part of the human psyche. Recent advances in the scientific fields of neurology and cognitive psychology have hammered home the significance of puzzles and mental exercise like never before.

We now understand that the brain continually builds, shapes and organises itself all through our lives. It is the only organ to be able to do so. Previously, we had assumed that the brain was constructed to optimise infant development, but the truth is that it continually rewrites its own operating instructions. It can route around physical damage, maximise its efficiency in dealing with commonly encountered situations and procedures, and alter its very structure in response to our experiences. This incredible flexibility is referred to as plasticity.

The most important implication of plasticity is that our mental abilities and cognitive fitness can be exercised at any age. Just like the muscles of the body, our minds can respond to exercise, allowing us to be more retentive and mentally fitter. Our early lives are the most important time, of course. Infants develop almost twice as many synapses

– the mental connections that are the building-blocks of the mind – as we retain as adults, to make sure that every experience can be learnt from and given its own space in the developing mental structure. The first thirty-six months are particularly vital, the ones which will shape the patterns of our intellect, character and socialisation for life. A good education through to adulthood – stretching the brain right through childhood – is one of the strongest indicators of late-life mental health, particularly when followed with a mentally challenging working life.

Just as importantly however, there is little difference between the brain at the age of 25 and the age of 75. As time passes, the brain optimises itself for the lifestyle we feed it. Circuits that are hardly ever used get re-adapted to offer greater efficiency in tasks we regularly use. Just as our body maximises available energy by removing muscle we don't use, the brain removes mental tone we're never stretching – and in the same way that working out can build up muscle, so mental exercise can restore a "fit" mind.

PUZZLE SOLVING AND BRAIN GROWTH

A surprising amount of mental decline in elders is now thought to be down to insufficient mental exercise. Where severe mental decline occurs, it is usually linked to the tissue damage of Alzheimer's Disease – although there is now even evidence that strong mental exercise lets the brain route around even Alzheimer's damage, lessening impairment. In other cases, where there is no organic damage, the main cause is disuse. Despite old assumptions, we do not significantly lose huge swathes of brain cells as we age. Better still, mental strength that has been allowed to atrophy may be rebuilt.

Research projects across the world have discovered strong patterns linking highly lucid venerable people. These include above-average education, acceptance of change, satisfying personal accomplishments, physical exercise, a clever spouse, and a strong engagement with life, including reading, social activity, travel, keeping up with new ideas, and regularly solving puzzles. Not all the things we assume to be engagement are actually helpful, however. Useful intellectual pursuits are the actively stimulating ones – such as solving jigsaws, crosswords and other puzzles, playing chess, and reading books that stimulate the imagination or require some mental effort to properly digest. However, passive intellectual pursuits may actually hasten the mind's decay. Watching television is the most damaging such pastime, but surprisingly anything that makes you "switch off" mentally can also be harmful, such as listening to certain types of music, reading very low-content magazines and even getting most of your social exposure on the telephone. For social interaction to be helpful, it may really need to be face to face.

THE COLUMBIA STUDY

A team of researchers from Columbia University in New York tracked more than 1,750 pensioners from the northern Manhattan region over a period of seven years. The subjects underwent periodic medical and psychological examination to assess both their mental health and the physical condition of their brains. Participants also provided the researchers with detailed information regarding their daily activities. The study found that even when you remove education and career attainment from the equation, leisure activity significantly reduced the risk of dementia.

The study's author, Dr Yaakov Stern, found that "Even when controlling for factors like ethnic group, education and occupation, subjects with high leisure activity had 38% less risk of developing dementia." Activities were broken into three categories: physical, social and intellectual. Each one was found to be beneficial, but the greatest protection came from intellectual pursuits. The more activity, the greater the protection – the cumulative benefit of each separate leisure pursuit was found to be 8%. Stern also found that leisure activity helped to prevent the physical damage caused by Alzheimer's from actually manifesting as dementia:

> "Our study suggests that aspects of life experience supply a set of skills or repertoires that allow an individual to cope with progressing Alzheimer's Disease pathology for a longer time before the disease becomes clinically apparent. Maintaining intellectual and social engagement through participation in everyday activities seems to buffer healthy individuals against cognitive decline in later life."

STAYING LUCID

There is strong evidence to back Stern's conclusion. Dr David Bennett of the Rush Alzheimer's Disease Centre in Chicago led a study that evaluated a group of venerable participants on a yearly basis, and then after death examined their donated brains for signs of Alzheimer's. The participants all led active lives mentally, socially and physically, and none of them suffered from dementia at the time of their death. It was

discovered that more than a third of the participants had sufficient brain-tissue damage to warrant diagnosis of Alzheimer's Disease, including serious lesions in the brain tissue. This group *had* recorded lower scores than other participants in episodic memory tests – remembering story episodes, for example – but performed identically in cognitive function and reasoning tests. A similar study took place with the aid of the nuns of the Order of the School Sisters of Notre Dame. The Order boasts a long average lifespan – 85 years – and came to the attention of researchers when it became clear that its members did not seem to suffer from any dementia either. The distinguishing key about the Order is that the nuns shun idleness and mental vacuity, taking particular effort to remain mentally active. All sorts of pursuits are encouraged, such as solving puzzles, playing challenging games, writing, holding seminars on current affairs, knitting and engaging with local government. As before, there was plenty of evidence of the physical damage associated with Alzheimer's Disease, but none of the mental damage that usually accompanied it, even in some nonagenarian participants.

MENTAL REPAIR

Other studies have also tried to enumerate the benefits of mental activity. A massive group study led by Michael Valenzuela from the University of New South Wales' School of Psychiatry tracked data from almost 30,000 people worldwide. The results were clear – as well as indicating the same clear relationship previously found between schooling, career and mental health, people of all backgrounds whose daily lives include a high degree of mental stimulation are 46% less likely to suffer dementia. This holds true even for people who take up mentally challenging activities as they get older – if you use your mind, the brain still adapts to protect it. If you do not use it, the brain lets it falter.

PUZZLE SOLVING TECHNIQUES

Puzzle solving is more of an art than a science. It requires mental flexibility, a little understanding of the underlying principles and possibilities, and sometimes a little intuition. It is often said of crosswords that you have to learn the writer's style to get really good at his or her puzzles, but the same thing applies to most other puzzle types to a certain extent, and that includes the many and various kinds you'll find in this book.

SEQUENCE PUZZLES

Sequence puzzles challenge you to find a missing value or item, or to complete a pattern according to the correct underlying design. In this type of puzzle, you are provided with enough previous entries in the sequence that the underlying logic can be worked out. Once the sequence is understood, the missing entry can be calculated. When the patterns are simple, the sequence will be readily visible to the naked eye. It is not hard to figure out that the next term in the sequence 1, 2, 4, 8, 16, ? is going to be a further doubling to 32. Numerical sequences are just the expression of a mathematical formula however, and can therefore get almost infinitely complex.

Proper recreational puzzles stay firmly within the bounds of human ability, of course. With the more complex puzzles, the best approach is often to calculate the differences between successive terms) in the sequences, and look for patterns in the way that those differences are changing. You should also be aware that in some puzzles, the terms of a sequence may not necessarily represent single items. Different parts or digits of each term may progress according to different calculations. For example, the sequence 921, 642, 383, 164 is actually three simple sequences stuck together - 9, 6, 2, 0 ; 2, 4, 8, 16; and 1, 2, 3, 4. The next term will be - 3325. Alternatively, in puzzles where the sequence terms are given as times, they may actually just represent the times they depict, but they might also be literal numbers, or pairs of numbers to be treated as totally different sequences, or even require conversion from hours: minutes to just minutes before the sequence becomes apparent.

For example, 11:14 in a puzzle might represent the time 11:14, or perhaps the time 23:14 - or the numbers 11 and 14, the numbers 23 and 14, the number 1114, the number 2314, or even the number 674 (11 * 60 minutes, with the remaining 14 minutes also added). As you can see, solving sequence puzzles requires a certain amount of trial and error as you test difference possibilities, as well as a degree of lateral thinking. It would be a very harsh puzzle setter who expected you to guess some sort of sequence out of context however. So in the absence of a clue

otherwise, 11:14 would be highly unlikely to represent 11 months and 14 days, or the value 11 in base 14, or even 11 hours and 14 minutes converted to seconds - unless it was given as 11:14:00, of course.

Letter-based sequences are all representational of course, as unlike numbers, letters have no underlying structure save as symbols. Once you deduce what the letters represent, the answer can be obvious. The sequence D, N, O, ? may seem abstract, until you think of months of the year in reverse order.

In visual sequences - such as pattern grids - the sequence will always be there for you to see, and your task is to look for repeating patterns. As with number sequences, easy grids can be immediately apparent. In harder puzzles, the sequences can become significantly long, and often be presented in ways that make them difficult to identify. Puzzle setters love to start grids of this type from the bottom right-hand square, and then progress in spirals or in a back-and-forth pattern - sometimes even diagonally.

Odd-one-out problems are a specialised case of sequence pattern where you are given the elements of a sequence or related set, along with one item that breaks the sequence. Like other sequence puzzles, these can range from very easy to the near-impossible. Spotting the odd one in 2, 4, 6, 7, 8 is trivial. It would be almost impossible to guess the odd item from the set of B, F,

H, N, O unless you already knew that the set in question was the physical elements on the second row of the standard periodic table. Even then, you might need a copy of the periodic table itself to notice that hydrogen, H, is on the first row. As with any other sequence problem, any odd-one-out should contain enough information in the puzzle, accompanying text and title to set the context for finding the correct answer. In the above case, a puzzle title along the lines of "An Elementary Puzzle" would probably be sufficient to make it fair game.

EQUATION PUZZLES

Equation puzzles are similar to sequences, but require a slightly different methodology. In these problems, you are given a set of mathematical calculations that contain one or more unknown terms. These may be represented as equations, as in the traditional form of $2x + 3y = 9$, or they may be presented visually, for example as two anvils and three iron bars on one side of a scale and nine horseshoes balancing on the other side of the scale. For each Unknown - x, y, anvils, etc - you need one equation or other set of values before you can calculate a definitive answer. If these are lacking, you cannot get the problem down to just one possible solution. Take the equation above, $2x + 3y = 9$. There are two unknowns, and therefore many

answers. For example, x can be 3 and y can be 1 - for x, 2 * 3 = 6; for y, 3 * 1 = 3, and overall, 6 + 3 = 9 - but x can also be 1.5 and y can be 2... and an infinite range of other possibilities. So when solving equation puzzles, you need to consider all the equations together before you can solve the problem.

To return to our example equation above, if you *also* knew that $x + 2y = 7$, you could then begin to solve the puzzle. The key with equation problems is to get your equation down to containing just one unknown term, which then lets you get a value for that term, and in turn lets you get the value of the other unknown/s. So, for example, in our previous equations ($2x + 3y = 9$ and $x + 2y = 7$) you could manipulate one equation to work out what x actually represents in terms of y ("How many Y is each X?") in one equation, and then replace the x in the other equation with it's value in y, to get a calculation that just has y as the sole unknown factor. It's not as confusing as it sounds so long as you take it step by step:

We know that

$x + 2y = 7$

Any change made to both sides of an equation balances out, and so doesn't change the truth of the equation. For example, consider 2 + 2 = 4. If you add 1 to each side, the equation is still true. That is, 2 + 2 + 1 = 4 + 1. We can use this cancelling out to get x and y on opposite sides of the equation, which will let us represent x in terms of y:

x + 2y - 2y = 7 - 2y.

Now the + 2y - 2y cancels out:

x = 7 - 2y.

Now we know x is a way of saying "7-2y", we can replace it in the other equation.

2x + 3y = 9 becomes:

2 * (7 - 2y) + 3y = 9.

Note 2x means that x is in the equation twice, so our way of re-writing x as y needs to be doubled to stay accurate. Expanding that out:

(2 * 7) - (2 * 2y) + 3y = 9, or

14 - 4y + 3y = 9.

The next step is to get just amounts of y on one side, and numbers on the other.

14 - 4y + 3y - 14 = 9 - 14.

In other words,

-4y + 3y = -5.

Now, -4 + 3 is -1, so:

-y = -5, and that means y=5.

Now you can go back to the first equation, x + 2y = 7, and replace y to find x.

x + (2 * 5) = 7

x + 10 = 7

x + 10 - 10 = 7 - 10

x = 7 - 10

and, finally.

x = -3.

As a last step, test your equations by replacing your number values for x and y in both at the same time, and making sure they balance correctly.

2x + 3y = 9 and x + 2y = 7.

(2 * -3) + (3 * 5) = 9 and -3 + (2 * 5) = 7

(-6 + 15) = 9; and (-3 + 10) = 7.

9 = 9 and 7 = 7.

The answers are correct.

Any equation-based puzzle you're presented with will contain enough information for you to work out the solution. If more than two terms are unknown, the technique is to use one equation to find one unknown as a value of the others, and then replace it in all the other equations. That gives you a new set of equations containing one less unknown term. You then repeat the process of working out an unknown again, until you finally get down to one unknown term and its numerical value. Then you replace the term you now know with its value in the equations for the level above to get the next term, and continue back on up like that. It's like a mathematical version of the old wooden Towers of Hanoi puzzle. As a final tip, remember that you should have one equation per unknown term, and that if one of your unknown variables is missing from an equation, the equation can be said to have 0 of that variable on either or both sides. That is, 4y + 2z = 8 is the same as 0x + 4y + 2z = 8.

Happy puzzling!

REFERENCES

Chronology of Recreational Mathematics; David Singmaster; http://www.eldar.org/~problemi/singmast/recchron.html

Pythagoras's theorem in Babylonian mathematics; J J O'Connor and E F Robertson; http://www-history.mcs.st-andrews.ac.uk/HistTopics/Babylonian_Pythagoras.html

The Rhind Mathematical Papyrus; http://en.wikipedia.org/wiki/Rhind_Mathematical_Papyrus

Puzzle Jug; http://en.wikipedia.org/wiki/Puzzle_jug

The Egyptian Labyrinth; http://www.amazeingart.com/seven-wonders/egyptian-labyrinth.html

The Ancient Egyptian Labyrinth; http://www.catchpenny.org/labyrin.html

Alzheimer's: Prevention, Treatment, and Slowing Down; Doug Russell, Jeanne Segal and Monika White; http://www.helpguide.org/elder/alzheimers_prevention_slowing_down_treatment.htm

The Human Brain; http://www.fi.edu/brain/exercise.htm

Power Up Your Brain; Terri Needels & Toby Bilanow; http://health.msn.com/guides/agingwell/articlepage.aspx?cp-documentid=100143902

Keeping Your Brain Fit For Life; Katherine Kam; http://www.positscience.com/newsroom/news/news/111406.php

Preliminary Results from PopCap Games and Games for Health; Peter Smith; http://www.gamesforhealth.org/archives/000125.html

Older Game Players Derive Mental Workouts, Stress Relief and Pain Distraction from Playing; Garth Chouteau; http://www.popcap.com/press/index.php?page=press_releases&release=survey_seniors_10-4-06

Complex Brain Circuits May Protect Against Alzheimer's; Susan Conova; http://www.cumc.columbia.edu/news/in-vivo/Vol3_Iss11_nov_dec_04/index.html

Use It or Lose It?; Beth Azar; http://www.apa.org/monitor/may02/useit.html

Fight Alzheimer's With an Active Brain; http://www.msnbc.msn.com/id/8292945

Want a Sharp Mind for your Golden Years? Start Now; Marilyn Elias; http://www.bri.ucla.edu/bri_weekly/news_050818.asp

How to Prevent Alzheimer's; http://www. sixwise.com/newsletters/05/08/24/how_to_ prevent_alzheimers_the_most_effective_ ways_to_avoid_this_rapidly_increasing_ disease.htm

Lifestyle May Be Key to Slowing Brain's Aging; Rob Stein; http://www.washingtonpost. com/wp-dyn/content/article/2005/08/13/ AR2005081300855.html

Disorder May Precede Alzheimer's; John Fauber; http://www.findarticles.com/p/ articles/mi_qn4196/is_20050308/ai_ n12411071

Mental Activities May Reduce Alzheimer's Risk; http://www.kirotv.com/health/1232090/ detail.html

Brain Savers; A. J. Mann; http:// www.time.com/time/magazine/ article/0,9171,1002535,00. html?internalid=ACA

Building a Better Brain; Daniel Golden & Alexander Tsiaras; http://www. enchantedmind.com/html/science/build_ better_brain.html

The Nuns Who Won't Sit Still; Marge Engelmann; http://www.agenet.com/ Category_Pages/document_display. asp?Id=12561&

Mental Exercise Nearly Halves Risk of Dementia; http://www.livescience.com/ humanbiology/060125_delay_dementia.html

Use Your Brain, Halve Your Risk of Dementia; Susi Hamilton; http://www. unsw.edu.au/news/pad/articles/2006/jan/ Dementia_brain_reserve.html

14-Day Health Plan Improves Memory; http://www.livescience.com/ humanbiology/051213_memory_exercise.html

The Happiness Manifesto; http://www. uofapain.med.ualberta.ca/documents/ manifesto1.pdf

Can We Live Happily Ever After?; Ron Horvath; http://www.australianreview.net/ digest/2006/10/horvath.html

Simple Lifestyle Changes May Improve Cognitive Function; http://www.news-medical. net/?id=18102

Effects of Self-Esteem on Age-Related Changes in Cognition; Sonia Lupien, Jens Pruessner, Catherine Lord and Michael Meaney; http://www.annalsnyas.org/cgi/ content/full/1032/1/186

Low Self-Esteem 'Shrinks Brain'; Pallab Ghosh; http://news.bbc.co.uk/2/hi/ health/3224674.stm

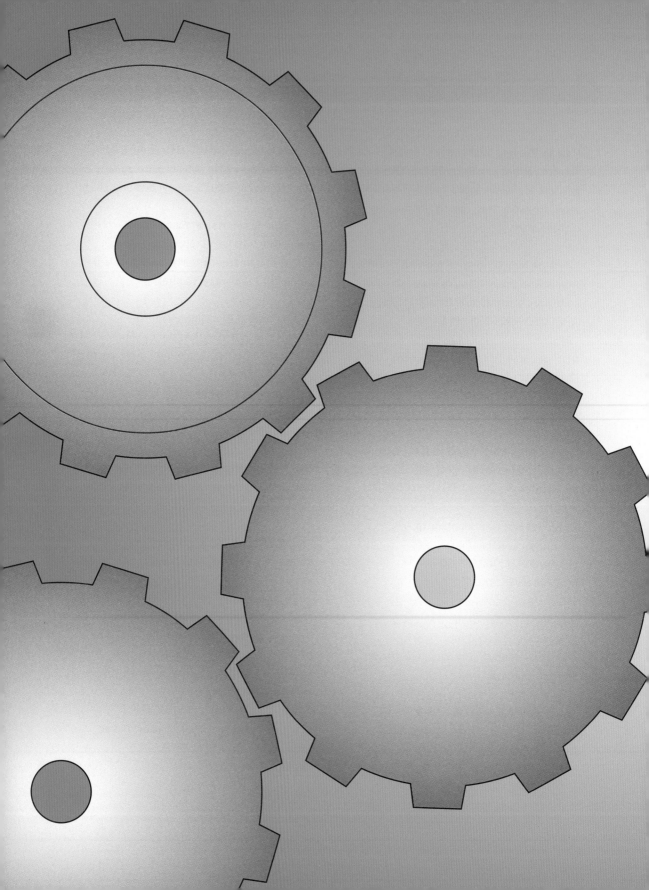

Easy Puzzles

If solving puzzles is a pleasurable activity – and all the evidence that we have suggests that it most certainly is – then this is the section that will let you sharpen your knife in preparation for the feast. The puzzles here represent the same types of problem that you'll find throughout this book. They'll certainly get you thinking, but not too hard – the answers to these problems are reassuringly straightforward, and you may find that many of them are readily apparent.

Don't get complacent, however. As well as warming up your mind for the challenges to come, this section also gives you an important chance to get used to the way that the puzzles work. You'll start to get a feeling for the way that the puzzle authors are thinking, and you'll also pick up a good intuitive grounding in the particular vagaries of the different puzzle types.

If you're new to puzzles, then it's probably going to be best for you to work your way through this entire section before moving on to the next one. Get a firm victory under your belt – and remember to pat yourself on the back – before moving on to some of the harsher problems. If you're more experienced in the ways of puzzling, you might prefer to dip into this section to warm yourself up, starting each of your puzzle sessions with a few of the problems here to get your brain in gear.

Whichever way you approach these problems however, remember one critical thing – to have fun!

PUZZLE 1

Which of these groups of triangles is the odd one out?

Answer see page **88**

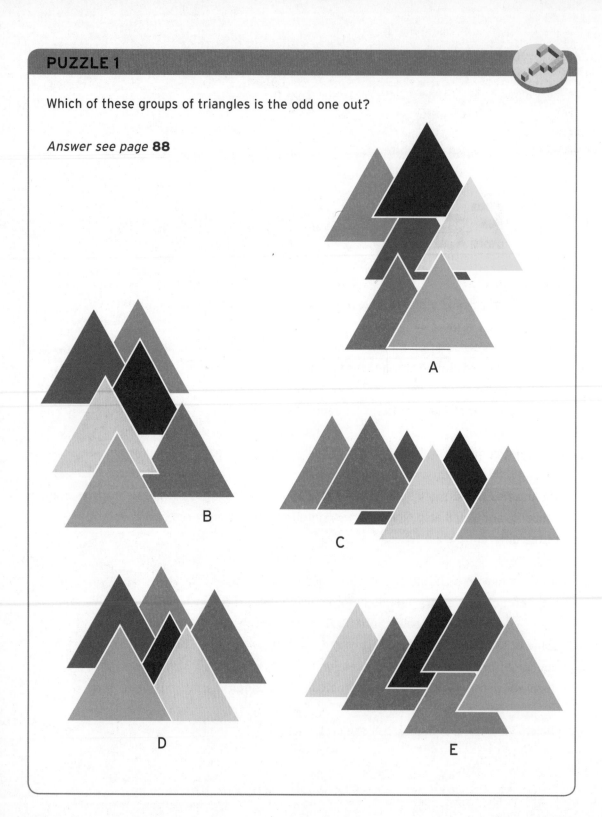

A

B

C

D

E

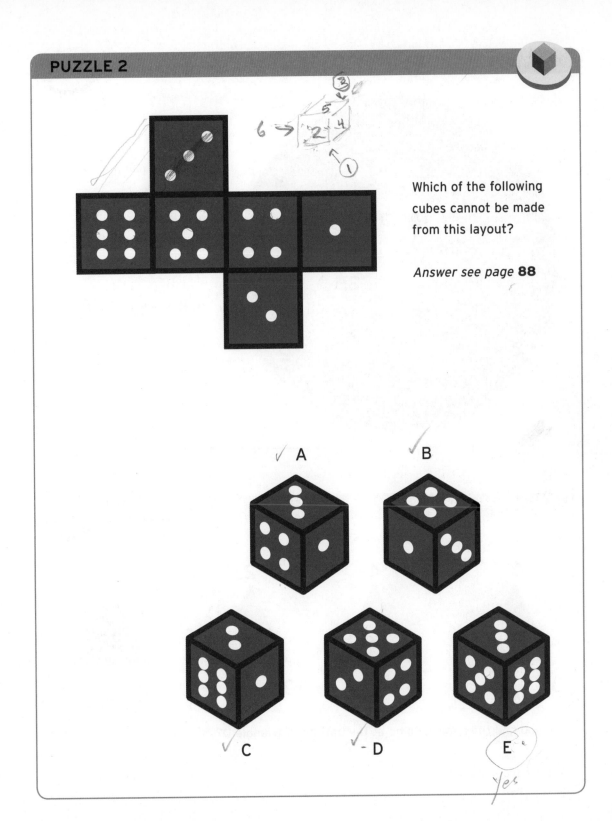

Which of the following cubes cannot be made from this layout?

Answer see page **88**

A

B

C

D

E

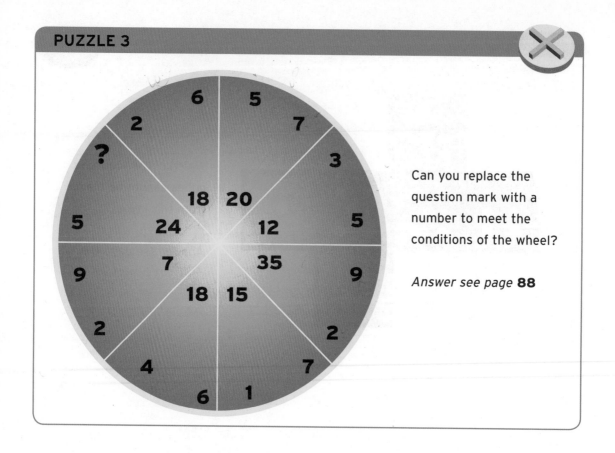

Can you replace the question mark with a number to meet the conditions of the wheel?

*Answer see page **88***

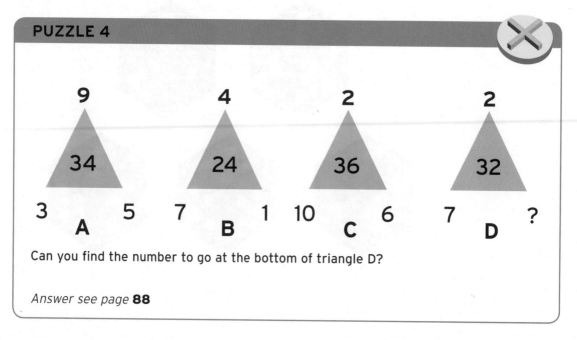

Can you find the number to go at the bottom of triangle D?

*Answer see page **88***

This diagram was constructed according to a certain logic. Can you work out what number should replace the question mark?

Answer see page **88**

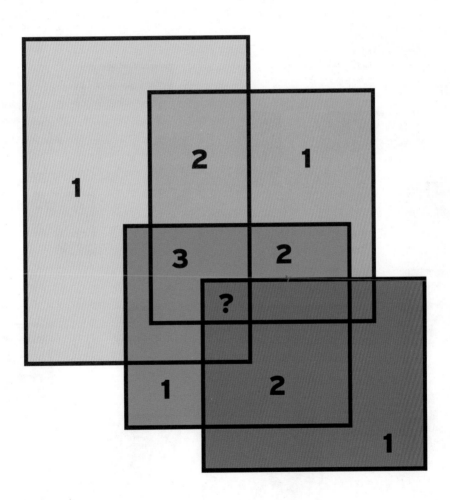

These tiles, when placed in the right order, will form a square in which the first horizontal line is identical with the first vertical line and so on. Can you successfully form the square?

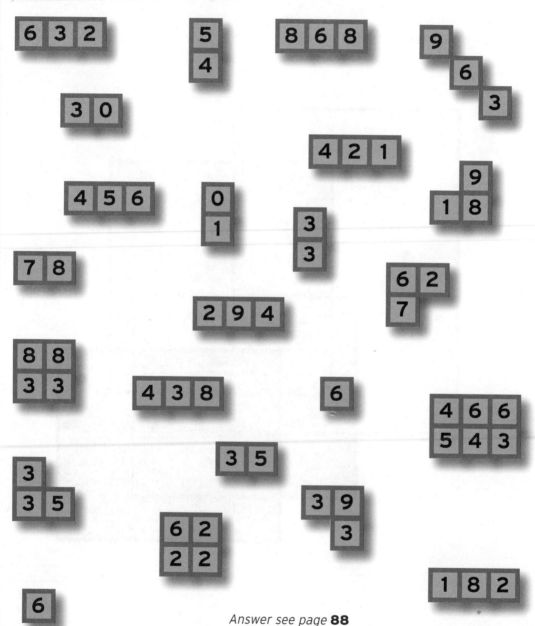

Answer see page **88**

PUZZLE 7

Can you work out how the numbers in the triangles are related and find the missing number?

Answer see page **88**

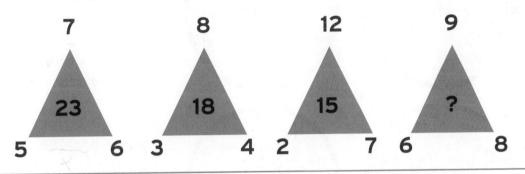

PUZZLE 8

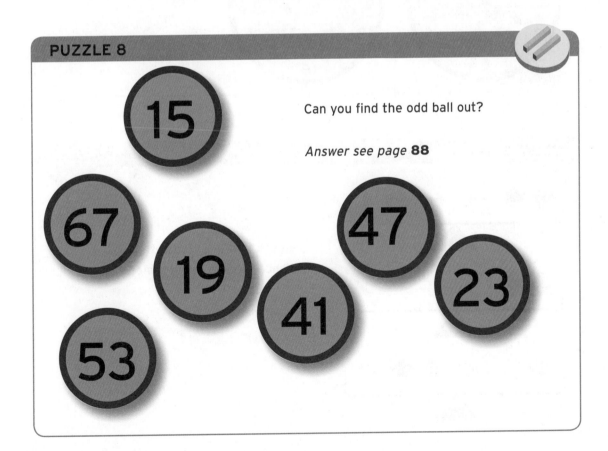

Can you find the odd ball out?

Answer see page **88**

1

2

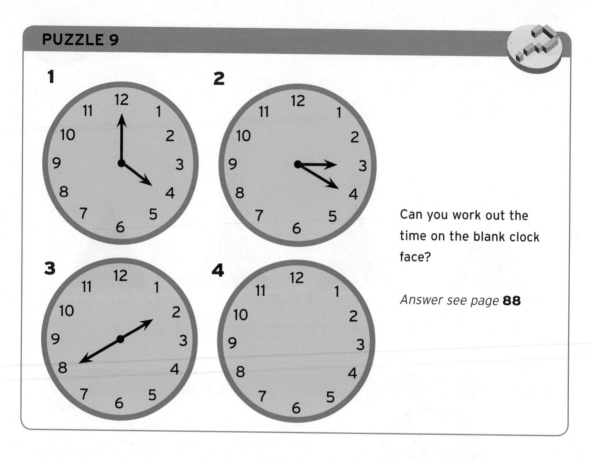

Can you work out the time on the blank clock face?

Answer see page **88**

3

4

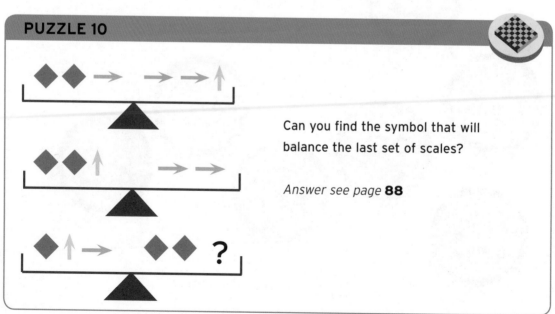

Can you find the symbol that will balance the last set of scales?

Answer see page **88**

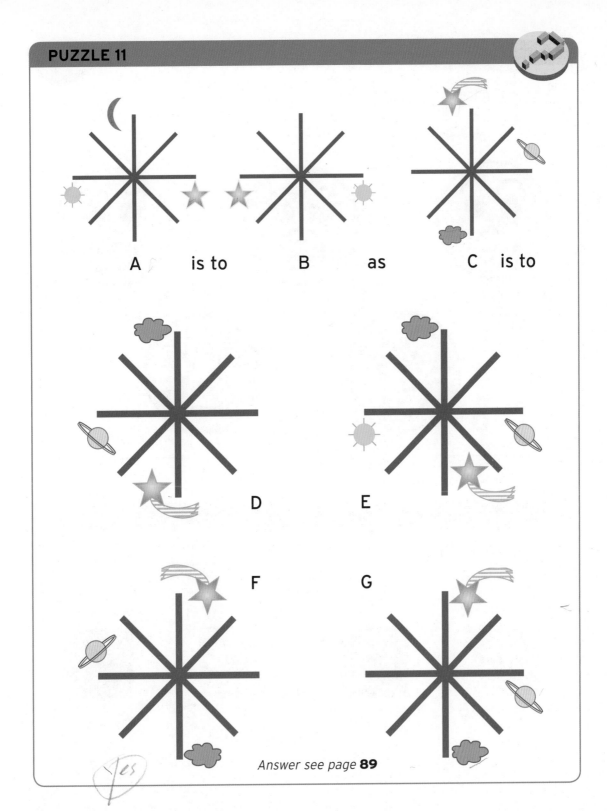

A   is to   B   as   C   is to

D

E

F

G

Answer see page **89**

PUZZLE 12

Can you find the odd face out?

Answer see page **89**

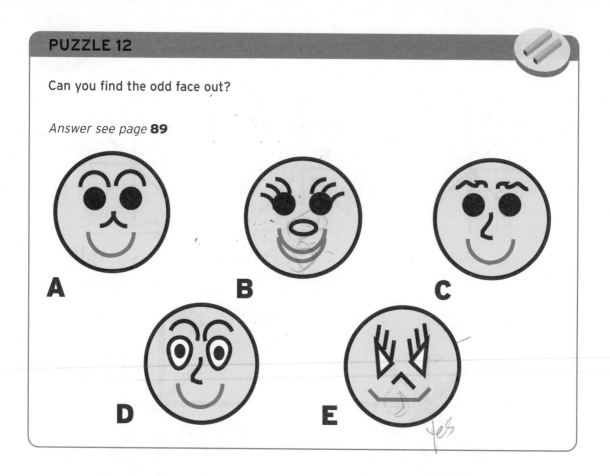

A

B

C

D

E

PUZZLE 13

Find the missing number.

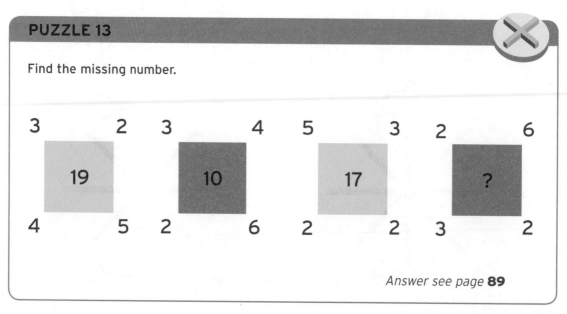

3	2	3	4	5	3	2	6
	19		10		17		?
4	5	2	6	2	2	3	2

Answer see page **89**

PUZZLE 14

Which matchstick man, G, H or I, would carry on the sequence?

Answer see page **89**

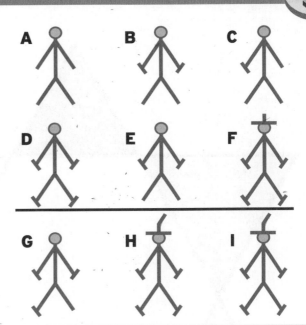

PUZZLE 15

 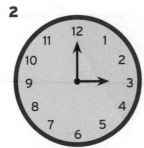

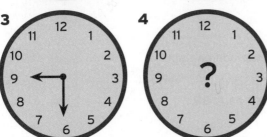

These clocks move in a certain pattern. Can you work out the time on the last clock?

Answer see page **89**

Which color is the odd one out?

Answer see page **89**

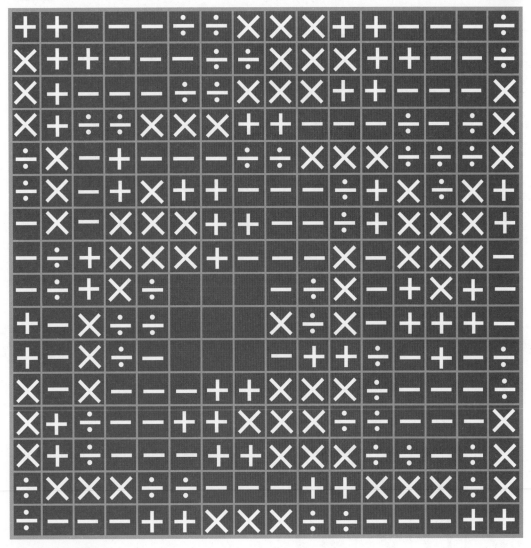

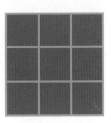

The symbols in the above grid follow a pattern. Can you work it out and find the missing section so that the logic of the grid is restored?

Answer see page **89**

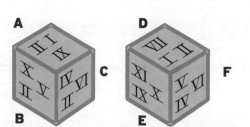

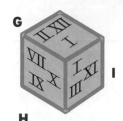

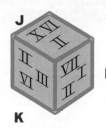

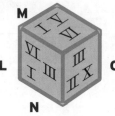

Can you work out which two sides on these cubes contain the same numbers?

Answer see page 89

24	63	24	21

✳	✳	✳	✓	33
✓	O	✓	‡	?
‡	O	‡	‡	33
✓	✓	✓	✳	27

Each symbol in this square represents a value. Can you work out how much the question mark is worth?

Answer see page 89

Two sides of these cubes contain the same
letters. Can you spot them?

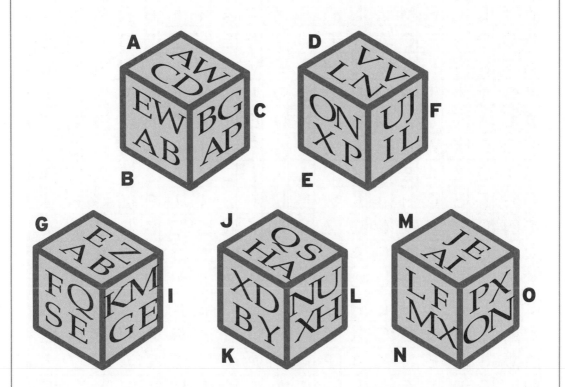

Answer see page **89**

```
C W C O A L M K W O E A C K L G O Z A N
L H E M I N G W A Y N E I Y L M O X A E
L E E C M O X K W A X F E X A N B K O S
C F A K K E N Z A E X L A E B L P E F B
A Y E L H M Z N O E X I A I F H R K L I
M O Q V T O A T E U I W E H T E O G M O
A T K V L A V C H A E M N O L E U A B C
F S I A T A M Q L S D I C K E N S S T A
A L S T V E M W M N O E I A C H T A C T
F O O X W A B E A L L E I T A W W A C G
G T O X A E A K F A K I L A A S T A W N
O N F B C H J K W L L T J I I E X G H I
E N O L F M G O Z X A Y N A E B E C W L
R V O L F I G A E Z I U I E J C C K T P
E W U V E C U O P T E G B P N H T S E I
C S E W X H L H J A L E C E K L T U Z K
U A T A E E C K U W P Q R A R A E P A Z
A U S T E N X A T A Q W A L E T A W V E
H A P E X E A B C B A C A E W W E X L E
C C W A O R W E L L K M N O P P E L T U
```

Austen	Hemingway	Michener
Chaucer	Huxley	Orwell
Chekhov	Ibsen	Proust
Dickens	Kafka	Tolstoy
Flaubert	Kipling	Twain
Goethe	Lawrence	Zola

In this grid are hidden the names of 18 famous authors. Can you detect them? You can go forward or in reverse, in horizontal, vertical and diagonal lines.

Answer see page 89

PUZZLE 22

These tiles, when placed in the right order, will form a square in which the first horizontal line is identical with the first vertical line, and so on. Can you successfully form the square?

Answer see page **90**

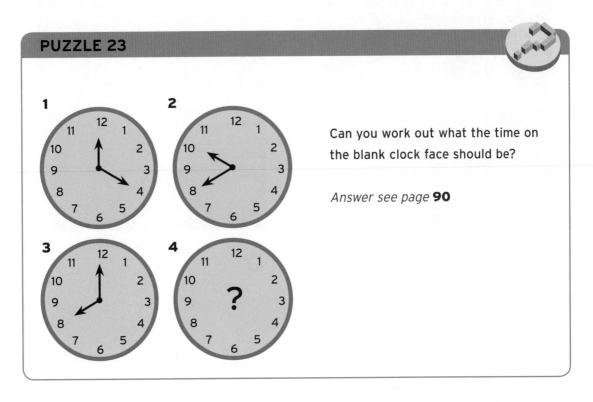

PUZZLE 23

1

2

3

4

?

Can you work out what the time on the blank clock face should be?

Answer see page **90**

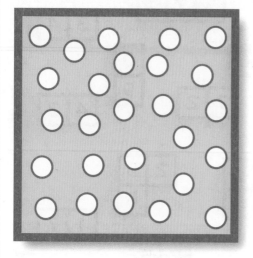

A

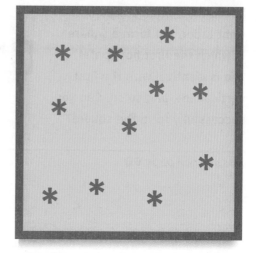

B

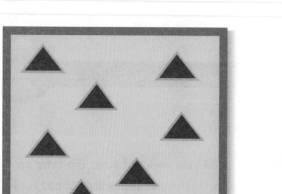

C

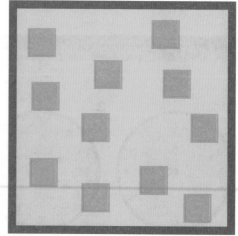

D

There is a logic to the patterns in these squares but one does not fit. Can you find the odd one out?

Answer see page **90**

30   50   42   38

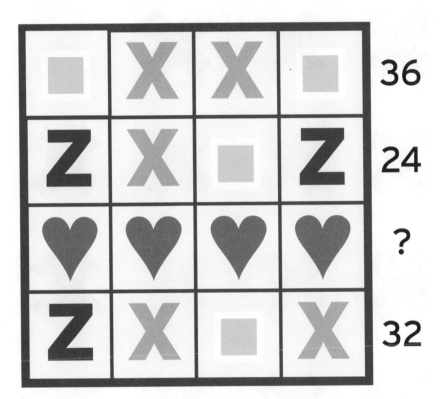

36

24

?

32

Each symbol in the square above represents a number. Can you find out how much the question mark is worth?

Answer see page **90**

Which of these is the odd one out?

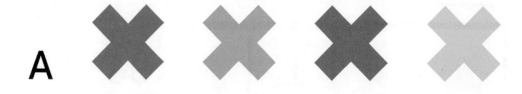

A

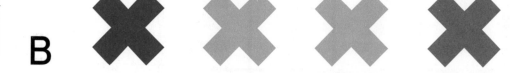

B

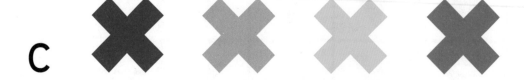

C

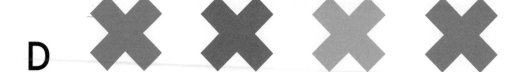

D

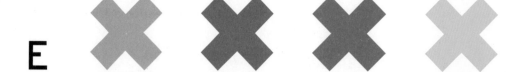

E

Answer see page 90

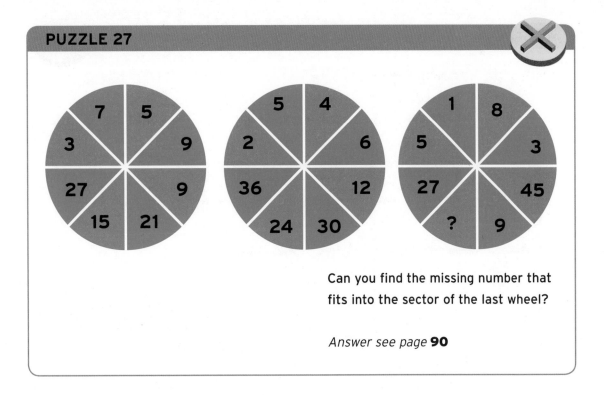

Can you find the missing number that fits into the sector of the last wheel?

Answer see page 90

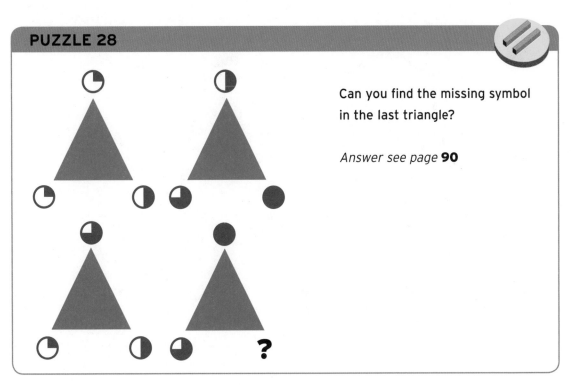

Can you find the missing symbol in the last triangle?

Answer see page 90

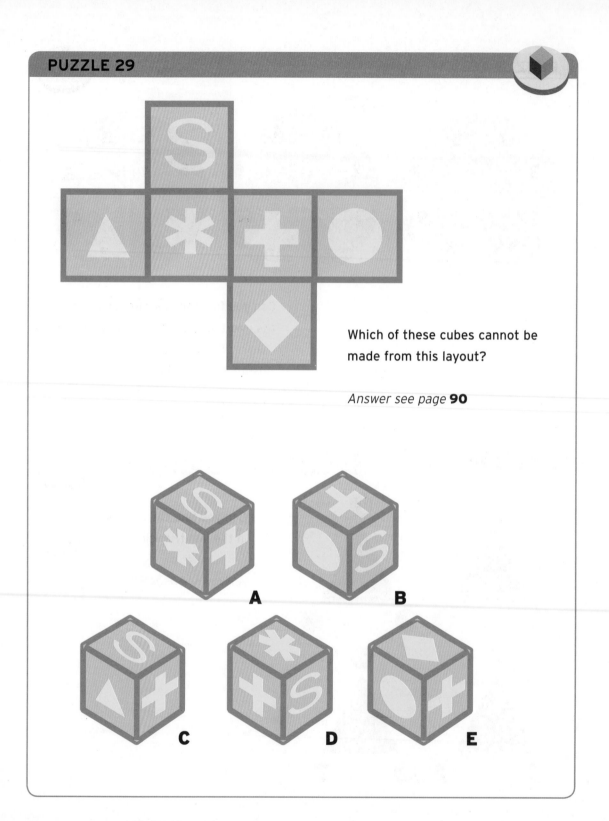

Which of these cubes cannot be made from this layout?

Answer see page **90**

A

B

C

D

E

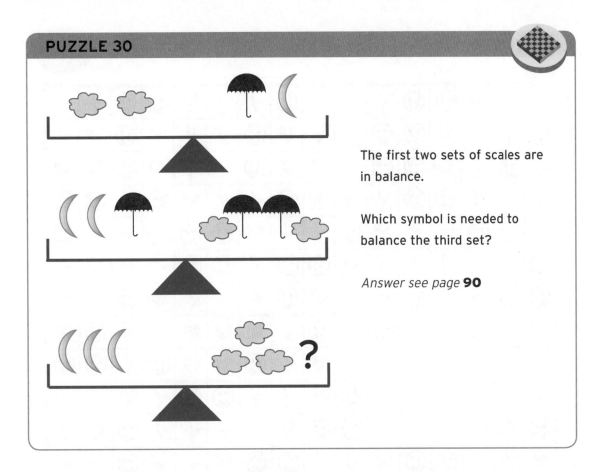

The first two sets of scales are in balance.

Which symbol is needed to balance the third set?

Answer see page **90**

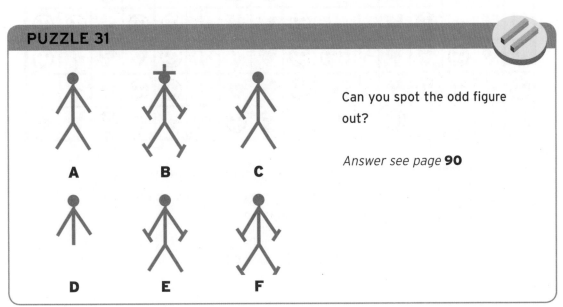

A   B   C

D   E   F

Can you spot the odd figure out?

Answer see page **90**

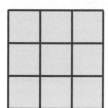

The symbols in the above grid follow a pattern. Can you work it out and find the missing section?

Answer see page **90**

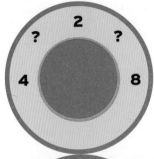

Can you work out what mathematical signs should replace the question marks so that both sections of the diagram arrive at the same value greater than 1. You have a choice between ÷ or x.

Answer see page **91**

36	40	50	23	
✳	✓	‡	0	38
✓	✓	✓	0	41
✳	✳	✓	0	?
✳	✳	‡	✳	37

Each symbol in this square represents a value. Can you find out what number should replace the question mark?

Answer see page **91**

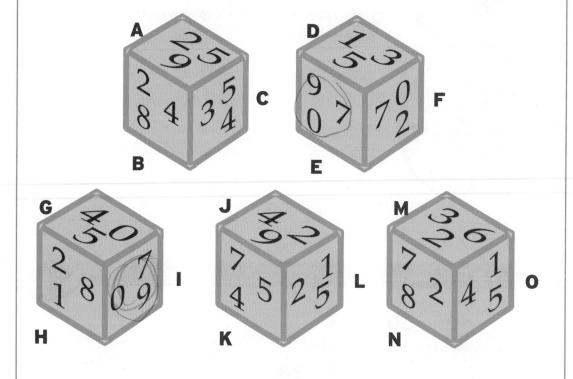

Two sides on these cubes contain the same numbers. Can you spot them?

Answer see page **91**

PUZZLE 36

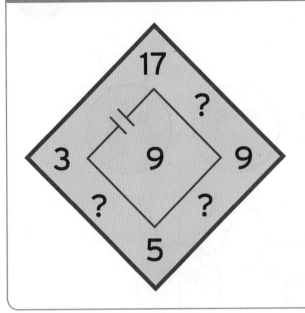

The mathematical signs in this diamond have been left out. Reading clockwise from the top can you work out what the question marks stand for?

Answer see page **91**

PUZZLE 37

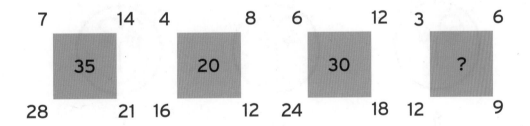

7	14	4	8	6	12	3	6
	35		20		30		?
28	21	16	12	24	18	12	9

Can you work out what number should go into the last square?

Answer see page **91**

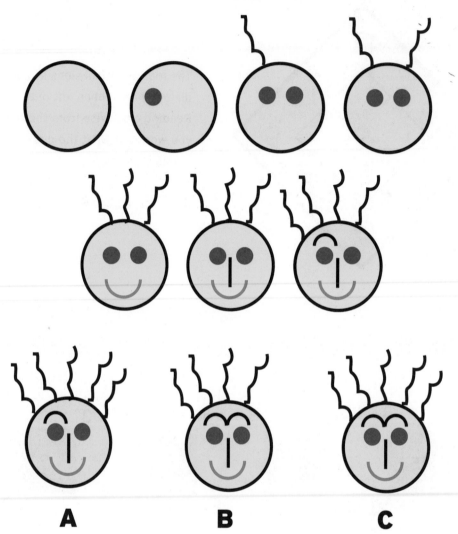

A   **B**   **C**

Which of the faces A, B or C would carry on
the sequence above?

Answer see page **91**

PUZZLE 39

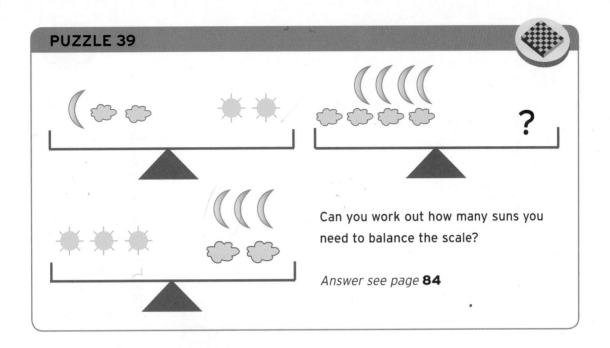

Can you work out how many suns you need to balance the scale?

Answer see page **84**

PUZZLE 40

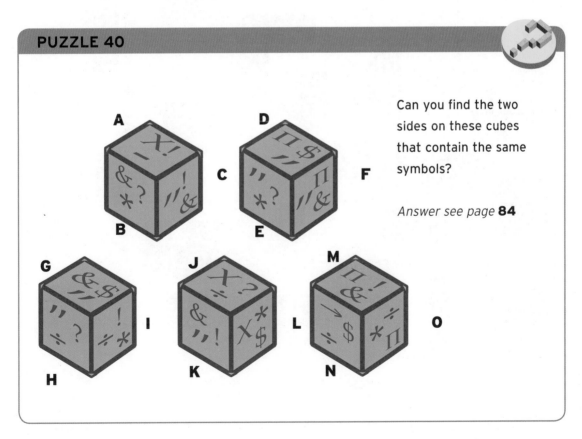

Can you find the two sides on these cubes that contain the same symbols?

Answer see page **84**

PUZZLE 41

These tiles when placed in the right order will form a square in which the first horizontal line is identical with the first vertical line, and so on. Can you successfully form the square?

Answer see page **91**

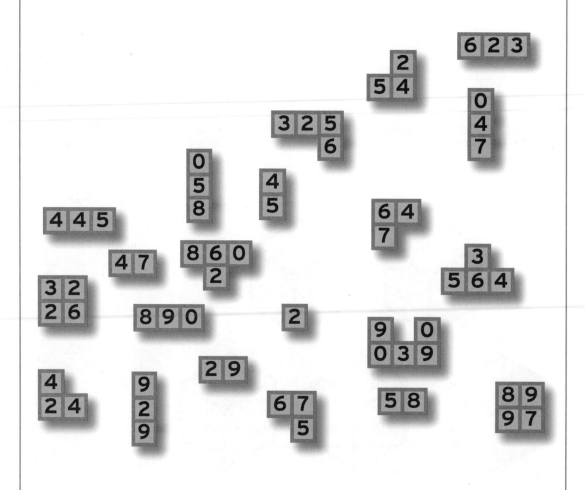

36   23   24   ?

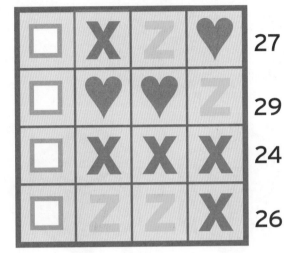

27

29

24

26

Each symbol in the grid has a numerical value. Work out what those values are and replace the question mark with a number.

Answer see page **91**

PUZZLE 43

Can you work out what number the question mark in the triangle stands for?

Answer see page **91**

PUZZLE 44

There are two sides on these cubes that contain exactly the same symbols. Can you spot them?

Answer see page 91

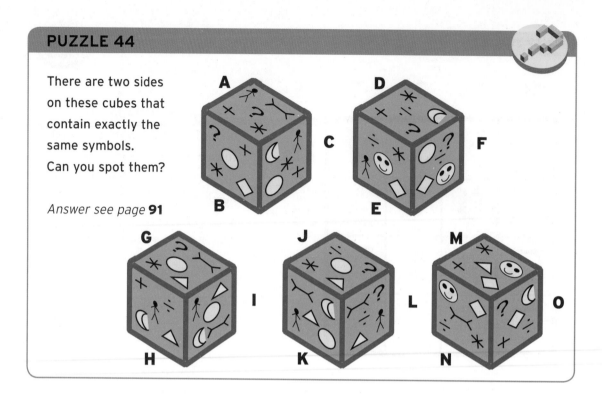

PUZZLE 45

44   46   44   44

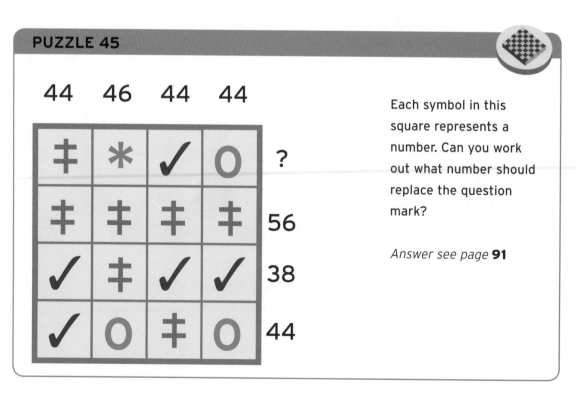

Each symbol in this square represents a number. Can you work out what number should replace the question mark?

Answer see page 91

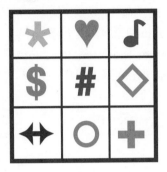
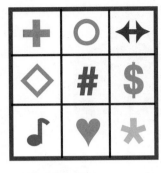
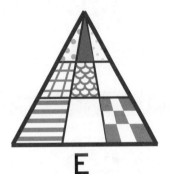

A   is to   B   as   C   is to

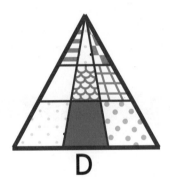
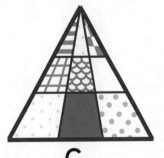

D

E

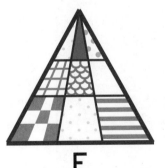

F

G

*Answer see page **91***

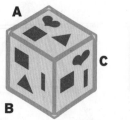
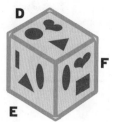
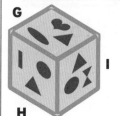
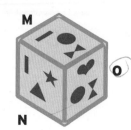
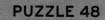
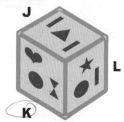

A
B
C
D
E
F
G
H
I
J
K
L
M
N
O

Can you find the two sides on these cubes that contain exactly the same symbols?

Answer see page **92**

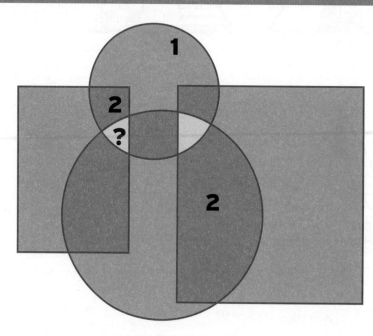

1

2

?

2

This diagram was constructed according to a certain logic. Can you work out what number should replace the question mark?

Answer see page **92**

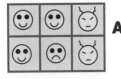 **A**
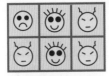 **B**

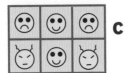 **C**
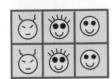 **D**

The symbols in the above grid follow a pattern. Can you work it out and find the missing section?

*Answer see page **92***

PUZZLE 50

Can you work out which two sides on these cubes contain the same symbols?

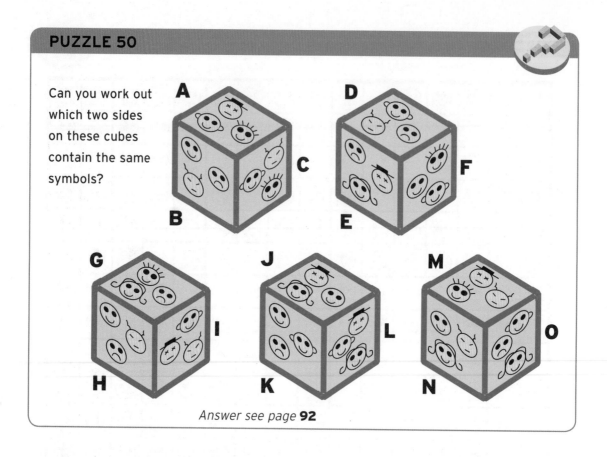

Answer see page **92**

PUZZLE 51

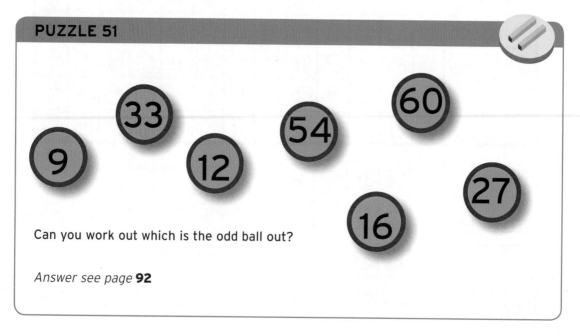

Can you work out which is the odd ball out?

Answer see page **92**

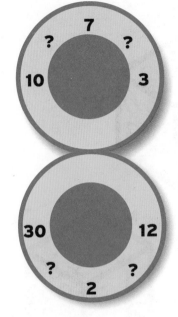

Can you replace the question marks with + or – so that both sections in this diagram add up to the same value?

Answer see page **92**

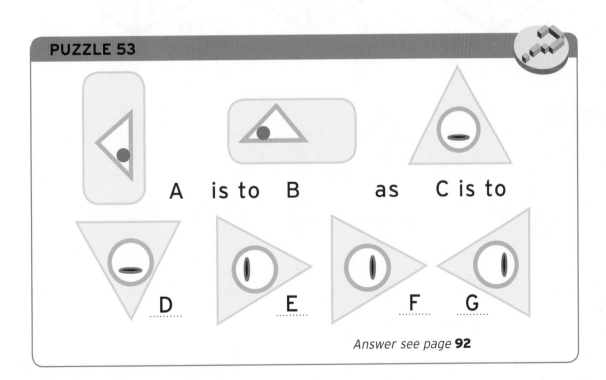

A   is to   B   as   C is to

D   E   F   G

Answer see page **92**

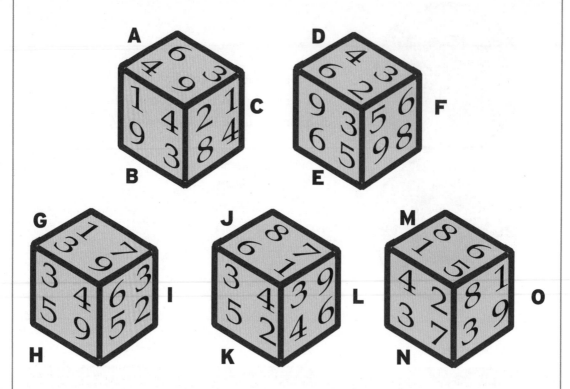

Two sides of these cubes contain
exactly the same numbers.
Can you spot them?

*Answer see page **92***

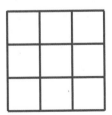

The symbols in this grid follow a pattern. Can you work it out and complete the missing section?

Answer see page **92**

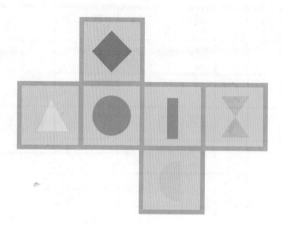

Which of these cubes cannot be made from this layout?

*Answer see page **92***

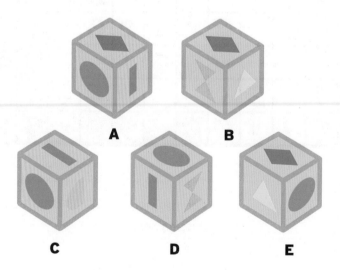

A

B

C

D

E

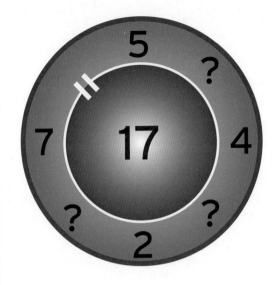

Can you find the mathematical signs that should replace the question marks in this diagram?

Answer see page **92**

The four triangles are linked by a simple mathematical formula.
Can you discover what it is and then find the odd one out?

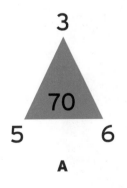

3

70

5   6

A

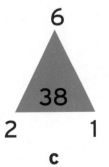

7

129

4   8

B

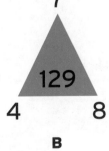

6

38

2   1

C

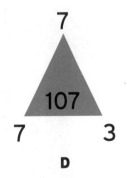

7

107

7   3

D

Answer see page **92**

PUZZLE 59

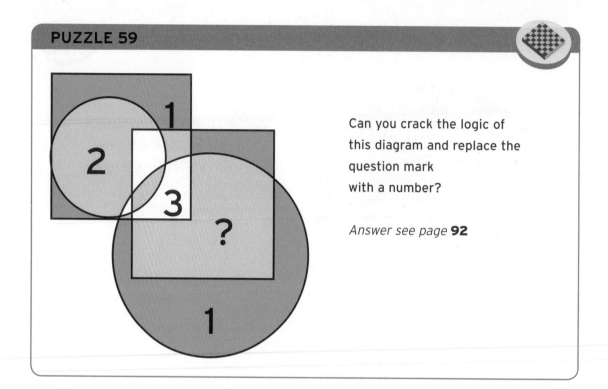

Can you crack the logic of this diagram and replace the question mark with a number?

*Answer see page **92***

PUZZLE 60

How would you continue this series?

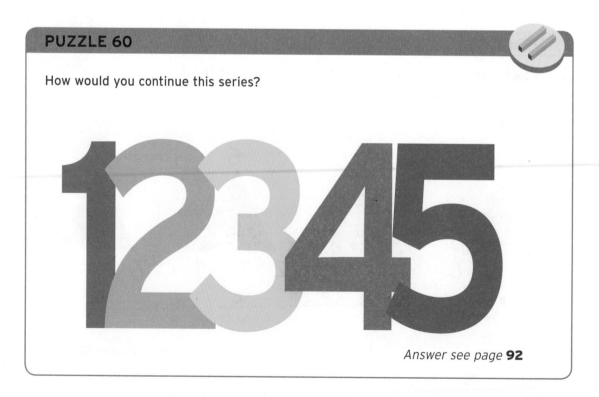

*Answer see page **92***

These tiles when placed in the right
order will form a square in which the first
horizontal line is identical with the first
vertical line, and so. Can you successfully
form the square?

Answer see page **93**

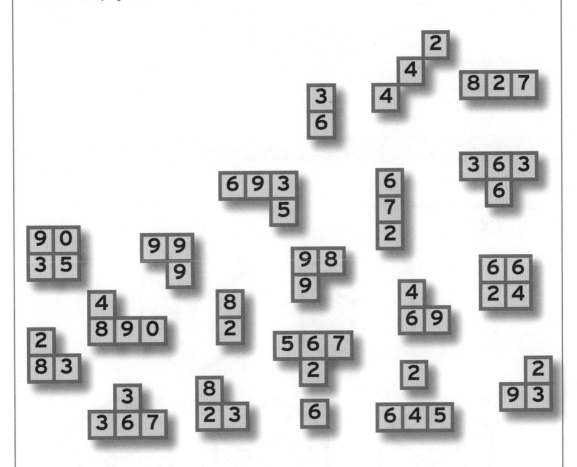

PUZZLE 62

Can you replace the question marks in this diagram with the symbols x and ÷ so that both sections arrive at the same value?

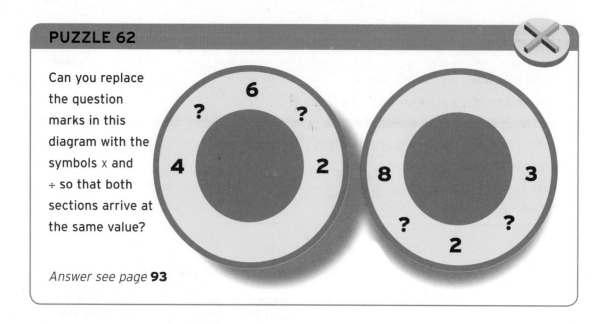

Answer see page 93

PUZZLE 63

Can you work out which three sides of these cubes contain the same symbols?

Answer see page 93

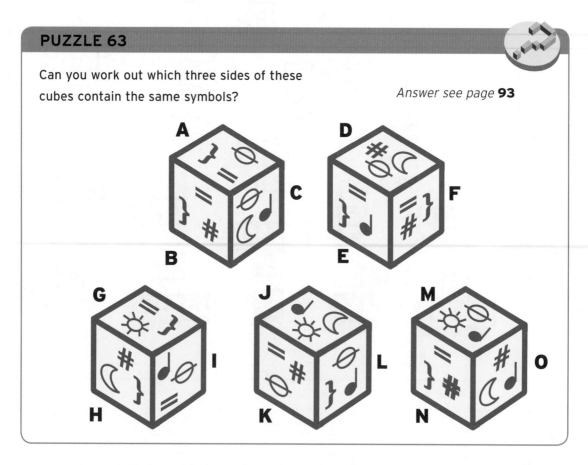

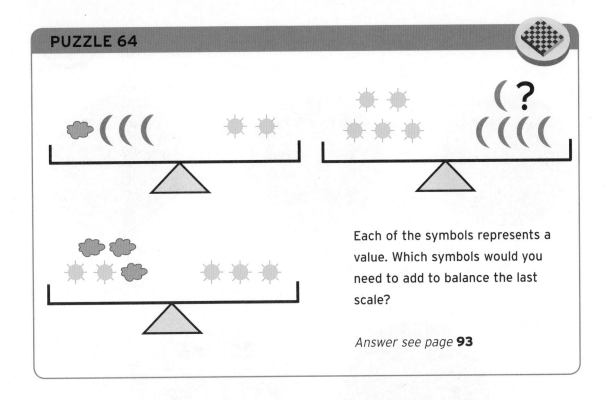

Each of the symbols represents a value. Which symbols would you need to add to balance the last scale?

Answer see page **93**

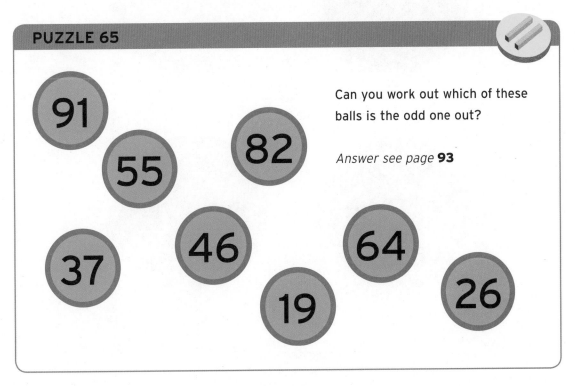

Can you work out which of these balls is the odd one out?

Answer see page **93**

PUZZLE 66

A: 68 57 15 31 26 42

B: 42 51 13 68 26 75

C: 24 59 93 46 82 13

A is to B as C is to

D: 42 95 63 31 28 39

E: 28 46 59 42 31 93

F: 95 24 39 31 82 46

G: 93 42 46 13 95 28

Answer see page **93**

PUZZLE 67

10   7   8   12   15   9   7   11

2   1   ?   4

4   3   3   8   5   7   1   9

Can you work out what number should replace the question mark in the square?

Answer see page **93**

PUZZLE 68

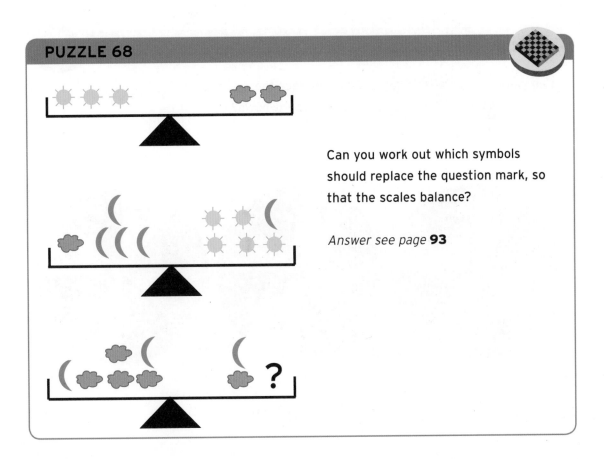

Can you work out which symbols should replace the question mark, so that the scales balance?

Answer see page **93**

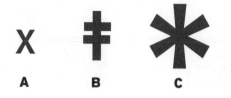

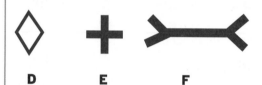

Can you find the odd one out of these symbols?

Answer see page **87**

Can you work out what number should replace the question mark to follow the rules of the other wheels?

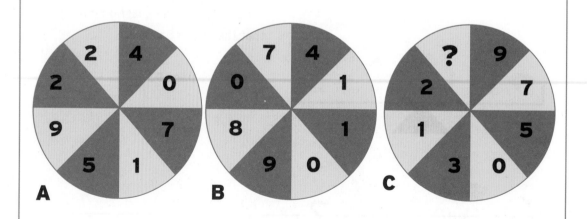

Answer see page **87**

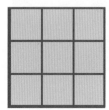

The symbols in this grid behave in a predictable manner. When you have discovered their sequence it should be possible to fill in the blank segment.

Answer see page **93**

The two pictures are very similar but not quite identical.

Find 11 ways in which A differs from B.

A

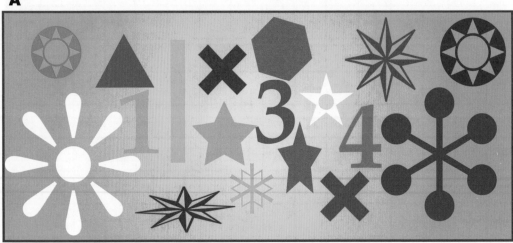

B

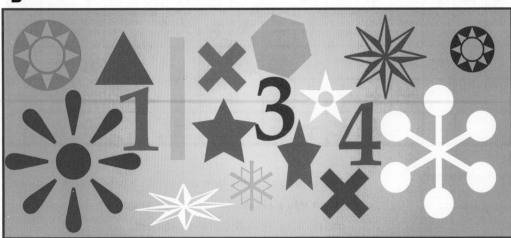

Answer see page **94**

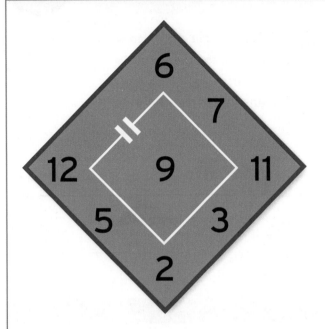

In this diagram, starting from the top of the diamond and working in a clockwise direction, the four basic mathematical signs (+, −, ×, ÷) have been omitted. Your task is to restore them so that the calculation, with the answer in the middle, is correct.

*Answer see page **94***

A

3 5
7 9
2 6
8 4

B

9 25
49 81
4 36
64 16

C

? 125
343 729
8 216
512 64

A curious logic governs the numbers in these circles. Can you discover what it is and then work out what the missing number should be?

*Answer see page **94***

PUZZLE 75

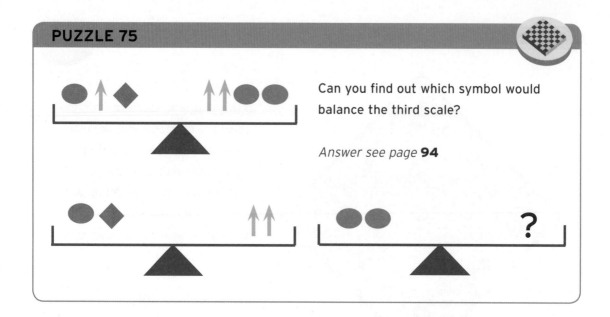

Can you find out which symbol would balance the third scale?

Answer see page 94

PUZZLE 76

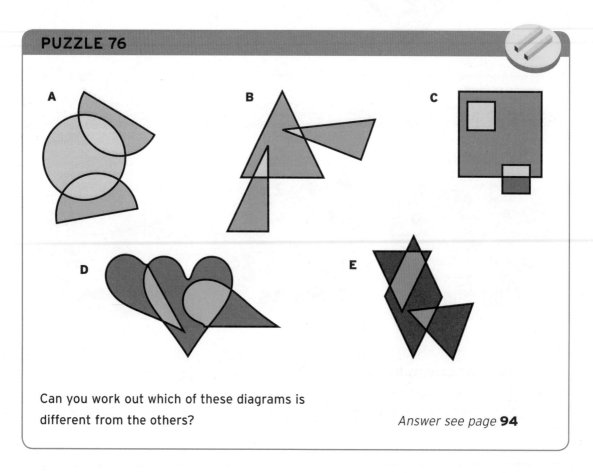

A

B

C

D

E

Can you work out which of these diagrams is different from the others?

Answer see page 94

Can you work out what the blank clockface should look like?

Answer see page **94**

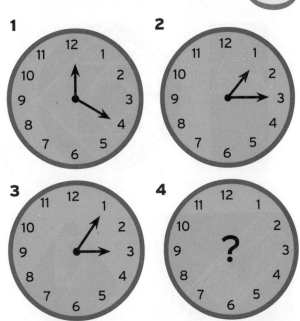

1   2

3   4

---

35   47   38   24

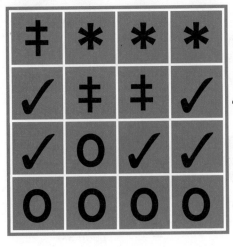

Can you work out what number each symbol represents and find the value of the question mark?

Answer see page **94**

PUZZLE 79

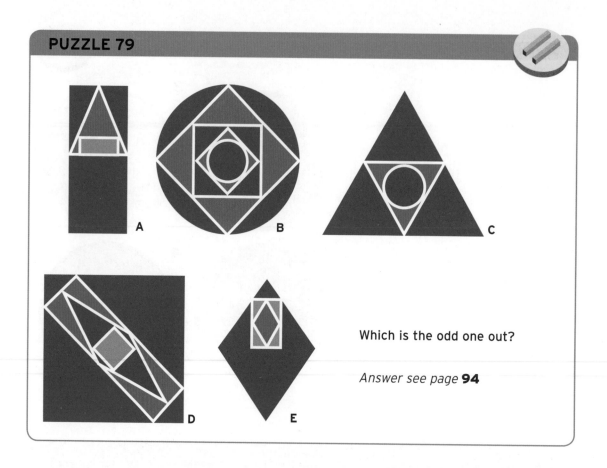

A **B** **C**

D **E**

Which is the odd one out?

Answer see page **94**

PUZZLE 80

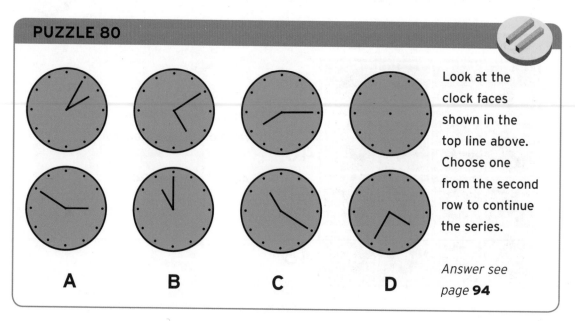

A **B** **C** **D**

Look at the clock faces shown in the top line above. Choose one from the second row to continue the series.

Answer see page **94**

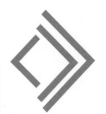 is to 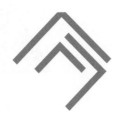 as 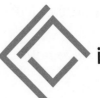 is to:

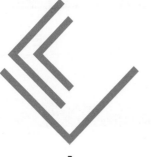

A

B

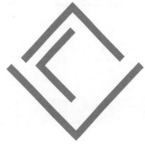

C

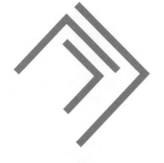

D

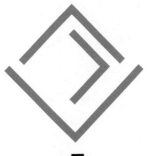

E

Answer see page **94**

PUZZLE 82

Which of the following shapes forms a perfect triangle when combined with the picture on the right ?

Answer see page **94**

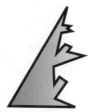

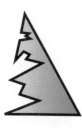 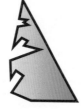 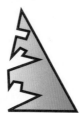 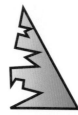 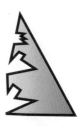

A   B   C   D   E

PUZZLE 83

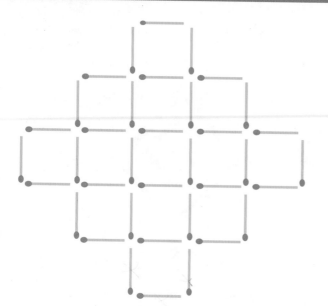

By taking away four matches from this diagram, leave eight small squares.

Answer see page **94**

PUZZLE 84

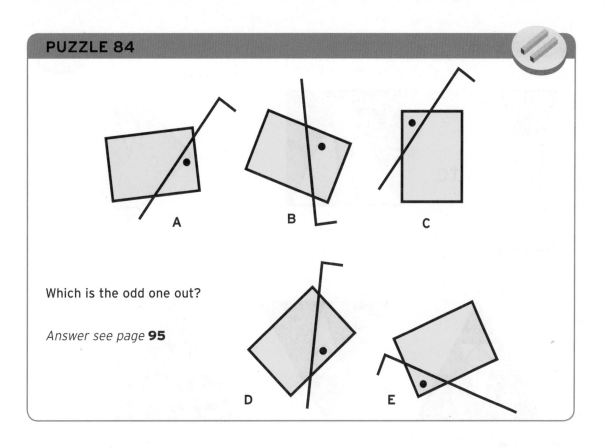

Which is the odd one out?

Answer see page **95**

PUZZLE 85

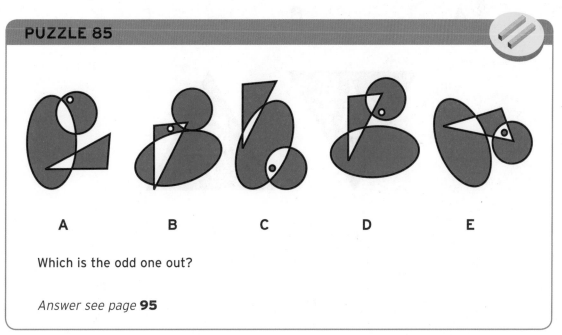

Which is the odd one out?

Answer see page **95**

PUZZLE 86

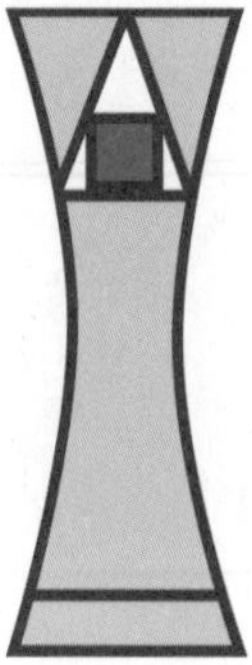

is to

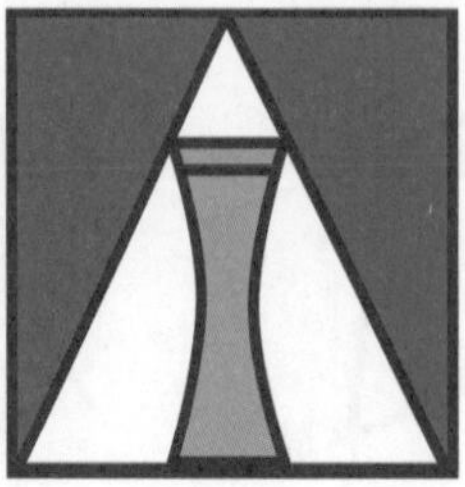

as

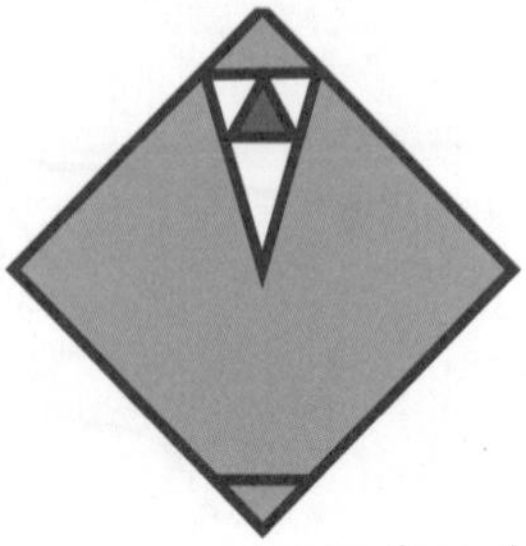

is to:

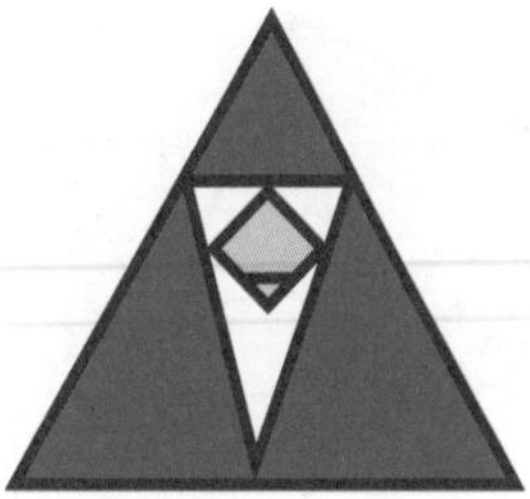

A

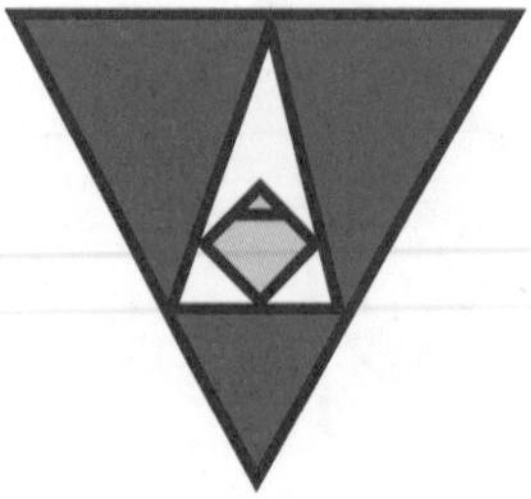

B

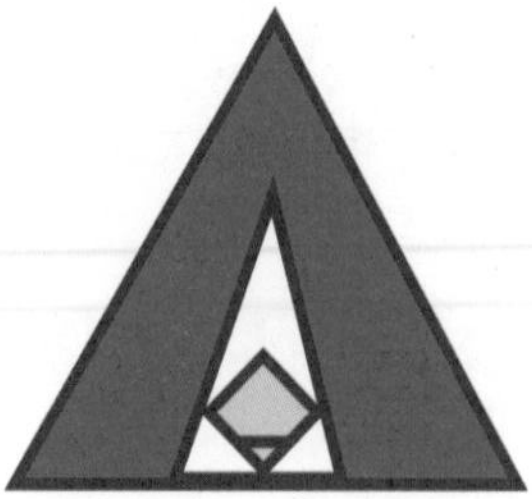

C

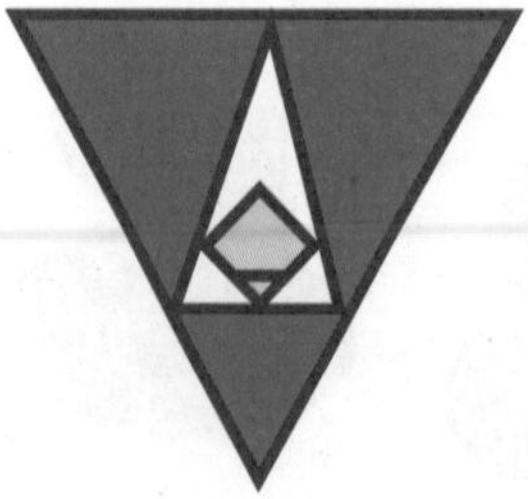

D

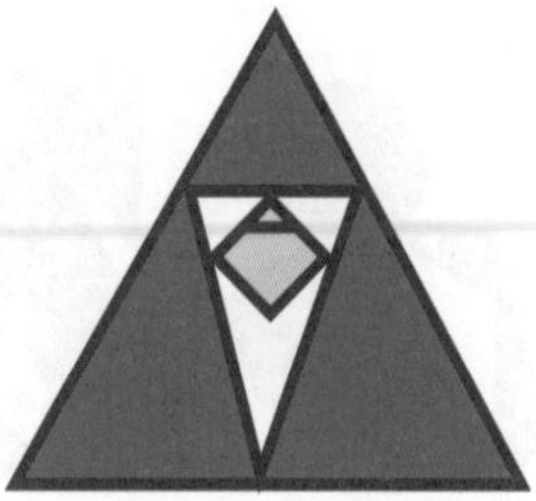

E

Answer see page **95**

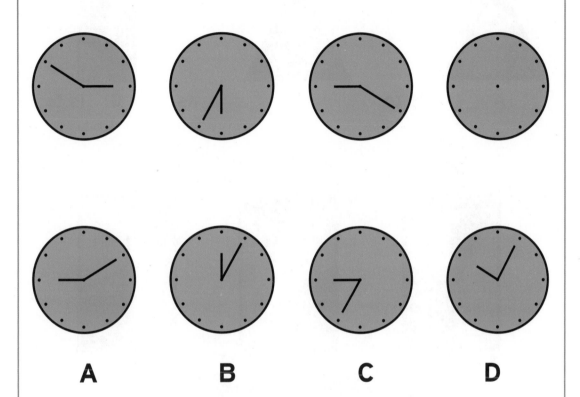

A **B** **C** **D**

Another series of clock faces. Again it is up to you to work out the logic behind the series in the top row and pick the clock from the bottom row that replaces the blank clock.

*Answer see page **95***

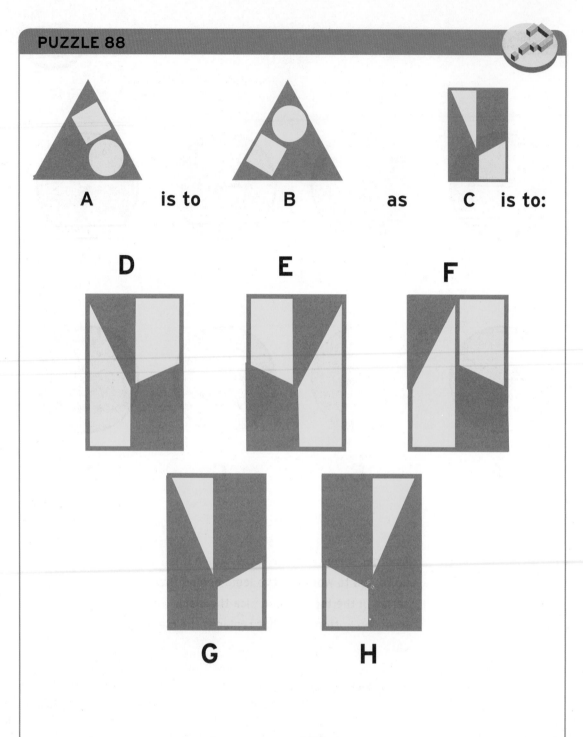

A   is to   B   as   C   is to:

D

E

F

G

H

*Answer see page **95***

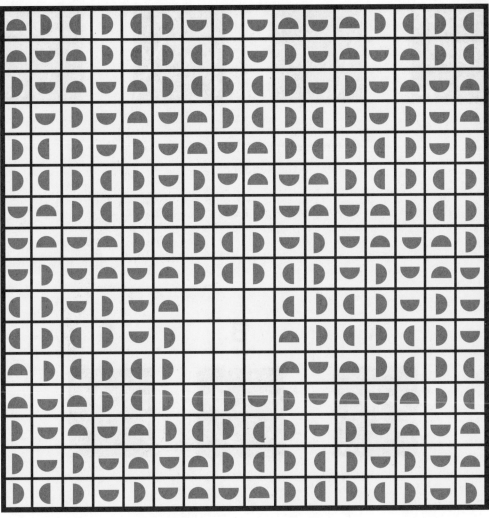

A

B

C

D

The symbols in the above grid follow a
pattern. Can you find the missing section?

*Answer see page **95***

   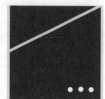

Which of the following comes
next in the sequence?

Answer see page **95**

A   **B**   **C**

 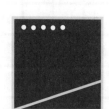 

 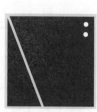

D   **E**

PUZZLE 91

Can you work out which sides on these cubes contain the same letters?

Answer see page **95**

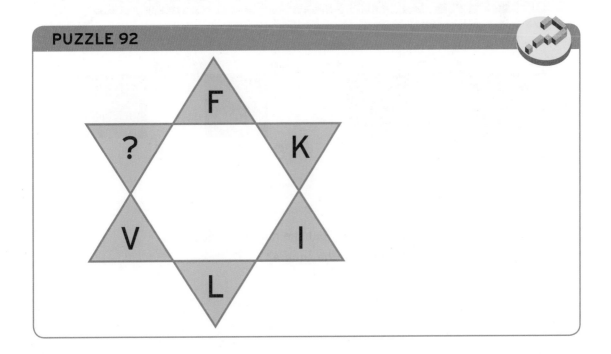

PUZZLE 92

PUZZLE 93

In this diamond the mathematical signs +, -, x and ÷ have been left out. Can you work out which sign fits between each pair of numbers to arrive at the number in the middle of the diagram? To start you off, three of the signs are each used twice.

Answer see page 95

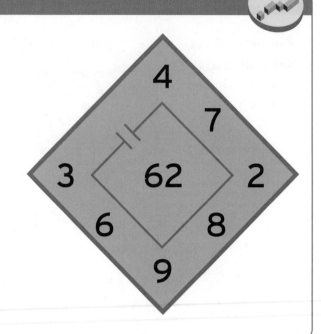

PUZZLE 94

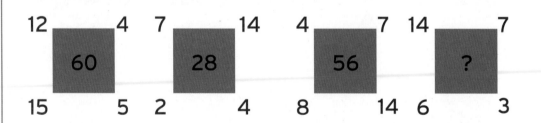

Can you work out the number needed to complete the square?

Answer see page 95

Someone has made a mistake decorating this cake. Can you correct the pattern?

Answer see page **95**

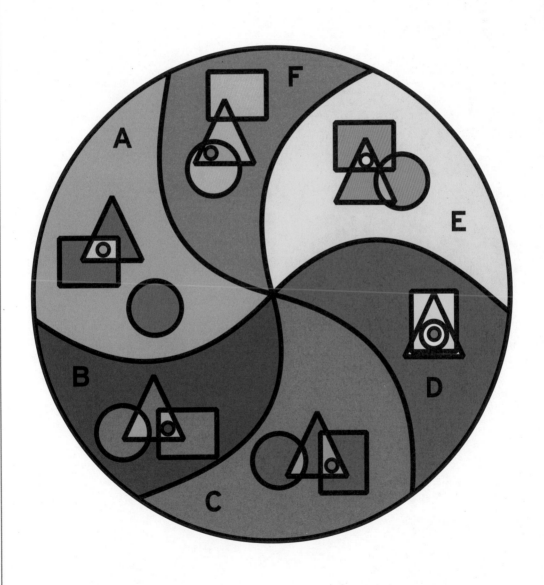

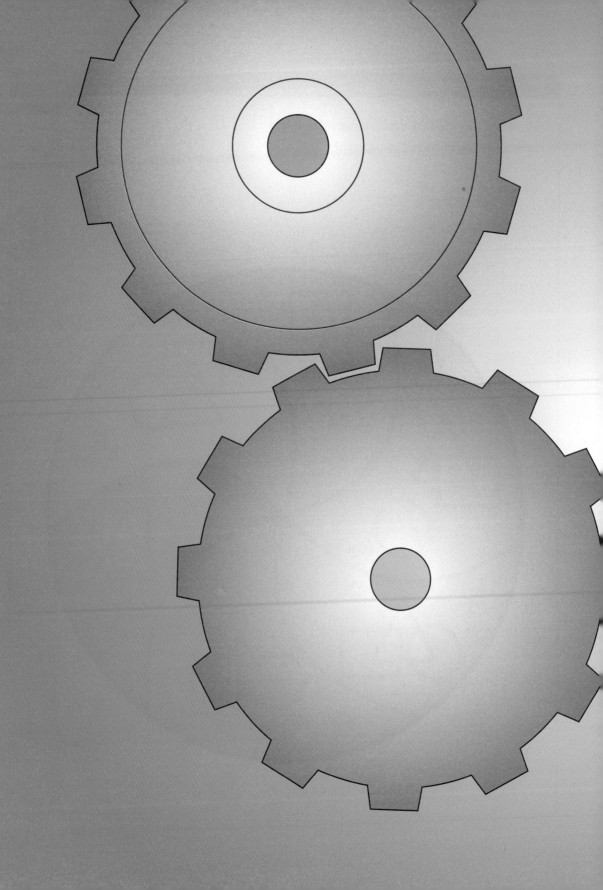

Easy Answers

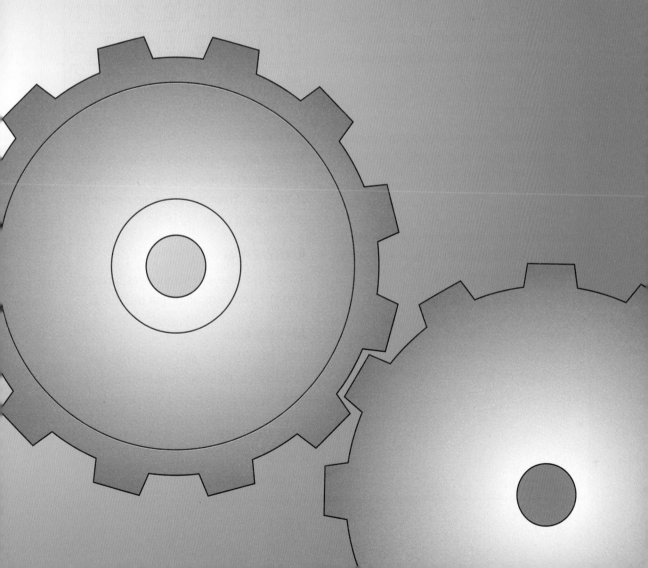

ANSWER 1

E. In all the others the colors follow the same sequence: light blue, red, dark blue, green, yellow, pink.

ANSWER 2

E.

ANSWER 3

4. Multiply the two numbers in the outer circle of each segment and place the product in the inner circle two segments away in a clockwise direction.

ANSWER 4

7. Add the three numbers at the corner of each triangle, multiply by 2, and place that number in the middle.

ANSWER 5

4. There are 4 boxes and the number relates to the number of boxes in which the number is enclosed.

ANSWER 6

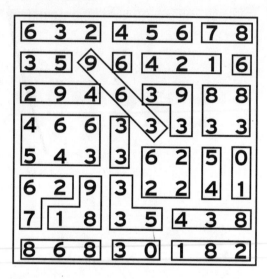

ANSWER 7

21. Add all the numbers of each triangle together and place the sum in the middle of the next triangle. When you reach D put the sum in A.

ANSWER 8

15. None of the other numbers have a divisor – they are all prime numbers.

ANSWER 9

1:00. The minute hand moves forward 20 minutes, the hour hand moves back 1 hour.

ANSWER 10

A diamond. (4 diamonds = 3 left/arrows = 6 up-arrows).

ANSWER 11

F. The symbols are reflected over a vertical line.

ANSWER 12

E. It contains no curved lines.

ANSWER 13

8. Add all the numbers together. In a yellow square you add 5 to the sum, in a green one you subtract 5.

ANSWER 14

G. Add 2 lines to the body, take away 1, add 3, take away 2, add 4, take away 3.

ANSWER 15

6:45. The minute hand moves back 15, 30 and 45 minutes. The hour hand moves forward 3, 6 and 9 hours.

ANSWER 16

Pink. All the other colors are either primary or secondary colors. Pink is a hue.

ANSWER 17

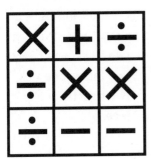

The order is 2 +, 3 -, 2 ÷, 3 x. The puzzle goes in an inward clockwise spiral starting from the top left corner.

ANSWER 18

D and L.

ANSWER 19

39. Tick = 6, star = 9, cross = 3, O = 24.

ANSWER 20

E and O. The letters are N, O, P and X.

ANSWER 21

Austen	Hemingway
Michener	Chaucer
Huxley	Orwell
Chekov	Ibsen
Proust	Dickens
Kafka	Tolstoy
Flaubert	Kipling
Twain	Goethe
Lawrence	Zola

```
C W C O A L M K W O E A C K L G O Z A N
L H E M I N G W A Y N E I Y L M O X A E
L E E C M O X K W A X F E X A N B K O S
C F A K K E N Z A E X L A E B L P E F B
A Y E L H M Z N O E X I A I F H R K L U
M O Q V T O A T E U I W E H T E O G M O
A T K V L A V C H A E M N O L E U A B C
F S I A T A M Q L S D I C K E N S S T A
A L S T V E M W M N O E I A C H T A C T
F O O X W A B E A L L E I T A W W A C G
G T O X A E A K F A K I L A A S T A W N
O N F B C H J K W L L T J I I E X G H I
E N O L F M G O Z X A Y N A E B E C W L
R V O L F I G A E Z I U I E J C C K T P
E W U V E C U O P T E G B P N H T S E I
C S E W X H L H J A L E C E K L T U Z K
U A T A E E C K U W P Q R A R A E P A Z
A U S T E N X A T A Q W A L E T A W V E
H A P E X E A B C B A C A E W W E X L E
C C W A O R W E L D K M N O P P E L T U
```

ANSWER 22

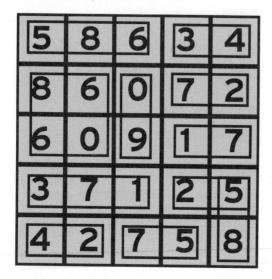

ANSWER 23

6:20. The minute hand advances 20 minutes each time, the hour hand goes back 2 hours each time.

ANSWER 24

B. The number of sides of the internal figures should increase by one each time. B is the odd one out because its internal figures should have 2 sides.

ANSWER 25

68. Square = 7; X = 11; Z = 3; Heart = 17.

ANSWER 26

C. In all other cases the first letters of the colors form words: gory, poor, prop, orgy.

ANSWER 27

72. Multiply all the numbers in the top sections to arrive at the number in the opposite bottom section. Multiply by 3 in the first circle, by 6 in the second one, and by 9 in the third circle.

ANSWER 28

A full circle. Go first along the top of the triangles, then along the bottoms. Each circle is filled one quarter at a time until the circle is complete, then reverts to one-quarter filled.

ANSWER 29

C.

ANSWER 30

One cloud. The values are: Cloud = 3; Umbrella = 2; Moon = 4.

ANSWER 31

C. It has an odd number of elements, the others all have an even number.

ANSWER 32

Start at the top right corner and work in a clockwise inward spiral. The pattern is:

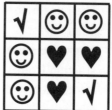 two ticks, one heart, two faces, one tick, two hearts, one face, etc.

ANSWER 33

Top half: ÷ x; bottom half: x x.

ANSWER 34

33. Star = 8; Tick = 12; Cross = 13; Circle = 5.

ANSWER 35

E and I.

ANSWER 36

- - x.

ANSWER 37

15. Start at the top left corner and add that number to each corner in a clockwise direction, eg. 7 + 7 = 14 + 7 = 21 + 7 = 28 + 7 = 35.

ANSWER 38

A. Add one new element to the face, then add one hair and an element to the face, then a hair, then a hair and an element to the face, repeat sequence.

ANSWER 39

Five suns. Moon = 2; Cloud = 3; Sun = 4.

ANSWER 40

C and K.

ANSWER 41

4	4	5	6	7	8	9	0
4	3	2	4	5	6	2	3
5	2	6	2	4	0	0	9
6	4	2	8	9	4	5	2
7	5	4	9	7	7	8	9
8	6	0	4	7	3	2	5
9	2	0	5	8	2	3	6
0	3	9	2	9	5	6	4

ANSWER 42

23. Square = 9; Cross = 5; Z = 6; Heart = 7.

ANSWER 43

2. The faces represent numbers, based on the elements in or around the face (excluding the head). Multiply the top number with the bottom right number and divide by the bottom left number. Place the answer in the middle.

ANSWER 44

I and K. The figures are: matchstick man, triangle, half-moon, circle, stile.

ANSWER 45

40. Star = 7; Tick = 8; Cross = 14; Circle = 11.

ANSWER 46

G. The internal patterns are rotated 180°.

ANSWER 47

K and O.

ANSWER 48

3. There are 4 shapes and the numbers refer to the number of shapes that surround each digit.

ANSWER 49

B. Start from top left corner and move in a vertical boustrophedon. Order is: 4 smiley face, 1 sad face, 3 straight mouth, 2 face with hair, etc.

ANSWER 50

B and H.

ANSWER 51

16. All the other numbers can be divided by 3.

ANSWER 52

Top half: + +; bottom half: + -.

ANSWER 53

E. Turn the diagram by 90° clockwise.

ANSWER 54

A and L. The numbers are 3, 4, 6 and 9.

ANSWER 55

Start at top left corner and move in a vertical boustrophedon. The order is two hearts, one square root, two crossed circles, one cross, one heart, two square roots, one crossed circle, two crosses, etc.

ANSWER 56

D.

ANSWER 57

5 x 4 ÷ 2 + 7 = 17.

ANSWER 58

C. The number in the middle is the sum of the squares of the numbers at the points of the triangles. C does not fit this pattern.

ANSWER 59

2. It relates to the number of shapes that enclose each figure.

ANSWER 60

Indigo and Violet (colors of the rainbow).

ANSWER 61

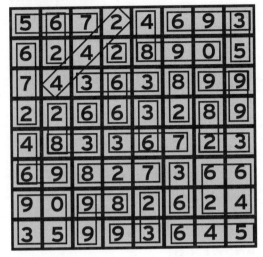

ANSWER 62

Top half: x ÷; bottom half: ⊕ x.

ANSWER 63

B, F and N.

ANSWER 64

4 moons. Sun = 9; Moon = 5; Cloud = 3.

ANSWER 65

26. The digits in each of the other balls add up to 10.

ANSWER 66

F. The numbers made up of odd numbers are reversed.

ANSWER 67

8. Subtract the bottom left corner from the top left corner. Now subtract the bottom right corner from the top right corner, then subtract this answer from the first difference and put the number in the middle.

ANSWER 68

Three clouds and a moon. Sun = 6; Moon = 7; Cloud = 9.

ANSWER 69

The diamond. It is a closed shape.

ANSWER 70

3. The numbers in each wheel add up to 30.

ANSWER 71

The pattern is a horizontal boustrophedon starting at the top left. The sequence is: 3 stars, 2 circles, 2 squares, 3 crosses, 2 stars, 3 circles, 3 squares, 2 crosses, etc.

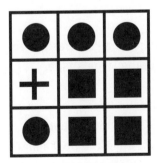

ANSWER 72

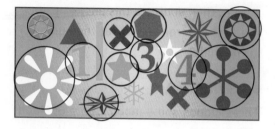

ANSWER 73

6 + 7 + 11 ÷ 3 x 2 + 5 - 12 = 9.

ANSWER 74

27. A number in the first circle is squared and the product is put in the corresponding segment of the second circle. The original number is then cubed and that product is put in the corresponding segment of the third circle.

ANSWER 75

One arrow. Oval = 1, Arrow = 2, Diamond = 3.

ANSWER 76

C. In the others the small shapes added together result in the large shape.

ANSWER 77

6:50. The minute hand moves back 5, 10 and 15 minutes, while the hour hand moves forward 1, 2 and 3 hours.

ANSWER 78

35. Star = 6; Tick = 3; Cross = 17; Circle = 12.

ANSWER 79

C. In all other cases, the biggest shape is also the smallest.

ANSWER 80

C. The minute hand moves forward 5 minutes and the hour hand moves forward 3 hours.

ANSWER 81

C. The smallest segment is rotated 90 degrees clockwise. The middle segment remains static. The largest segment is rotated 90º anti-clockwise.

ANSWER 82

B.

ANSWER 83

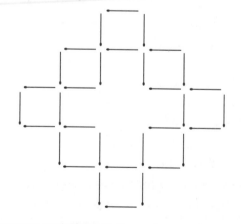

ANSWER 84

B. There is no triangle intersection on this one.

ANSWER 85

B. In all other cases the smaller circle is within the larger circle.

ANSWER 86

E. Largest shape is reflected horizontally and the size order is reversed.

ANSWER 87

B. The minute hand moves back 15 minutes and the hour hand moves forward 3 hours.

ANSWER 88

H.

ANSWER 89

A. Pattern is: 2 by arch on top, 4 by arch at right, 3 by arch on bottom, 2 by arch at left. Start at the top left corner and move down
the grid in vertical lines, reverting to the top of the next column when you reach the bottom.

ANSWER 90

B. The sequence here is minus one dot, plus two dots; the box rotates one place clockwise for each dot added or subtracted.

ANSWER 91

E and M.

ANSWER 92

R. Multiply the value of the three earliest letters, based on their value in the alphabet, by 2. The answer goes in the opposite triangle.
I (9) x 2 = 18 (R).

ANSWER 93

4 x 7 ÷ 2 + 8 + 9 x 6 ÷ 3 = 62.

ANSWER 94

42. Multiply the top top right number by the bottom left number or the top left number by the bottom right number.

ANSWER 95

D is wrong because the dot is in 3 shapes. In all the others the dot is in 2 shapes.

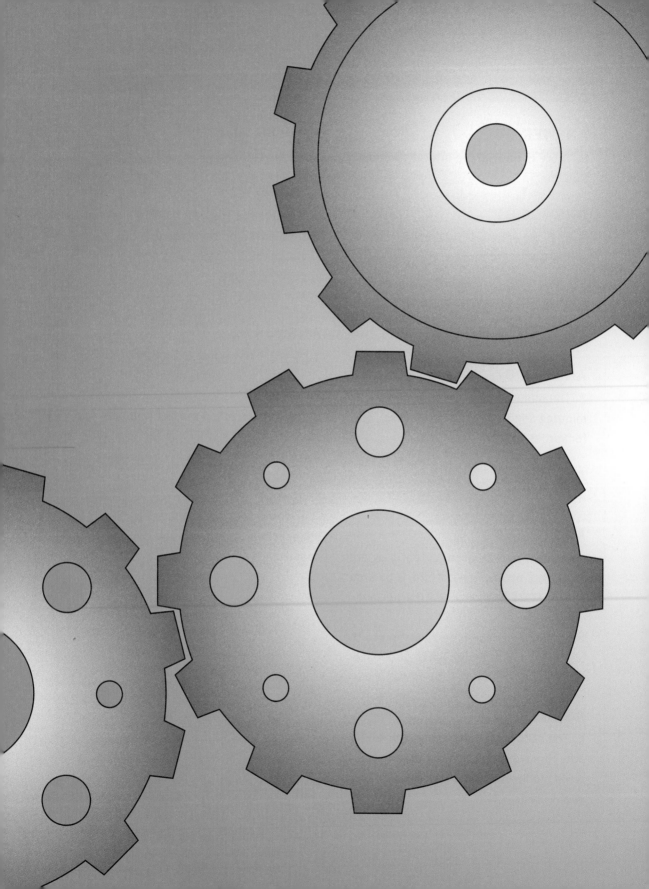

Medium Puzzles

This is where things start to warm up. By this point, you should have developed a reasonable feel for the types of puzzle in this book, and the basic ways in which they work. You also ought to be getting some idea about the devious minds of the puzzle authors, which will prove invaluable in the pages to come. In the pages that follow, we'll challenge you to push your brain up a gear and really start getting to grips with the puzzles.

These problems are going to test your logic, deduction, arithmetic and ingenuity. The answers in this section are not obvious. They're designed to make you think seriously about the possible answers. You may need to forget about being able to spot solutions, and fall back on the first principles for each puzzle - how to analyse each problem, break it down to its essential components, squeeze all the information you need out of it, and put it back together again in such a way as to let you glean the answer.

Don't be disheartened if you find this section slower going than the one before. Everyone will need to take this section more seriously than the one before. Even the most hardened puzzle supremos will find themselves breaking stride to examine these problems carefully. This is where you'll find the meat of your mental workout - a few sets of these problems will leave your mind well and truly pumped.

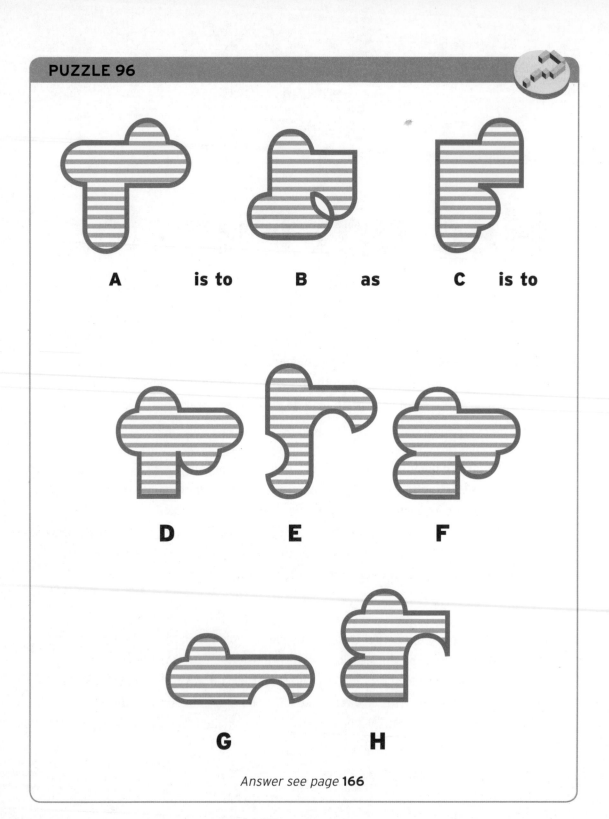

A   is to   B   as   C   is to

D   E   F

G   H

*Answer see page **166***

PUZZLE 97

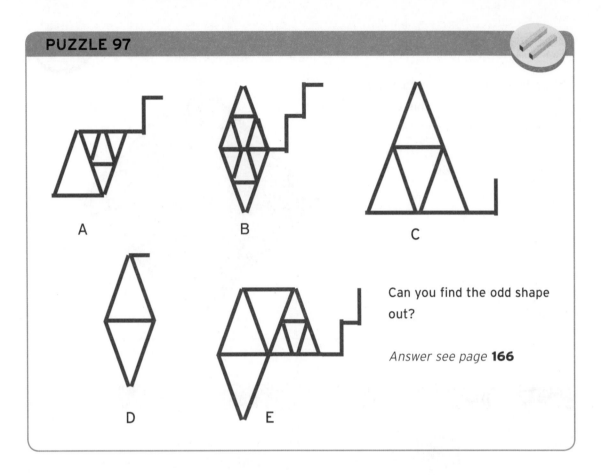

A

B

C

D

E

Can you find the odd shape out?

Answer see page **166**

PUZZLE 98

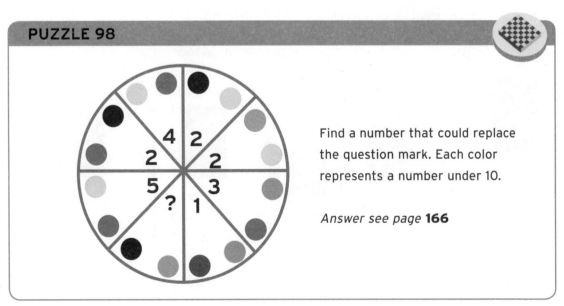

Find a number that could replace the question mark. Each color represents a number under 10.

Answer see page **166**

PUZZLE 99

The four main mathematical signs have been left out of this equation. Can you replace them?

Answer see page **166**

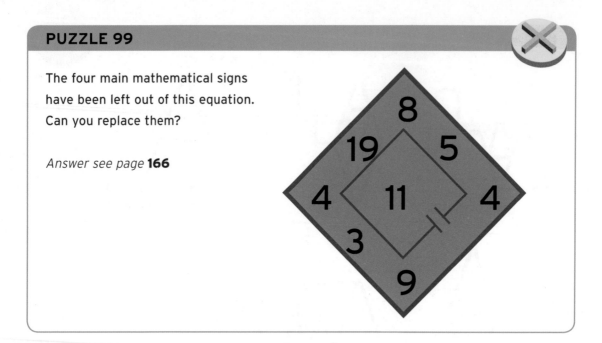

PUZZLE 100

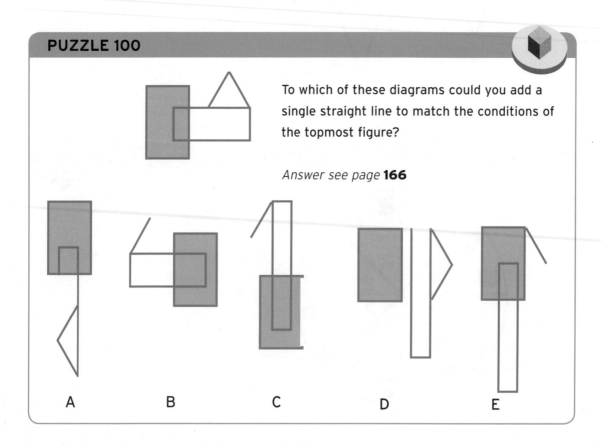

To which of these diagrams could you add a single straight line to match the conditions of the topmost figure?

Answer see page **166**

A   B   C   D   E

What is yellow worth?

Answer see page **166**

 + =

 +  =

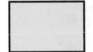 - =

 - =

 - =

 + + = **9**

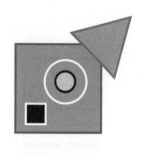 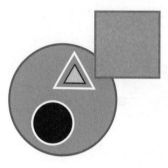 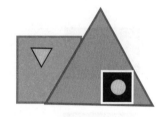

A is to **B** as **C** is to

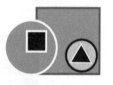 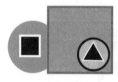 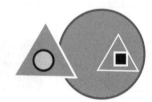

D **E** **F**

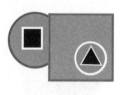

G **H**

Answer see page **166**

PUZZLE 103

Can you work out which number the missing hand on clock 4 should point to?

Answer see page **166**

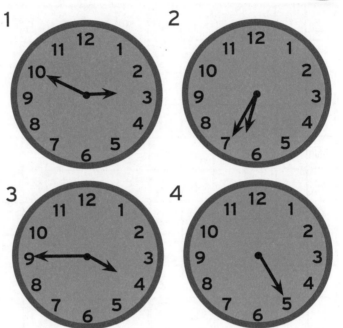

PUZZLE 104

Can you work out the logic behind this square and fill in the missing section?

Answer see page **166**

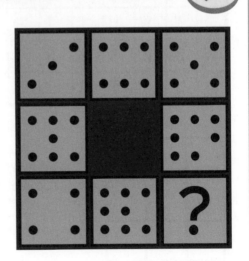

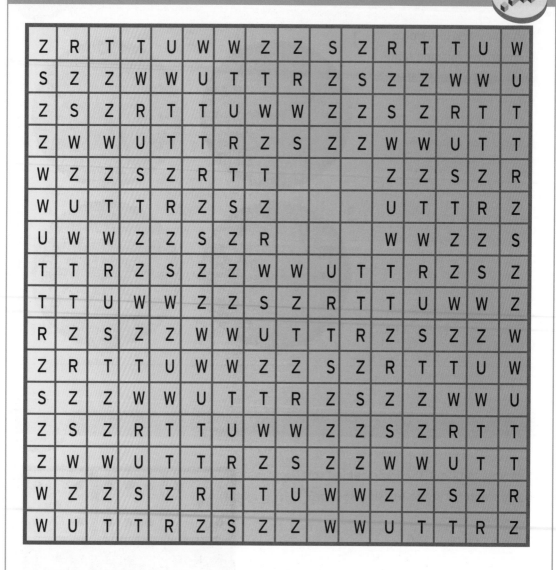

Z	R	T	T	U	W	W	Z	Z	S	Z	R	T	T	U	W
S	Z	Z	W	W	U	T	T	R	Z	S	Z	Z	W	W	U
Z	S	Z	R	T	T	U	W	W	Z	Z	S	Z	R	T	T
Z	W	W	U	T	T	R	Z	S	Z	Z	W	W	U	T	T
W	Z	Z	S	Z	R	T	T				Z	Z	S	Z	R
W	U	T	T	R	Z	S	Z				U	T	T	R	Z
U	W	W	Z	Z	S	Z	R				W	W	Z	Z	S
T	T	R	Z	S	Z	Z	W	W	U	T	T	R	Z	S	Z
T	T	U	W	W	Z	Z	S	Z	R	T	T	U	W	W	Z
R	Z	S	Z	Z	W	W	U	T	T	R	Z	S	Z	Z	W
Z	R	T	T	U	W	W	Z	Z	S	Z	R	T	T	U	W
S	Z	Z	W	W	U	T	T	R	Z	S	Z	Z	W	W	U
Z	S	Z	R	T	T	U	W	W	Z	Z	S	Z	R	T	T
Z	W	W	U	T	T	R	Z	S	Z	Z	W	W	U	T	T
W	Z	Z	S	Z	R	T	T	U	W	W	Z	Z	S	Z	R
W	U	T	T	R	Z	S	Z	Z	W	W	U	T	T	R	Z

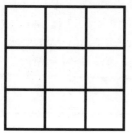

Can you spot the pattern of this grid and complete the missing section?

Answer see page **166**

PUZZLE 106

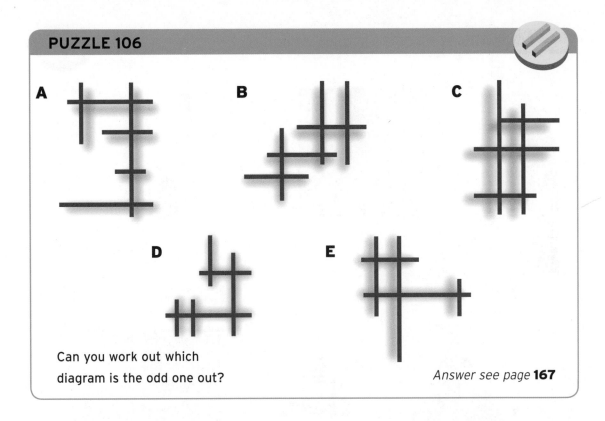

A

B

C

D

E

Can you work out which diagram is the odd one out?

Answer see page 167

PUZZLE 107

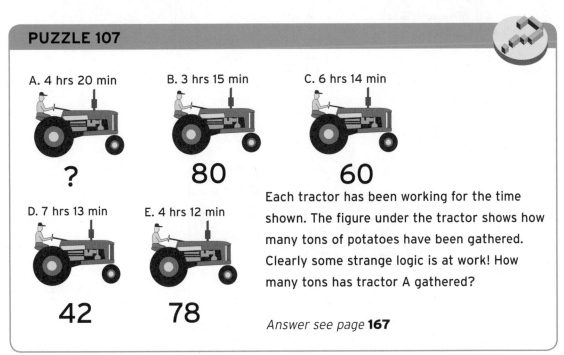

A. 4 hrs 20 min

?

B. 3 hrs 15 min

80

C. 6 hrs 14 min

60

D. 7 hrs 13 min

42

E. 4 hrs 12 min

78

Each tractor has been working for the time shown. The figure under the tractor shows how many tons of potatoes have been gathered. Clearly some strange logic is at work! How many tons has tractor A gathered?

Answer see page 167

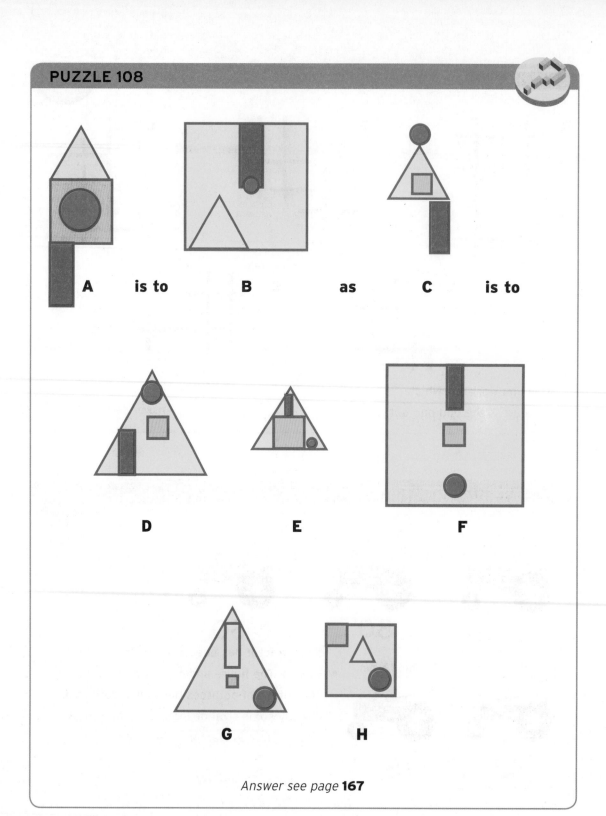

A   is to   B   as   C   is to

D   E   F

G   H

Answer see page **167**

PUZZLE 109

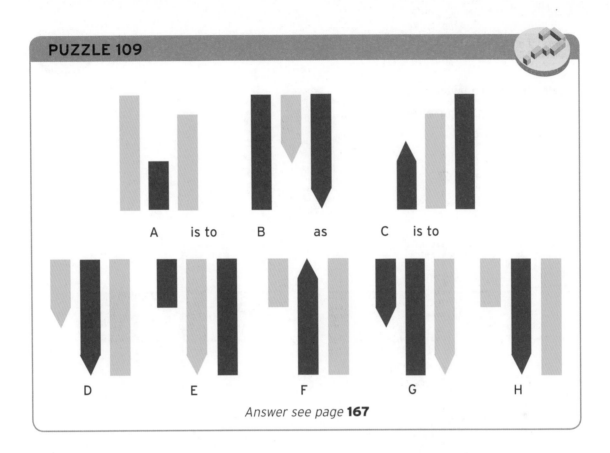

A   is to   B   as   C   is to

D   E   F   G   H

Answer see page 167

PUZZLE 110

Can you spot the cube that cannot be made from the layout below?

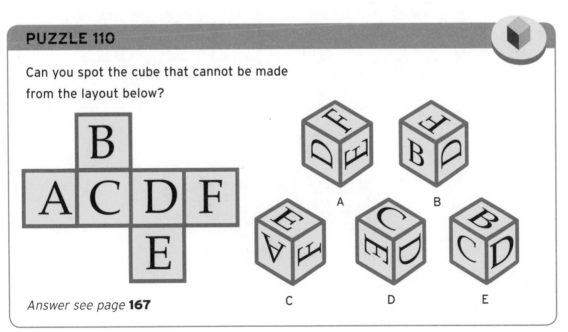

Answer see page 167

Which of these layouts could be used to make the cube to the right?

Answer see page **167**

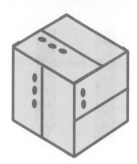

A

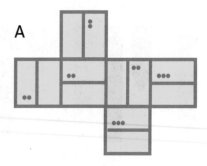

B

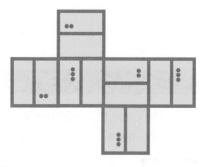

C

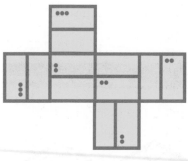

D

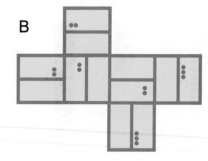

E

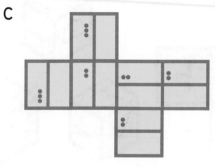

PUZZLE 112

If you know that the answer forms a well-known sequence, can you work out how much each shape is worth?

Answer see page **167**

15	♥	1	♦
15	3	5	7
15	♣	9	♠
	15	15	15

PUZZLE 113

Can you work out what the next matchstick man in this series should look like?

Answer see page **167**

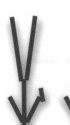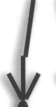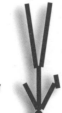

?

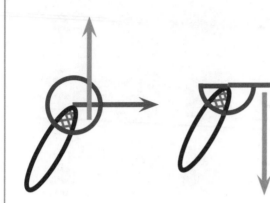

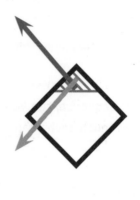

A   is to   **B**   as   **C**   is to

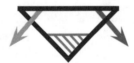

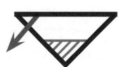

D

E

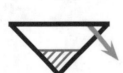

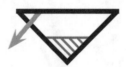

F

G   *Answer see page* **167**

PUZZLE 115

Which of these columns would continue the sequence to the right?

Answer see page **167**

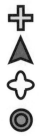

A B C D E

PUZZLE 116

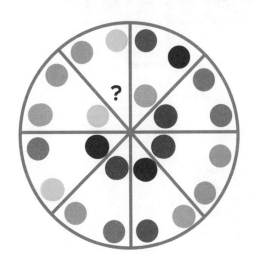

Find a number that could replace the question mark. Each color represents a number under 10.

Answer see page **167**

Which of the following layouts could
be used to make the above cube?

Answer see page **167**

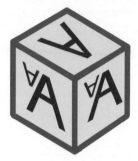

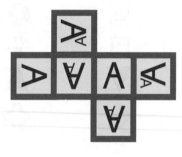

A

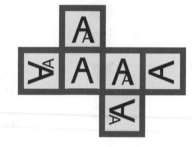

B

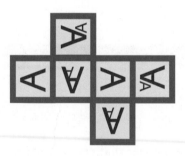

C

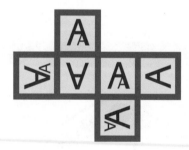

D

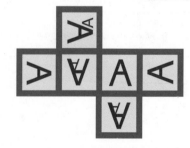

E

PUZZLE 118

Can you work out which symbol is
the odd one out?

Answer see page **167**

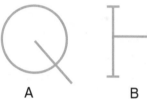 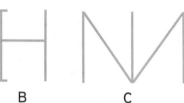 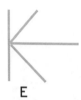 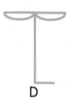

A   B   C   D   E

PUZZLE 119

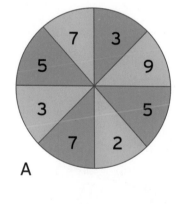 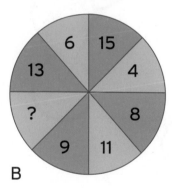 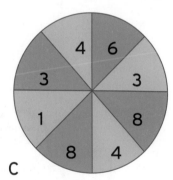

A   B   C

Can you replace the question mark with a
number?

Answer see page **167**

Can you work out which is
the odd diagram out?

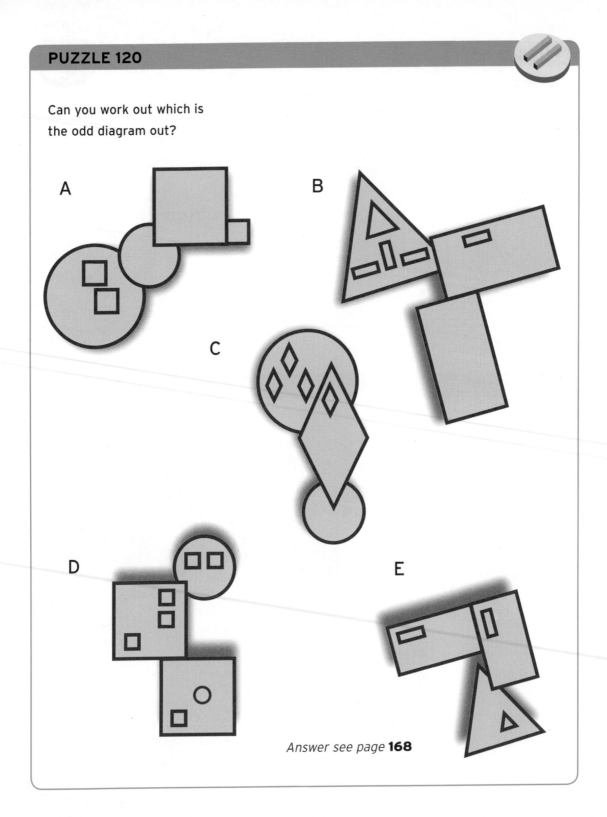

A

B

C

D

E

Answer see page **168**

Can you work out which of these symbols comes next in this sequence?

Answer see page **168**

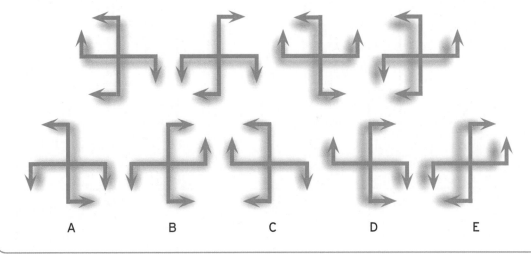

A   B   C   D   E

Can you work out the logic behind this square and find the missing number?

Answer see page **168**

24	?	21
22		45
5	38	17

Can you work out what pattern this grid follows and complete the missing section?

Answer see page **168**

Can you work out the reasoning behind this
grid and complete the missing section?

Answer see page **168**

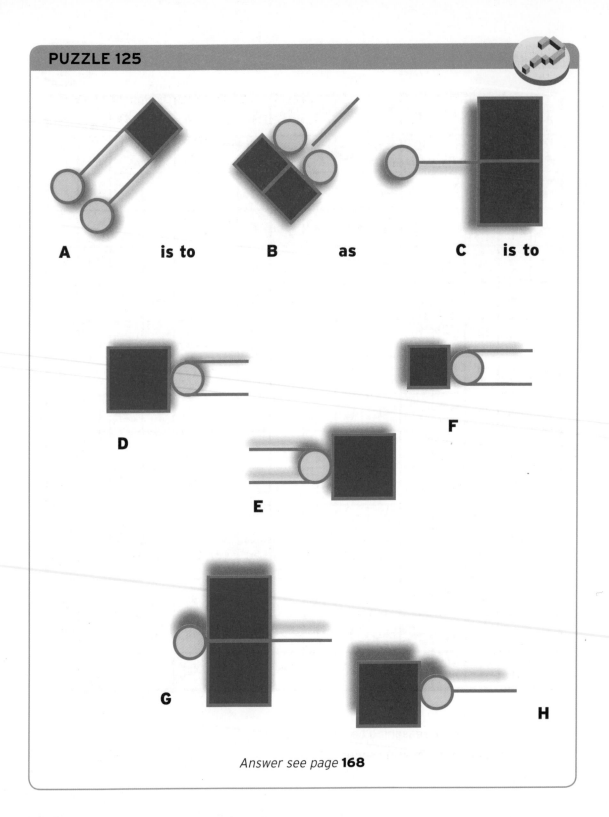

PUZZLE 125

A is to B as C is to

D

E

F

G

H

Answer see page **168**

PUZZLE 126

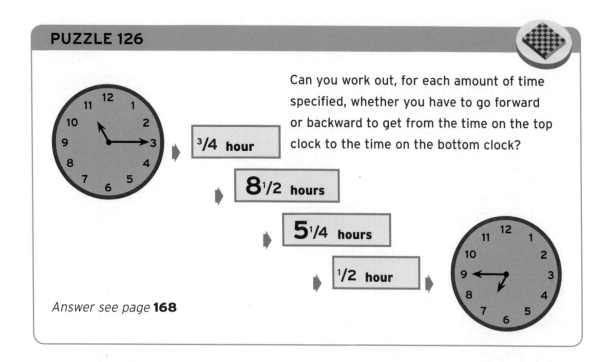

Can you work out, for each amount of time specified, whether you have to go forward or backward to get from the time on the top clock to the time on the bottom clock?

³/4 hour

8¹/2 hours

5¹/4 hours

¹/2 hour

Answer see page **168**

PUZZLE 127

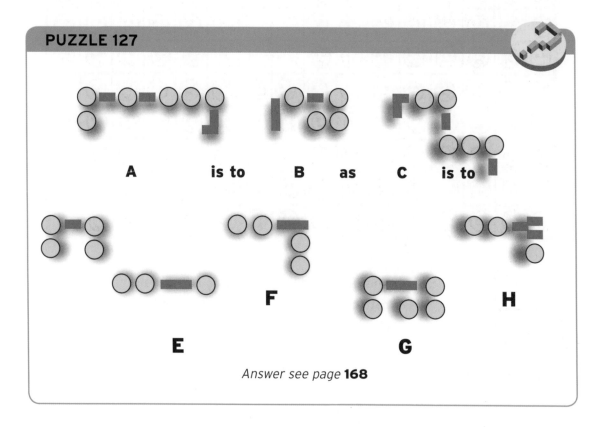

A   is to   B   as   C   is to

E

F

G

H

Answer see page **168**

This grid is made up according to a certain pattern. Can you work it out and fill in the missing section?

Answer see page **168**

PUZZLE 129

Can you work out how many rectangles altogether can be found in this diagram?

Answer see page **169**

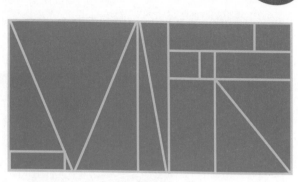

PUZZLE 130

Can you work out which shape is the odd one out?

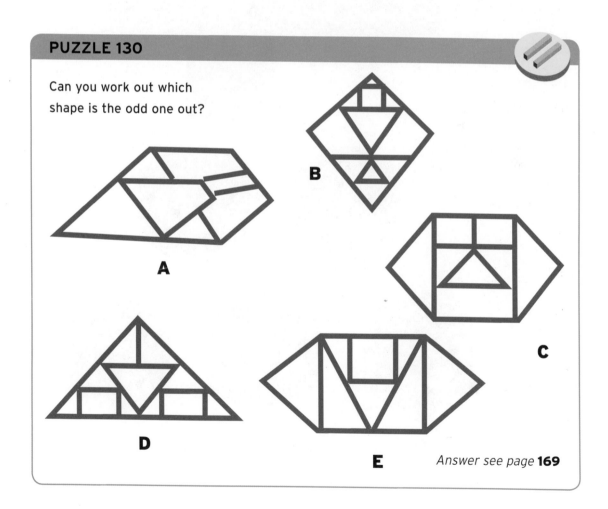

A

B

C

D

E

Answer see page **169**

Can you work out which of these cubes
cannot be made from the layout below?

Answer see page **169**

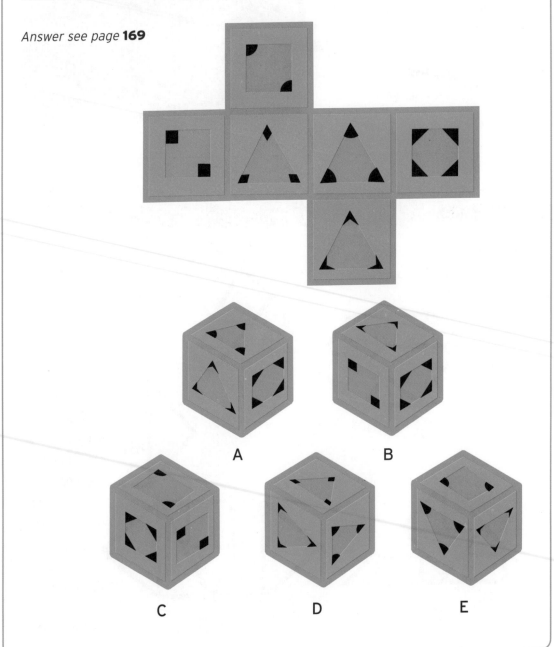

A

B

C

D

E

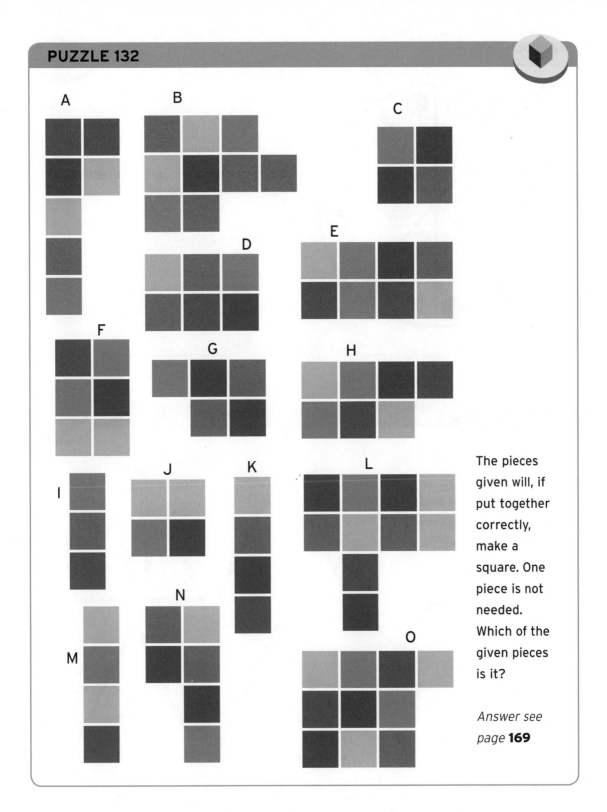

The pieces given will, if put together correctly, make a square. One piece is not needed. Which of the given pieces is it?

Answer see page **169**

PUZZLE 133

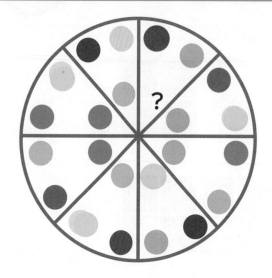

Which color is the circle that replaces the question mark?

Answer see page **169**

PUZZLE 134

Find a number that could replace the question mark. Each color represents a number under 10.

Answer see page **169**

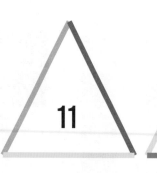
11

13

14

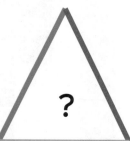
?

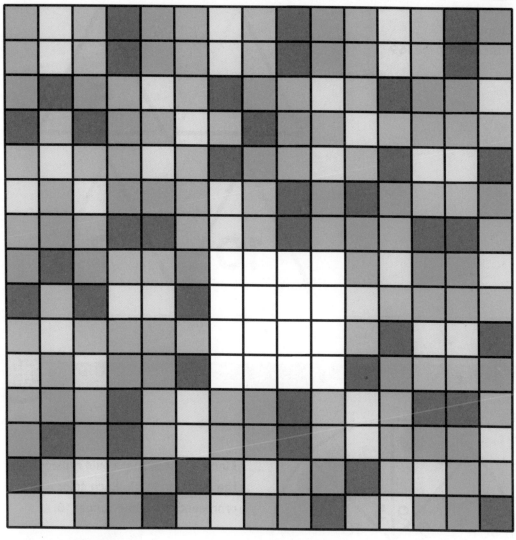

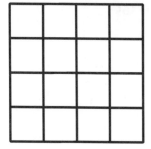

This square is drawn according to a certain logic. If you can work out what the system is you should be able to fill in the missing area.

Answer see page **169**

PUZZLE 136

Find the missing number.

Answer see page **169**

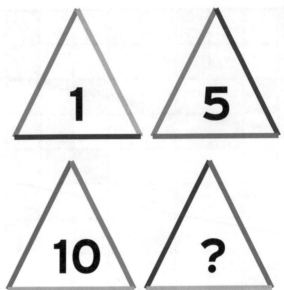

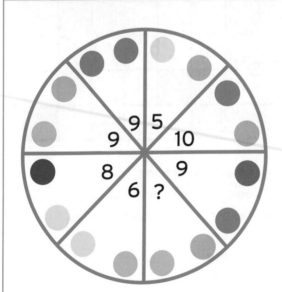

PUZZLE 137

Find a number that could replace the question mark. Each color represents a number under 10.

Answer see page **169**

5	6	9
4	3	2
2	7	1

8	4	12
2	6	0
0	10	4

4	9	6
22	7	11
2	14	1

A   is to   B   as   C   is to

8	18	12
44	14	22
4	28	2

D

7	7	9
25	5	9
5	17	0

E

7	12	9
25	10	14
5	17	4

F

2	12	4
20	10	14
0	12	4

G

Answer see page 169

2	2	3	1	1	7	1	4	5	5	2	2	3	1	1	7
5	3	1	1	7	1	4	5	5	2	2	3	1	1	7	1
5	2	3	1	1	7	1	4	5	5	2	2	3	1	1	4
4	2	2	2	2	3	1	1	7	1	4	5	5	2	7	5
1	5	2	5	1	4	5	5	2	2	3	1	1	2	1	5
7	5	5	5	7	2	2	3	1	1	7	1	7	3	4	2
1	4	5	4	1	5	3	1	1	7	1	4	1	1	5	2
1	1	4	1	1	5	2	3	1	1	4	5	4	1	5	3
3	7	1	7	3	4	2	2	2	7	5	5	5	7	2	1
2	1	7	1	2	1	5	5	4	1	5	2	5	1	2	1
2	1	1	1	2	7	1	1	3	2	2	2	2	4	3	7
5	3	1	3	5	5	4	1	7	1	1	3	2	5	1	1
5	2	3	2	2	5	5	4	1	7	1	1	3	5	1	4
4	2	2	2	5	5	4	1	7	1	1	3	2	2	7	5
1	4	5	4	1	7	1	1	3	2	2	5	5	4	1	5
1	1	1	3	2	2	5	5	4	1	7	1	1	3	2	2

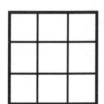

Can you work out the reasoning behind this grid and complete the missing section?

Answer see page **169**

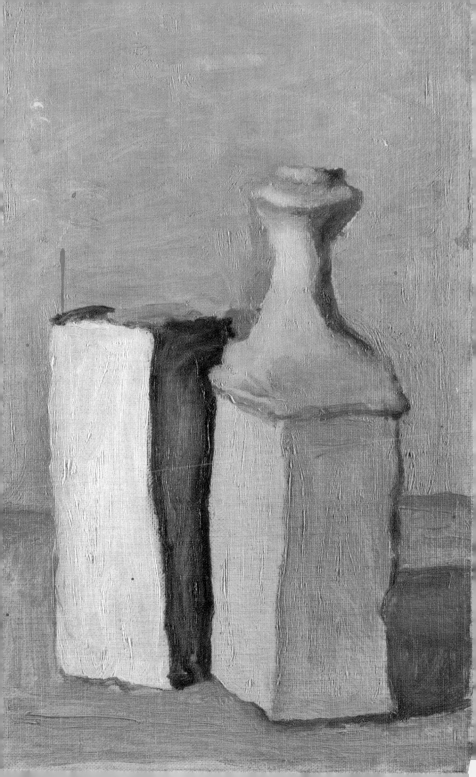

PUZZLE 140

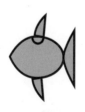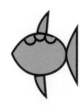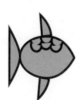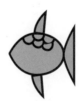

?

Can you find the column that comes next in the sequence?

Answer see page **169**

 A   B   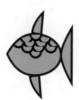 C   D    E

PUZZLE 141

Can you work out what the next fish in this sequence should look like?

Answer see page **170**

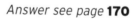

?

5	÷	2	=	6
−				X
13				5
+				−
?	÷	7	+	21

Can you work out what number should replace the question mark?

*Answer see page **170***

The weight of each suitcase is shown.
Which is the odd one out?

*Answer see page **170***

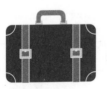 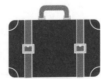 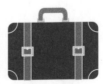 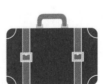

A 33 kg   B 35 kg   C 60 kg   D 42 kg   E 15 kg

PUZZLE 144

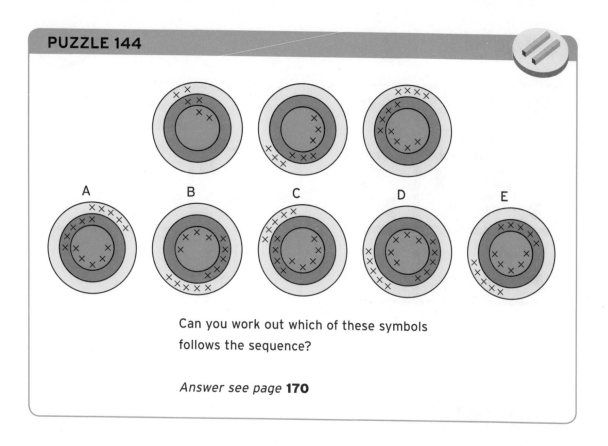

Can you work out which of these symbols follows the sequence?

Answer see page **170**

PUZZLE 145

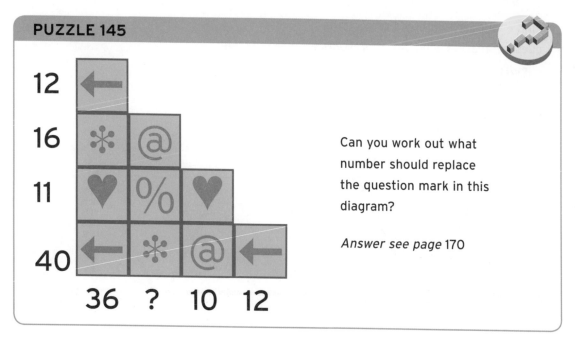

Can you work out what number should replace the question mark in this diagram?

Answer see page 170

PUZZLE 146

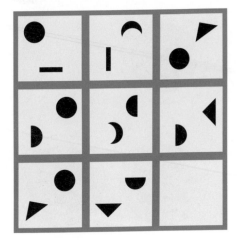

Can you work out which of these squares would complete the above diagram?

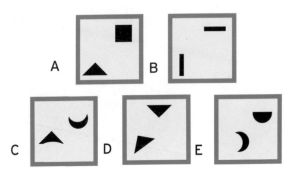

A   B   C   D   E

Answer see page **170**

PUZZLE 147

Find a number that could replace the question mark. Each color represents a number under 10.

Answer see page **170**

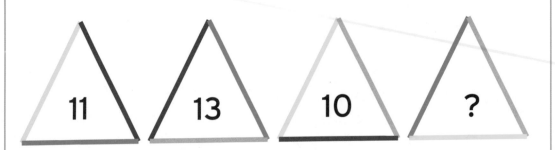

11   13   10   ?

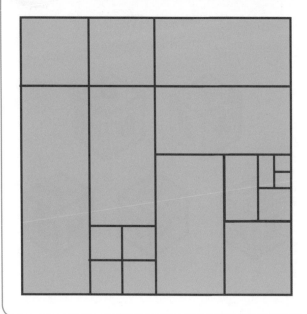

How many squares can you find altogether in this diagram?

Answer see page **170**

Which of these triangles is the odd one out? Their color is a factor.

Answer see page **170**

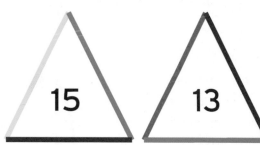

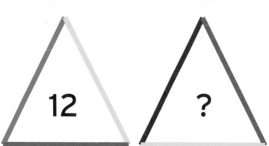

PUZZLE 150

Can you spot the cube that cannot be made from the layout below?

Answer see page **170**

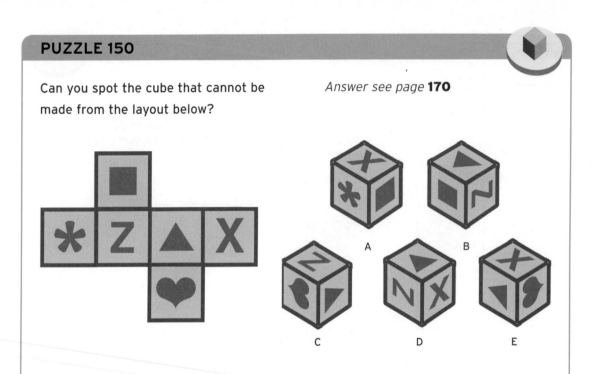

PUZZLE 151

Find a number that could replace the question mark. Each color represents a number under 10.

Answer see page **170**

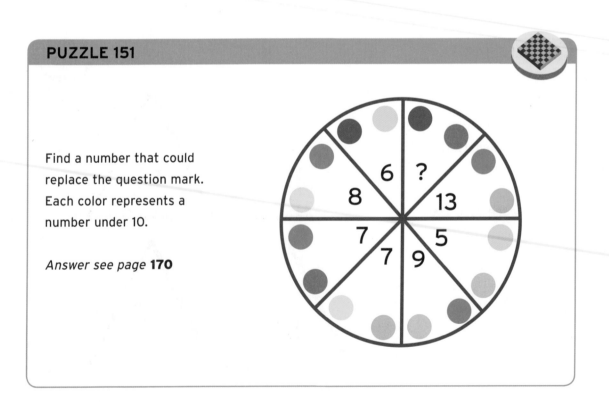

PUZZLE 152

12   19

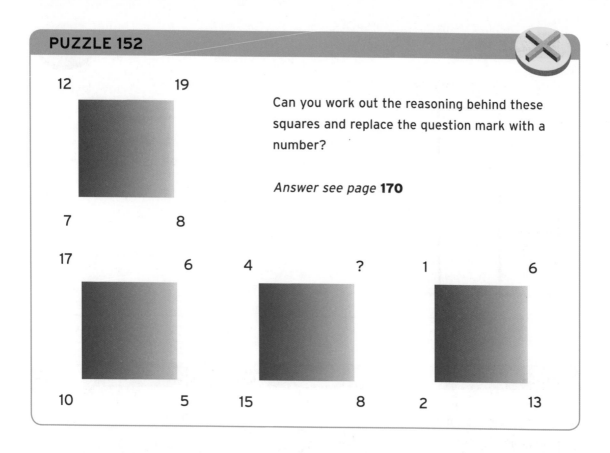

7   8

17   6   4   ?   1   6

10   5   15   8   2   13

Can you work out the reasoning behind these squares and replace the question mark with a number?

Answer see page **170**

PUZZLE 153

Can you find the number that should replace the question mark?

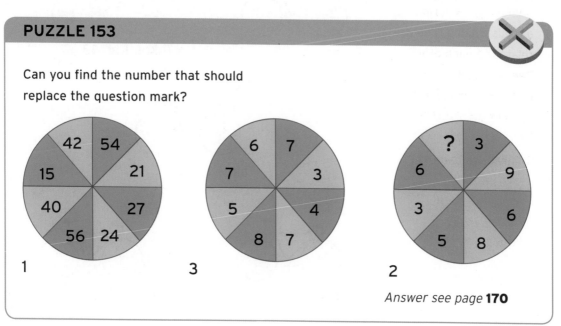

1   3   2

Answer see page **170**

PUZZLE 154

1   2   3

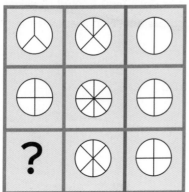

Can you work out the reasoning behind this square and replace the question mark with the correct shape?

Answer see page **170**

PUZZLE 155

Five cyclists are taking part in a race. The number of each rider and his cycling time are related to each other. Can you work out the number of the last cyclist?

Answer see page **171**

No. 9

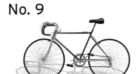

Takes 1 hr 35

No. 10

Takes 1 hr 43

No. 11

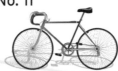

Takes 1 hr 52

No. 14

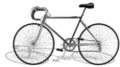

Takes 2 hr 27

No. ?

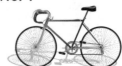

Takes 2 hr 33

PUZZLE 156

Can you work out which diagram would continue the series?

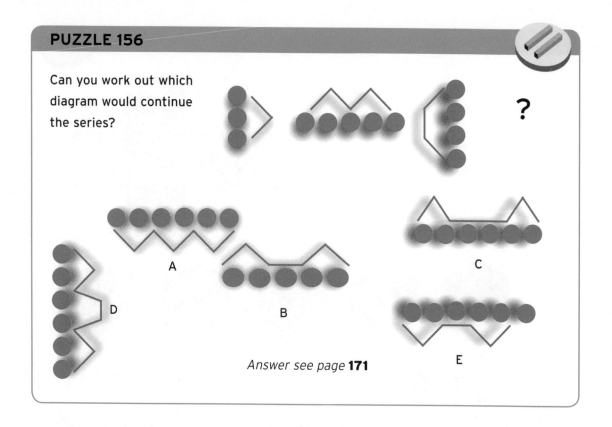

*Answer see page **171***

PUZZLE 157

Find the missing number.

*Answer see page **171***

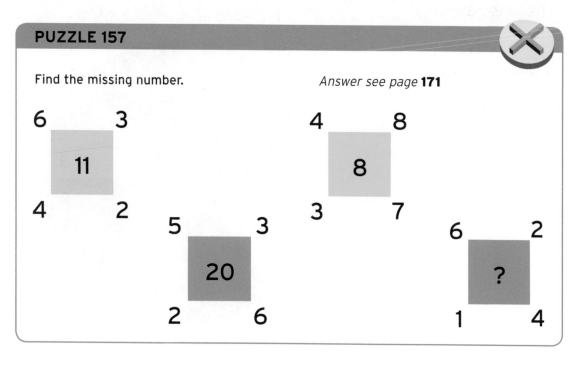

PUZZLE 158

Which of these cubes can be made from the above layout?

Answer see page **171**

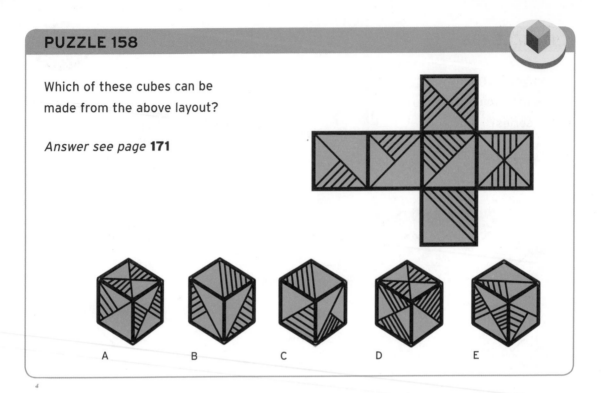

A   B   C   D   E

PUZZLE 159

Can you work out the reasoning behind this wheel and replace the question mark with a number?

Answer see page **171**

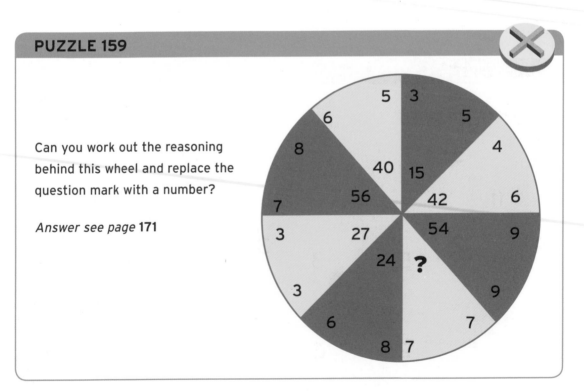

A   is to   B   as   C   is to

D

E

F

G

H

*Answer see page **171***

PUZZLE 161

Can you work out what the next grid in the sequence below should look like?

Answer see page **171**

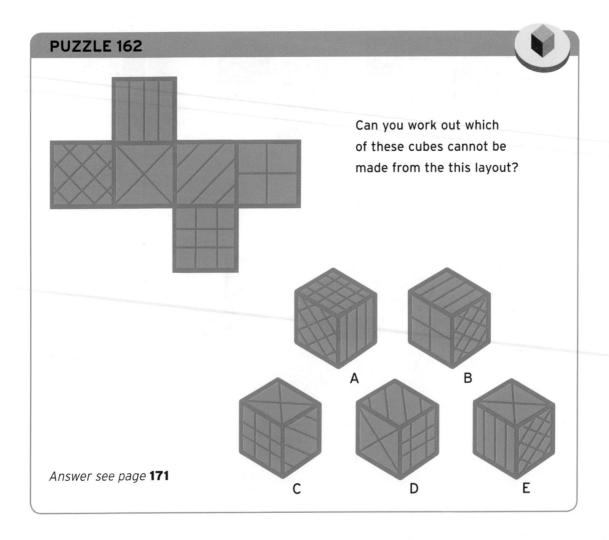

PUZZLE 162

Can you work out which of these cubes cannot be made from the this layout?

Answer see page **171**

A   B   C   D   E

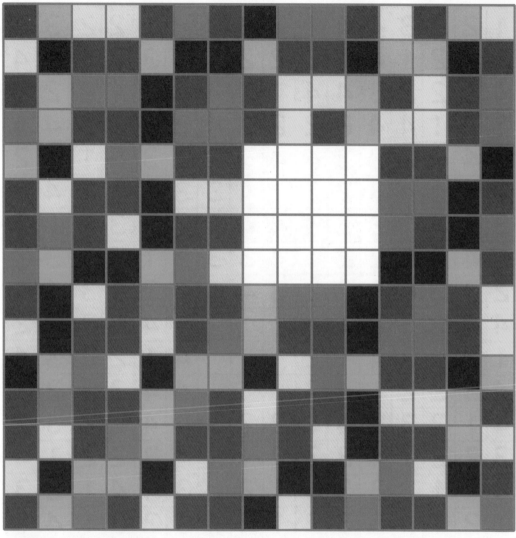

The small squares form a logical sequence. If you can discover what that sequence is you should be able to complete the missing section.

Answer see page 171

1	2	2	3	4	4	1	2	3	3	4	1	2	2	3	4
3	3	2	1	4	4	3	2	2	1	4	3	3	2	1	4
4	1	2	2	3	4	4	1	2	3	3	4	1	2	2	3
3	2	1	4	4	3	2	2	1	4	3	3	2	1	4	4
3	4	1	2	2	3	4	4	1	2	3	3	4	1	2	2
2	1	4	4	3	2	2	1	4	3	3	2	1	4	4	3
3	3	4	1	2	2	3	4	4	1	2	3	3	4	1	2
1	4	4	3	2	2	1	4	3	3	2	1	4	4	3	2
2	3	3	4	1	2	2	3	4	4	1	2	3	3	4	1
4	4	3	2	2	1	4				1	4	4	3	2	2
1	2	3	3	4	1	2				4	1	2	3	3	4
4	3	2	2	1	4	3				4	4	3	2	2	1
4	1	2	3	3	4	1	2	2	3	4	4	1	2	3	3
3	2	2	1	4	3	3	2	1	4	4	3	2	2	1	4
4	4	1	2	3	3	4	1	2	2	3	4	4	1	2	3
2	2	1	4	3	3	2	1	4	4	3	2	2	1	4	3

Can you work out the reasoning behind this grid and complete the missing section?

Answer see page 171

142

PUZZLE 165

```
      3
   5  ◆  4
      9
```

A

is to

```
      8
  14 (21) 7
     13
```

B

as

```
      4
   2  ◆  8
     11
```

C

is to

```
      6
 13 (25) 12
     19
```

D

```
      7
  5 (44) 11
     14
```

E

```
     12
 13 (16) 19
     15
```

F

```
     12
  6 (25) 19
     13
```

G

Answer see page 172

PUZZLE 166

Each horse carries a weight handicap.

Can you work out the number of the final horse?

Answer see page 172

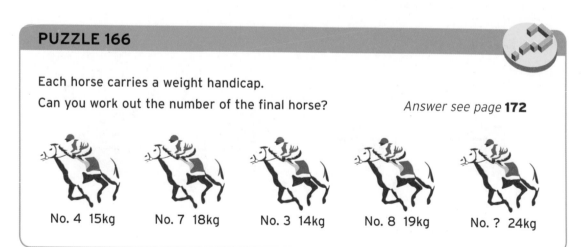

No. 4 15kg   No. 7 18kg   No. 3 14kg   No. 8 19kg   No. ? 24kg

143

PUZZLE 167

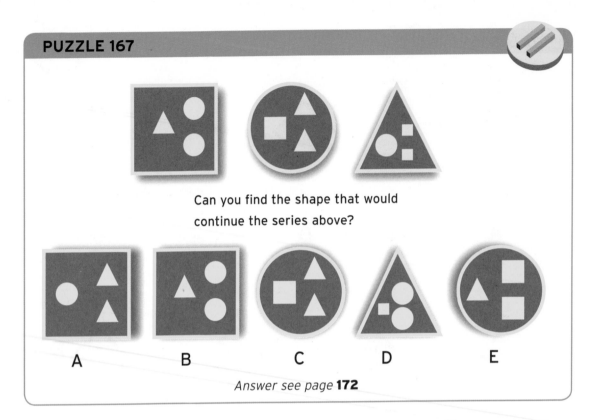

Can you find the shape that would continue the series above?

A   B   C   D   E

Answer see page **172**

PUZZLE 168

Can you work out the reasoning behind these squares and find the missing number?

Answer see page **172**

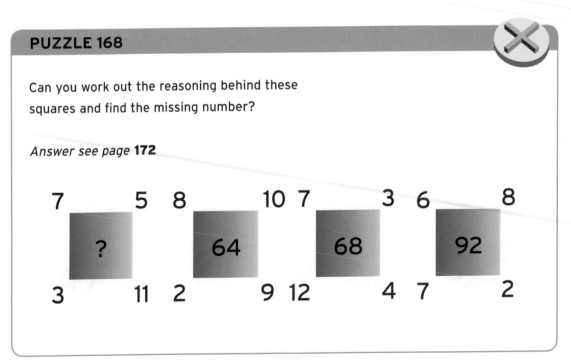

144

PUZZLE 169

All these bikes took part in an overnight race. Something really weird happened! The start and finish times of the bikes became mathematically linked. If you can discover the link you should be able to decide when bike D finished.

Answer see page **172**

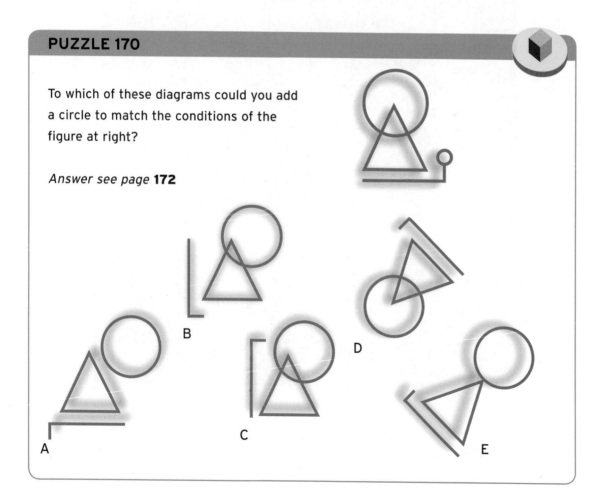

A START 3:15
FINISH 2:06

B START 3:20
FINISH 1:09

C START 5:24
FINISH 2:11

D START 7:35
FINISH ?

E START 6:28
FINISH 4:22

PUZZLE 170

To which of these diagrams could you add a circle to match the conditions of the figure at right?

Answer see page **172**

A

B

C

D

E

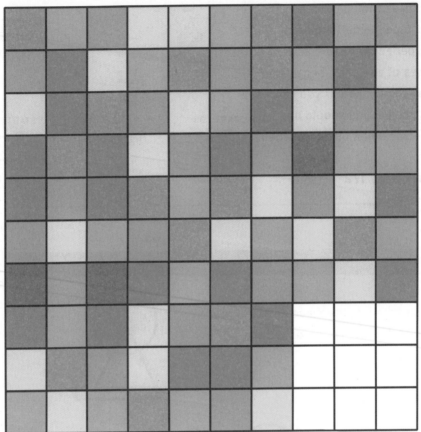

A   B   C

Which of the sections shown would
logically complete the puzzle?

Answer see page **172**

PUZZLE 172

Which of these shapes fits to complete the polygon?

Answer see page **172**

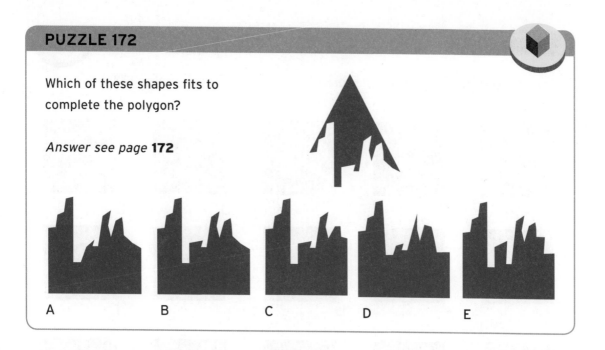

A   B   C   D   E

PUZZLE 173

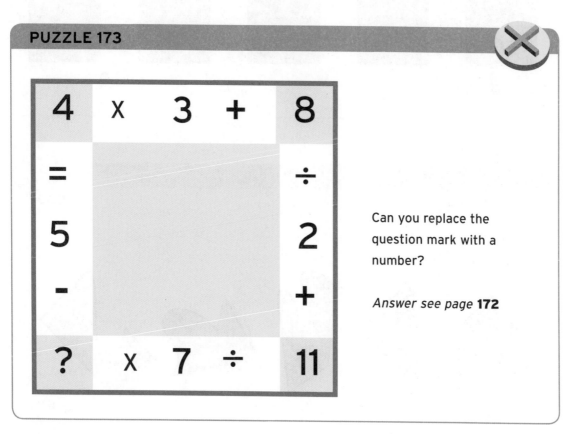

Can you replace the question mark with a number?

Answer see page **172**

PUZZLE 174

Can you work out which of these squares is the odd one out?

Answer see page **172**

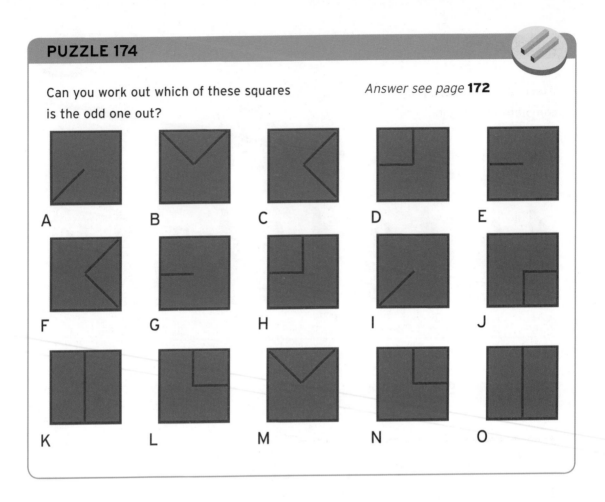

A   B   C   D   E

F   G   H   I   J

K   L   M   N   O

PUZZLE 175

Can you find the odd shape out?

Answer see page **172**

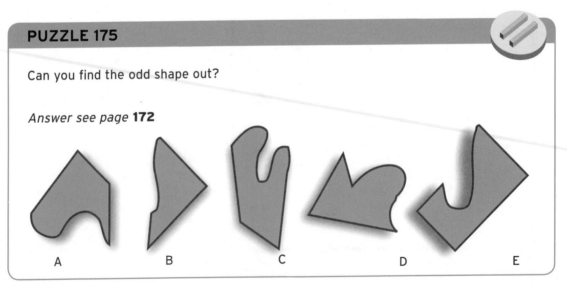

A   B   C   D   E

&	&	%	*	%	@	@	%	*	&	&	%	*	%	@	@
*	@	@	%	*	&	&	%	*	%	@	@	%	*	&	&
%	%	&	&	%	*	%	@	@	%	*	&	&	%	*	%
@	*	*	*	%	@	@	%	*	&	&	%	*	%	%	*
@	%	%	%	@				&	&	%	*	%	@	@	%
%	&	@	&	%				&	&	%	*	@	@	@	@
*	&	@	&	*				*	&	&	%	@	%	%	@
%	*	%	*	%	%	@	@	@	%	%	@	%	*	*	%
&	%	*	%	&	*	%	%	*	*	*	@	*	&	&	*
&	@	%	@	&	%	*	%	&	&	%	%	&	&	&	&
*	@	&	@	*	&	&	*	%	@	@	*	&	%	%	&
%	%	&	%	%	@	@	%	*	%	&	&	%	*	*	%
@	*	*	*	%	&	&	*	%	@	@	%	*	%	%	*
@	%	%	@	@	%	*	%	&	&	*	%	@	@	@	%
%	&	&	*	%	@	@	%	*	%	&	&	*	%	@	@
*	%	&	&	*	%	@	@	%	*	%	&	&	*	%	@

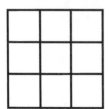

Can you work out the pattern sequence and fill in the missing section?

*Answer see page **172***

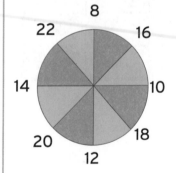

?	−	5	x	4
÷				÷
14				6
+				−
8	=	5	+	1

Can you work out what number should replace the question mark?

Answer see page **173**

Can you work out what number should replace the question mark?

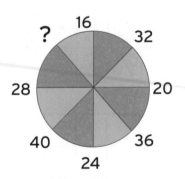

Circle 1: 8, 16, 10, 18, 12, 20, 14, 22

Circle 2: 12, 24, 15, 27, 18, 30, 21, 33

Circle 3: 16, 32, 20, 36, 24, 40, 28, ?

Answer see page **173**

PUZZLE 179

Which cube can be made from this layout?

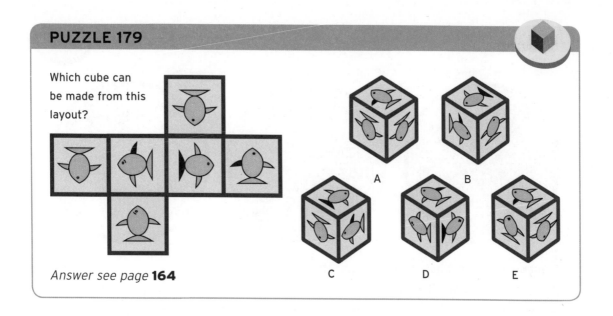

Answer see page **164**

PUZZLE 180

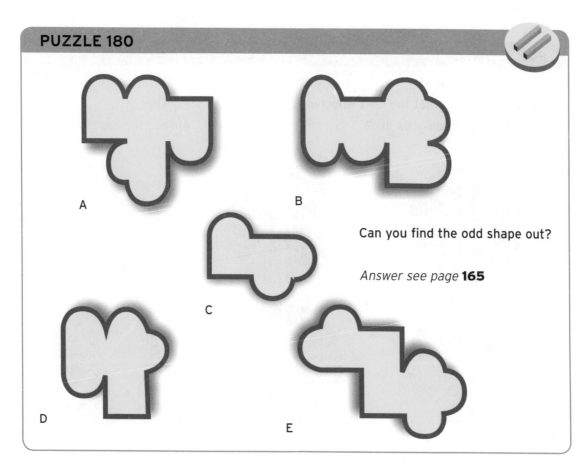

Can you find the odd shape out?

Answer see page **165**

PUZZLE 181

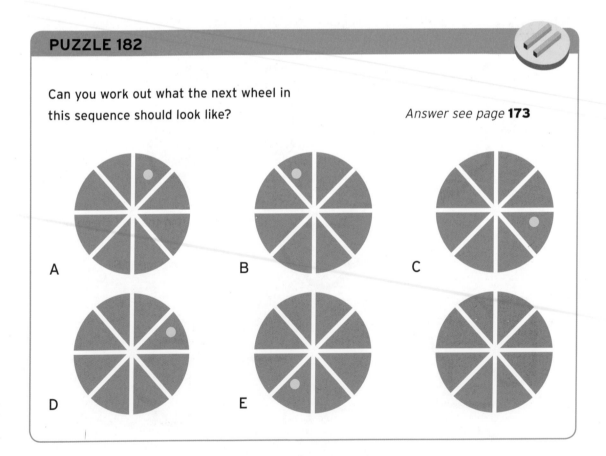

Can you work out what the missing section in the last wheel should look like?

Answer see page **173**

PUZZLE 182

Can you work out what the next wheel in this sequence should look like?

Answer see page **173**

A

B

C

D

E

152 ●●●

PUZZLE 183

A is to   B as   C is to

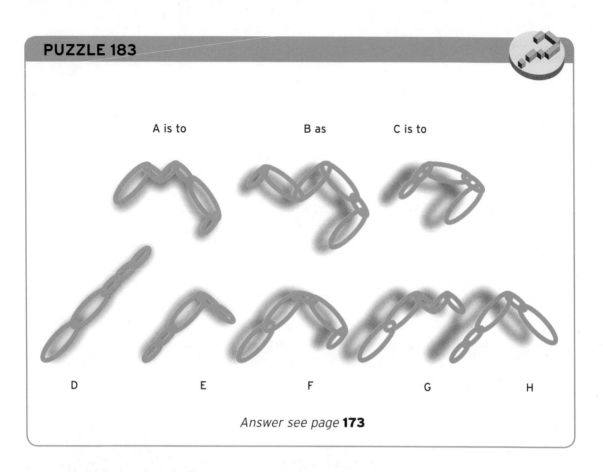

D   E   F   G   H

Answer see page 173

PUZZLE 184

Can you work out the reasoning behind these
squares and find the number that should
replace the question mark?

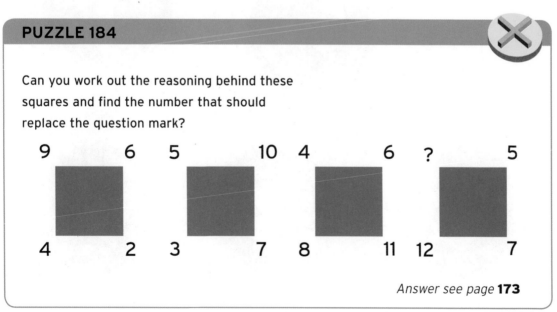

9   6   5   10   4   6   ?   5

4   2   3   7   8   11 12   7

Answer see page 173

PUZZLE 185

Can you find the odd shape out?

Answer see page **173**

A   B   C   E   D

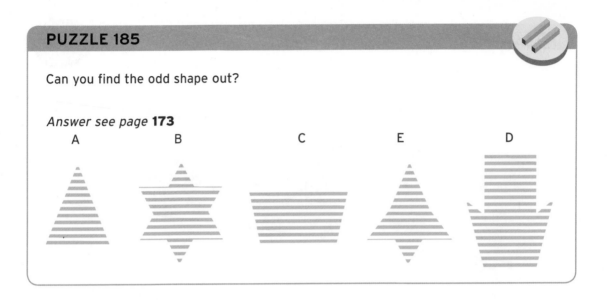

PUZZLE 186

Can you find the odd diagram out?

Answer see page **173**

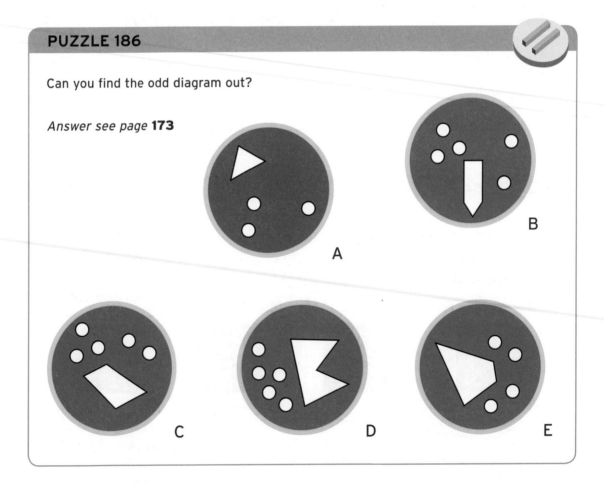

A

B

C

D

E

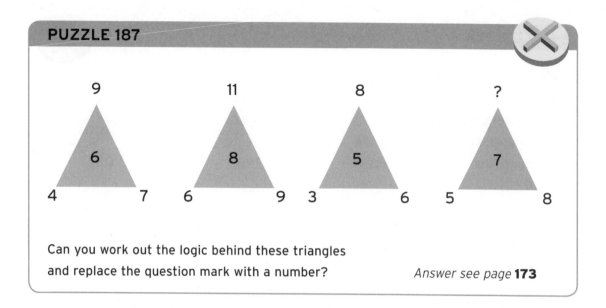

Can you work out the logic behind these triangles
and replace the question mark with a number?

Answer see page **173**

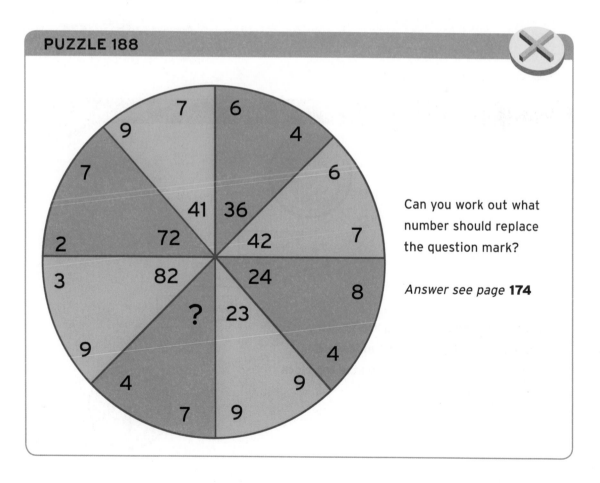

Can you work out what
number should replace
the question mark?

Answer see page **174**

PUZZLE 189

Five cyclists are taking part in a race. The number of each rider and its arrival time are in some way related. Can you work out the number of the rider who arrives at 2:30?

No. 10

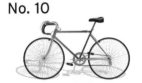

Arrives 2:15

No. 2

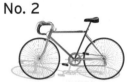

Arrives 3:02

No. 30

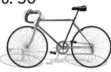

Arrives 2:45

No. 8

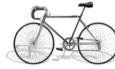

Arrives 3:08

No. ?

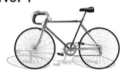

Arrives 2:30

Answer see page **1674**

PUZZLE 190

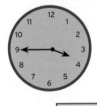

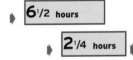

1 hour

3¹/2 hours

6¹/2 hours

2¹/4 hours

Using the amounts of time specified, can you work out whether you have to go forward or backward to get from the time on the top clock to that on the bottom clock?

Answer see page **174**

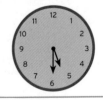

PUZZLE 191

Can you work out the reasoning behind this square and replace the question mark with a number?

Answer see page **174**

5	3	8	7
12	15	49	56
3	9	4	12
18	27	36	?

PUZZLE 192

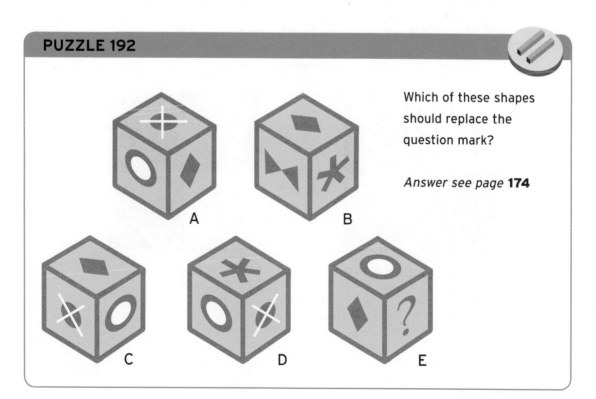

Which of these shapes should replace the question mark?

Answer see page **174**

What colour replaces the
question mark?

Answer see page **174**

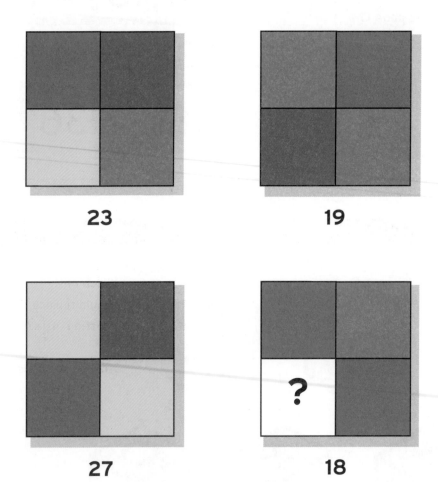

23

19

27

18

PUZZLE 194

Can you work out which of these symbols follows the sequence above?

Answer see page **174**

A   B   C   D   E

PUZZLE 195

Can you work out the reasoning behind these triangles and replace the question mark with a number?

Answer see page **174**

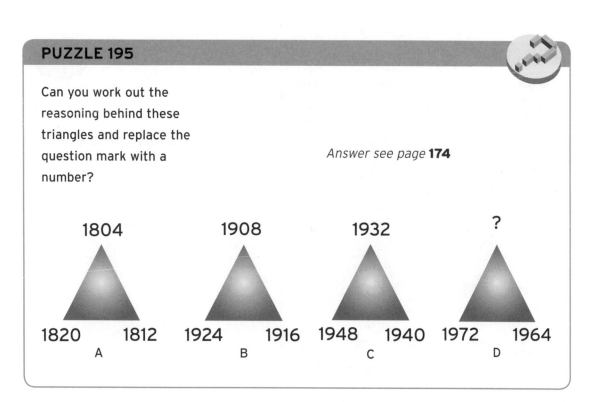

1804

1908

1932

?

1820   1812
       A

1924   1916
       B

1948   1940
       C

1972   1964
       D

PUZZLE 196

The following clock faces are in some way related. Can you work out what the time on clock No. 3 should be?

Answer see page 174

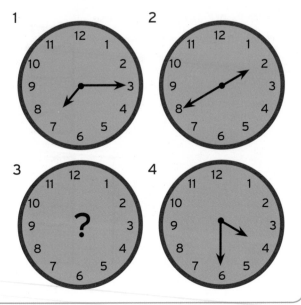

PUZZLE 197

?	-	9	x	5
=				÷
7				2
+				-
3	÷	12	+	4

Can you work out what number should replace the question mark in this square?

Answer see page 174

Which diagram is the odd
one out?

Answer see page **174**

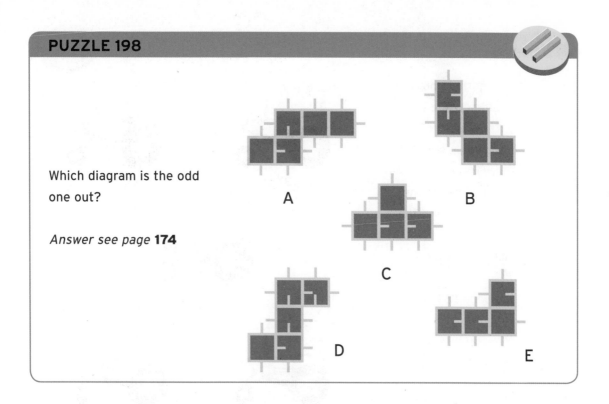

A

B

C

D

E

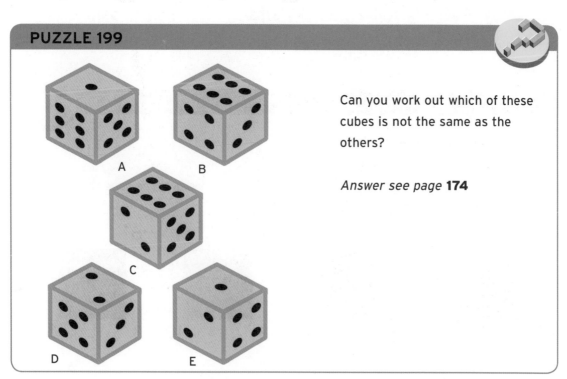

Can you work out which of these
cubes is not the same as the
others?

Answer see page **174**

A

B

C

D

E

PUZZLE 200

Each tractor gathers potatoes over a certain acreage (shown in brackets). The weight of potatoes in kilos is shown under each tractor. There is a relationship between the number of the tractor, the acreage and the weight gathered. What weight should tractor B show?

Answer see page **174**

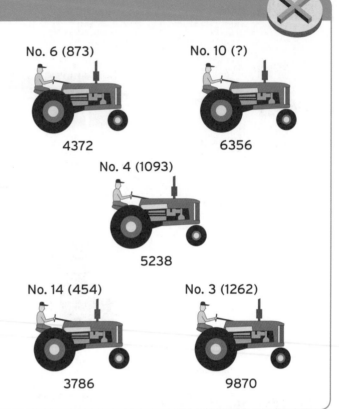

No. 6 (873)

4372

No. 10 (?)

6356

No. 4 (1093)

5238

No. 14 (454)

3786

No. 3 (1262)

9870

PUZZLE 201

Can you unravel the logic behind these squares and find the missing number?

Answer see page **174**

10   5   4   7   9   1   6   2

25   10   17   ?

3   1   6   2   3   10   3   6

1536	48	96	3
384	192	24	12
768	96	48	6
192	?	12	24

Can you find the missing number in this square?

Answer see page **175**

Can you work out what the next flower in this series should look like?

Answer see page **175**

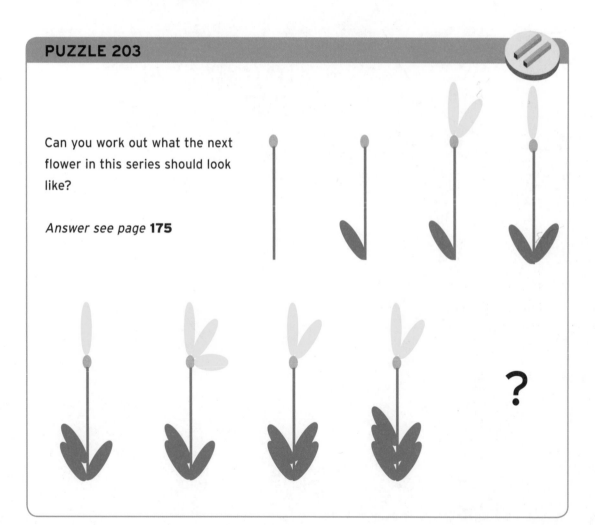

?

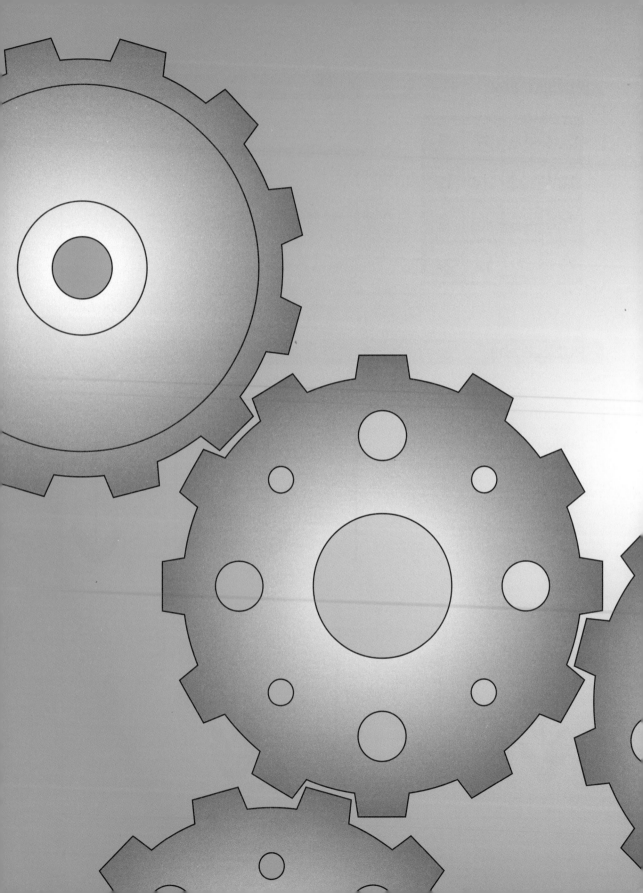

Medium
Answers

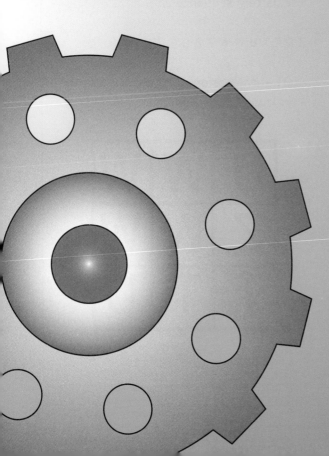

ANSWER 96

F. A curve turns into a straight line and a straight line into a curve.

ANSWER 97

C. It is the only one that does not have half as many 'step' lines as there are triangles.

ANSWER 98

2. The colors are worth Pink 1, Green 2, Orange 3, Yellow 4, Red 5, Purple 6. In each segment subtract the smaller outer number from the larger and put the difference in the center of the next segment clockwise.

ANSWER 99

- x + - ÷ +.
9 - 3 x 4 + 19 - 8 ÷ 5 + 4 = 11.

ANSWER 100

B. It is the only figure that, with an additional line, has a triangle adjoining the rectangle that overlaps the square.

ANSWER 101

7

ANSWER 102

E. A square becomes a circle, a circle a triangle, and a triangle a square of similar proportions and positions.

ANSWER 103

8. The sum of hands on each clock is 13.

ANSWER 104

It should have two dots. Add together the corner squares of each row or column and put the sum in the middle square of the opposite row or column.

ANSWER 105

The pattern sequence is:

Z R T T U W W Z Z S

Start at the bottom right and work up in a horizontal boustrophedon.

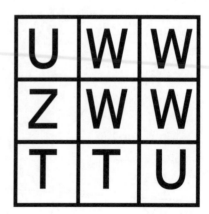

ANSWER 106

B. It is the only one with the same number of vertical and horizontal lines.

ANSWER 107

84. Multiply the hours of A by the minutes of B to get the tonnage of C, then B hours by C minutes to get D, C hours by D minutes to get E, D hours by E minutes to get A, and E hours by A minutes to get the tonnage of B.

ANSWER 108

G. The top and bottom elements swap position, the smaller central element becomes smaller still, and all three elements move inside the larger central shape.

ANSWER 109

E.

ANSWER 110

C.

ANSWER 111

B.

ANSWER 112

Spade = 2, Club = 4, Diamond = 6, Heart = 8.

ANSWER 113

The pattern is +1 lines, +2, +3, -2, -1, +1, +2, +3, etc. A figure with an even number of lines (ignoring the head) is turned upside down.

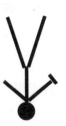

ANSWER 114

E. The shape has been folded along a horizontal line. A shaded piece covers an unshaded one.

ANSWER 115

D. Each column of elements alternates and moves up two rows.

ANSWER 116

6. The colors are worth Red 1, Orange 2, Green 3, Yellow 4, Pink 5, Purple 6, Brown 7. Add the outer numbers and put the sum in the center of the opposite segment.

ANSWER 117

D.

ANSWER 118

D. All the others are symmetrical.

ANSWER 119

12. Add together the values in the same segments in wheels A and C and put the answer in the opposite segment in wheel B.

ANSWER 120

C. It is the only one to have an odd number of one element.

ANSWER 121

D. Alternate between rotating the pattern 90° anti-clockwise, and swapping the direction of each individual arrow.

ANSWER 122

29. Add together the corner squares of each row or column in a clockwise direction. Put the sum in the middle of the next row or column.

ANSWER 123

The pattern sequence is: 1:00, 2:00, 2:00, 1:00, 3:00, 3:00, 2:00, 4:00, 4:00. 3:00, 5:00, 5:00, 4:00, 6:00, 6:00. Starting at the bottom left, work upwards in a vertical boustrophedon.

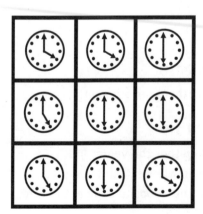

ANSWER 124

The pattern sequence is as follows.

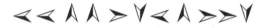

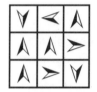 and spirals in a clockwise direction from the bottom left.

ANSWER 125

D. A circle becomes a square, a line a circle, and a square a line, all in the same size and position as the original.

ANSWER 126

Back, back, forward, back.

ANSWER 127

F. Circles and rectangles interchange except for strings of 3 circles, which disappear.

ANSWER 128

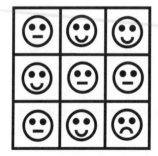

The faces pattern sequence is smiley, smiley, straight, sad, sad, smiley, straight, straight, sad, etc. Start at the bottom left and work in a horizontal boustrophedon.

ANSWER 129

23.

ANSWER 130

B. It consists of 14 straight lines, the rest of 13.

ANSWER 131

E.

ANSWER 132

B.

ANSWER 133

Yellow. The colors are worth Pink 2, Yellow 3, Orange 4, Green 5, Purple 6, Red 7, Brown 8. In each segment subtract the smaller of the outer numbers from the larger and put the result in the center of the next segment clockwise.

ANSWER 134

10. The colors are worth Orange 2, Red 3, Green 5, Yellow 6. The formula is 'add all three sides together'.

ANSWER 135

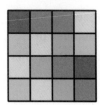 The colors are in the sequence Orange, Yellow, Pink, Red, Green and form an inward spiral starting at the top left.

ANSWER 136

The colors are worth Green 4, Purple 5, Red 6, Orange 8. The formula is left side plus base, minus right side.

ANSWER 137

6. The colors are worth Yellow 1, Green 3, Pink 4, Orange 5, Red 6, Purple 9. Add the outer numbers and put the result in the opposite segment.

ANSWER 138

G. Add 3 to odd numbers, subtract 2 from even numbers.

ANSWER 139

The pattern sequence is 7, 1, 1, 3, 2, 2, 5, 5, 4, 1. It starts at the top right and works in an anti-clockwise spiral.

4	2	2
1	5	5
7	1	1

ANSWER 140

A. Each shape increases by one of the same until there are three and it then becomes one. The image is reflected for a shape with two elements.

ANSWER 141

The pattern is +2 scales, +3 scales, –1 scale. A fish with an even number of scales faces the other way.

ANSWER 142

4.

ANSWER 143

B. The digits of all the others add up to 6.

ANSWER 144

A. Each ring contains one cross more than the previous example, and the first and last cross in each adjacent circle are level.

ANSWER 145

21. ← = 12, * = 9, ♥ = 3, % = 5, @ = 7.

ANSWER 146

D. The number of edges of the shapes in each square increases by 1 in each column, starting from the top.

ANSWER 147

14. Colors are worth Purple 2, Yellow 3, Orange 5, Green 6. Add sides together and put sum in center of triangle.

ANSWER 148

16.

ANSWER 149

14. The colors are worth Red 5, Yellow 3, Green 6, Blue 4. Add the sides together and swap the results within horizontally adjacent triangles.

ANSWER 150

D.

ANSWER 151

11. The colors are worth Brown 1, Green 2, Orange 3, Yellow 4, Pink 5, Red 6, Purple 7. Add the outer numbers in each segment and place in the center of the next segment clockwise.

ANSWER 152

3. The numbers rotate anti-clockwise from one square to the next and decrease by 2 each time.

ANSWER 153

9. Multiply the values in the same segments in wheels 2 and 3 and put the answer in the next segment in wheel 1, going clockwise.

ANSWER 154

Add the number of segments in column 1 to the number of segments in column 3. Draw this number of segments into column 2.

ANSWER 155

15. Take the number of minutes in the hours, add the minutes and divide by 10. Ignore the remainder.

ANSWER 156

E. Add two circles and two lines, take away one of each, repeat. The pattern is also rotated by 90° anti-clockwise each time.

ANSWER 157

27. Add all the numbers for each square. For Yellow add 5, for Green subtract 5. Then swap the numbers in adjacent Yellow and Green squares.

ANSWER 158

C.

ANSWER 159

21. Multiply each number by the number on the opposite side of the wheel on the same side of the spoke and put the product in that segment next to the center.

ANSWER 160

F. The circles and squares become squares and circles, respectively. The largest element loses all internal elements.

ANSWER 161

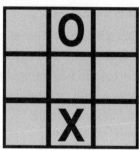

Starting at opposite ends the symbols move alternately 1 and 2 steps to the other end of the grid in a boustrophedon.

ANSWER 162

A.

ANSWER 163

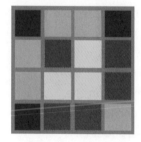

The sequence is Brown, Orange, Yellow, Brown, Purple, Green. It forms a diagonal boustrophedon (or ox plough pattern) starting in the bottom left corner.

ANSWER 164

The pattern sequence is 1, 2, 2, 3, 4, 4, 1, 2, 3, 3, 4. Start at the top left and work in a horizontal boustrophedon.

ANSWER 165

D. Add consecutive clockwise corners of the diamond and place the sum on the corresponding second corner. Add the four numbers together and place the sum in the middle.

ANSWER 166

No. 2. Take the first digit of the weight from the second to arrive at new number.

ANSWER 167

B. Each time the square becomes the circle, the triangle the square, and the circle the triangle.

ANSWER 168

92. Multiply the numbers on the diagonally opposite corners of each square and add the products. Put the sum in the third square along.

ANSWER 169

3:13. Start time A minus Finish A equals Finish B. Start time B minus Finish B equals Finish C, etc.

ANSWER 170

D. It is the only one to which a circle can be added where the triangle overlaps the circle and a right-angled line runs parallel to the whole of one side of the triangle.

ANSWER 171

C. Each row and column must contain two Orange and two Green squares.

ANSWER 172

B.

ANSWER 173

3.

ANSWER 174

J. All of the others have a matching partner.

ANSWER 175

E. All elements consist of 3 straight lines except 'E', which consists of 4 straight lines.

ANSWER 176

The pattern sequence is @, @, %, *, %, &, &, *, %. It starts at the top right and works inwards in an anti-clockwise spiral.

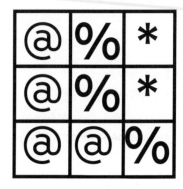

ANSWER 177

2.

ANSWER 178

44. The numbers increase clockwise first missing one spoke, then two at the fourth step. Each circle increases by a different amount
(2, 3, 4).

ANSWER 179

B.

ANSWER 180

B. The others all have an equal number of straight lines and curves.

ANSWER 181

The corresponding sections in each wheel should contain a black section in each compartment.

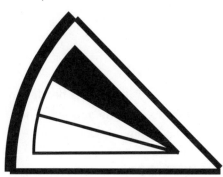

ANSWER 182

Starting with a vertical line reflect the dot first against that line and then each

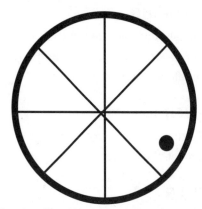

following line in a clockwise direction.

ANSWER 183

F. The small and large elements become large and small, respectively.

ANSWER 184

9. The numbers rotate clockwise and increase by 1 each time.

ANSWER 185

B. It is the only one to have an odd number of horizontal lines.

ANSWER 186

C. The number of small circles equals the number of edges of the shape, except for 'C', where there is one more circle than edges.

ANSWER 187

10. Add 2 to each value, place sum in corresponding position in next triangle, then subtract 3, and add 2 again.

ANSWER 188

18. Multiply the numbers in the outer section, reverse the product and put it in the middle of the next section.

ANSWER 189

20. Multiply hours by minutes and divide by 3 to get the number of the rider.

ANSWER 190

Forward, back, forward, back.

ANSWER 191

48. In each box of four numbers, multiply the top two numbers, put the product in the bottom right box, then subtract the top right number from the bottom right one and put
the difference in the bottom left box.

ANSWER 192

ANSWER 193

Yellow (the numbers are added to give the totals).

ANSWER 194

B. Each arch moves closer to its opposite end by an equal amount each time.

ANSWER 195

1956. The numbers represent the leap years clockwise around the triangles starting at the apex. Miss one leap year each time.

ANSWER 196

9:05. The minute hand goes forward 25 minutes, the hour hand back by 5 hours.

ANSWER 197

13.

ANSWER 198

B. It is the only figure that does not have three boxes in one row.

ANSWER 199

C.

ANSWER 200

987. The tractor number is divided into the weight to give the acreage. The weights have been mixed up.

ANSWER 201

6. In each square, multiply the top and bottom left together, then multiply the top and bottom right. Subtract this

second product from the first and put this number in the middle.

ANSWER 202

384. Starting at the top right-hand corner work through the square in a vertical boustrophedon, multiplying by 4 and dividing by 2 alternately.

ANSWER 203

Add one leaf. Add two petals. Deduct 1 petal and add 1 leaf. Repeat.

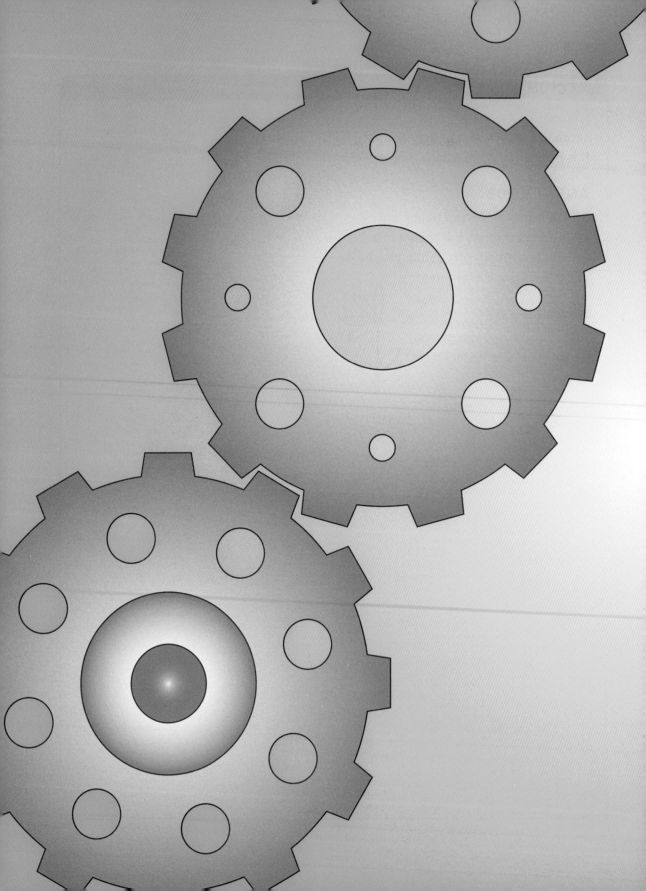

Hard Puzzles

Prepare to really feel your mind sweat! The puzzles in this section have all been carefully devised to push your mental functions to the absolute maximum. There are no easy solutions here, no quick gimmes – just lots and lots of really good, seriously challenging problems to test your capabilities. You'll need to use every trick you've learned to master the brain-benders in these pages – and you'll have to draw on some serious resolve and creativity, to boot.

But if the difficulty level of these problems is set to high, then so is the reward. The puzzles in this section are the ones that will really help you build new mental muscle. By stretching yourself beyond the point of everyday comfort, you are forced to strengthen and grow. That's as true of the mind as it is of the body. In a gym, these puzzles would be the final two or three extra-heavy lifts – the ones that do you as much good (or more) as all the workouts that went before them.

That's not all, either. These puzzles are a real challenge, and that means that solving them is a real achievement. As you work through the problems in this section, you'll feel the deep satisfaction of genuinely proving yourself against a serious obstacle. Every one you beat will become a badge of pride – another item to add to the stack of things you can feel good about. And that's every bit as important as the really great mental exercise you'll be doing. Play on: mind fitness awaits!

PUZZLE 204

Can you work out what the
missing symbol should look like?

Answer see page **246**

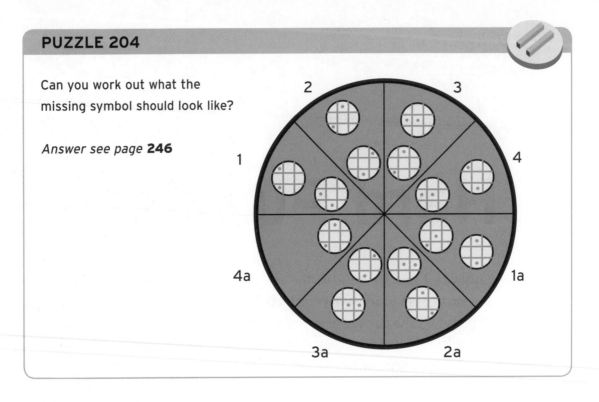

PUZZLE 205

Can you work out which symbol follows the
series?

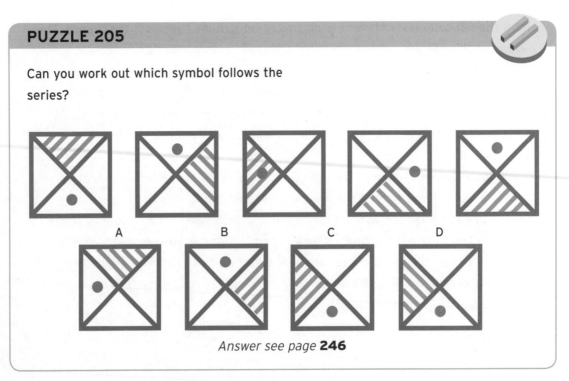

Answer see page **246**

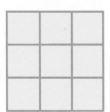

Can you work out the reasoning behind this grid and complete the missing section?

Answer see page 246

PUZZLE 207

Can you find the number that should replace the question mark?

Answer see page **246**

12	19		5	7
11			2	6

16	4		3	14
11	9		3	10

PUZZLE 208

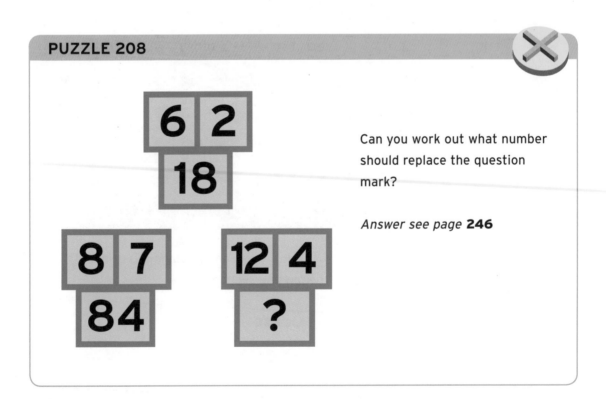

Can you work out what number should replace the question mark?

Answer see page **246**

Which two of these butterflies are identical?

Answer see page **242**

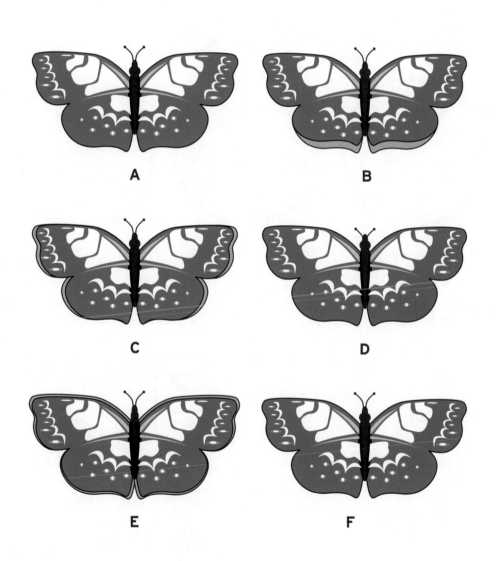

A

B

C

D

E

F

PUZZLE 210

A

Can you find the odd one out?

Answer see page **246**

B

C

D

E

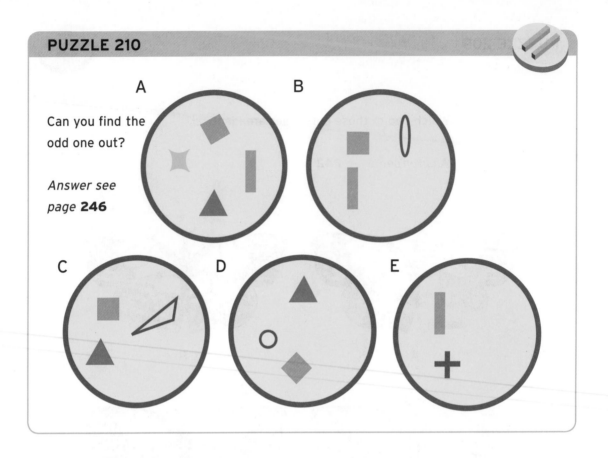

PUZZLE 211

Can you unravel the reasoning behind this grid and complete the missing square?

Answer see page **246**

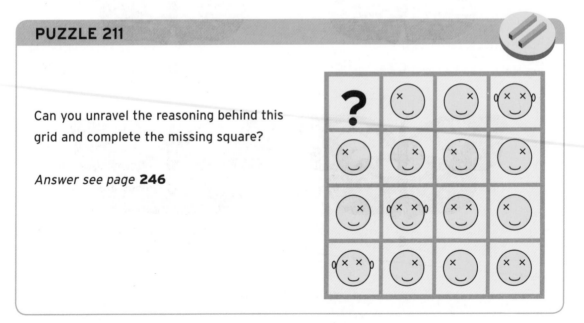

		2	7	3	8	4	9		2	7	3	8	4	9
9	9								2	7	3	8	4	9
4	4	3	8	4	9									
8	8	7				2	7	3	8	4	9			
3	3	2		4	9									
7	7			8	7	3	8	4	9				2	
2	2			3	2								7	
				7									3	
				2									8	2
													4	7
9													9	3
4														8
8					9	4	8	3	7	2				4
3					9	4	8	3	7	2				9
7		9	4	8	3	7	2							
2					9	4	8	3	7	2				

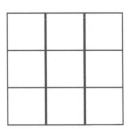

The numbers in this grid occur in the following order: 9, 4, 8, 3, 7, 2 and run in an anti-clockwise spiral starting at the top right. It is complicated by the addition of spaces and repeats according to a pattern.

Can you complete the missing section?

Answer see page 247

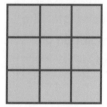

Can you work out the reasoning behind this grid and complete the missing section?

Answer see page **247**

PUZZLE 214

Which of the following is the odd one out?

Answer see page **247**

A

B

C

D

PUZZLE 215

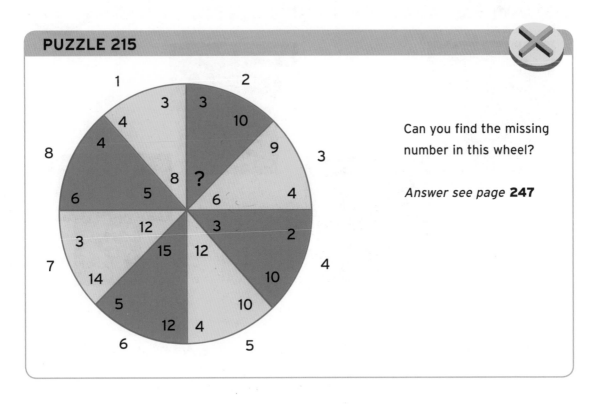

Can you find the missing number in this wheel?

Answer see page **247**

Can you work out what the
missing number is?

Answer see page 247

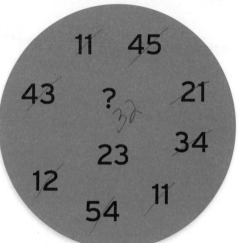

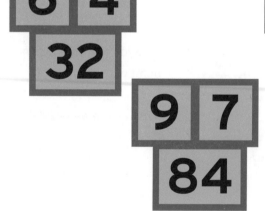

Can you work out what number should
go into the square with the question mark?

Answer see page 247

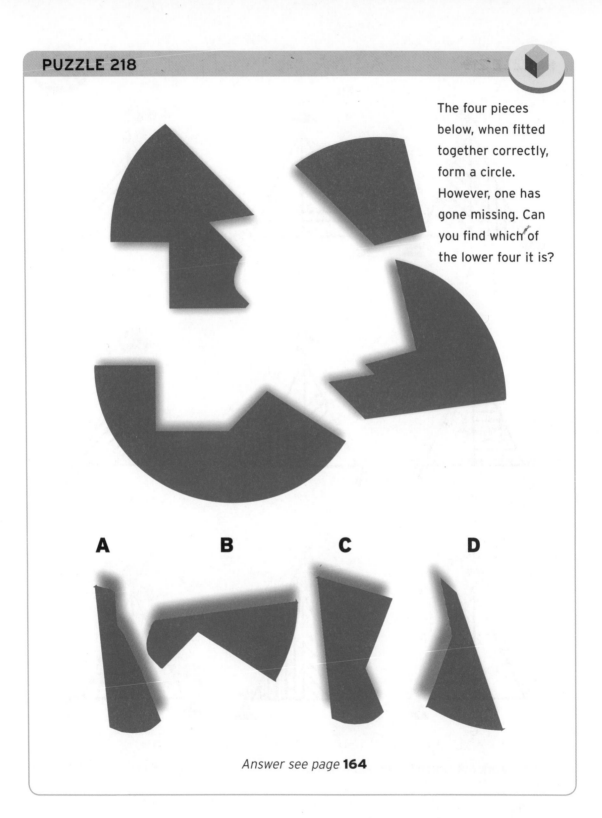

The four pieces below, when fitted together correctly, form a circle. However, one has gone missing. Can you find which of the lower four it is?

A   **B**   **C**   **D**

Answer see page **164**

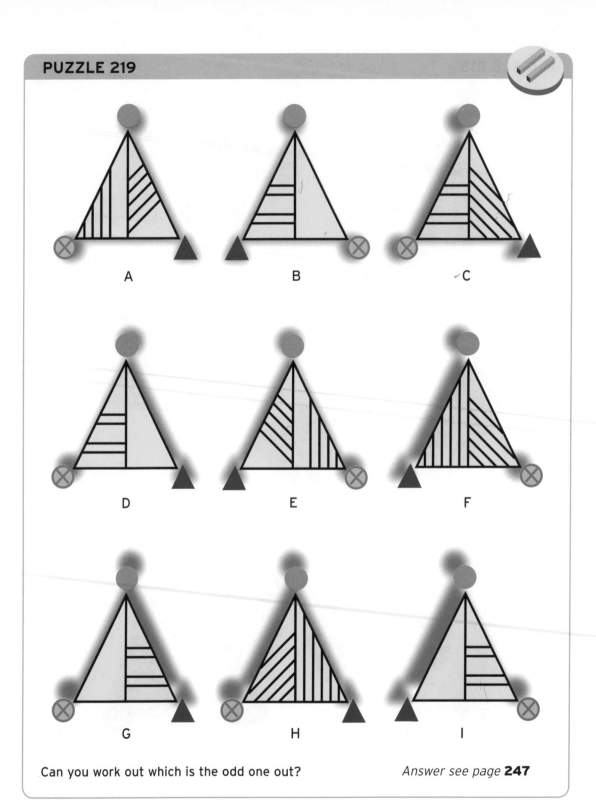

Can you work out which is the odd one out?

Answer see page **247**

PUZZLE 220

Can you work out the reasoning behind this wheel and fill in the missing number?

Answer see page **247**

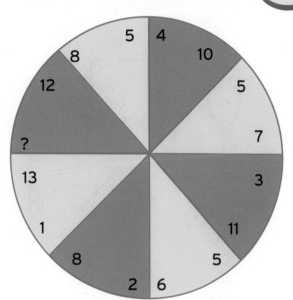

PUZZLE 221

3	6	3	5
4	12	11	1
3	?	15	5
1	6	7	2

Can you unravel the reasoning behind this square and replace the question mark with a number?

Answer see page **247**

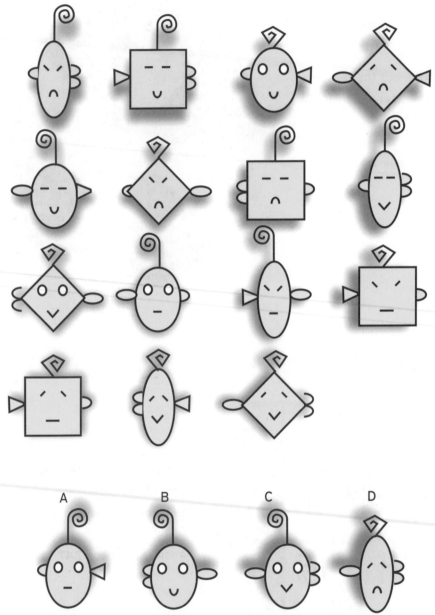

Can you work out which face would fit the missing space?

Answer see page **248**

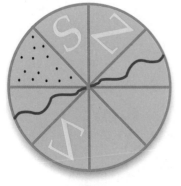

A

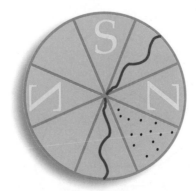

B

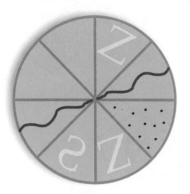

C

Can you work out which is the odd diagram out?

Answer see page **248**

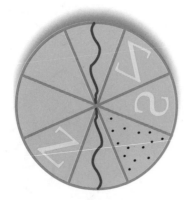

D

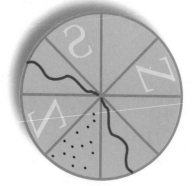

E

Can you work out which two models cannot
be made from the above layout?

Answer see page **248**

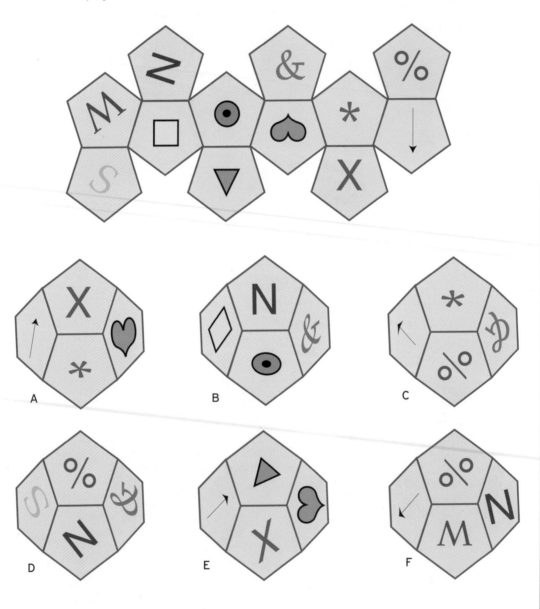

PUZZLE 225

Find a number that could replace the question mark. Each color represents a number under 10.

Answer see page **248**

103	131	135	107	
				?
				121
				142
				72

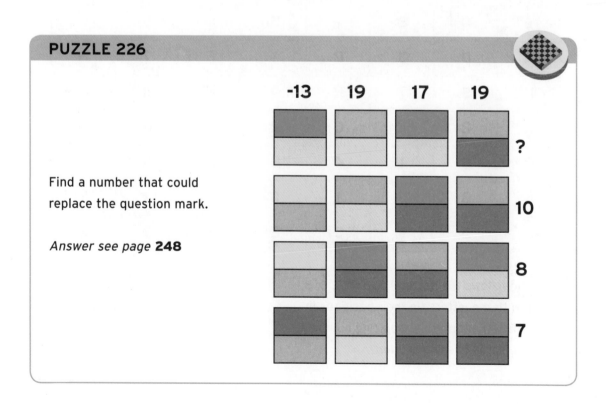

PUZZLE 226

Find a number that could replace the question mark.

Answer see page **248**

-13	19	17	19	
				?
				10
				8
				7

6	G	B	6	2	G	F	5
5	D	3	9	D	I	3	4
1	F	7	H	A	7	1	H
9	E	4	C	2	5	C	E
2	A	6	G	8	I	F	8
8	I	5			B	1	4
3	B	1			H	9	E
7	H	9	E	4	C	2	A
4	C	2	A	6	G	8	I
6	G	8	I	5	D	3	B
A	D	3	B	1	F	7	H
H	5	7	H	9	E	4	C
6	2	F	C	2	A	6	G
8	D	I	4	8	I	5	D
A	B	7	1	G	B	1	F
F	5	9	C	E	3	9	E

This grid follows the pattern: 5, 6, 4, 7, 3, 8, 2, 9, 1, with the letters (in their positions in the alphabet) alternately replacing numbers. Can you fill the missing section?

Answer see page **248**

PUZZLE 228

5		3		1		4		6		2		7		3
	32				**11**				**38**				**20**	
6		2		3		4		7		3		4		1

6		7		3		4		7		3		7		3
	60				**54**				**35**				**29**	
4		9		2		1								

(columns)

5 ... 6 ... 5 ... 2 ... 4 ... 8

3		5		8		3		5		6		4		3
6		7		5		9		2		3		8		4
	?				**?**				**?**				**?**	
3		4		6		5		7		6		3		6

What numbers should replace the question marks?

*Answer see page **248***

PUZZLE 229

Find a number that could replace the question mark.

*Answer see page **248***

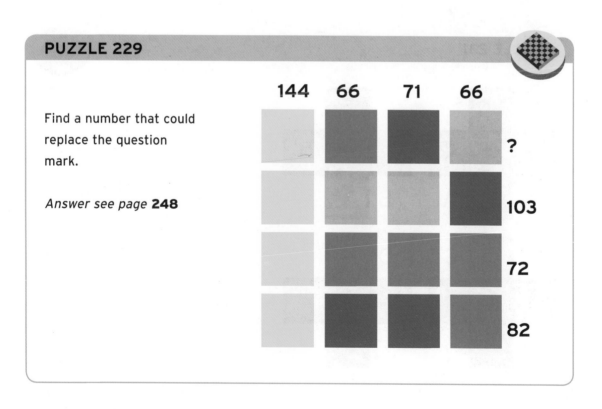

144	66	71	66	
				?
				103
				72
				82

Can you work out what the last clockface should look like?

Answer see page **248**

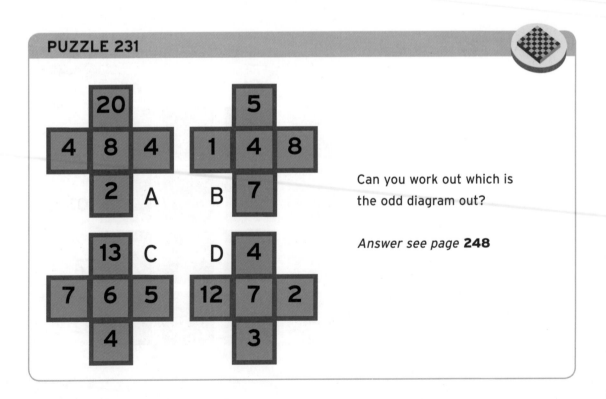

Can you work out which is the odd diagram out?

Answer see page **248**

5	3	6	4	4	3	5	7	5	7	9	2	2	5	8	3
9	8	9	6	1	5	8	6	6	8	3	7	6	7	4	4
2	1	5	7	8	3	1	3	5	1	6	6	8	9	8	6
7	6	2	9	1	1	8	3	1	5	1	7	5	3	4	1
8	5	6	6	2	4	4	8	3	8	4	7	1	6	1	8
7	6	2	2	5	2	3	7	4	5	8	5	7	6	3	1
7	9	3	1	8	4	5	4	7	7	9	4	8	5	6	3
3	6	8	8	2	9	8	8	2	5	7	2	1	8	3	5
5	6	9	6	5	3	4	7	4	7	4	2	6	6	5	5
1	6	3	2	3	4	5	8	1	1	2	4	9	3	2	7
5	8	9	7	1	8	3	6	9	3	6	3	5	4	9	4
8	4	5	6	7	1	5	1	8	5	8	3	1	2	5	7
7	2	2	9	2	2	4	7	4	9	4	1	8	6	7	8
2	4	3	9	5	6	7	8	5	8	3	2	7	5	6	1
5	9	4	3	4	2	6	1	7	3	4	9	2	6	9	1
3	2	5	8	1	3	2	5	3	8	3	5	3	1	2	7

Look at this grid carefully and you will
find pairs of numbers that add up to 10,
in a either horizontal, vertical or diagonal
direction. How many can you spot?

Answer see page 249

PUZZLE 233

How many yellow spotted tiles are missing from this design?

Answer see page **249**

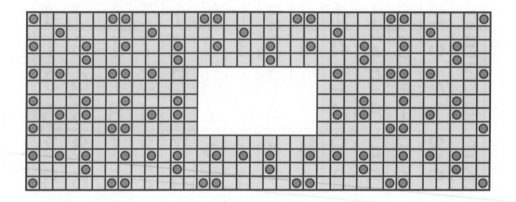

PUZZLE 234

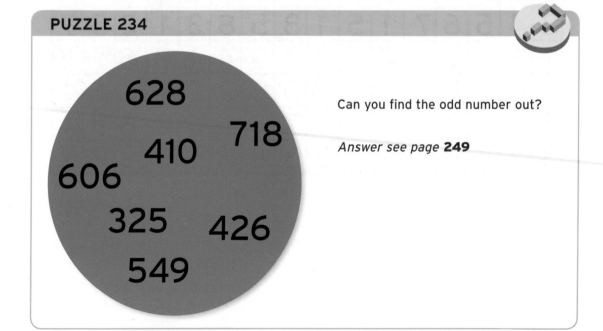

Can you find the odd number out?

Answer see page **249**

6	7	3	8	2	4	1	6	9	5	91
3	4	6	2	9	7	7	6	3	4	111
5	9	6	8	3	2	4	7			74
9	8	2	3			6	8			51
8	7	3	4			6	1	4	6	68
2	9	5	4	8	3	6	2	7	8	97
4	3	2	9	1	4	5	6	8	3	85
6	2	4	3	1	7	9	6	3	8	91
2	4	7	6			1	2			36
3	5	6	8			2	4			45

90 108 89 100 36 44 94 82 52 ?

Find a number that could replace the question mark. Each color represents a number under 10. Some may be negative numbers.

Answer see page **249**

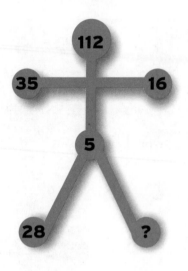

Can you unravel the reasoning behind this diagram and find the missing number?

Answer see page **249**

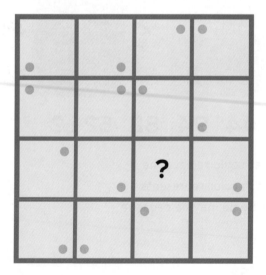

Can you work out what the square with the question mark should look like?

Answer see page **249**

3	4	6	9	7	2	5	8	3	9	?
6	5	2	7	3	4	5	1	2	6	71
3	8	2	1	9	7	8	6	1	3	82
5	4	3	4	1	2	9	8	6	5	85
6	8	9	3	5	4	8	3	6	2	91
4	1	9	8	6	3	2	2	4	5	74
7	6	3	5	2	4	6	8	9	7	93
8	4	6	5	3	6	2	1	3	8	83
9	2	1	4	3	7	8	9	6	3	88
1	3	7	6	4	3	8	6	2	4	77

89 75 77 87 79 86 81 93 67 102

Find a number that could replace the question mark. Each
color represents a number under 10.

Answer see page **249**

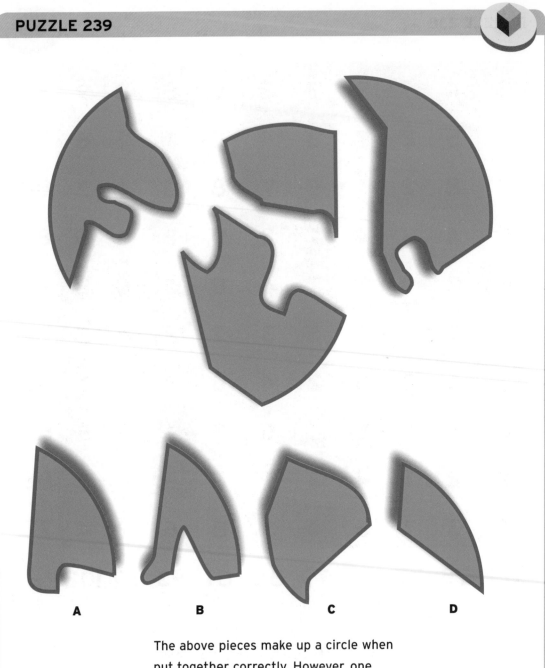

A   **B**   **C**   **D**

The above pieces make up a circle when
put together correctly. However, one
piece is missing. Which is it?

Answer see page **249**

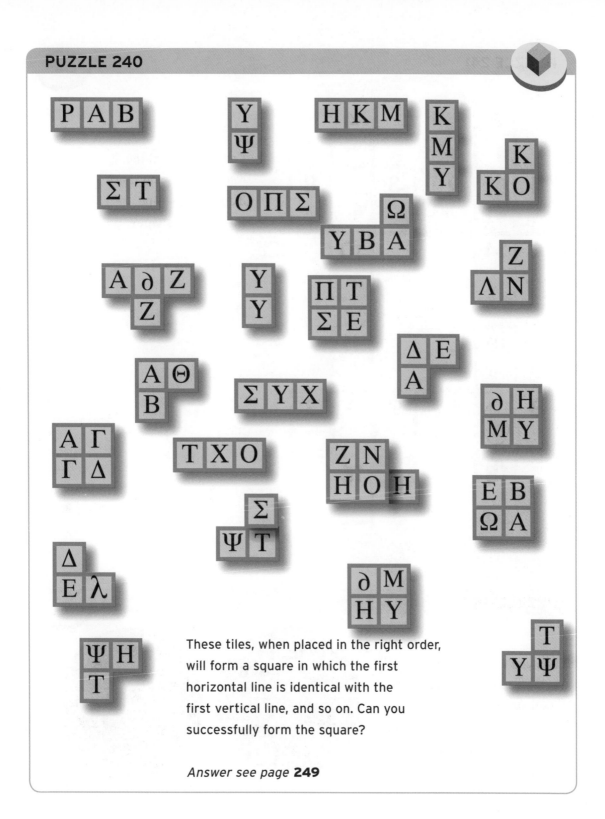

These tiles, when placed in the right order, will form a square in which the first horizontal line is identical with the first vertical line, and so on. Can you successfully form the square?

*Answer see page **249***

PUZZLE 241

8

4 (9

14

4

3 (8

10

16

8) 5

18

11

9 ? 3

16

Can you unravel the reasoning behind these diagrams and find the missing shape?

Answer see page **250**

PUZZLE 242

Can you work out which is the odd number out in each circle?

Answer see page **250**

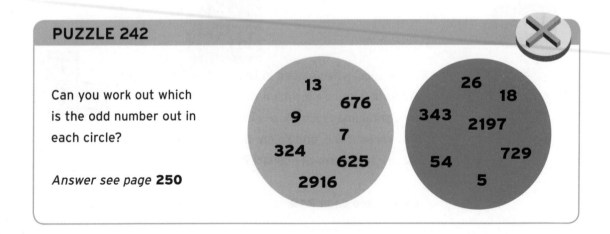

13
676
9
7
324
625
2916

26
18
343
2197
54
729
5

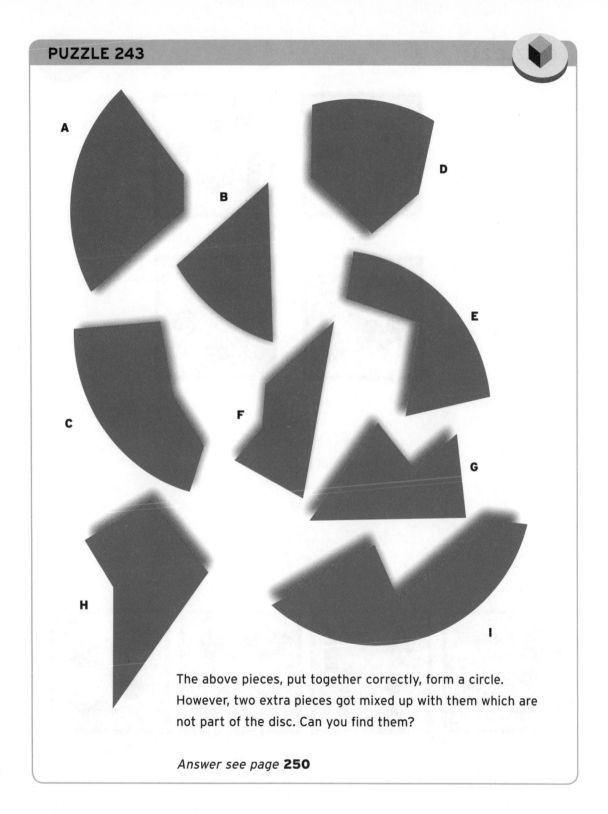

A

D

B

E

C

F

G

H

I

The above pieces, put together correctly, form a circle. However, two extra pieces got mixed up with them which are not part of the disc. Can you find them?

Answer see page 250

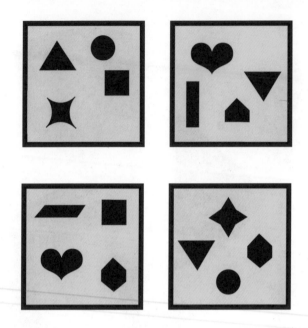

Can you work out which diagram would follow
the series above?

Answer see page **250**

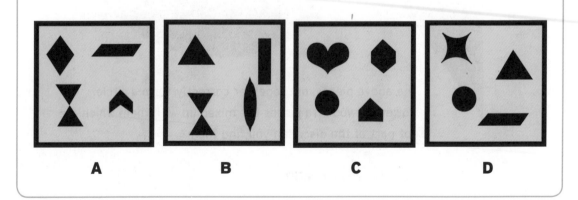

A   B   C   D

PUZZLE 245

Can you find the missing number?

Answer see page **250**

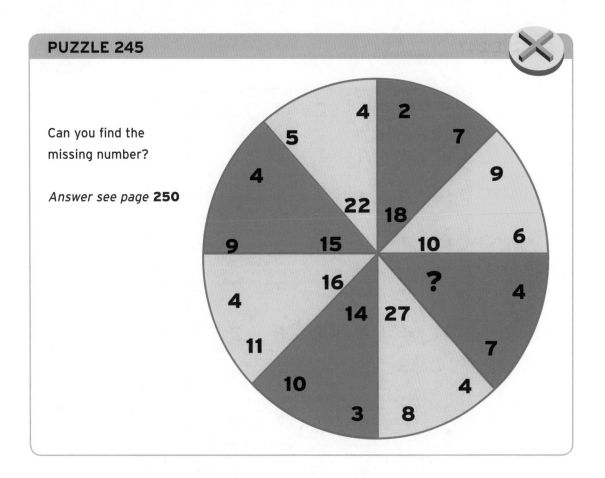

PUZZLE 246

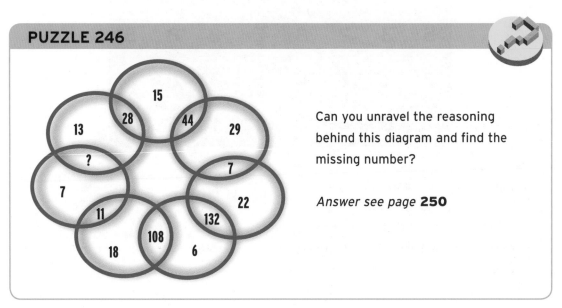

Can you unravel the reasoning behind this diagram and find the missing number?

Answer see page **250**

1	1	5	2	1	8	4	3
1	4	4	1	8	3	5	1
1	4	2	2	5	6	7	1
1	4	2	3	3	1	1	2
1	4	2	3	7	7	3	4
4	4	2	4	8	2	2	7
3	1	2	3	7	2	8	8
8	7	4	3	7	2	8	5
1	5	3	7	7	2	8	5
5	3	2	8	2	2	8	5
2	1	7	4	5	8	8	5
7	8	4	2	1	1	5	5

This grid follows the pattern: 3, 1, 4, 1, 5, 8, 2, 7. As a complication you will find some numbers have been increased by one. If you highlight these numbers you will discover a letter. What is it?

*Answer see page **250***

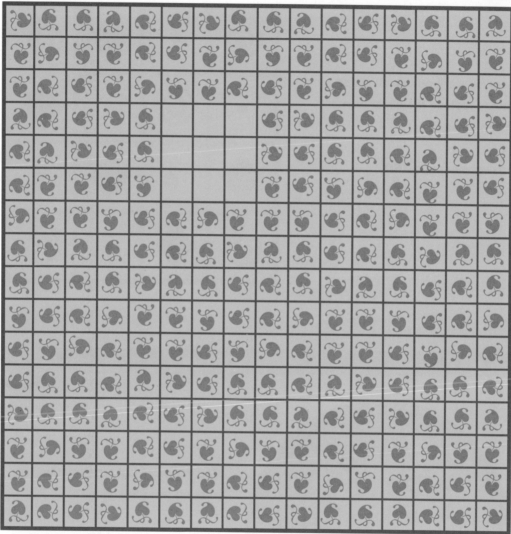

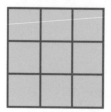

Can you work out the reasoning behind this grid and fill in the missing section?

Answer see page **250**

Can you work out which shape should replace the question mark in this square?

Answer see page **250**

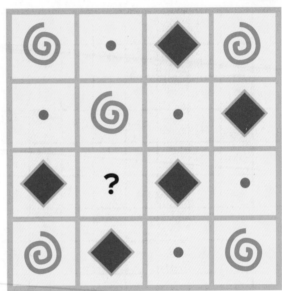

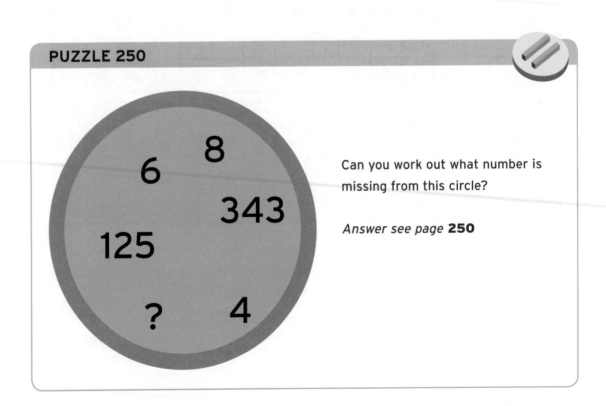

Can you work out what number is missing from this circle?

Answer see page **250**

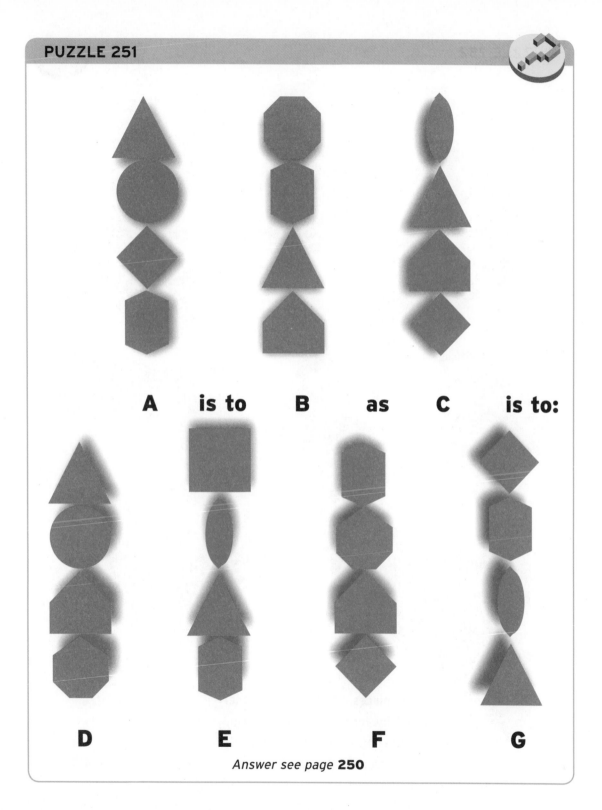

A   is to   B   as   C   is to:

D   E   F   G

Answer see page 250

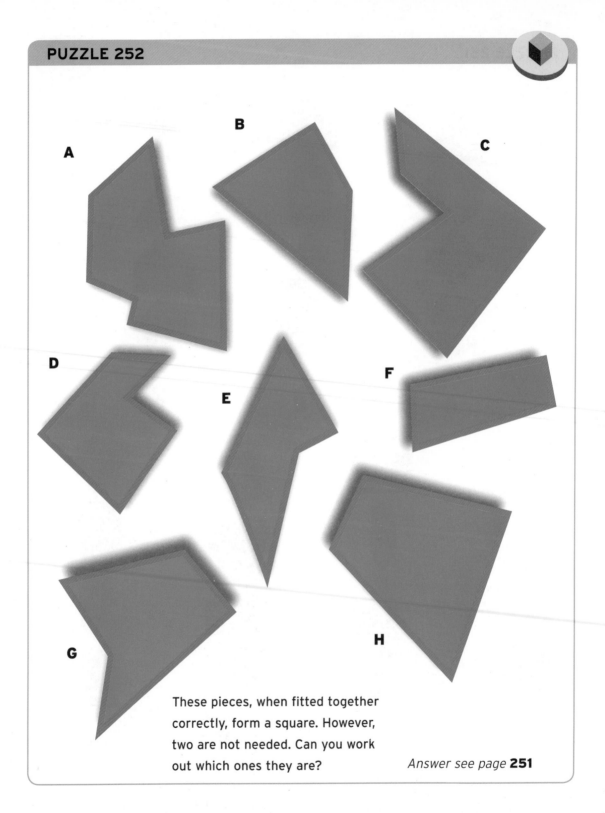

These pieces, when fitted together correctly, form a square. However, two are not needed. Can you work out which ones they are?

Answer see page 251

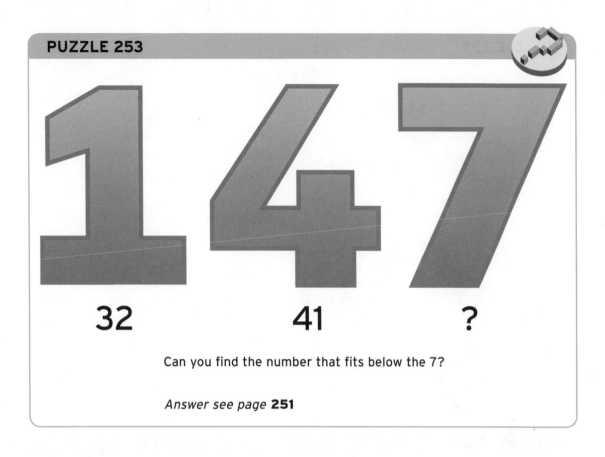

32   41   ?

Can you find the number that fits below the 7?

Answer see page 251

Can you unravel the reasoning behind this wheel and replace the question mark with a number?

Answer see page 251

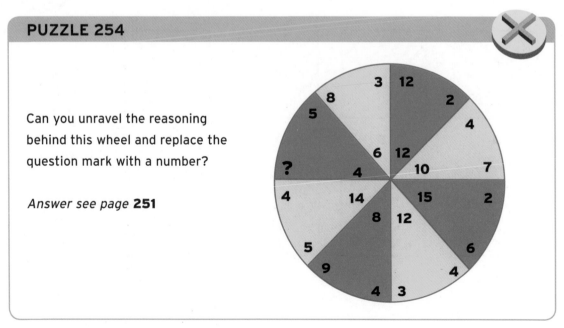

PUZZLE 255

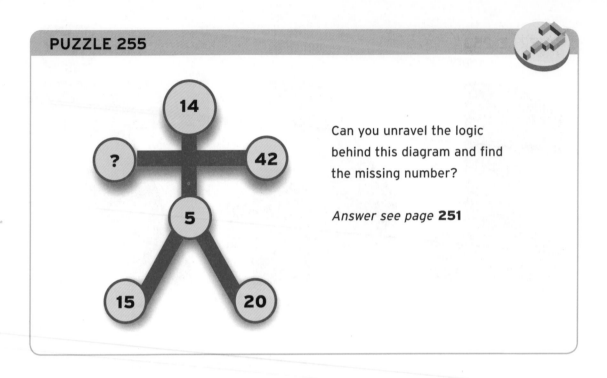

Can you unravel the logic behind this diagram and find the missing number?

Answer see page **251**

PUZZLE 256

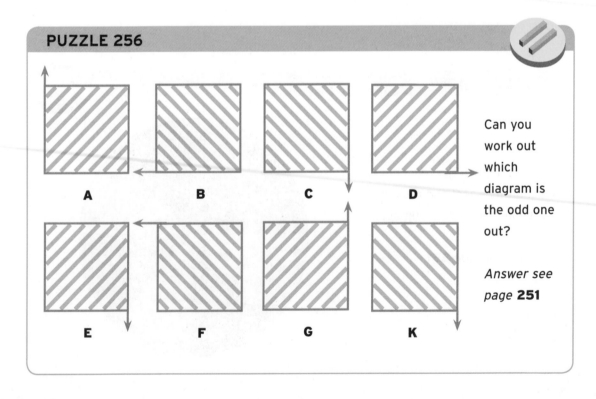

Can you work out which diagram is the odd one out?

Answer see page **251**

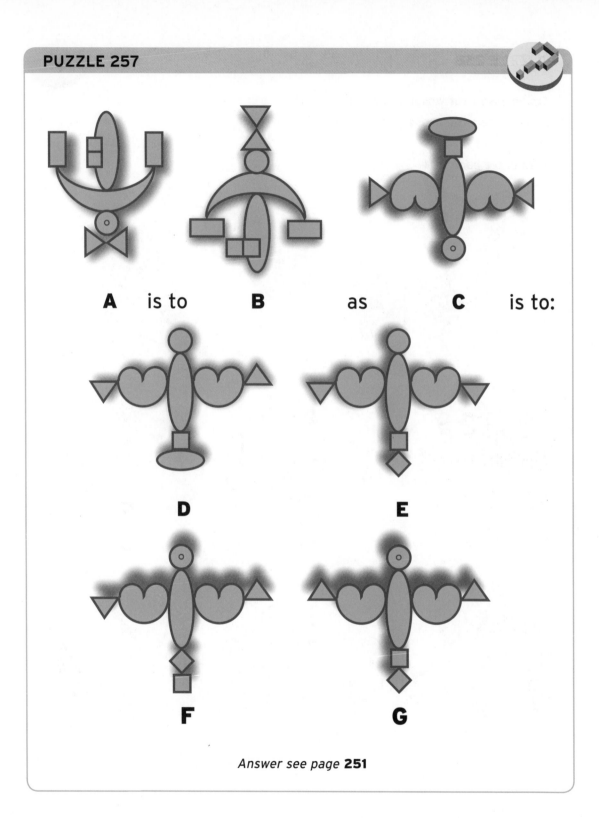

A is to **B** as **C** is to:

D

E

F

G

Answer see page **251**

Can you work out which two models cannot
be made from the above layout?

Answer see page 251

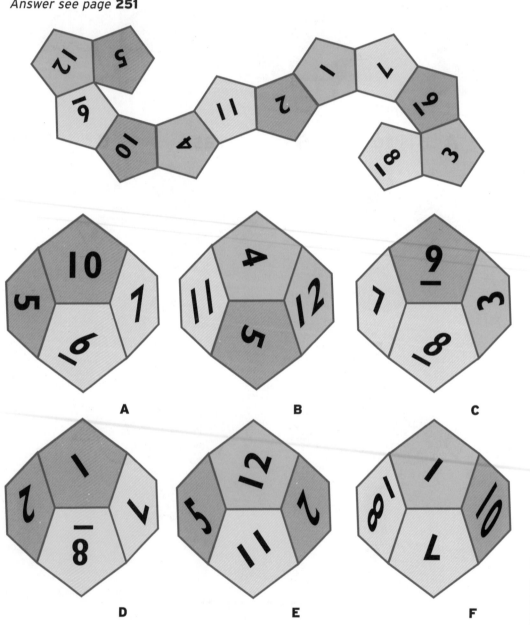

A

B

C

D

E

F

PUZZLE 259

These pieces, when fitted together correctly, make up a square.
However, one piece is not needed. Can you work out which one it is?

Answer see page **251**

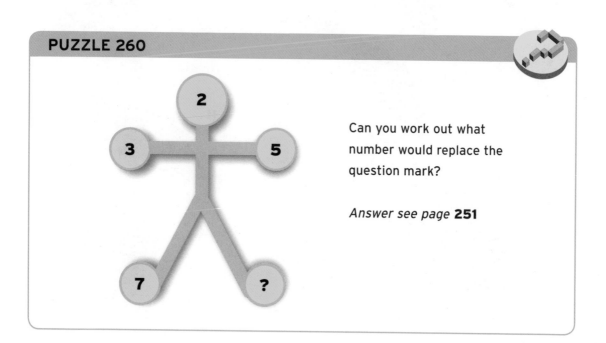

PUZZLE 260

Can you work out what number would replace the question mark?

Answer see page **251**

The above pieces, when fitted together correctly, form a square. However, one wrong piece is among them. Can you work out which one it is?

Answer see page **251**

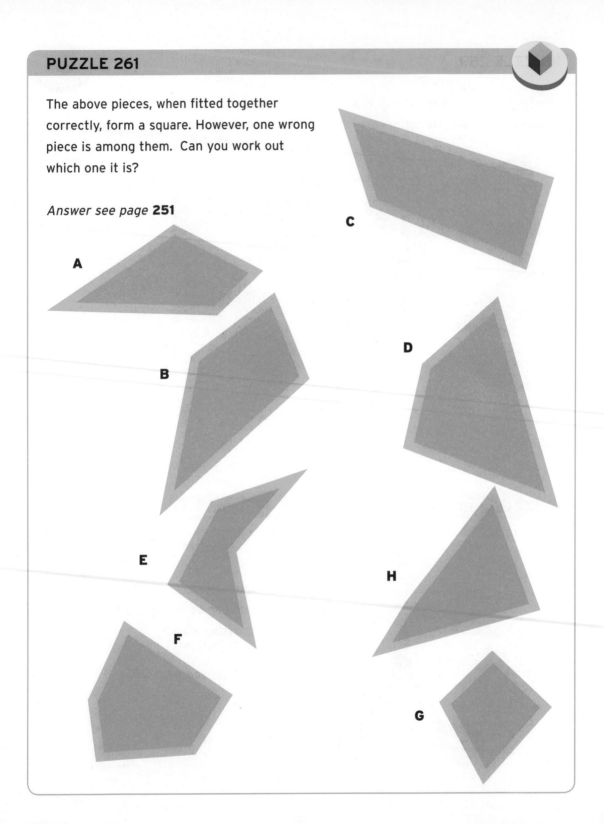

Can you find the odd number out?

Answer see page **251**

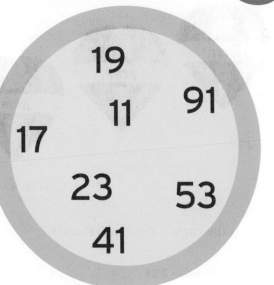

3	3	9	3
5	8	2	1
4	3	8	1
8	2	1	?

This square follows a pattern. Can you unravel it and replace the question mark with a number?

Answer see page **251**

PUZZLE 264

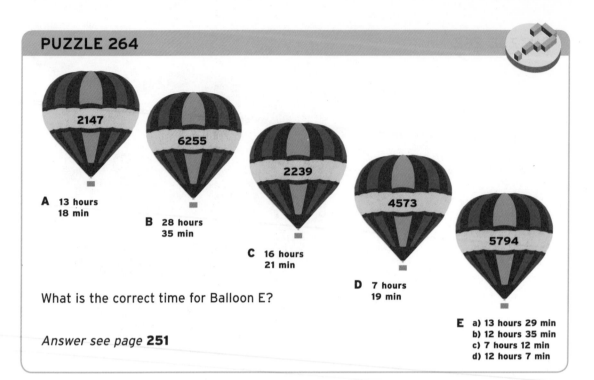

A 13 hours 18 min

B 28 hours 35 min

C 16 hours 21 min

D 7 hours 19 min

E a) 13 hours 29 min
b) 12 hours 35 min
c) 7 hours 12 min
d) 12 hours 7 min

What is the correct time for Balloon E?

Answer see page **251**

PUZZLE 265

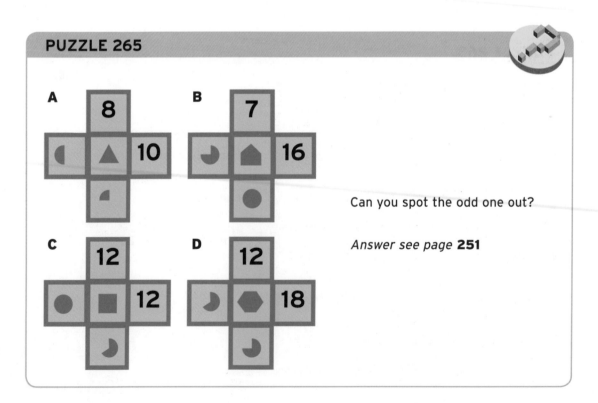

Can you spot the odd one out?

Answer see page **251**

What comes next in this series?

Answer see page **252**

A

B

C

D

4	8	3	2	7	5	6	1	9	4	?
2	3	7	6	2	4	1	5	3	7	90
8	7	3	2	4	6	9	1	4	2	101
4	3	6	8	2	9	7	6	8	7	115
3	2	1	6	9	8	8	7	3	4	101
6	2	3	8	4	1	9	7	2	6	104
7	3	4	2	1	9	4	5	3	5	100
6	5	4	3	2	8	4	7	6	1	103
3	5	2	1	8	6	9	4	3	7	106
6	8	7	3	2	4	5	9	5	6	109

103 98 99 100 81 117 121 109 99 107

Find a number that could replace the question mark. Each color represents a number under 10.

Answer see page 252

13   14   18   24

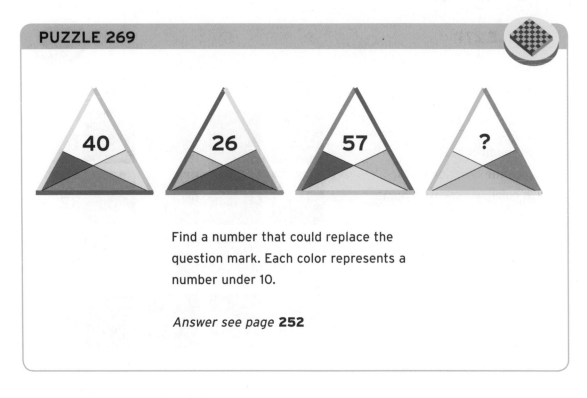

?

19

17

14

Find a number that could replace the question mark. Each color represents a number under 10.

Answer see page **252**

40   26   57   ?

Find a number that could replace the question mark. Each color represents a number under 10.

Answer see page **252**

PUZZLE 270

41 35 37 35

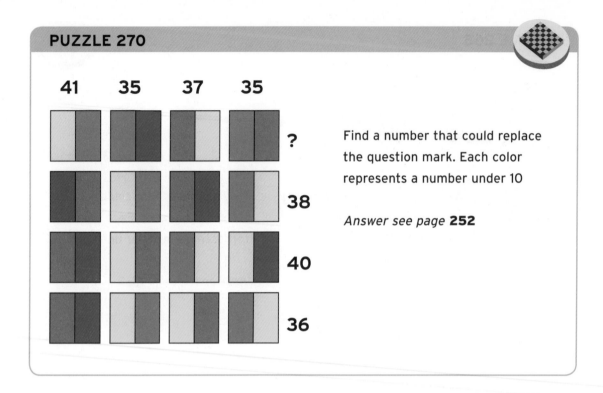

?
38
40
36

Find a number that could replace the question mark. Each color represents a number under 10

Answer see page 252

PUZZLE 271

Find a number that could replace the question mark. Each color represents a number under 10.

Answer see page 252

28 28 29 32

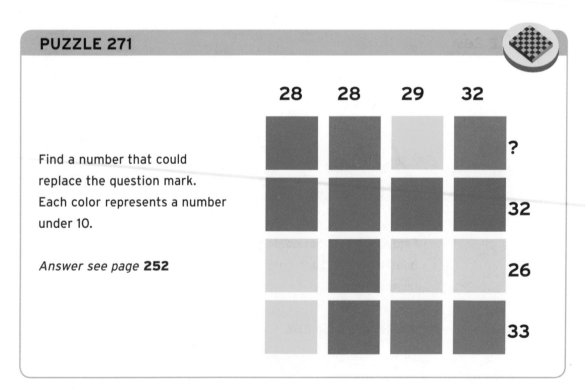

?
32
26
33

If the black arrow pulls in
the direction indicated,
will the load rise or fall?

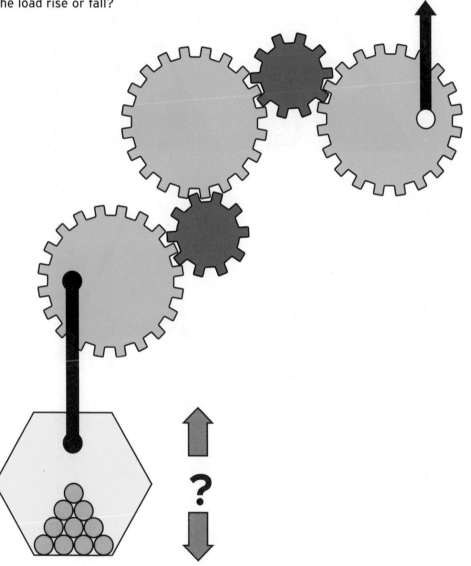

Answer see page **252**

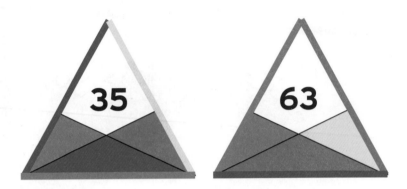

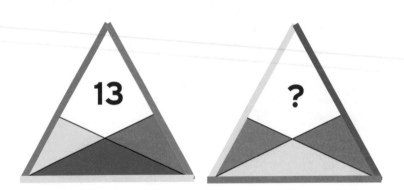

Find a number that could replace the question mark. Each color represents a number under 10.

Answer see page 252

Take 9 matches or toothpicks and lay them out in 3 triangles. By moving 3 matches try to make 5 triangles.

Answer see page **252**

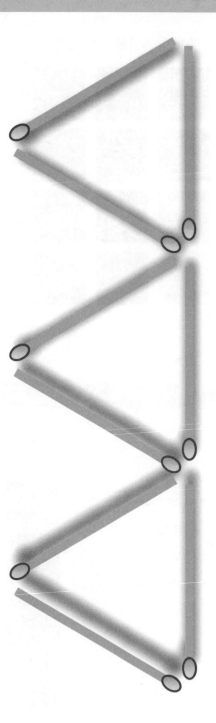

PUZZLE 275

13   14   18   24

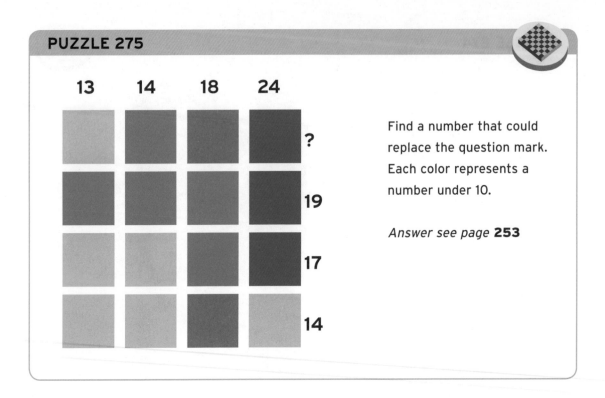

?
19
17
14

Find a number that could replace the question mark. Each color represents a number under 10.

*Answer see page **253***

PUZZLE 276

35   28   34   34

Find a number that could replace the question mark. Each color represents a number under 10.

*Answer see page **253***

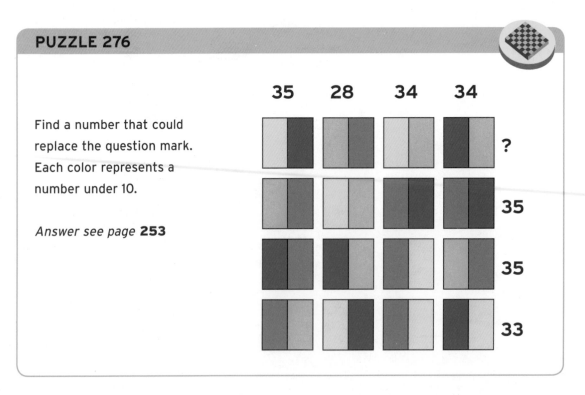

?
35
35
33

Have a look at the strange watches below. By cracking the logic that connects them you should be able to work out what time should be shown on the face of the fifth watch.

Answer see page **253**

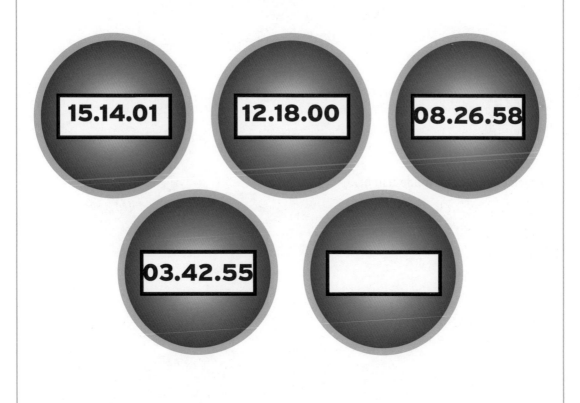

PUZZLE 278

Which of the following forms a perfect circle when combined with the diagram on the right?

Answer see page **253**

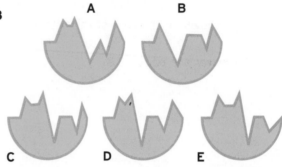

A

B

C

D

E

PUZZLE 279

Which cube can be made using:

Answer see page **253**

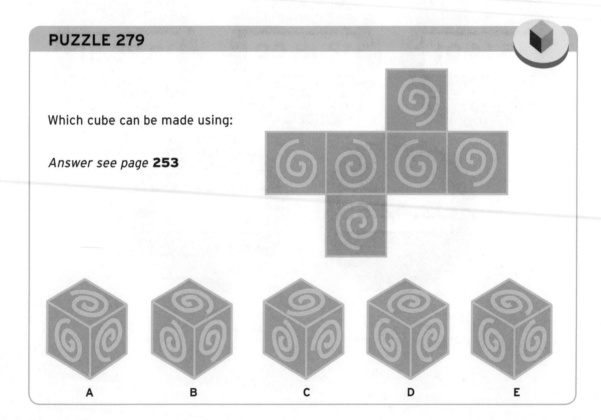

A   B   C   D   E

When old gardener Lincoln died, he left his grandchildren 19 rose bushes each. The grandchildren, Agnes (A), Billy (B), Catriona (C) and Derek (D), hated each other, and so decided to fence off their plots as shown. Who had to build the greatest run of fence?

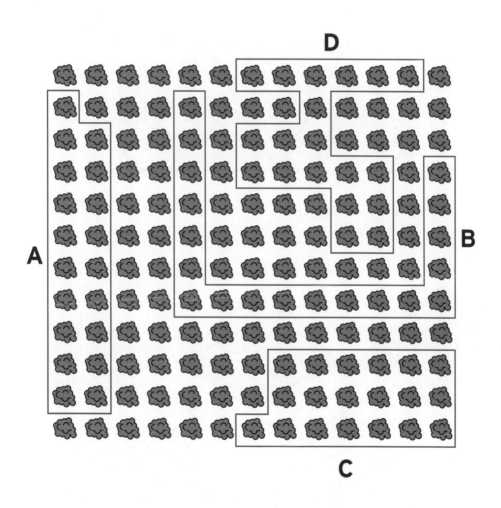

Answer see page **253**

Which of the following can be constructed
using this layout?

Answer see page **253**

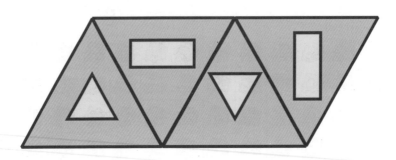

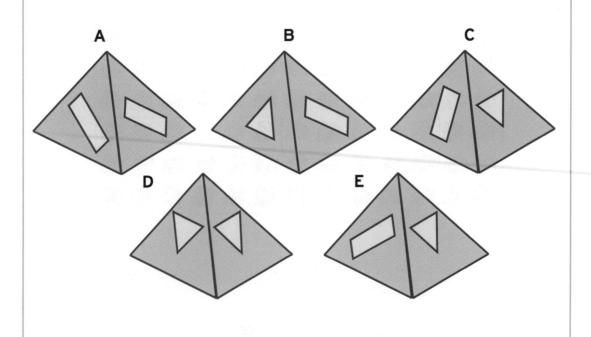

A

B

C

D

E

PUZZLE 282

Which is the odd one out?

Answer see page **253**

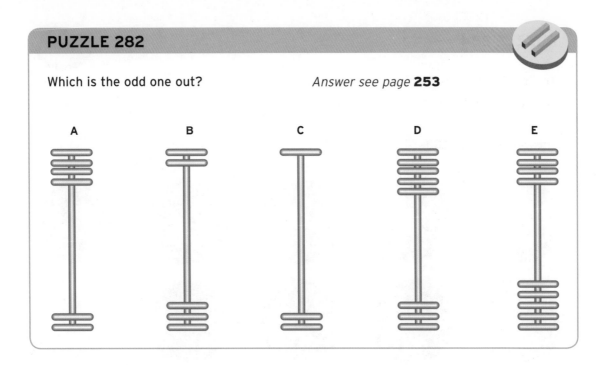

A   B   C   D   E

PUZZLE 283

What comes next in the sequence?

Answer see page **253**

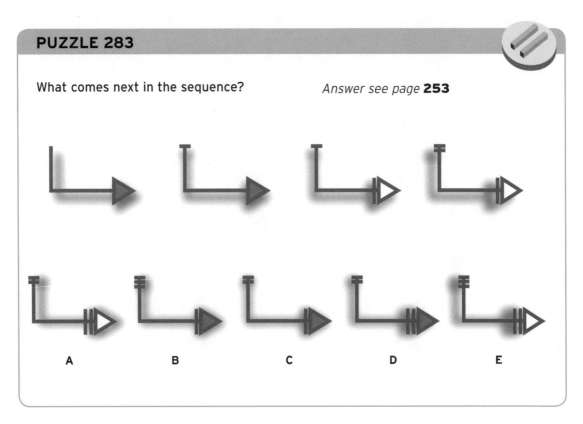

A   B   C   D   E

PUZZLE 284

Try to work out the fiendish logic behind this series of
clocks and replace the question mark.

Answer see page **253**

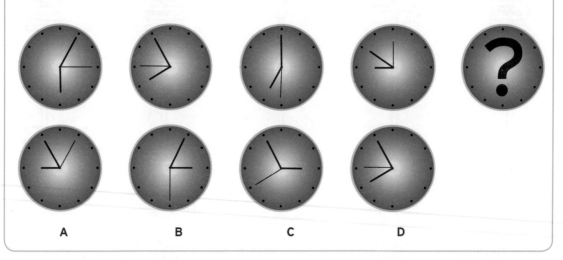

A   B   C   D

PUZZLE 285

Which is the odd one
out?

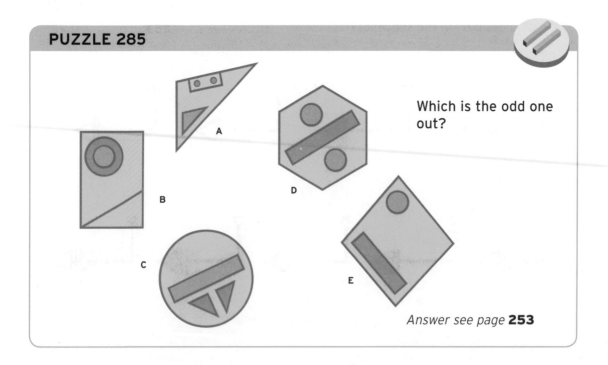

Answer see page **253**

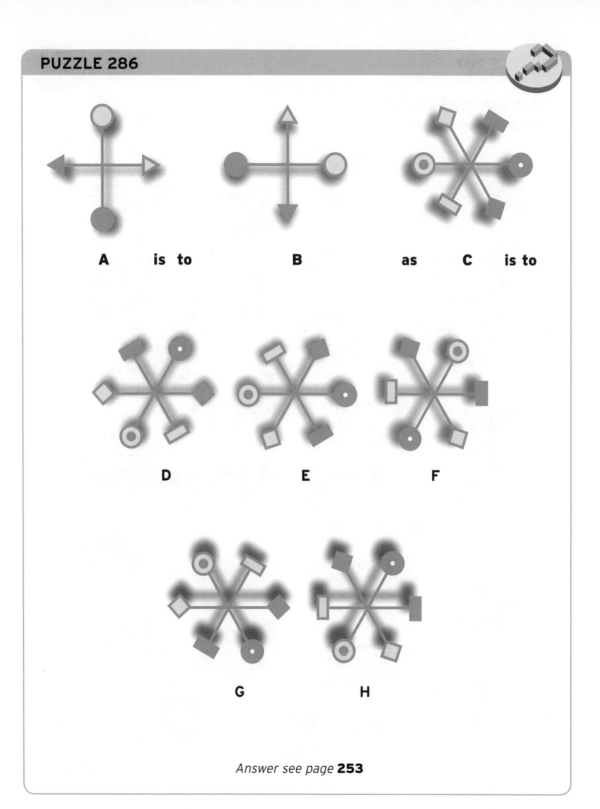

A   is to   B   as   C   is to

D   E   F

G   H

*Answer see page **253***

Only two of these butterflies
are identical. Which are they?

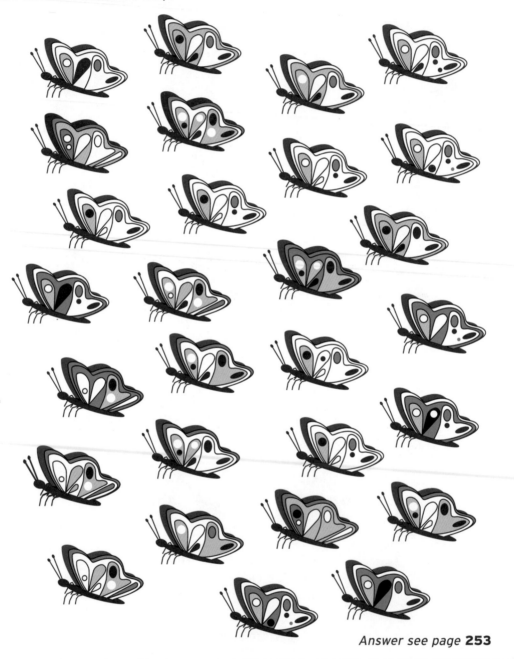

Answer see page **253**

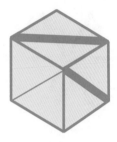 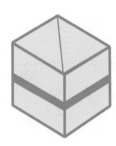 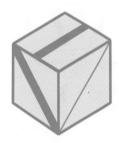 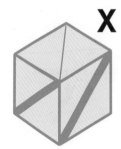

The pictures illustrate different views of one cube. What does the hidden side indicated by the X look like?

Answer see page **254**

A   B   C   D   E

    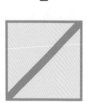

Which of the following comes next in the sequence?

Answer see page **254**

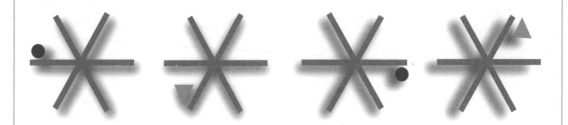

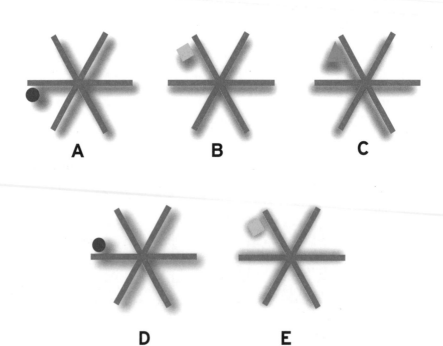

A   B   C

D   E

The values of the segments are 3 consecutive numbers under 10. The yellow is worth 7 and the sum of the segments equals 50. What do the blue and green segments equal?

Answer see page **254**

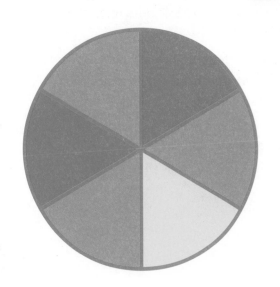

63

49

33

64

61

57

?

How much is the question mark worth?

Answer see page **254**

Look at these triangles. What geometrical shape should logically be placed in the fourth triangle?

Answer see page **254**

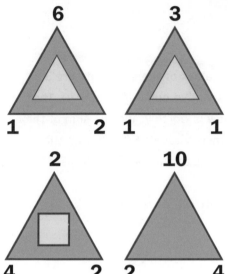

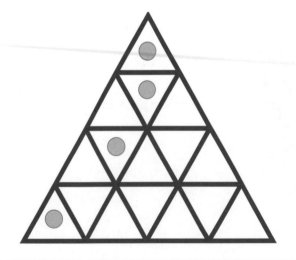

Where should another dot belong?

Answer see page **254**

PUZZLE 294

Which comes next in the sequence?

Answer see page **254**

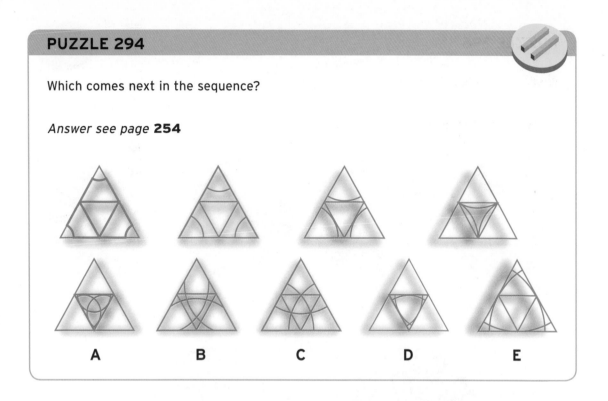

A B C D E

PUZZLE 295

Which is the odd one out?   *Answer see page* **254**

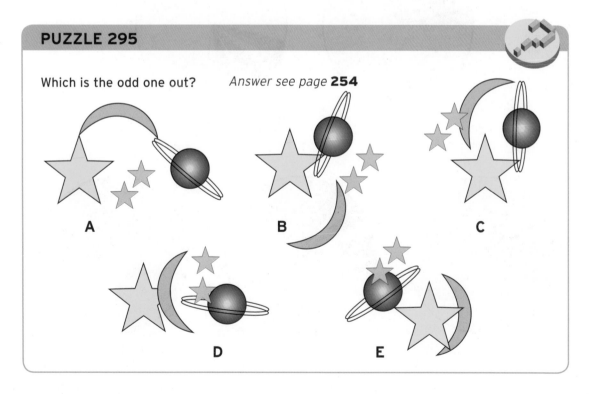

A   B   C

D   E

What comes next in the sequence?

Answer see page **254**

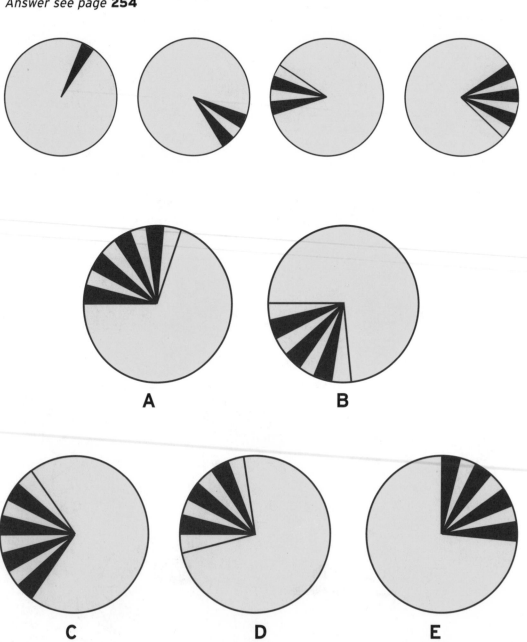

A

B

C

D

E

Answer see page **254**

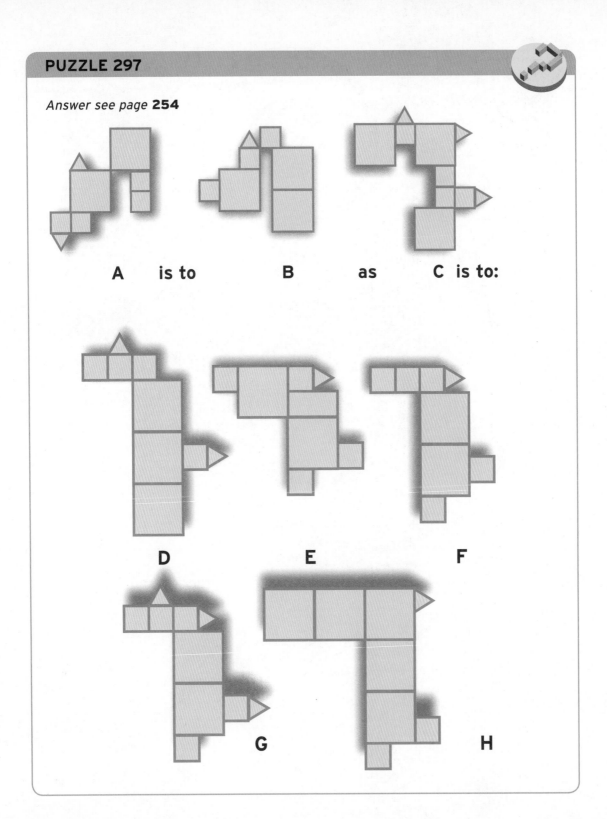

A   is to   B   as   C is to:

D

E

F

G

H

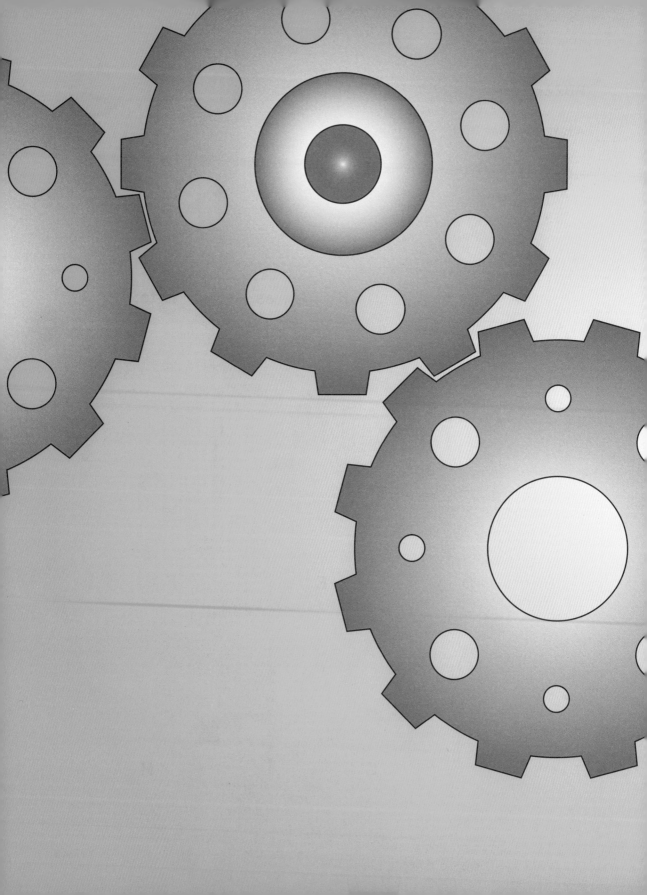

Hard
Answers

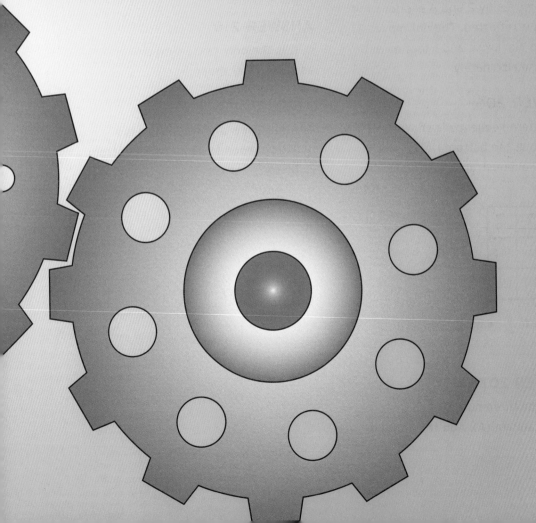

ANSWER 204

Reading across segments 1 and 1a, 2 and 2a, etc, the dots move around the circle in a vertical boustrophedon.

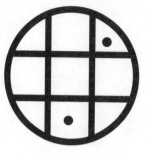

ANSWER 205

D. The striped section moves clockwise by 1, 2, 3 and 4 sections (repeat). Each time it moves by 2 and 4 sections the pattern is reflected. The dot moves 2 sections clockwise and 1 section anticlockwise alternately.

ANSWER 206

The pattern sequence is shown below. Starting at the bottom right, work in a diagonal boustrophedon (clockwise start).

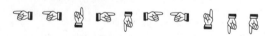

ANSWER 207

7. Add the three numbers on the outside of each square (A). Add the digits of the sum (B). Divide A by B and place in the small square.

ANSWER 208

72. Halve the number on the top left, multiply the number on the top right by 3. Multiply the two resulting numbers with each other, and put the product in the bottom square.

ANSWER 209

A and F.

ANSWER 210

C. It is the only circle with an asymmetrical shape.

ANSWER 211

The pattern is and the puzzle is a boustrophedon starting in the bottom right-hand corner.

ANSWER 212

		2
9		7
4	8	3

ANSWER 213

The pattern sequence is shown below. It starts at the top right and works down in a diagonal boustrophedon (anti-clockwise start).

ANSWER 214

B. This is a mirror image of the other shapes.

ANSWER 215

10. Multiply the two numbers on the outside of each segment, divide the product by 1,2,3 ...8 respectively and put the new number in the middle of the opposite segment.

ANSWER 216

32. All the others have a partner, with the digits being reversed.

ANSWER 217

56. Take 2/3 of the number in the top left square and multiply it by twice the number in the top right square. Put the new number in the bottom square.

ANSWER 218

B.

ANSWER 219

C. All the others, when reflected on a vertical line, have an identical partner.

ANSWER 220

5. Add both numbers in one segment, add the digits of that sum and place new number in the next segment, going clockwise.

ANSWER 221

8. Starting at the top left corner add the first three numbers and place the sum below, beside or above the second number as appropriate. Moving around the square in a clockwise spiral, repeat with the next three numbers, etc.

ANSWER 222

B. Each column contains faces with 4 different types of hair, pairs of ears, eyes, mouths and face shapes.

ANSWER 223

C. A and D, and B and E are pairs. When reflected against a vertical line and turned, they are identical.

ANSWER 224

D and E.

ANSWER 225

141. The colors are worth Red 2, Green 4, Orange 7, Yellow 9. Multiply the numbers in each square together.

ANSWER 226

17. The colors are worth Red 6, Yellow 7, Green 10, Orange 12. In each square subtract the lower color from the upper. The colors represent numbers but are NOT necessarily under 10.

ANSWER 227

The pattern starts at the top right and goes in diagonal stripes from left to right.

D	3
F	7

ANSWER 228

57, 71, 53, 45. The colors are worth Blue 3, Yellow 5, Orange -4, Green -5. Multiply the two top numbers in each square and add them to the product of the two bottom numbers. Then add or subtract according to the color of the square.

ANSWER 229

90. Colors are worth Orange 25, Purple 17, Yellow 36, Green 12.

ANSWER 230

The minute hand should be on the 4, the hour hand on the 8. The numbers the hands are pointing to are doubles of each other. The lower number moves forward by 1 each time, with the hands being reversed.

ANSWER 231

D. The formula is: left + (middle x right) = top + (middle x bottom), but in D, the answers are 26 and 25 respectively.

ANSWER 232

There are 43 pairs.

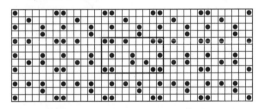

ANSWER 233

14 spotted tiles

ANSWER 234

410. In all the others the first two digits added equal the third.

ANSWER 235

54. The colors are worth Pink 3, Orange 4, Yellow 5, Green 6, Purple -2, Red -4. Add the value of the colors to the number in each square.

ANSWER 236

20. Left hand x right hand ÷ waist = head. Left foot x right foot ÷ waist = head.

ANSWER 237

Start at the top right and move in an anti-clockwise spiral. The dot moves clockwise around the square.

ANSWER 238

96. The colors are worth Pink 2, Yellow 3, Green 4, Orange 5.

ANSWER 239

A.

ANSWER 240

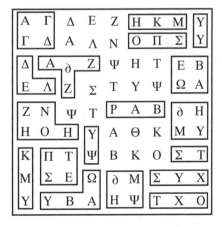

ANSWER 241

The formula is (right x left – top) x black fraction of circle = bottom.

ANSWER 242

625 and 5. The cubes of 7, 9 and 13 go into the right-hand circle, the squares of 18, 26 and 54 go into the left-hand circle.

ANSWER 243

C and F.

ANSWER 244

A. The edges of all the symbols in one square added together, increase by 2 with each square (i.e. 12, 14, 16, 18, 20).

ANSWER 245

7. Multiply the two numbers on the outside of each segment, divide their product by 2 and place the new number two segments ahead in the middle.

ANSWER 246

20. Take two numbers in adjacent circles. If both are odd, add them. If both are even, multiply them. If one number is odd and one is even take the difference. Put the new number in the overlapping section.

ANSWER 247

The hidden letter is F. The pattern is diagonal stripes starting from the top right and going up from right to left.

ANSWER 248

The pattern sequence is shown below. It starts at the top left and works downwards in a vertical boustrophedon.

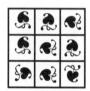

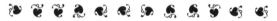

ANSWER 249

 The pattern sequence is:

Start at top left and follow the pattern in a clockwise spiral.

ANSWER 250

27 or 729. The numbers are part of a sequence that alternates A^3, B, C^3, D, E^3, ...

ANSWER 251

F. Each shape changes into a shape with 2 extra sides. The order of shapes is reversed.

ANSWER 252

B and E.

ANSWER 253

11. Multiply the number of sides of each number by 3, and then subtract the number printed.

ANSWER 254

9. Multiply the two outer numbers in each segment, and divide the product by 2 and 3 alternately. Place the new number in the middle of the opposite segment.

ANSWER 255

56. (Head x left foot) ÷ waist = right hand; (head x right foot) ÷ waist = left hand).
(14 x 15) ÷ 5 = 42; (14 x 20) ÷ 5 = 56.

ANSWER 256

E. The squares with lines from the bottom left to the top right have arrows pointing up or right. Squares with lines from the bottom right to the top left have arrows pointing down or left.

ANSWER 257

D. The whole figure is reflected on a horizontal line. Any shape with straight lines is then rotated by 90° clockwise and a dot in a round shape disappears.

ANSWER 258

B and F.

ANSWER 259

G.

ANSWER 260

11. It is a series of prime numbers.

ANSWER 261

D.

ANSWER 262

91. All the others are prime numbers.

ANSWER 263

5. Three numbers in a horizontal line add up to the fourth number.

ANSWER 264

A. Multiply first and last digits. Subtract second digit for hours and add third for minutes.

ANSWER 265

D. The formula is: (right x shaded fraction of left) - (top x shaded fraction of bottom) = middle shape's number of sides. Therefore, in example D: (18 x $\frac{2}{3}$ [12]) - (12 x $\frac{3}{4}$ [9]) = 3. The answer shape should be 3-sided, so it is the odd one out.

ANSWER 266

D. The symbols turn by 180° and 90° alternately. The circle and square swap places, the diamond and rectangle swap shading.

ANSWER 267

105. The colors are worth Yellow 4, Pink 5, Green 6, Orange 7. Add the value of the color to the number in each square.

ANSWER 268

19. Colors are worth Orange 3, Green 4, Red 5, Purple 7.

ANSWER 269

77. The colors are worth Purple 3, Green 4, Yellow 6, Orange 9. Add the left side to the right side and multiply by the base. This is Result 1. Now add the two upper internal colors and subtract the lower. This is Result 2. Then subtract Result 2 from Result 1.

ANSWER 270

34. The colors are worth Green 3, Red 4, Yellow 5, Purple 7. Add colors in each square together.

ANSWER 271

26. The colors are worth Red 3, Yellow 6, Purple 8, Green 9.

ANSWER 272

It will fall.

ANSWER 273

27. The colors are worth Yellow 2, Red 3, Green 4, Purple 6. Multiply the sides of the triangle together to get Result 1. Add the inner numbers together to get Result 2. Now subtract R2 from R1 to get the answer.

ANSWER 274

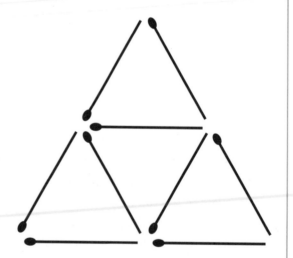

ANSWER 275

19. The colors are worth Orange 3, Red 5, Purple 7, Green 4. Add colors in the same square together.

ANSWER 276

28. Colors are worth Purple 5, Orange 2, Yellow 3, Green 6. Add colors in each square together.

ANSWER 277

The hours move back 3, 4, 5, and 6 hours. The minutes move forward 4, 8, 16, and 32 minutes. The seconds move back 1, 2, 3, and 4 seconds. The time on the fifth watch should be 21:14:51.

ANSWER 278

C.

ANSWER 279

A.

ANSWER 280

B. Billy's plot has the greatest perimeter.

ANSWER 281

A.

ANSWER 282

D. In all other cases the number of cross pieces on top of each vertical line is multiplied by the number of cross pieces on the bottom. All give even answers apart from D.

ANSWER 283

D. Add a cross piece each time, alternating between adding them vertically and horizontally. A vertical cross piece changes the color of the arrow head.

ANSWER 284

D. The second hand moves forward 30 and back 15 seconds alternately, the minute hand moves back 10 and forward 5 minutes alternately, and the hour hand moves forward 2 hours and back 1 hour alternately.

ANSWER 285

D.

ANSWER 286

H. Rotate one place clockwise and then reflect across a horizontal line through the middle of the figure.

ANSWER 287

The third on the second column and the fifth on the third column.

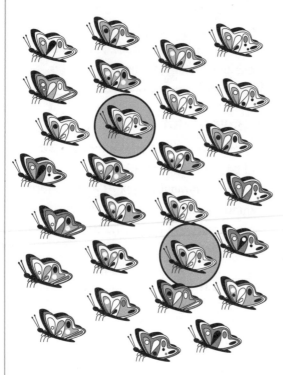

ANSWER 288

D.

ANSWER 289

D. Circle and triangle alternate. After a circle the next figure moves around 1 space, staying on the same side of the line. After a triangle it moves on 2.

ANSWER 290

Blue = 8; Green = 9.

ANSWER 291

1. Starting with 64, subtract 1, 2, 4, 8, 16, 32, missing a number each time and working in a clockwise direction.

ANSWER 292

A square. If the three numbers around the triangle add to an even number the shape is a square; if it is odd, then it is another triangle.

ANSWER 293

Penultimate triangle on the bottom row. Sequence, starting from the top and working from left to right, of dot, miss 1 triangle, dot, miss 2, dot, miss 3, dot, miss 4.

ANSWER 294

C. Curved lines gradually encroach on space within triangle.

ANSWER 295

D. One tip of the star is missing.

ANSWER 296

C.

ANSWER 297

F. Small square becomes a big square and vice versa. A small square with a triangle goes to small square alone. A triangle on big square remains a triangle.